ADULT RESPIRATORY DISTRESS SYNDROME

LUNG BIOLOGY IN HEALTH AND DISEASE

Executive Editor: **Claude Lenfant**

Director, National Heart, Lung, and Blood Institute
National Institutes of Health
Bethesda, Maryland

Volume 1 IMMUNOLOGIC AND INFECTIOUS REACTIONS IN THE LUNG, *edited by Charles H. Kirkpatrick and Herbert Y. Reynolds*

Volume 2 THE BIOCHEMICAL BASIS OF PULMONARY FUNCTION, *edited by Ronald G. Crystal*

Volume 3 BIOENGINEERING ASPECTS OF THE LUNG, *edited by John B. West*

Volume 4 METABOLIC FUNCTIONS OF THE LUNG, *edited by Y. S. Bakhle and John R. Vane*

Volume 5 RESPIRATORY DEFENSE MECHANISMS (in two parts), *edited by Joseph D. Brain, Donald F. Proctor, and Lynne M. Reid*

Volume 6 DEVELOPMENT OF THE LUNG, *edited by W. Alan Hodson*

Volume 7 LUNG WATER AND SOLUTE EXCHANGE, *edited by Norman C. Staub*

Volume 8 EXTRAPULMONARY MANIFESTATIONS OF RESPIRATORY DISEASE, *edited by Eugene Debs Robin*

Volume 9 CHRONIC OBSTRUCTIVE PULMONARY DISEASE, *edited by Thomas L. Petty*

Volume 10 PATHOGENESIS AND THERAPY OF LUNG CANCER, *edited by Curtis C. Harris*

Volume 11 GENETIC DETERMINANTS OF PULMONARY DISEASE, *edited by Stephen D. Litwin*

Volume 12 THE LUNG IN THE TRANSITION BETWEEN HEALTH AND DISEASE, *edited by Peter T. Macklem and Solbert Permutt*

Volume 13 EVOLUTION OF RESPIRATORY PROCESSES: A COMPARATIVE APPROACH, *edited by Stephen C. Wood and Claude Lenfant*

Volume 14 PULMONARY VASCULAR DISEASES, *edited by Kenneth M. Moser*

Volume 15 PHYSIOLOGY AND PHARMACOLOGY OF THE AIRWAYS, *edited by Jay A. Nadel*

Volume 16 DIAGNOSTIC TECHNIQUES IN PULMONARY DISEASE (in two parts), *edited by Marvin A. Sackner*

Volume 17 REGULATION OF BREATHING (in two parts), *edited by Thomas F. Hornbein*

Volume 18 OCCUPATIONAL LUNG DISEASES: RESEARCH APPROACHES AND METHODS, *edited by Hans Weill and Margaret Turner-Warwick*

Volume 19 IMMUNOPHARMACOLOGY OF THE LUNG, *edited by Harold H. Newball*

Volume 20 SARCOIDOSIS AND OTHER GRANULOMATOUS DISEASES OF THE LUNG, *edited by Barry L. Fanburg*

Volume 21 SLEEP AND BREATHING, *edited by Nicholas A. Saunders and Colin E. Sullivan*

Volume 22 *PNEUMOCYSTIS CARINII* PNEUMONIA: PATHOGENESIS, DIAGNOSIS, AND TREATMENT, *edited by Lowell S. Young*

Volume 23 PULMONARY NUCLEAR MEDICINE: TECHNIQUES IN DIAGNOSIS OF LUNG DISEASE, *edited by Harold L. Atkins*

Volume 24 ACUTE RESPIRATORY FAILURE, *edited by Warren M. Zapol and Konrad J. Falke*

Volume 25 GAS MIXING AND DISTRIBUTION IN THE LUNG, *edited by Ludwig A. Engel and Manuel Paiva*

Volume 26 HIGH-FREQUENCY VENTILATION IN INTENSIVE CARE AND DURING SURGERY, *edited by Graziano Carlon and William S. Howland*

Volume 27 PULMONARY DEVELOPMENT: TRANSITION FROM INTRAUTERINE TO EXTRAUTERINE LIFE, *edited by George H. Nelson*

Volume 28 CHRONIC OBSTRUCTIVE PULMONARY DISEASE, second edition, revised and expanded, *edited by Thomas L. Petty*

Volume 29 THE THORAX (in two parts), *edited by Charis Roussos and Peter T. Macklem*

Volume 30 THE PLEURA IN HEALTH AND DISEASE, *edited by Jacques Chrétien, Jean Bignon, and Albert Hirsch*

Volume 31 DRUG THERAPY FOR ASTHMA: RESEARCH AND CLINICAL PRACTICE, *edited by John W. Jenne and Shirley Murphy*

Volume 32 PULMONARY ENDOTHELIUM IN HEALTH AND DISEASE, *edited by Una S. Ryan*

Volume 33 THE AIRWAYS: NEURAL CONTROL IN HEALTH AND DISEASE, *edited by Michael A. Kaliner and Peter J. Barnes*

Volume 34 PATHOPHYSIOLOGY AND TREATMENT OF INHALATION INJURIES, *edited by Jacob Loke*

Volume 35 RESPIRATORY FUNCTION OF THE UPPER AIRWAY, *edited by Oommen P. Mathew and Giuseppe Sant'Ambrogio*

Volume 36 CHRONIC OBSTRUCTIVE PULMONARY DISEASE: A BEHAVIORAL PERSPECTIVE, *edited by A. John McSweeny and Igor Grant*

Volume 37 BIOLOGY OF LUNG CANCER: DIAGNOSIS AND TREATMENT, *edited by Steven T. Rosen, James L. Mulshine, Frank Cuttitta, and Paul G. Abrams*

Volume 38 PULMONARY VASCULAR PHYSIOLOGY AND PATHOPHYSIOLOGY, *edited by E. Kenneth Weir and John T. Reeves*

Volume 39 COMPARATIVE PULMONARY PHYSIOLOGY: CURRENT CONCEPTS, *edited by Stephen C. Wood*

Volume 40 RESPIRATORY PHYSIOLOGY: AN ANALYTICAL APPROACH, *edited by H. K. Chang and Manuel Paiva*

Volume 41 LUNG CELL BIOLOGY, *edited by Donald Massaro*

Volume 42 HEART-LUNG INTERACTIONS IN HEALTH AND DISEASE, *edited by Steven M. Scharf and Sharon S. Cassidy*

Volume 43 CLINICAL EPIDEMIOLOGY OF CHRONIC OBSTRUCTIVE PULMONARY DISEASE
edited by Michael J. Hensley and Nicholas A. Saunders

Volume 44 SURGICAL PATHOLOGY OF LUNG NEOPLASMS
edited by Alberto M. Marchevsky

Volume 45 THE LUNG IN RHEUMATIC DISEASES
edited by Grant W. Cannon and Guy A. Zimmerman

Volume 46 DIAGNOSTIC IMAGING OF THE LUNG
edited by Charles E. Putman

Volume 47 MODELS OF LUNG DISEASE: MICROSCOPY AND STRUCTURAL METHODS
edited by Joan Gil

Volume 48 ELECTRON MICROSCOPY OF THE LUNG
edited by Dean Schraufnagel

Volume 49 ASTHMA: ITS PATHOLOGY AND TREATMENT
edited by Michael A. Kaliner, Peter J. Barnes, and Carl G. A. Persson

Volume 50 ADULT RESPIRATORY DISTRESS SYNDROME
edited by Warren M. Zapol and François Lemaire

Additional Volumes in Preparation

PULMONARY PHYSIOLOGY AND THE PATHOPHYSIOLOGY OF EXERCISE
edited by Brian J. Whipp and Karlman Wasserman

LUNG DISEASE IN THE TROPICS
edited by Om P. Sharma

DEVELOPMENTAL NEUROBIOLOGY OF BREATHING
edited by Gabriel G. Haddad and Jay P. Farber

ADULT RESPIRATORY DISTRESS SYNDROME

Edited by

Warren M. Zapol
Massachusetts General Hospital
Harvard Medical School
Boston, Massachusetts

François Lemaire
Hôpital Henri Mondor
University of Paris XII
(Paris-Val-de-Marne)
Créteil, France

MARCEL DEKKER, INC. New York • Basel • Hong Kong

Library of Congress Cataloging--in--Publication Data

Adult respiratory distress syndrome / edited by Warren M. Zapol,
Francois Lemaire.
p. cm. -- -- (Lung biology in health and disease; v. 50)
Includes bibliographical references and index.
ISBN 0-8247-8359-X
1. Respiratory distress syndrome, Adult. I. Zapol, Warren M.
II. Series.
[DNLM: 1. Respiratory Distress Syndrome, Adult. W1 LU62 v. 50 /
WF 140 A24315]
RC776.R38A286 1991
616.2-- --dc20
DNLM/DLC
for Library of Congress 90-14094
CIP

Marcel Dekker, Inc.
270 Madison Avenue, New York, New York 10016

Current printing (last digit):
10 9 8 7 6 5 4 3 2 1

Printed in the United States of America

INTRODUCTION

In 1985, the twenty-fourth volume in the Lung Biology in Health and Disease series was published: its title was *Acute Respiratory Failure* and the editors were Dr. Warren M. Zapol and Konrad J. Falke. This volume, *Adult Respiratory Distress Syndrome*, is edited by Warren Zapol and François Lemaire.

The term *adult respiratory distress syndrome* (ARDS) was coined by Ashbaugh, Bigelow, Petty, and Levine in 1967. Since that time, this condition has received much attention from clinicians and researchers. Undoubtedly, such interest stems from the public health importance of the syndrome, even though the manifold causes and protean clinical manifestations of the syndrome are often reported instead of ARDS, making it difficult to obtain good statistical data. Although the morbidity and mortality statistics from ARDS are imprecise, everyone agrees that its incidence is very high. In 1972, a United States Public Health Service Report estimated that nearly 150,000 cases of ARDS occur in the United States each year.

Recently, some authors have preferred to use the term *increased permeability pulmonary edema* when referring to ARDS.

> Increased permeability pulmonary edema is encountered clinically in the many forms of acute lung injury that are collectively lumped together under the generic name of ARDS. The syndrome occurs most often in patients hospitalized for a serious medical or surgical problem that does not involve the lungs initially. . . . (Murray, 1988)*

The future will show whether this proposed new way of looking at the condition will simplify matters or create more confusion. Regardless, it is clear that ARDS, or increased permeability pulmonary edema, is a major clinical and research concern.

---

*Murray, J. F. (1988). In *Textbook of Respiratory Medicine*. Edited by J. F. Murray and J. A. Nadel. Philadelphia, W.B. Saunders Co., p. 1293.

Since the publication of Zapol and Falke's volume, much work has been done and much progress has been accomplished. This new volume provides a timely and important review of the current state of the art of ARDS. It is timely because the many ongoing investigations are developing new information that must be widely communicated. This volume is an important new landmark in a field that is changing quickly.

Drs. Zapol and Lemaire have assembled a roster of contributors that represents a wide spectrum of interest and expertise. I am most appreciative of their participation in this volume as well as their commitment to producing a monograph that adds much to the Lung Biology in Health and Disease series.

Claude Lenfant, M.D.
Bethesda, Maryland

PREFACE

Adult Respiratory Distress Syndrome (ARDS) covers recent advances in the scientific understanding of acute inflammatory respiratory failure, extending the coverage of volume 24 in this series, *Adult Respiratory Failure*, which was published in 1985. Because the vast number of clinical and laboratory studies of this complex syndrome could not be addressed in anything less than an encyclopedia, we selected the contents of this volume primarily with an eye toward clinical relevance. We begin with the definition, incidence, and prediction of ARDS and then summarize the results of therapy. Next, we turn to clinical problems of infection in the lungs and elsewhere, tissue oxygen delivery, and cardiovascular function during acute respiratory failure. A review of mechanical ventilation in respiratory failure follows. The basis of respiratory mechanics measurements is also analyzed.

A discussion of new lung imaging techniques should bring the reader up to date on computed tomography scanning and nuclear magnetic resonance in ARDS and will highlight important clinical implications. For example, because postural changes are shown to alter the distribution of collapsed lung early in this disease (see the cover illustration, courtesy of Dr. L. Gattinoni, Milan) we may need to change our routines of clinical care. A number of novel therapies, both proven and disproven, are covered in this volume. Some, such as the use of monoclonal antibodies against the core lipids of endotoxin and surfactant therapy, are just beginning to be evaluated and only an outline of how they might work is available. On the other hand, details are provided on the effects of antiproteases in acute lung injury and on the failure of corticosteroids to alter the progression of septic ARDS in a recent clinical trial.

The use of extracorporeal membrane oxygenation (ECMO) in acute respiratory failure is not included. The benefits to adults of this therapy are uncertain, and although a number of researchers remain optimistic about artificial lungs, in ARDS there is little proof of their efficacy over conventional ventilator therapy. For ECMO enthusiasts, the chapter on barotrauma (really volume trauma) should further convince them of the righteousness of the extracorporeal gas exchange route. ARDS patients who fail to improve on ECMO and develop 100% shunt and little hope of recovery of lung function may now be treated with unilateral lung transplantation. This, the topic of our final chapter, is an important new treatment that provides hope for future severe ARDS patients.

A number of these chapter authors attended a conference at the Chateau of Seillac in the Loire Valley. This conference was given as a memorial to Dr. Maurice Rapin, the first clinician to describe ARDS in France and the leader of a world-class group of ARDS researchers. The editors wish to thank the Rapin Foundation, in particular Mrs. Marie Claude Rapin, for guidance, assistance, and sponsorship of this conference. The editors would also like to thank their wives, Nikki Jane Zapol and Ivana Fulli-Lemaire, for their assistance and support with this endeavor.

Warren M. Zapol
François Lemaire

CONTENTS

Introduction *iii*

Preface *v*

Contributors *xv*

1. Clinical Risks Associated with the Adult Respiratory Distress Syndrome **1**

Richard J. Maunder and Leonard D. Hudson

I. Introduction 1
II. Definition of ARDS 2
III. Rationale for Identifying Patients at Risk for ARDS 4
IV. Prediction of ARDS by Physiologic Measurements 6
V. Prediction of ARDS by Clinical Predispositions 7
VI. Prediction of ARDS in Cellular and Biochemical Markers 13
VII. Summary 18
References 18

2. Adult Respiratory Distress Syndrome: Definition, Risk Factors, and Outcome **23**

Thomas M. Hyers

I. Introduction 23
II. Incidence 24
III. Definition 24
IV. Risk Groups 26
V. Outcome 30
VI. New Directions in Clinical Studies of ARDS 32
References 33

3. Clinical Presentation, Prognostic Factors, and Outcome of ARDS in the European Collaborative Study (1985-1987): A Preliminary Report **37**

A. Artigas, J. Carlet, J. R. Le Gall, C. L. Chastang, L. Blanch, and R. Fernández

I. Introduction 37
II. Diagnosis of ARDS 38
III. Etiology 42
IV. Mortality and Prognostic Factors 44
V. Severity Scoring Indices 50
VI. Long-Term Recovery 53
VII. Summary 57
VIII. Appendix 58
References 59

4. Tissue Oxygen Delivery and Utilization in Patients with the Adult Respiratory Distress Syndrome **65**

David R. Dantzker

I. Introduction 65
II. Normal Response to Reduced To_2 66
III. To_2-Vo_2 Relationships in ARDS 69
References 73

5. Bacterial Infection in Adult Respiratory Distress Syndrome **77**

Waldemar G. Johanson, Jr.

I. Introduction 77
II. Pneumonia as the Source of Sepsis in ARDS 80
III. The Gastrointestinal Tract as the Source of Sepsis in ARDS 83
IV. Mechanisms of MOF Related to Sepsis 86
V. Summary 86
References 87

6. Prognostic Factors in the Intensive Care Unit with Special Emphasis on Acute Respiratory Failure **91**

William A. Knaus

I. Introduction 91
II. Source of Patient Information: Validation of APACHE II 92

III. Results 97
IV. Discussion 100
V. Summary 102
References 103

7. Measurement of Respiratory Elastance and Resistance in Mechanically Ventilated Patients 105

Anne M. Lorino and Alain Harf

I. Introduction 105
II. Respiratory Models 107
III. Methods for Measuring Respiratory Mechanics 113
IV. Comparison of the Methods 126
V. The Limits of Models and Methods 130
VI. Conclusion 133
References 134

8. Lung Mechanics in ARDS: Compliance and Pressure-Volume Curves 139

Laurent Beydon, François Lemaire, and Björn Jonson

I. Introduction 139
II. Titration of PEEP 140
III. Measurement of the Total Thoracopulmonary Compliance (Static and Dynamic) 142
IV. Recent Concepts of P-V Loops 147
V. Methodologic Limitations 154
VI. Conclusion 155
References 156

9. Minimizing Breathing Effort During Mechanical Ventilation 163

John J. Marini

I. Introduction 163
II. Quantifying Breathing Effort 164
References 194

10. Computed Tomography Scanning in Acute Respiratory Failure 199

Luciano Gattinoni and Antonio Pesenti

I. Introduction 199
II. Lung Morphology 200

III. A Quantitative Analysis of CT Scan Images 208
IV. Comparing Physiologic Measurements with CT Scan Anatomy 211
V. Alterations in Lung Anatomy and Function with Changing Conditions 214
VI. A Model of the ARDS Lung Derived from CT Scans of the Lung 217
VII. Appendix: Calculations for Estimating Pulmonary Weight 218
References 219

11. Cardiorespiratory Interactions 223

James L. Robotham and Jürgen Peters

I. Introduction 223
II. Lung Volume and Intrathoracic Pressure 224
III. The Circulatory System 224
IV. Spontaneous Ventilation and the Left Ventricle 225
V. The Cardiac Cycle 228
VI. Spontaneous Ventilation: Mitral and Aortic Flows 228
VII. Transient Analysis of a Negative ITP 238
VIII. Transient Analysis Techniques 238
IX. Positive Pressure Ventilation and Cardiopulmonary Resuscitation 246
X. Conclusion 249
References 249

12. Cardiovascular Function During Acute Respiratory Failure 253

William E. Hurford and Jean-Louis Teboul

I. Introduction 253
II. Assessing Cardiac Function During ARDS 254
III. Effect of Acute Pulmonary Artery Hypertension 259
IV. Effect of Sepsis 262
V. Positive-Pressure Ventilation and PEEP 265
VI. Cardiovascular Function During Weaning from Mechanical Ventilation 270
VII. Summary 273
References 274

13. Corticosteroids in Adult Respiratory Distress Syndrome **285**

Kenneth L. Brigham

I. Introduction 285
II. Actions of Corticosteroids That May Be Beneficial in ARDS 286
III. Evidence of Efficacy of Corticosteroids in Animal and Organ Models 288
IV. In Vitro Versus In Vivo Effects of Corticosteroids 293
V. Clinical Trial of High-Dose Methylprednisolone in ARDS 296
VI. Summary and Conclusions 300
References 302

14. Proteases and Antiproteases in the Adult Respiratory Distress Syndrome **305**

G. Deby-Dupont, M. Lamy, M. E. Faymonville, A. Adam, P. Damas, C. Deby, and P. Franchimont

I. Introduction 305
II. Proteases Involved in ARDS 306
III. Regulation of Protease Activity: Role of Antiproteases 321
IV. Is a Protease-Antiprotease Imbalance Present During ARDS? 327
References 330

15. Capillary Pressure Measurement in Human Lungs **353**

Aubrey E. Taylor, Doris K. Cope, Ronald C. Allison, and Scott A. Barman

I. Introduction 353
II. Capillary Pressure and Its Relation to Transcapillary Fluid Exchange 354
III. Measurement of Pulmonary Capillary Pressure in Isolated Lungs 356
IV. Measurement of Pulmonary Capillary Pressure Using Only Arterial Occlusion 360
V. Measurement of Pulmonary Capillary Pressure in Humans 361
References 365

16. **The Adult Respiratory Distress Syndrome at Massachusetts General Hospital: Etiology, Progression, and Survival Rates 1978-1988** **367**

Warren M. Zapol, Mark J. Frikker, Henning Pontoppidan, Roger S. Wilson, and Karen E. Lynch

I. Introduction 367
II. Results 370
III. Discussion 376
References 378

17. **Abnormalities of Lung Surfactant Function in Patients with Acute Lung Injury: Implications for Therapy** **381**

Roger G. Spragg

I. Introduction 381
II. Surfactant System of the Healthy Lung: Composition and Structure 382
III. Function 383
IV. Abnormalities of Lung Surfactant in ARDS 385
V. Possible Causes of Surfactant Abnormalities in Patients with ARDS 385
VI. Surfactant Replacement in Patients with IRDS 386
VII. Animal Models for Evaluation of Surfactant Therapy of Acute Adult Lung Injury 387
VIII. Surfactants Available for Therapeutic Administration 388
IX. Use of Exogenous Surfactants in the Therapy of ARDS 390
X. Conclusion 391
References 391

18. **Humoral Aspects of Endotoxin Neutralization** **397**

H. Shaw Warren

I. Introduction 397
II. Neutralization of Endotoxin by Normal Serum 399
III. Neutralization of Endotoxin by Immunoglobulins 400
IV. Neutralization of Endotoxin by Inflammatory Factors in Serum 403
V. Conclusions 405
References 405

19. **Pulmonary Nuclear Magnetic Resonance: Potential Applications in ARDS** 411

Alan H. Morris, Antonio G. Cutillo, David C. Ailion, Carl H. Durney, and Krishnamurthy Ganesan

I. Introduction 411
II. Basic NMR Phenomena 413
III. NMR Imaging: Frequency Encoding of Position 415
IV. NMR of Lung Water: An Absolute Standard? 416
V. Unique NMR Behavior of Inflated Lung and the Difference Signal D 417
VI. Nonspatial Distributions of Lung Water 422
VII. Geometric Information About Lung Structure Without Requiring Optical Resolution 423
VIII. Relaxation Times T_1 and T_2 424
IX. Potential Applications in ARDS 426
References 428

20. **Lung Overinflation: Physiologic and Anatomic Alterations Leading to Pulmonary Edema** 433

Didier Dreyfuss and Georges Saumon

I. Introduction 433
II. Pathways for Pulmonary Edema Due to Lung Distention 433
III. Pulmonary Edema Due to Mechanical Ventilation 437
References 446

21. **Adverse Heparin-Protamine Neutralization Interactions and the Lung** 451

Erni Kreil, Gilles Montalescot, Dwight R. Robinson, Warren M. Zapol, Edward Lowenstein, and Karen E. Lynch

I. Introduction 451
II. Overview 452
III. Animal Models of Heparin-Protamine-Associated Pulmonary Vasoconstriction 452
IV. Heparin-Protamine, Lipopolysaccharide, and Lung Injury in Sheep 471
V. The Clinical Syndrome of Heparin-Protamine-Associated Acute Pulmonary Vasoconstriction in Humans 472

VI. Summary 482
References 482

22. Lung Transplantation 491

Larry R. Kaiser and Joel D. Cooper

I. Introduction 491
II. History of Lung Transplantation 492
III. Indications for Lung Transplantation 495
IV. Evaluation and Management of Potential Candidates 500
V. The Pulmonary Donor 502
VI. Retrieval of the Donor Lung 506
VII. Lung Preservation 509
VIII. Technique of Lung Transplantation 513
IX. Postoperative Course Following Lung Transplantation 518
X. Clinical Results of Lung Transplantation 522
XI. Summary and Conclusions 528
References 529

Author Index 539

Subject Index 579

CONTRIBUTORS

A. Adam, Ph.D. Faculty of Pharmacy, University of Montreal, Montreal, Quebec, Canada

David C. Ailion, Ph.D. Professor, Department of Physics, University of Utah, Salt Lake City, Utah

Ronald C. Allison, M.D. Associate Professor, Departments of Physiology and Medicine, University of South Alabama College of Medicine, Mobile, Alabama

A. Artigas, M.D. Director, Intensive Care Department, Hospital de Sabadell, Sabadell, and Associate Professor, Medical Physiology, Universidad Autonoma de Barcelona, Barcelona, Spain

Scott A. Barman, Ph.D. Instructor, Department of Physiology, University of South Alabama College of Medicine, Mobile, Alabama

Laurent Beydon, M.D. Department of Anesthesia III, Hôpital Henri Mondor, Paris Val-de-Marne University, Créteil, France

L. Blanch, M.D. Attending Physician, Intensive Care Department, Hospital de Sabadell, Sabadell, Spain

Kenneth L. Brigham, M.D. Professor of Medicine, Division of Pulmonary and Critical Care Medicine, Center for Lung Research, Vanderbilt University School of Medicine, Nashville, Tennessee

J. Carlet, M.D. Director, Intensive Care Department, Hôpital Saint Joseph, Paris, France

C. L. Chastang, M.D. Professor, Department of Biomathematics, Hôpital Saint Louis, Paris, France

Joel D. Cooper, M.D. Professor of Surgery, Division of Cardiothoracic Surgery, Washington University School of Medicine, St. Louis, Missouri

Doris K. Cope, M.D. Assistant Professor of Physiology, Department of Anesthesiology, University of South Alabama College of Medicine, Mobile, Alabama

Antonio G. Cutillo, M.D. Professor, Division of Respiratory, Critical Care, and Occupational Pulmonary Medicines, Department of Internal Medicine, University of Utah, Salt Lake City, Utah

P. Damas, M.D. Clinical Staff, Department of Anesthesiology, University of Liège, Liège, Belgium

David R. Dantzker, M.D.* Professor and Director, Division of Pulmonary Medicine, Department of Internal Medicine, The University of Texas Health Science Center at Houston, Houston, Texas

C. Deby, M.D. Head, Department of Oxygen Metabolism, Laboratory of Biochemistry and Radiobiology, Institute of Chemistry, University of Liège, Liège, Belgium

G. Deby-Dupont, Ph.D. Clinical Staff, Department of Anesthesiology and Laboratory of Radioimmunology, University of Liège, Liège, Belgium

Didier Dreyfuss, M.D. Intensive Care Unit, Hôpital Louis Mourier, Columbes, and INSERM U82, Faculté Xavier Bichat, Paris, France

Carl H. Durney, Ph.D. Professor, Departments of Electrical Engineering and Bioengineering, University of Utah, Salt Lake City, Utah

M. E. Faymonville, M.D. Clinical Staff, Department of Anesthesiology, University of Liège, Liège, Belgium

R. Fernández, M.D. Attending Physician, Intensive Care Department, Hospital de Sabadell, Sabadell, Spain

P. Franchimont, M.D. Professor and Head, Department of Endocrinology, Laboratory of Radioimmunology, University of Liège, Liège, Belgium

Mark J. Frikker, M.D.† Clinical Fellow, Harvard Medical School, Massachusetts General Hospital, Boston, Massachusetts

Present affiliations:
*Long Island Jewish Medical Center, New Hyde Park, New York
†William Beaumont Hospital, Royal Oak, Michigan

Krishnamurthy Ganesan, Ph.D. Assistant Professor, Department of Physics, University of Utah, Salt Lake City, Utah

Luciano Gattinoni, M.D. Associate Professor in Intensive Care, Institute of Anesthesiology, Università di Milano, Milano and Director, Anesthesia and Intensive Care Department, Ospedale Nuovo S. Gerardo, Monza, Italy

Alain Harf, M.D. Associate Professor, Department of Physiology and INSERM U 296, Hôpital Henri Mondor, Créteil, France

Leonard D. Hudson, M.D. Professor and Head, Division of Pulmonary and Critical Care Medicine, Department of Medicine, Harborview Medical Center and University of Washington, Seattle, Washington

William E. Hurford, M.D. Assistant Professor in Anesthesia, Department of Anesthesiology, Harvard Medical School and Assistant in Anesthesia, Massachusetts General Hospital, Boston, Massachusetts

Thomas M. Hyers, M.D. Director, Division of Pulmonology, Department of Internal Medicine, St. Louis University Medical Center, St. Louis, Missouri

Waldemar G. Johanson, Jr., M.D. Professor and Chair, Department of Internal Medicine, University of Texas Medical Branch, Galveston, Texas

Björn Jonson, M.D. Professor of Clinical Physiology, Department of Clinical Physiology, University Hospital, Lund, Sweden

Larry R. Kaiser, M.D. Assistant Professor of Surgery, Division of Cardiothoracic Surgery, Washington University School of Medicine, St. Louis, Missouri

William A. Knaus, M.D. Director and Professor, ICU Research Unit, Department of Anesthesiology, The George Washington University Medical Center, Washington, D.C.

Erni Kreil, M.D. Instructor in Anesthesia, Harvard Medical School and Massachusetts General Hospital, Boston, Massachusetts

M. Lamy, M.D. Professor and Head, Department of Anesthesiology, University of Liège, Liège, Belgium

J. R. Le Gall, M.D. Professor of Intensive Care Medicine and Director, Medical Intensive Care Department, Hôpital Saint Louis, Paris, France

François Lemaire, M.D. Chief, Medical Intensive Care Unit, Hôpital Henri Mondor and Professor of Medical Intensive Care, University of Paris XII (Paris-Val-de-Marne), Créteil, France

Anne M. Lorino, Ph.D. Assistant Professor, Department of Physiology, INSERM U 296, Hôpital Henri Mondor, Créteil, France

Edward Lowenstein, M.D. Professor of Anesthesia, Harvard Medical School and Beth Israel Hospital, Boston, Massachusetts

Karen E. Lynch, B.S.N. Research Nurse Clinician, Department of Anesthesia, Massachusetts General Hospital, Boston, Massachusetts

John J. Marini, M.D. Professor of Medicine, University of Minnesota, Minneapolis and St. Paul Ramsey Medical Center, Department of Pulmonary and Critical Care Medicine, Jackson University, St. Paul, Minnesota

Richard J. Maunder, M.D. Assistant Professor of Medicine, Division of Pulmonary and Critical Care Medicine, Harborview Medical Center and University of Washington, Seattle, Washington

Gilles Montalescot Research Fellow in Anesthesia, Harvard Medical School and Massachusetts General Hospital, Boston, Massachusetts

Alan H. Morris, M.D. Professor, Division of Pulmonary/Critical Care, Department of Internal Medicine, University of Utah and LDS Hospital, Salt Lake City, Utah

Antonio Pesenti, M.D. Research Fellow, Institute of Anesthesiology, Università di Milano, Milan, and Ospedale Nuovo S. Gerardo, Monza, Italy

Jürgen Peters, M.D. Zentrum fur Anaesthesiologie, Universitat Dusseldorf, Dusseldorf, Federal Republic of Germany

Henning Pontoppidan, M.D. Professor of Anesthesia, Harvard Medical School and Massachusetts General Hospital, Boston, Massachusetts

Dwight R. Robinson Professor of Medicine, Harvard Medical School and Massachusetts General Hospital, Boston, Massachusetts

James L. Robotham, M.D. Associate Professor, Department of Anesthesiology and Critical Care Medicine, The Johns Hopkins University Medical Institutions, Baltimore, Maryland

Georges Saumon, M.D. Intensive Care Unit, Hôpital Louis Mourier, Columbes, and INSERM U82, Faculté Xavier Bichat, Paris, France

Roger G. Spragg, M.D. Professor of Medicine, Division of Pulmonary and Critical Care Medicine, Department of Medicine, University of California, San Diego, California

Aubrey E. Taylor, Ph.D. Professor and Chairman, Department of Physiology, University of South Alabama College of Medicine, Mobile, Alabama

Jean-Louis Teboul, M.D. Assistant Professor of Medical Intensive Care, Department de Réanimation Médicale, INSERM U 296 and Université Paris XII, Hôpital Henri Mondor, Créteil, France

H. Shaw Warren, M.D. Assistant Professor, Infectious Disease Units, Departments of Pediatrics and Medicine, Shriners Burns Institute, Massachusetts General Hospital, and Harvard Medical School, Boston, Massachusetts

Roger S. Wilson, M.D. Associate Professor of Anesthesia, Harvard Medical School and Massachusetts General Hospital, Boston, Massachusetts

Warren M. Zapol, M.D. Professor of Anesthesia, Department of Anesthesia, Harvard Medical School and Massachusetts General Hospital, Boston, Massachusetts

ADULT RESPIRATORY DISTRESS SYNDROME

1

Clinical Risks Associated with the Adult Respiratory Distress Syndrome

RICHARD J. MAUNDER and LEONARD D. HUDSON

Harborview Medical Center and University of Washington
Seattle, Washington

I. Introduction

From the earliest reports of the adult respiratory distress syndrome (ARDS), it was clear that such clinical predispositions as traumatic injury or sepsis commonly preceded the onset of respiratory failure and appeared to act as a "trigger," initiating a complex sequence of events that culminated in the physiologic abnormalities by which we define ARDS. Early research into the pathophysiology and treatment of ARDS focused on the disordered respiratory physiology, seeking to re-establish alveolar stability, reduce the accumulation of edema fluid, and improve gas exchange. Despite improvements in respiratory supportive care, however, this approach has had little impact on natural history or outcome. More recently, as the importance of inflammatory pathways has been recognized and earlier intervention is discussed, attention has been redirected to the initial events in the lung injury process, including the clinical events predisposing to ARDS as well as cellular and biochemical mediators of inflammation.

This chapter deals with the ability of these initial events to predict the development of ARDS. The predictive ability of clinical risk factors associated with ARDS is particularly emphasized. First, a working definition of ARDS is discussed. Next, methods for the prediction or early detection of

ARDS are reviewed. These methods include identification of the clinical risk factors or the clinical settings of ARDS; available data for the incidence of ARDS associated with each clinical risk are reviewed. Finally the overall incidence of ARDS is briefly discussed.

II. Definition of ARDS

ARDS represents a pathophysiologic concept in which the lung abnormalities are due to diffuse acute lung injury (Ashbaugh et al., 1967; Pontoppidan et al., 1972). The lung injury is manifest by several clinical findings making up the clinical syndrome. Since both the clinical syndrome and the concept that acute lung injury is the cause are both important to the definition, a succinct definition is difficult. Most definitions describe the clinical syndrome and then attempt to exclude other etiologies for these findings. This was the approach of the Denver group in their original 1967 definition (Ashbaugh et al., 1967). Their clinical definition of the syndrome includes obvious respiratory distress with tachypnea, severe hypoxemia (with intrapulmonary shunting as the major pathophysiologic mechanism), decreased total respiratory compliance, and diffuse infiltrates on chest roentgenogram. They hypothesized that the pathophysiology involved acute diffuse lung injury with (1) increased permeability pulmonary edema and (2) surfactant depletion or inactivation leading to diffuse microatelectasis (Ashbaugh et al., 1967). Subsequent investigations have supported this hypothesis (Anderson et al., 1979; Backofen and Weibel, 1982; Fein et al., 1986; Hallman et al., 1982; Holter et al., 1986; Mason, 1987; Meyrick, 1986; Petty et al., 1977, 1979; Rinaldo et al., 1986; Sibbald et al., 1981; von Wichert and Kohl, 1977).

Several other terms have been applied to the same syndrome. These include descriptive pathologic terms, such as congestive atelectasis or diffuse alveolar damage, terms implying pathogenesis, such as alveolar capillary leak syndrome, or a combination of the two (increased permeability edema). Several others name the syndrome for the specific clinical situation in which it occurs, such as shock lung, pump lung, posttraumatic pulmonary insufficiency, and DaNang lung, used during the Vietnam war for posttraumatic ARDS.

The notion of acute widespread lung injury in a variety of clinical settings was the foundation for understanding ARDS. A second important concept has recently been emphasized by several authors, that ARDS is best thought of as representing a spectrum of lung injury (Murray et al., 1988; Petty, 1988; Rinaldo, 1986; Rocker et al., 1989). Thus any given definition that involves a specific blood gas or any radiographic criteria may not include all patients having some degree of acute lung injury. Despite this concept, the use of the term ARDS has usually been reserved for patients with some threshold level of physiologic or clinical effects in order to compare patients clinically.

Most definitions of ARDS include the minimum of (1) a degree of hypoxemia and (2) a chest radiograph criteria. Additional components of some definitions include (3) respiratory symptoms or signs, (4) clinical setting known to be associated with ARDS, and (5) an attempt to exclude other possible causes of this clinical picture, especially a major component of congestive heart failure. Criteria for the diagnosis of ARDS that are widely used are included in Table 1.

Common blood gas criteria have included a Pa_{O_2}/FI_{O_2} ratio less than 150 (Pepe et al., 1987), a Pa_{O_2}/FI_{O_2} ratio less than 200 (Calindrino et al., 1988), or a Pa_{O_2}/PA_{O_2} ratio less than 0.20 (Fowler et al., 1983). Most definitions have required bilateral alveolar-filling infiltrates, and some have required infiltrates involving all four quadrants of the lung fields (Calindrino et al., 1988; Fowler et al., 1983; Pepe et al., 1984). Although it is usually required that the process be generalized on chest radiograph, computed tomography has shown that the process may be patchy with regional inhomogeneity (Maunder et al., 1986). Some definitions have required a normal pulmonary artery wedge pressure or at least one that was not increased sufficiently to explain the abnormalities solely on the basis of left-sided conges-

Table 1 Criteria for the Diagnosis of ARDS

1. Respiratory distress (judged clinically)
   Respiratory rate > 20
   Labored breathing
2. Severe hypoxemia
   $Pa_{O_2}/FI_{O_2} \leqslant 150$ without PEEP or $\leqslant 200$ with PEEP
3. Generalized infiltrates on chest radiograph
4. Clinical setting consistent with ARDS (underlying illness or injury known to be associated with ARDS)
5. Exclusion of other diseases that could be associated with 1-3, especially cardiogenic pulmonary edema, that is, either no clinical evidence or likelihood of left heart failure or pulmonary artery wedge pressure $\leqslant$ 18 mmHg if pulmonary artery catheter present

Optional

6. Total respiratory compliance < 50 ml/cmH_2O
7. Response to PEEP with improved oxygenation

tive heart failure (Calindrino et al., 1988; Pepe et al., 1984). Since the placement of a pulmonary artery balloon flotation catheter may not be justified in many patients, the definition should be modified to require either a normal pulmonary artery wedge pressure or no clinical evidence or setting that would suggest left heart failure (Murray et al., 1988; Petty, 1988).

The common clinical settings associated with ARDS are discussed below in the review of clinical risk factors for the development of ARDS. Several clinical settings are associated with pulmonary abnormalities that might qualify for the preceding definition of ARDS, but controversy exists whether the designation of ARDS is warranted. High-altitude pulmonary edema (HAPE) is one such example. HAPE fits all the criteria; however, the course of the illness differs markedly from ARDS associated with most other clinical situations. In HAPE patients, rapid improvement occurs on either breathing a supplemental oxygen mixture or taking the victim to low altitude (Schoene, 1985). Because of this difference in clinical course, it does not seem to be clinically useful to include HAPE as a classic form of ARDS. Whether to include diffuse infections, such as *Pneumocystis carinii* pneumonia, as a form of ARDS is also controversial. Certainly, the clinical presentation may meet all the defined criteria and the hypoxemia may respond to the application of PEEP.

The term ARDS probably should be further modified by the suspected etiology or associated condition for any given clinical situation. Thus, it should be stated that the patient has ARDS secondary to aspiration of gastric contents, ARDS associated with septic shock, or ARDS associated with severe blunt trauma to the lower extremities and the abdomen. This allows each clinical practitioner to make a decision as to whether the use of the term ARDS is consistent with their own understanding and usage.

III. Rationale for Identifying Patients at Risk for ARDS

Although specific criteria and definitions may vary, we are certainly capable of identifying patients *after* the onset of ARDS. There are several reasons, however, for seeking a method to identify patients at an earlier stage. These fall into four categories.

A. Assuring Appropriate Diagnosis of ARDS

Many ARDS definitions require that the clinical syndrome occur in a clinical setting known to be associated with ARDS. A thorough understanding of these clinical settings is important to assure a correct diagnosis and also to avoid inappropriate exclusions leading to underdiagnosis of ARDS.

B. Understanding the Epidemiology and Pathogenesis of ARDS

Initial attempts to understand ARDS epidemiology adopted a retrospective approach, describing "risk factors" on the basis of a population that had already developed ARDS. Studies of inflammatory mediators or early markers of lung injury suffered from the same limitation. Using the retrospective approach, investigators could discover features that distinguished the ARDS population from normal patients or volunteers, describing, for example, the proportion of ARDS patients with antecedent sepsis or the number of ARDS patients with evidence of complement activation. A prospective approach, on the other hand, allows one to ask: How many patients with sepsis or trauma, for example, will subsequently develop ARDS? In examining the role of circulating inflammatory mediators, the prospective approach offers the advantage of an earlier look at inflammatory pathways and simultaneously selects a "control" population of patients with similar injury or illness who do not subsequently develop ARDS.

C. Triage and Clinical Management

The development of methods for predicting ARDS offers the potential for improvements in decision-making at the patient care level. Not only would this be useful in discussing prognosis with patients and their families, those found to be at particularly high risk could be targeted for more intensive monitoring and therapy.

D. Application to Clinical Trials

As the basic mechanisms underlying acute lung injury become better understood, clinical trials have already been designed to examine the application of anti-inflammatory agents and other therapeutic interventions in ARDS. The careful identification of a high-risk population is crucial for a variety of reasons: (1) from the statistical point of view, a significant beneficial effect of therapy may be missed if an unselected study population is used and the overall incidence of ARDS is low; (2) early (or prophylactic) institution of therapy may be necessary to demonstrate an effect; and (3) for ethical reasons, it may be inappropriate to subject patients to the potential side effects of an experimental agent unless a substantial risk of ARDS has been established.

This chapter reviews three approaches to the prediction or early detection of ARDS. The first involves measurement of physiologic changes in patients at risk for ARDS. The second approach is to screen patients for certain clinical predispositions known to be associated with ARDS. A third approach involves the measurement of circulating inflammatory mediators or markers of lung injury.

IV. Prediction of ARDS by Physiologic Measurements

Based upon the observation that established ARDS is associated with a variety of abnormalities in cardiorespiratory physiology, Shoemaker et al. (1980) postulated that certain changes might occur prior to the development of respiratory failure. These investigators performed a detailed analysis of cardiorespiratory patterns in 152 patients hospitalized because of sustained hemorrhagic or traumatic shock. Of these patients, 39% developed respiratory failure, defined by the following criteria: (1) Pa_{O_2} less than 59 torr on mask oxygen; (2) failure of response to conservative measures; and (3) need for mechanical ventilation. When compared to those without respiratory complications, the group that subsequently developed respiratory failure showed no consistent differences in hemodynamics or gas exchange. As a group, patients with subsequent respiratory failure did have a significantly greater reduction in blood volume and red cell mass, particularly in the late stages of shock, and average oxygen delivery was lower in the group developing respiratory failure. Several other variables tended to be different between the two groups, but the differences were not statistically significant. Despite some differences in group means for several of the 26 variables tested at various time points, the usefulness of this approach to prediction in the *individual* patient is severely limited.

Pepe et al. (1982) examined the relationship between the initial oxygenation, assessed as the Pa_{O_2}/FI_{O_2} ratio on admission to the hospital, and subsequent development of ARDS. Compared to patients with normal oxygenation, those with impaired oxygenation early in their hospital course were at significantly greater risk for development of ARDS. Two shortcomings of this approach must be mentioned. First, the analysis represents data for groups of patients, and extrapolation of findings to the individual patient at risk may be inappropriate. Second, by selecting hypoxemia as a predictor of a syndrome that is itself defined in terms of hypoxemia, there is the possibility that successful "prediction" actually represents early detection of lung injury.

Weigelt et al. (1981) selected 73 patients with traumatic injury, abdominal sepsis, or aspiration of gastric contents, examining the value of various physiologic parameters in predicting respiratory failure. A total of 10 patients were excluded because they developed hypoxemia within 12 hr of selection, providing insufficient time for evaluation. Of the remaining 59 patients, 22 developed pulmonary failure and 39 had minimal pulmonary difficulties. When these two groups were compared, there were minor differences in static pulmonary compliance, venous admixture, and chest roentographic findings. In contrast to Shoemaker, however, Weigelt found that *sequential* measurements of arterial oxygen tension were useful in distinguishing those patients who would eventually develop pulmonary failure. Hypoxemia demonstrated by a Pa_{O_2} of less than 100 torr on 40% oxygen *and* less than 350 torr on 100% oxygen, indicated a 95% probability of pulmonary deterioration. When the Pa_{O_2} was above these levels, the probability of pulmonary deterioration was extremely low. The study is limited by the fact that ARDS was ambiguously defined; some patients had low shunt fractions, some had normal static compliance, and many did not have bilateral pulmonary infiltrates. Nonetheless, the approach appears very promising in that the reported predictive value is higher than for any prediction methods reported to date in the literature.

A variety of other physiologic approaches to the early detection of lung injury and edema have emerged in the last few years. These include techniques that measure the clearance of radiolabeled aerosols by the lung, leakage of labeled macromolecules by the pulmonary microvasculature, and sophisticated imaging techniques that allow the early detection of excess lung water and labeled solutes. Although much of this investigation has been performed in animals during experimental lung injury, most of the techniques employed are appropriate for use in humans and show promise of being useful in the early detection of pulmonary vascular and epithelial injury.

V. Prediction of ARDS by Clinical Predispositions

Initially, the clinical risk factors associated with ARDS were determined in a retrospective fashion (Hudson, 1982). Although this approach could allow determination of the most common clinical settings associated with ARDS, it does not allow assessment of the true incidence of development of ARDS with any particular disease process. These retrospective studies or reviews generated lists of clinical "causes" of ARDS (Hudson, 1982) that were helpful but failed to address the incidence of ARDS with these associated disorders. Generally, disorders associated with ARDS were divided into three categories by probable route of injury: (1) inhalation or airway source (including aspiration of gastric contents, near-drowning, and inhalation of toxic gases); (2) vascular or blood-borne source (including sepsis syndrome or septic shock and multiple trauma); and (3) direct or physical lung injury (lung contusion, radiation, and re-expansion edema).

In 1982 and 1983, investigators at the University of Washington (Pepe et al., 1982) and the University of Colorado (Fowler et al., 1983) reported studies of the application of clinical criteria in the identification of patients at risk for ARDS. After carefully defining a panel of risk factors believed to be associated with ARDS, patients meeting the criteria were identified as soon as possible after admission and followed for the subsequent development of ARDS. In both studies, ARDS was defined as a syndrome of acute respiratory failure characterized by generalized bilateral pulmonary infiltrates on the chest roentgenogram, normal capillary wedge pressure, and profound hypoxemia.

Fowler and co-workers (1983) at the University of Colorado used relatively broad entry criteria, enrolling 993 patients with one or more of the predispositions outlined in Table 2. Of these, 68 patients (6.8%) developed ARDS. During the study period an additional 20 patients developed ARDS without meeting the specified risk criteria (77% sensitivity).

The study by Pepe et al. (1982) at the University of Washington included only intubated patients and used purposely restrictive entry criteria designed to select a higher risk population. For example, only patients with sepsis syndrome (evidence of serious infection with a deleterious systemic response) were selected rather than all those with bacteremia. In addition, patients with serious head injury, drug overdose, liver disease, chronic lung disease, or bronchopleural fistula were excluded. Overall, 46 of the 136 patients (34%) developed ARDS. During the study period, 30 additional patients developed ARDS but did not meet the specified risk criteria (61% sensitivity) and another 33 patients with ARDS met the specific exclusion criteria.

These studies are important because they represent the first attempt to examine ARDS risk in a prospective fashion. The study populations are well-defined, patients are identified before they develop ARDS, and "control" populations (those with identical illness or injury who do not develop ARDS) are simultaneously identified for comparison. The two studies are quite different in purpose and methodology but taken together provide important new information on clinical prediction of ARDS. The University of Colorado study attempted to identify all patients with a clinical risk of ARDS and thus was much more inclusive with virtually no exclusion criteria (Fowler et al., 1983). Although 77% of those developing the syndrome were successfully identified in the Colorado study, it has the disadvantage of using entry criteria that define a relatively low risk of subsequent ARDS (6.8%). By applying this methodology in a clinical trial, a large number of patients with minimal risk for ARDS would be included, creating problems with data analysis, study duration, and exposure of non-ARDS subjects to potential side effects. The University of Washington study attempted to identify risk factors associated with a high incidence of ARDS for the purpose of planning a clinical intervention trial (Pepe et al., 1982). The yield of ARDS patients was considerably higher (34%), but over half the patients with ARDS were either excluded or actually missed by applying the rigidly specified entry and exclusion criteria.

In subsequent work, we have attempted to draw upon the most successful and effective aspects of these two studies, expanding the study population by eliminating the many exclusions while utilizing entry criteria that define a substantial risk for ARDS. The study population and the specific criteria

Table 2 Clinical Condition and Incidence of ARDS

	University of Colorado,	University of Washington		
	single-risk data	Single-risk data	Multiple-risk data	Total (%)
Sepsis				
Bacteremia	9/239 (4%)	—	—	—
Sepsis syndrome	—	39/94 (41%)	15/31 (48%)	43
Pneumonia in ICU	10/84 (12%)	—	—	—
Aspiration of gastric contents	16/45 (36%)	6/62 (10%)	15/45 (33%)	20
Drug overdose in ICU	—	8/76 (11%)	7/18 (39%)	16
Fractures[a]	2/38 (5%)	5/52 (10%)	18/48 (38%)	23
Multiple transfusions				
10 units/24 hr	9/197 (5%)	—	—	—
15 units/24 hr	—	18/53 (34%)	18/36 (50%)	40
Pulmonary contusion	—	13/72 (18%)	23/65 (35%)	26
Cardiopulmonary bypass	4/237 (2%)	—	—	—
Burn	2/87 (2%)	—	—	—
Disseminated intravascular coagulation	2/9 (22%)	—	—	—
Near-drowning	—	3/6 (50%)	4/6 (67%)	58
Head injury	—	6/100 (6%)	8/28 (29%)	11
Total	68/993 (6.8%)[b]	98/520 (19%)	58/138 (42%)	156/658 = 24%

[a]Includes single fractures in Colorado series, only multiple fractures requiring ICU care in Washington series.
[b]Includes both single-risk and multiple-risk patients.

defining clinical predispositions are described in detail elsewhere (Maunder, 1985; Maunder and Hudson, 1986). The research staff is notified of potentially eligible patients by emergency room, operating room, and intensive care unit personnel. After the collection of demographic, clinical, and physiologic data, patients are monitored for a variety of outcome variables, including the development of ARDS.

Results of this ongoing study are summarized in Table 2 and displayed graphically in Figure 1 for patients with a single risk event (Fig. 1, open boxes) or those with multiple risks (Fig. 1, shaded boxes). Two additional risk categories have been examined in the study but have resulted in low numbers of patients at risk (near-drowning) or a low incidence of ARDS following a risk (head injury). Altogether, the incidence of ARDS in patients meeting specific criteria for one or more of these clinical predispositions is 24%, and the sensitivity of this approach exceeds 80%.

Some important differences in definitions used by the Colorado and Washington groups should be noted. The Colorado group examined patients with bacteremia determined by two or more positive blood culture, whereas the Washington study examined sepsis syndrome or septic shock, requiring not only clinical evidence of infection or inflammation but also a deleterious systemic effect consisting of significant hypotension, otherwise unexplained metabolic acidosis, or a low systemic vascular resistance. Correspondingly, the incidence of ARDS associated with bacteremic patients was only 3.8%

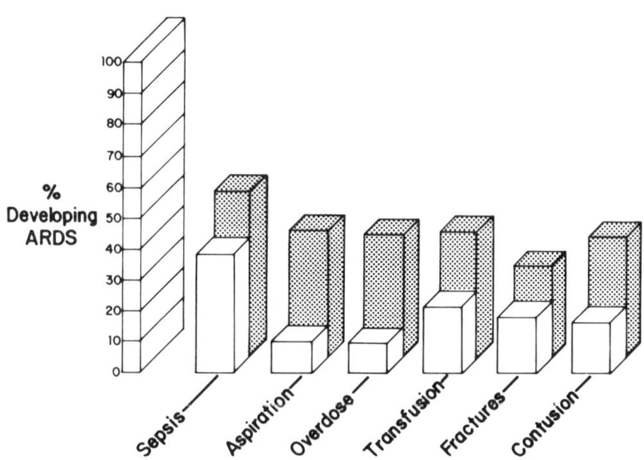

Figure 1 The incidence of ARDS in patients meeting predefined criteria for various risk factors, either alone (open boxes) or in combination with other risk factors (shaded boxes).

but was 43% in patients with sepsis syndrome. The category of "pneumonia in intensive care unit" in the Colorado study was not examined in the University of Washington study, although most of these patients were probably included in the sepsis syndrome category. Also, disseminated intravascular coagulation (DIC) used as a clinical risk in the Colorado study was not examined in Seattle because it was considered that this was probably another complication of the true underlying clinical risk, just as ARDS was a complication. (This does not negate the usefulness of DIC as a risk factor, however.) Also, burn patients were included in the Colorado study but excluded in the Washington series.

Several impressions can be gained from examining the results of the Colorado study by Fowler et al. together with our continuing series from the University of Washington (see Table 2). First, sepsis syndrome is both the most common single cause of ARDS and is also associated with the highest incidence of ARDS, whereas bacteremia without clinical sepsis is rarely associated with ARDS. Aspiration of gastric contents was frequently associated with ARDS in the Colorado study but much less frequently so in the Washington series. In the University of Washington study, aspiration and drug overdose were associated with a similar risk of developing ARDS (10 and 11%, respectively). However, when these conditions were combined, the incidence of ARDS more than tripled. When a definition of multiple transfusions was 10 units per 24 hr, the ARDS incidence was relatively low (5%) but rose significantly when the value was increased to 15 units per 24 hr in the Washington study (34% as a single risk and 40% overall). This difference may also reflect differing reasons for the blood transfusions. Harborview Medical Center, the site of the University of Washington study, is a major regional trauma center, and the majority of the patients receiving multiple emergency transfusions receive them as a resuscitative measure for management of multiple trauma. On the other hand, in that study when 15 units of blood per 24 hr was given in nontrauma patients, the incidence of ARDS was even higher than in trauma victims. The largest number of patients in this group were patients with upper gastrointestinal hemorrhage and underlying liver disease with clotting abnormalities.

In the Harborview series, nearly half the patients had multiple trauma with multiple emergency transfusions, pulmonary contusion, and/or multiple major fractures as the marker of severe trauma. Weigelt looked prospectively at 73 surgical patients with emergency admission to a surgical intensive care unit and found that the diagnosis of major trauma, abdominal sepsis, and aspiration of gastric contents all carried a high risk of the development of ARDS (Weigelt et al., 1981). Presumably, in the Harborview series the diagnosis of abdominal sepsis would have been identified under the category of sepsis syndrome.

Table 3 Current Study Population

Sepsis syndrome (must have both)
1. Evidence of serious infectious process (≥two of the following)
   Temperature ≤35 °C or ≥39 °C
   WBC count < 3000 μl or >12,000 μl[1] (or >20% band neutrophils)
   Known or strongly suspected source of infection
   Positive blood culture for a recognized pathogen
2. Deleterious systemic response (≥one of the following)
   Unexplained hypotension (systolic BP < 80 for at least 30 min)
   Systemic vascular resistance <800 dyne sec/cm^5
   Unexplained metabolic acidosis (anion gap ≥ 20 mEq/liter)

Major trauma (must have at least two):
1. Long bone or pelvic fracture
2. Significant intra-abdominal injury (requiring laparotomy)
3. Significant thoracic injury (pulmonary contusion, flail chest, or intrathoracic injury requiring thoracotomy)
4. Hypertransfusion (≥8 units over 12 hr)

Limitations of prospective studies at a single institution include that underlying causes that are seen more frequently at that institution compared to others may be overrepresented as a risk. Also, problems that are seen infrequently may be underrepresented. In addition, these studies may misrepresent illnesses that are clearly but infrequently associated with ARDS. This could either include such diseases as near-drowning that might be seen infrequently at a given institution but almost by definition is associated with a high incidence of ARDS. The same is true for certain toxic inhalations. On the other hand, pancreatitis may be a frequent problem seen in a given institution but might be associated with a low incidence of ARDS even though such an association is unquestionably present.

In summarizing current data available regarding the risk of ARDS associated with various clinical predispositions, we conclude that sepsis syndrome or septic shock and severe multiple trauma are disorders that carry the highest risk of developing ARDS. Aspiration of gastric contents and drug overdose requiring endotracheal intubation and admission to an intensive care unit have a somewhat lower but still substantial incidence of ARDS. A variety of other conditions carry a significantly lower risk of developing ARDS.

There are several advantages to using clinical predispositions for the identification of patients at risk. First, because of the high degree of sensitivity, the approach is relatively comprehensive and therefore well-suited to the epidemiologic study of ARDS. Since risk criteria are carefully and specifically defined, the technique is objective and reproducible. Finally, it is noninvasive. There are some limitations, however. The specificity remains relatively low, largely due to the inclusion of certain risk categories associated with a relatively low incidence of ARDS. In addition, the population selected is heterogeneous, both with respect to the pathogenesis of lung injury (e.g., sepsis versus aspiration) and with respect to the incidence of ARDS. Such heterogeneity is a potentially serious confounding factor in therapeutic clinical trials. The variable incidence of ARDS offers difficult problems for design and data analysis. Additionally, if there are differences in presumed pathogenesis between the risk groups, the treatment being investigated may selectively benefit one group but have no effect (or even an adverse effect) on another. We are currently collecting data from a more homogeneous population of patients (criteria outlined in Table 3) who have either sepsis syndrome or major traumatic injury, both of which are associated with a 40-50% incidence of subsequent ARDS.

VI. Prediction of ARDS in Cellular and Biochemical Markers

Extensive research efforts have been directed at clarifying the cellular and biochemical events responsible for lung tissue damage following sepsis, trauma, and other precipitants of ARDS. A logical extension of this work is the effort to identify circulating mediators or markers of lung injury that might be useful in predicting those at greatest risk for the development of ARDS. Table 4 summarizes the blood-borne factors that have attracted the greatest interest as potential predictors of acute lung injury. Space does not permit a comprehensive review of the recent work in this area. The topic is more thoroughly covered elsewhere (Maunder, 1985; Maunder and Hudson, 1986; Rinaldo and Rogers, 1982).

The majority of studies examining inflammatory mediators in ARDS are flawed by the fact that patients have been entered only after the development of full-blown lung injury. Using this approach, investigators have generally compared the ARDS population to either normal volunteers or hospitalized patients with other forms of respiratory failure. Not only do such studies fail to directly address the question of ARDS *prediction*, the control groups selected may be inappropriate for comparison. A handful of prospective studies have been performed in patients at risk for ARDS, prior to the development of respiratory failure. The question of complement activation in patients at risk for ARDS has been the most widely studied and is chosen as a focus here, not because of any particular success in predicting

Table 4 Circulating Mediators or Markers of Acute Lung Injury

Formed blood elements
Neutrophils
Platelets
Chemoattractants
Complement fragments
Lipoxygenase products
Platelet-activating factor
Bacterial peptides
Mediators of cell damage
Toxic oxygen intermediates
Proteolytic enzymes
Phospholipase products
Markers of cell damage
Prostacyclin
Factor VIII
Miscellaneous markers
Angiotensin-converting enzyme
Fibronectin
Fibrin degradation products
Phospholipase A_2

ARDS but because these studies illustrate some important principles about design and interpretation of investigation in this area.

A. Complement Activation and ARDS

The theory of complement-mediated pulmonary leukostasis as a primary mechanism in the pathogenesis of acute lung injury gained wide acceptance after the report of Hammerschmidt et al. (1980) describing evidence of complement activation in patients with established ARDS. There was also the strong implication from their work that the detection of complement activation may be valuable in *predicting* ARDS. Subsequent attempts to confirm this hypothesis have met with limited success (Duchateau et al., 1984; Maunder et al., 1984; Weinberg et al., 1984). At Harborview Medical Center, we studied 110 high-risk patients with sepsis syndrome, aspiration of gastric contents, or multiple trauma, collecting plasma samples shortly after admission or as close to risk onset as possible. Plasma $C3a_{desarg}$ and $C5a_{desarg}$ were measured by radioimmunoassay using commercially available kits. As illustrated in Figure 2, levels of $C5a_{desarg}$ were actually normal in the majority of patients

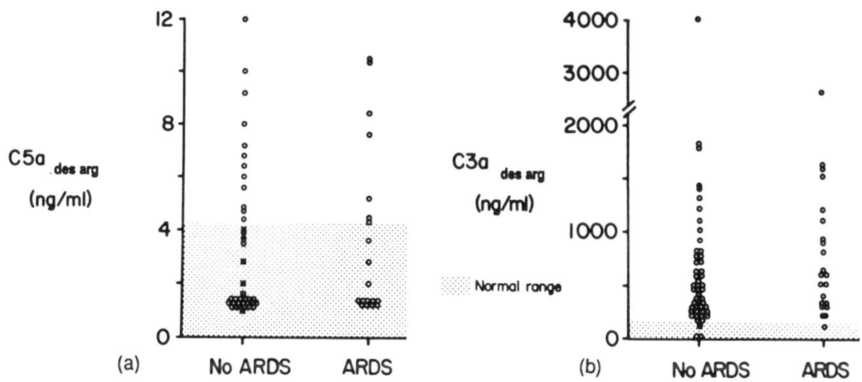

Figure 2 Plasma levels of $C5a_{desarg}$ and $C3a_{desarg}$ in patients with sepsis syndrome, major trauma, or aspiration of gastric contents. Although plasma $C3a_{desarg}$ was elevated in virtually all patients at risk (indicating evidence of complement activation), neither metabolite was useful in distinguishing those who would subsequently develop ARDS.

whether or not ARDS occurred. This phenomenon was not expected based upon the earlier results of Hammerschmidt et al. but is probably explained by the extremely short half-life of C5a (and the desarg metabolite) and the avid binding of this molecule to neutrophils and monocytes within the bloodstream. $C3a_{desarg}$ levels were elevated in most patients, indicating that complement activation had occurred. Again, there was no difference between those who subsequently developed ARDS and those with similar illness or injury who did not develop the syndrome.

Similar observations have been made by two other groups of investigators. In a closely related study of 40 patients with sepsis syndrome, Weinberg et al. (1984) found high levels of both $C3a_{desarg}$ and $C5a_{desarg}$ measured by radioimmunoassay. Although levels tended to be higher when sepsis was complicated by hypotension and/or acidemia, there was no relationship between complement levels and the subsequent development or worsening of acute respiratory failure. In this study, neutrophil aggregating activity was also examined, using a technique similar to that used by Hammerschmidt in the earlier study. Not only did aggregometry fail to predict acute lung injury, the technique was also found to be insensitive as an index of complement activation. Duchateau and colleagues (1984) evaluated 50 patients with a variety of risks predisposing to ARDS, measuring neutrophil aggregation and the C3d/C3 ratio as indicators of complement activation. Neutrophil aggregating activity was found in 86% of the patients at risk, but consistent with the findings of Weinberg, there was no difference between the ARDS and non-

ARDS groups. C3 consumption was assessed by measuring the C3d/C3 ratio. The ratio was elevated in 84% of those at risk, but levels did not distinguish those who subsequently developed ARDS.

These observations suggest that complement activation, although common in patients with developing or established ARDS, is a nonspecific finding, apparently more related to the underlying illness or injury than to lung inflammation and ARDS. Yet studies in experimental animals indicate a potentially important role for complement in the lung injury process (Hosea et al., 1980; Till et al., 1982). The available data suggest that perhaps complement activation is "necessary, but not sufficient" to produce the degree of inflammatory injury to the lung seen in ARDS. Based on the available information, two hypotheses could be constructed: certain patients are rendered more susceptible to the adverse consequences of complement activation (1) through depletion (or functional inactivation) of endogenous regulatory proteins, such as chemotactic factor inactivator, or (2) through prior exposure of the neutrophil to a "priming agent," such as endotoxin. Both hypotheses recently have been tested.

Robbins and co-workers (1986) found functional loss of chemotactic factor inactivator (CFI) in the bronchoalveolar lavage (BAL) fluid of patients with ARDS. CFI functional activity was similar in patients at risk who subsequently developed ARDS compared to similar patients who did not. CFI activity was not measured in BAL of at-risk patients without subsequent ARDS. Therefore, functional loss of CFI in the lung may play a mechanistic role in some patients developing ARDS but it does not allow prediction of ARDS development at the present time.

Parsons and co-workers (1989) tested the hypothesis that both endotoxin and complement are necessary for development of ARDS by measuring both in patients with appropriate clinical risks. The results for the complement measurements alone are similar to the findings of others, discussed above (Duchateau et al., 1984; Maunder et al., 1984; Weinberg et al., 1984). Endotoxin was present in 74% of the samples from patients who subsequently developed ARDS and only 22% of the samples from at-risk patients without subsequent ARDS. (The patients had more than one sample drawn, and data are given for the percentage of samples positive rather than for patients.) However, the range of values in those patients with measurable endotoxin was similar in both groups, limiting the predictive value in an individual patient. Their data on both substances are limited to patients at risk without subsequent ARDS and the patients with ARDS. Data for the ARDS patients prior to their development of the syndrome are not given. Of the 24 ARDS patients, 15 (62%) had both endotoxin and activated complement present while but 16 of the 56 at-risk patients without subsequent ARDS (29%) did. This lends support to the notion that endotoxin may serve as a priming agent in the presence of activated complement (or vice versa). Regarding prediction of ARDS, one can only surmise that the percentage of at-risk patients with both endotoxin and activated complement who would subsequently develop ARDS would be no greater than 62% (unless endotoxemia was transient). Thus, this phenomenon may be important as a mechanism in the etiology of lung injury but is unlikely to provide a highly sensitive or specific prediction of ARDS development. It is possible, although not likely, that these newly proposed methods will eventually be useful in predicting patients at risk.

B. Other Blood-Borne Mediators or Markers

Of the mediators and markers outlined in Table 4, only a few have shown recent promise as predictors of ARDS. Thommasen et al. (1984) prospectively studied patients with trauma, sepsis, and miscellaneous risk conditions, performing serial leukocyte counts and observing patients for the subsequent development of ARDS. Peripheral leukopenia, defined as a white blood cell count of less than 40000 cells/μl, occurred in 8 of the ARDS patients (80%) but in only 4 of 30 patients in whom ARDS did not develop (13%). Overall, the sensitivity of leukopenia for prediction of ARDS was 80%, and specificity was 87%. However, it should be noted that "prediction" was not always possible since ARDS was diagnosed *after* leukopenia in 5 patients, simultaneously in 3 patients, and *before* leukopenia in 2 patients. The predictive value of leukopenia was best in the subgroup with trauma. False-positive results were seen only in patients with sepsis.

Hallgren et al. (1984) presented results of a study examining serum lactoferrin levels in high-risk patients. Although lactoferrin levels were elevated in the study group as a whole, the patients who subsequently developed ARDS had significantly higher serum levels than did non-ARDS patients. The predictive value in individual patients remains to be established.

Studying patients with septic shock, Vadas (1984) found significantly higher levels of circulating phospholipase A_2 in those patients whose course was complicated by ARDS. A total of 34 surgical patients with gram-negative septic shock were included, of whom 11 (32%) developed ARDS during the course of their illness. Phospholipase A_2 levels were elevated in all patients when compared with normal controls. In addition, those with concurrent ARDS had a mean plasma phospholipase A_2 activity of 4332 $\pm$ 701 U/ml, and those who did not develop ARDS had a mean level of 3002 $\pm$ 474 U/ml ($p = 0.05$). The difference was even more striking when only those with positive blood cultures were included in the analysis. Again, from the data presented, it is not possible to determine the sensitivity and specificity of a particular level of enzyme for predicting ARDS.

Finally, Rubin, Matthay, and co-workers (1985) and Carvalho et al. (1982) have measured plasma concentrations of factor VIII-related antigen in patients with sepsis, finding that those with subsequent progression of lung injury have significantly higher levels. Furthermore, in the small group of patients reported thus far, sensitivity and specificity appear to be excellent, using a cutoff value of 450 U/ml.

Despite these few encouraging results, a reliable blood test for predicting ARDS is not yet available. We agree with Simon's observation (1987) that "only a better understanding of the various pathogenetic mechanisms of ARDS will lead to the development of accurate, clinically applicable (biochemical) predictors of the syndrome." Even then, there is the problem of availability and rapid turnaround times in applying sophisticated assay techniques such as these in the clinical management and decision-making process. It is likely that such techniques, if they are found to be useful, will have greater value in predicting outcome and complications.

VII. Summary

The rationale for developing methods of prediction or early detection of ARDS has been reviewed. Although the application of prediction methods to patient management is a reasonable goal, at this time application should be limited to epidemiologic research and clinical trials. Physiologic measurements, clinical predispositions, and measurement of circulating mediators or markers of inflammation have all been studied by various investigators. Surveillance for the presence of clinical predispositions to ARDS has been used successfully to identify a high-risk population. Further refinements to assure population homogeneity are essential. Recently developed techniques for detecting changes in vascular or epithelial permeability and lung water are certain to be applied in this population over the next several years. The measurement of circulating inflammatory mediators or markers of lung injury, however, shows greater promise in clarifying mechanisms of lung injury than in predicting ARDS. ARDS represents a spectrum of disease, rather than a yes/no phenomenon.

References

Anderson, R. R., Holliday, R. L., Driedger, A. A., Lefcoe, M., Reid, B., and Sibbald, W. J. (1979). Documentation of pulmonary capillary permeability in the adult respiratory distress syndrome accompanying human sepsis. *Am. Rev. Respir. Dis.,* **119**:869-877.

Ashbaugh, D. G., Bigelow, D. B., Petty, T. L., and Levine, B. E. (1967). Acute respiratory distress in adults. *Lancet,* **2**:319-323.

Bachofen, M., and Weibel, E. R. (1982). Structural alterations of lung parenchyma in the adult respiratory distress syndrome. *Clin.Chest Med.,* **3**:35-56.

Calindrino, F. S., Jr., Anderson, D. L., Mintun, M. A., and Schuster, D. P. (1988). Pulmonary vascular permeability during the adult respiratory distress syndrome: A positron emission tomographic study. *Am. Rev. Respir. Dis.,* **138**:421-428.

Carvalho, A. C. A., Bellman, S. M., Saullo, V. J., and Zapol, W. M. (1982). Altered Factor VIII in acute respiratory failure. *N. Engl. J. Med.,* **307**: 1113-1119.

Duchateau, J., Haas, M., Schreyen, H., et al. (1984). Complement activation in patients at risk of developing the adult respiratory distress syndrome. *Am. Rev. Respir. Dis.,* **130**:1058-1064.

Fein, A., Weiner-Kronish, J. P., Niederman, M., and Matthay, M. A. (1986). Pathophysiology of the adult respiratory distress syndrome: What have we learned from human studies? *Crit. Care Clin.,* **2**:429-453.

Fowler, A. A., Hamman, R. F., Good, J. T., et al. (1983). Adult respiratory distress syndrome: Risk with common predispositions. *Ann. Intern. Med.,* **98**:593-597.

Hallgren, R., Borg, T., Venge, P., et al. (1984). Signs of neutrophil and eosinophil activation in adult respiratory distress syndrome. *Crit. Care Med.,* **12**:14-18.

Hallman, M., Spragg, R., Harrell, J. H., et al. (1982). Evidence of lung surfactant abnormality in respiratory failure: Study of bronchoalveolar lavage phospholipids, surface activity, phospholipase activity and plasma myoinositol. *J. Clin. Invest.,* **70**:673-683.

Hammerschmidt, D. E., Weaver, L. J., Hudson, L. D., et al. (1980). Association of complement activation and elevated plasma C5a with adult respiratory distress syndrome. *Lancet,* **1**:947-949.

Holter, J. F., Weiland, J. E., Pacht, E. R., Gadek, J. E., Davis, W. B. (1986). Protein permeability in the adult respiratory distress syndrome: Loss of size selectivity of the alveolar epithelium. *J. Clin. Invest.,* **78**:1513-1522.

Hosea, S., Brown, E., Hammer, C., et al. (1980). Role of complement activation in a model of adult respiratory distress syndrome. *J. Clin. Invest.,* **66**:375-382.

Hudson, L. D. (1982). Causes of the adult respiratory distress syndrome: Clinical recognition. *Clin. Chest Med.,* **3**:195-212.

Mason, R. J. (1987). Surfactant in adult respiratory distress syndrome. *Eur. J. Respir. Dis.,* **71**(Suppl. 153):229-236.

Maunder, R. J. (1985). Clinical prediction of the adult respiratory distress syndrome. *Clin. Chest Med.,* **6**:413-426.

Maunder, R. J., and Hudson, L. D. (1986). The adult respiratory distress syndrome. In *Current Pulmonology*. Vol. 7. Edited by D. H. Simmons. Chicago, Year Book Medical Publishers, Chap. 4, pp. 97-116.

Maunder, R. J., Harlan, J. M., Talucci, R. C., et al. (1984). Measurement of C3a and C5a in high-risk patients does not predict ARDS (abstract). *Am. Rev. Respir. Dis.*, **129**:A104.

Maunder, R. J., Shuman, W. P., McHugh, J. W., Marglin, S. I., and Butler, J. (1986). Preservation of normal lung regions in the adult respiratory distress syndrome: Analysis by computed tomography. *JAMA*, **255**: 2463-2465.

Meyrick, B. (1986). Pathology of the adult respiratory distress syndrome. *Crit. Care Clin.*, **2**:405-428.

Murray, J. F., Matthay, M. A., Luce, J. M., and Flick, M. R. (1988). An expanded definition of the adult respiratory distress syndrome. *Am. Rev. Respir. Dis.*, **138**:720-723.

Parsons, P. E., Worthen, G. S., Moore, E. E., Tate, R. M., and Henson, P. M. (1989). The association of circulating endotoxin with the development of the adult respiratory distress syndrome. *Am. Rev. Respir. Dis.*, **140**:294-301.

Pepe, P. E., Potkin, R. T., Holtman-Reus, D., Hudson, L. D., and Carrico, C. J. (1982). Clinical predictors of the adult respiratory distress syndrome. *Am. J. Surg.*, **144**:124-130.

Pepe, P. E., Hudson, L. D., and Carrico, C. J. (1984). Early application of positive end-expiratory pressure in patients at risk for the adult respiratory distress syndrome. *N. Engl. J. Med.*, **311**:281-286.

Petty, T. L. (1988). ARDS: Refinement of concept and redefinition. *Am. Rev. Respir. Dis.*, **138**:724.

Petty, T. L., Reiss, O. K., Paul, G. W., et al. (1977). Characteristics of pulmonary surfactant in adult respiratory distress syndrome associated with trauma and shock. *Am. Rev. Respir. Dis.*, **115**:531-536.

Petty, T. L., Silvers, G. W., Paul, G. W., et al. (1979). Abnormalities in lung elastic properties and surfactant function in adult respiratory distress syndrome. *Chest*, **75**:571-574.

Pontoppidan, H., Geffin, B., and Lowenstein, E. (1972). Acute respiratory failure in the adult. *N. Engl. J. Med.*, **287**:690, 743, 799.

Rinaldo, J. E. (1986). The prognosis of the adult respiratory distress syndrome: Inappropriate pessimism? *Chest*, **96**:470-471.

Rinaldo, J. E., and Rogers, R. M. (1982). Adult respiratory distress syndrome: Changing concepts of lung injury and repair. *N. Engl. J. Med.*, **306**:900-908.

Rinaldo, J. E., Borovetz, H. S., Mancini, M. C., Hardesty, R. L., and Griffith, B. P. (1986). Assessment of lung injury in the adult respiratory distress syndrome using multiple indicator dilution curves. *Am. Rev. Respir. Dis.,* **133**:1006-1010.

Robbins, R., Maunder, R., Grossman, G., Kendall, T., Hudson, L., and Rennard, S. (1986). Functional loss of chemotactic factor inactivator in the adult respiratory distress syndrome (abstract). *Am. Rev. Respir. Dis.,* **133**:A277.

Rocker, D. M., Pearson, D., Wiseman, M. S., and Shale, D. J. (1989). Diagnostic criteria for adult respiratory distress syndrome: Time for reappraisal. *Lancet,* **1**:120-123.

Rubin, D. B., Matthay, M. A., Weinberg, P. F., and Murray, J. F. (1985). Factor VIII antigen: Possible plasma marker of progressive acute lung injury in patients with sepsis. *Am. Rev. Respir. Dis.,* **131**:A142.

Schoene, R. B. (1985). Pulmonary edema at high altitude: Review, pathophysiology, and update. *Clin. Chest Med.,* **6**:256-263.

Shoemaker, W. C., Appel, P., Czer, L. S. C., et al. (1980). Pathogenesis of respiratory failure (ARDS) after hemorrhage and trauma. I. Cardiorespiratory patterns preceding the development of ARDS. *Crit. Care Med.,* **8**:504-512.

Sibbald, W. J., Driedger, A. A., Hoffat, J. D., Myers, M. L., Reid, B. A., and Holliday, R. L. (1981). Pulmonary microvascular clearance of radiotracers in human cardiac and noncardiac pulmonary edema. *J. Appl. Physiol.,* **50**(6):1337-1347.

Simon, R. H. (1987). Predictors of the adult respiratory distress syndrome (editorial). *J. Crit. Care,* **2**:81-85.

Thommasen, H. V., Russell, J. A., Boyko, W. J., et al. (1984). Transient leucopenia associated with adult respiratory distress syndrome. *Lancet,* **1**:809-812.

Till, G. O., Johnson, K. J., Kunkel, R., et al. (1982). Intravascular activation of complement and acute lung injury. *J. Clin. Invest.,* **69**:1126-1135.

Vadas, P. (1984). Elevated plasma phospholipase A_2 levels: Correlation with the hemodynamic and pulmonary changes in gram-negative septic shock. *J. Lab. Clin. Med.,* **104**:873-881.

von Wichert, P., and Kohl, F. V. (1977). Decreased dipalmitoyllecithin content found in lung specimens from patients with so-called shock lung. *Intensive Care Med.,* **3**:27-30.

Weigelt, J. A., Snyder, W. H., III, and Mitchell, R. A. (1981). Early identification of patients prone to develop adult respiratory distress syndrome. *Am. J. Surg.,* **142**:687-691.

Weinberg, P. F., Matthay, M. A., Webster, R. O., et al. (1984). Biologically active products of complement and acute lung injury in patients with the sepsis syndrome. *Am. Rev. Respir. Dis.,* **130**:791-796.

2

Adult Respiratory Distress Syndrome: Definition, Risk Factors, and Outcome

THOMAS M. HYERS

St. Louis University Medical Center
St. Louis, Missouri

I. Introduction

The syndrome of acute respiratory failure associated with traumatic shock or sepsis has been known for many decades (Petty, 1981). Most obvious in battle field casualties, the syndrome was linked by a number of synonyms that usually identified a locale and battle (Buford and Burbank, 1945). Ashbaugh and colleagues gave the syndrome its first coherent medical description in 1967. These authors described explosive respiratory failure that accompanied trauma, sepsis, or certain drug overdoses. They defined the syndrome by the presence of severely decreased oxygenation, widespread pulmonary infiltrates on chest roentgenogram in the absence of cardiac failure, and decreased pulmonary compliance in the absence of cardiac failure. They subsequently proposed the name "adult respiratory distress syndrome" because this respiratory failure in adults had similarities to the neonatal respiratory distress syndrome (Petty and Ashbaugh, 1971). These authors hypothesized that the adult syndrome might also involve a deficiency of surfactant production or function. Since those seminal reports, a great deal of research has been conducted to clarify pathogenesis, risk factors, clinical course, and outcome. However, the mortality rate remains high and treatment is still only supportive despite some advances in the understanding of pathogenesis (Bell et al., 1983; Fowler et al., 1983; Pepe et al., 1982). In this chapter the current definition and descriptions of risk factors, natural history, and outcome are developed.

II. Incidence

It has been estimated that some 150,000 cases of ARDS occur in the United States yearly. Although this number is imprecise, it is a reasonable estimate based on recent prospective studies in defined populations (Fowler et al., 1983; Pepe et al., 1982). Furthermore, in the absence of specific therapy it is likely that the incidence of ARDS will not decrease, since the ever-increasing use of immunosuppressive regimens in oncology and organ transplantation enhances the proclivity of these patients to develop severe bacterial infections.

III. Definition

The earliest detailed definition of the syndrome included widespread pulmonary infiltrates on chest roentgenogram and defects of oxygenation and pulmonary compliance in the absence of cardiac failure (Petty and Ashbaugh, 1971). Since that time, various refinements or minor changes in the definition have been proposed (Murray, 1975, 1977; Petty, 1985; Rinaldo, 1986). Despite minor revisions in the definition of ARDS, all such definitions have nearly uniformly identified a group of individuals who, taken as a whole, require mechanical ventilation with a high fraction of inspired oxygen and have an expected mortality rate of 50-70%.

Recently it has been proposed that the definition of ARDS be broadened and made more inclusive so that more patients with respiratory failure can be included for purposes of research. A more inclusive definition would also allow identification of many more patients for epidemiologic purposes (Rinaldo, 1986). Although this approach has some superficial appeal, it has a number of drawbacks as well. First, the stringent requirements for widespread pulmonary infiltrate and severe oxygenation defect select a more uniform group of patients with an expected high mortality. Such requirements stay faithful to the original description of the syndrome and have been shown repeatedly to be useful in selecting patients with a poor prognosis for trials of pharmaceutical interventions (Bernard et al., 1987; Luce et al., 1988). The argument is frequently made that many patients with ARDS go through an early period of less severe respiratory failure first and that a more liberal definition would identify patients with the syndrome earlier. However, it is the author's experience that many patients develop the syndrome explosively and that progression to severe respiratory failure is often rapid. Recent studies of the relationship between sepsis and ARDS support this position (Montgomery et al., 1985; Seidenfeld et al., 1986). Having made this assertion, it must also be emphasized that many lesser cases of enhanced pulmonary microvascular permeability never progress to ARDS as it is defined here. Many such patients have only been identified by serial studies of bronchoalveolar lavage in high-risk patients. These patients do not develop significant clinical respiratory failure and have a much better prognosis than patients with ARDS.

Similarly, it has been proposed that the requirement for measurement of pulmonary arterial occlusion pressure be eliminated from the definition of ARDS. In fact, it is common clinical practice to diagnose ARDS without measuring the occlusion pressure, relying instead on the physical examination and the chest roentgenogram to exclude left heart dysfunction. However, for purposes of research the elimination of the pulmonary artery occlusion pressure measurement will invariably dilute a group of ARDS patients with other groups, notably with patients suffering from congestive heart failure. This latter group has a much better prognosis and is decidedly easier to treat (Da Luz et al., 1975). Consequently, the "contamination" of the ARDS group by less severely ill groups will only confuse studies of the pathogenesis and treatment of ARDS.

In contrast to the continued insistence on widespread, bilateral pulmonary infiltrates, severe oxygenation defect, and normal pulmonary arterial occlusion pressure, the requirement for low pulmonary compliance has largely been dropped from most current definitions of ARDS. Measurements of pulmonary compliance are highly dependent on the type and mode of mechanical ventilation and on the elastic properties of an individual's lungs. Consequently, the compliance criterion has proved to be the most variable of the components of the definition of ARDS and is currently not widely utilized.

The current definition used by investigators in the Specialized Center of Research of the Lung Division of the National Heart, Lung and Blood Institute is given in Table 1. The requirement for bilateral widespread infiltrates of onset within 7 days helps to eliminate patients with subacute forms of respiratory failure, such as accelerated interstitial lung disease (Hamman-Rich syndrome) or lymphangiocarcinomatosis of the lung. The utilization of a ratio of Pa_{O_2} to FI_{O_2} (P/F) simplifies the calculation of the oxygenation defect and probably minimizes the effect of ambient altitude on the calculation as well. Since the positive end-expiratory pressure (PEEP) may alter gas exchange, the requirement is liberalized for any patient receiving any amount of PEEP at the time of entry. Finally, the allowable pulmonary arterial occlusion pressure has been set at 17 mmHg or below. It is emphasized that

Table 1 Definition of ARDS

Widespread, bilateral pulmonary infiltrates of less than 7 days' duration
Pa_{O_2}/FI_{O_2} < 150 off PEEP < 200 on PEEP
Pulmonary artery occlusion pressure < 18 mmHg

this pressure should be carefully measured at end-expiration from a paper tracing, not directly from an electronic monitor or oscilloscope. Although the choice of 17 mmHg as the allowable limit to exclude hydrostatic contributions to edema is somewhat arbitrary, a number of experimental and clinical studies support this division (Fein et al., 1979; Staub, 1974).

It will be noted that no mention of risk group or causation is given in this definition. Risk groups or clinical predispositions are very important and should always be identified and managed in any patient with ARDS. However, ARDS is a syndrome, not a disease, and its manifestations are nonspecific enough that this or a similar definition will suffice for all patients, no matter what the risk group.

IV. Risk Groups

The three risk groups of aspiration of gastric contents, trauma, and sepsis account for nearly 75% of cases of ARDS. Sepsis alone accounts for approximately one-half of all cases. Altogether, scores of conditions have been associated with ARDS, but many of these lesser risk groups are epidemiologically unimportant as causes of acute respiratory failure (Table 2).

A. Sepsis

Bacterial sepsis, especially with gram-negative aerobic bacilli, is the most common infectious cause of ARDS (Fowler et al., 1983; Montgomery et al., 1985; Pepe et al., 1982; Seidenfeld et al., 1986). *Staphylococcus aureus*, other bacteria, viruses, rickettsiae, and parasites have also been implicated.

Bacterial sepsis, defined roughly as bacteremia, hypotension, fever, and evidence of end-organ dysfunction, results in ARDS and multiple organ failure in as much as 30-50% of cases (Bell et al., 1983; Fowler et al., 1983; Pepe et al., 1982). Sepsis syndrome or clinical sepsis, defined as the typical patient response in the absence of documented bacteremia, results in a similar incidence of ARDS and multiple organ failure, even in the absence of an obvious site of infection. The finding that sepsis syndrome or clinical sepsis is

Table 2 Some Clinical Predispositions to ARDS

1. Infections
   Bacterial (mostly gram-negative aerobic rods and *S. aureus*)
   Fungal and *Pneumocystis carinii*
   Viruses
   Mycobacteria
   Rickettsiae
2. Aspiration
   Gastric acid
   Near-drowning
   Hydrocarbons and other caustic liquids
3. Trauma (usually associated with shock and multiple blood transfusions)
   Fractures and soft tissue
   Burns
   Head trauma
   Lung contusion
   Fat embolism syndrome
4. Drugs and other chemicals
   Opiates
   Salicylates
   Paraquat
   Paraldehyde
   Ethchlorvynol (Placidyl)
   Colchicine
   Thiazides
   Tricyclic antidepressants
   Benzodiazepines
5. Disseminated intravascular coagulation (DIC)
   Thrombotic thrombocytopenic purpura (TTP)
   Hemolytic uremic syndrome (HUS)
   Other vasculitic syndromes
   Heat stroke
6. Pancreatitis
7. Inhaled
   Smoke from combustion
   Gases (NO_2, NH_3, Cl_2, cadmium, phosgene, oxygen)
8. Metabolic
   Ketoacidosis
   Uremia

Table 2 (continues)

Table 2 Continued

9. Miscellaneous
   Amniotic fluid embolism
   Retained products of conception
   Eclampsia
   Bowel infarction
   Subarachnoid or intracerebral hemorrhage
   Leukagglutin reaction

as menacing and lethal as sepsis strongly suggests that mediators of sepsis and the patient's response to infection are as important as the bacteria in the genesis of ARDS and organ injury.

B. Aspiration of Gastric Contents

This second most frequent cause of ARDS can be explosive when it occasionally occurs immediately following endotracheal extraction in the postoperative state, or it may be more surreptitious. The etiologic agent is thought to be hydrochloric acid. Animal studies indicate that the pH of the gastric content must be <2.5 to induce significant lung injury (Ribaudo and Grace, 1971). In some cases the event can be documented by suctioning gastric contents from the trachea or measuring a low pH in the tracheal secretions, but these findings are not necessary for the syndrome of respiratory failure to occur. When aspiration of gastric contents is witnessed, ARDS has been seen to occur in approximately one in three patients (Fowler et al., 1983; Pepe et al., 1982). Generally, cases of ARDS that follow gastric aspiration occur quickly, with a median time to onset of less than 3 hr from the witnessed event.

C. Trauma

Trauma without hypotension or blood transfusions results in a low incidence of ARDS unless the trauma impinges directly on the thorax, as in pulmonary contusion. However, when trauma is associated with significant hypotension and more than 10 units of whole blood or packed red blood cells transfused within 24 hr, the incidence of ARDS is considerable (Fowler et al., 1983). There is some evidence to suggest that the incidence of ARDS is directly related to the amount and frequency of blood transfused (Fowler et al., 1983). Other studies have not shown such a close relationship (Collins et al., 1978). It is more likely that the incidence of the syndrome is in some way related to the severity of the trauma. At any rate it is generally appreciated that cases of ARDS resulting from trauma are easier to manage than those that result from sepsis or aspiration of gastric contents. Furthermore, the mortality rate of patient with ARDS resulting from trauma, although considerable, appears to be significantly lower than that seen in ARDS resulting from sepsis or aspiration of gastric contents (Schonfeld et al., 1983). Furthermore, only in fat embolism syndrome, a peculiar subtype of ARDS associated with trauma, has glucocorticoid prophylaxis or treatment been shown to be effective (Schonfeld et al., 1983).

D. Other Causes of ARDS

The recognition that capillary pressure can be estimated from the pulmonary arterial occlusion pressure tracing has aided in our understanding and separation of cases of pulmonary edema caused by enhanced permeability from those caused by increased hydrostatic presence. For example, many drugs, including the opiates and aspirin, appear to cause pulmonary edema by raising capillary pressure, not by enhancing microvascular permeability. The various causes of neurogenic pulmonary edema all seem to work by increasing capillary pressure. In contrast, pancreatitis and disseminated intravascular coagulation seem to be the causes of enhanced permeability pulmonary edema (Table 3). The clinical syndrome of disseminated intravascular coagulation, when it occurs in conjunction with marked metabolic perturbations, such as heat stroke, seems to be a harbinger of ARDS. The finding that many conditions that were previously thought to cause enhanced pulmonary microvascular permeability actually cause pulmonary edema by raising pulmonary capillary pressure emphasizes even more the major etiologic roles of sepsis, trauma, and aspiration of gastric contents in the enhanced microvascular permeability that is ARDS.

Although ARDS is a syndrome, not a disease, the designation of ARDS should not be allowed to become a wide net into which every case of acute respiratory failure falls. For instance, acute lupus pneumonia can fulfill the criteria for ARDS but the underlying condition is chronic and the pathogenesis of lung injury is probably quite different (Haupt et al., 1981). Similarly, *Pneumocystis carinii* pneumonia in a patient with the acquired immunodeficiency syndrome can also meet the criteria for ARDS but again the underlying condition is chronic. It is again important to emphasize that the designation of ARDS implies an acute process causing severe respiratory failure with an expected high mortality rate. In every case the clinical predisposition or risk group must be specified.

E. High-Risk Groups

Early epidemiologic studies of ARDS indicated that clinical predispositions, such as trauma or sepsis, seemed to be risk factors, since not every patient

Table 3 Noncardiac Causes of Pulmonary Edema (Animal and Human Studies)

Enhanced permeability	Increased capillary pressure
Acid aspiration	High altitude
Sepsis	Fibrin degradation products
Trauma, thermal burns	Hemorrhagic shock
Microembolism (glass beads, air, thrombin)	Opiates
Complement activation	Histamine
Macrophage and neutrophil activation	Lung re-expansion
Pancreatitis	Neurogenic
Oleic acid	Salicylates
Hyperoxygen	Serotonin
Free radicals	
Chemicals	
Paraquat	
Ethchlorvynol	
Alloxan	

with a clinical predisposition developed the syndrome and combinations of clinical predispositions increased the incidence of the syndrome. In this way trauma alone resulted in a low incidence of ARDS, but trauma and multiple blood transfusions followed by sepsis resulted in a very high incidence of the syndrome (Fowler et al., 1983; Pepe et al., 1982). Furthermore, it has become evident that individuals who have the clinical predispositions but who do not develop the syndrome still manifest lesser amounts of lung injury (Fowler et al., 1987; Hyers and Fowler, 1986). Although these subclinical permeability changes only become evident in prospective studies utilizing bronchoalveolar lavage in high-risk patients, the findings imply that the clinical predispositions may be repetitively and cumulatively associated with subclinical lung injury. Consequently, these subclinical changes should not be termed early or pre-ARDS, since ARDS is not an invariable result. These conditions are better considered high-risk states that may lead to ARDS through cumulative lung injury that remains poorly understood.

V. Outcome

Just as ARDS is an occasional severe manifestation of a subclinical lung injury that occurs in many high-risk patients, subclinical injury of other organs also occurs frequently (Kreuzfelder et al., 1988). In fact, ARDS often represents the most obvious type of organ injury in multiple organ failure (MOF). Multiple organ failure is frequently seen in patients with sepsis (Montgomery et al., 1985; Seidenfeld et al., 1986), but it also develops in patients with ARDS from noninfectious causes because this group frequently becomes nosocomially infected (Montgomery et al., 1985; Seidenfeld et al., 1986).

The syndrome of multiple organ failure has been recognized for decades, particularly in the surgical literature (Blaisdell, 1973; Fry et al., 1980; Meakins et al., 1980). More recently, efforts to quantify the risk of mortality in multiple organ failure have been published (Knaus et al., 1985). These schemes incorporated descriptions of the patient's underlying physiologic status and number of organs failing. Although such efforts are still immature, they have advanced our efforts to prognosticate outcome in acute organ failure.

In ARDS, early prognostic studies have also pointed to the importance of underlying organ failure and poor host response to injury (Fowler et al., 1985).

Infection with gram-negative aerobic bacteria has been shown to be particularly important in ARDS both as cause and complication. In this way abdominal infection with gram-negative rods often leads to ARDS. In contrast, in those with noninfectious causes of ARDS, pulmonary nosocomial infections with these organisms often complicates the syndrome. After the first 3 days of the syndrome nearly all subsequent deaths occur from sepsis and multiple organ failure (Da Luz et al., 1975; Seidenfeld et al., 1986). Consequently, nosocomial lung infection in a patient with ARDS is a dire prognostic sign, and the avoidance of lung infection favors recovery. This problem is further complicated by our poor ability to diagnose lung infection in mechanically ventilated patients with underlying respiratory failure (Faling, 1988a). Improvements in our ability to diagnose pulmonary infection in these patients using quantitative cultures of protected brush and bronchoalveolar lavage specimens should aid in prognostication and in evaluation of various treatment and prophylaxis regimens (Fagar et al., 1988; Johanson et al., 1988; Torres et al., 1988). However, the clinical adage is widely appreciated that in cases of ARDS and multiple organ injury associated with bacterial infection, the organ injury does not begin to resolve until the infection is successfully treated.

Approximately 90% of all deaths in cases of ARDS occurs within 2-3 weeks following the onset of the syndrome. In the first few days of the syndrome, deaths tend to occur from the underlying clinical predisposition, and after 3 days the majority of deaths occur from sepsis and multiple organ failure. Survivors for more than 2-3 weeks have a good long-term outlook for recovery, although up to a year may be required for maximum recovery of lung function. A minority of survivors will develop significant restrictive or obstructive lung dysfunction or some combination of the two. Predictors and determinants of who will develop permanent lung dysfunction and of which type are not well described.

VI. New Directions in Clinical Studies of ARDS

Since the syndrome continues to be lethal in 50-70% of patients and treatment remains only supportive, emphasis must be placed on prevention and developing new modes of treatment (Bernard et al., 1987; Luce et al., 1988). There is now reasonable agreement on what constitutes high-risk groups and on the definition of the syndrome. However, early clinical predictors of sepsis need to be identified so that prophylactic regimens and antibiotics can be started as early as possible. In this regard more general agreement on a definition of the sepsis syndrome or clinical sepsis is needed, since it has been mistaken for documentable sepsis in approximately 30-50% of prospective treatment studies.

The word *sepsis* implies infection and a characteristic systemic pathophysiologic response. Under this broad rubric the term "bacteremia" means the documented presence of bacteria in the blood. It has become apparent that in suspected infection, the presence of deleterious host responses, such as hypotension, metabolic acidosis, and a lowered systemic vascular resistance, are important clinical markers of subsequent organ failure. Consequently, the terms "sepsis syndrome" or "clinical sepsis" have been used to describe host changes associated with suspected sepsis that occur in the absence of documented bacteremia. The definition of clinical sepsis usually includes some combinations of fever and leukocytosis associated with hypotension, acidosis, and a lowered systemic vascular resistance. Septic shock is the extreme example of clinical sepsis. If one waits to define sepsis until bacteremia is documented, hours to days are lost and the clinical syndrome has either cleared or progressed to such extensive damage that current therapy is ineffective. Consequently, in most recent studies of pharmacologic interventions, patients are entered at the time of recognition of clinical sepsis. Several interesting corollaries have emerged from the clinical definition of sepsis. First, when sepsis is suspected based on the presence of the deleterious host response, bacterial cultures of blood are often negative (Fowler et al., 1983; Montgomery et al., 1985; Pepe et al., 1982; Seidenfeld et al., 1986). Second, clinical sepsis can be evident without an obvious focus of infection (Seidenfeld et al., 1986). Third and perhaps most important, in the setting of clinical sepsis the outcome is comparable whether or not blood cultures subsequently turn positive for pathogenic bacteria (Bone et al., 1987; VA Study Group, 1987). Fourth, the presence of clinical sepsis *and* organ failure in the form of ARDS doubles the observed mortality rate of clinical sepsis alone

(Bone et al., 1987; Montgomery et al., 1985; VA Study Group, 1987). This increased mortality rate seems to be closely linked to ongoing infection. These findings strongly suggest that bacterial products, such as endotoxin, are as toxic as are live bacteria. Furthermore, it appears that a deleterious host response, for example, sepsis syndrome, to bacteremia or their nonviable components leads to a worse outcome.

Consequently, clinical investigators working in this field must distinguish bacteremia from sepsis and arrive at a common definition of sepsis syndrome or clinical sepsis. These distinctions will be useful in describing the relationship of sepsis to organ failure. On a more mechanistic level, consensus on clinical definitions will aid in understanding the intermediate links between dissemination of bacterial components and tissue damage. This clinical work is now ready to proceed because of the advent of more sensitive assays for bacterial endotoxin and because of the availability of more accurate tests for nosocomial pneumonia in the mechanically ventilated patient (Fagon et al., 1988; Johanson et al., 1988a; Torres et al., 1988). In this regard the incidence of nosocomial pneumonia may be decreased by the use of enteral or topical antibiotic application to the mouth (Faling, 1988; Johanson et al., 1988b). Human trials of this prophylaxis are in progress.

Finally, the relationship of ARDS to other organ failure needs further study both in cases of sepsis and in the noninfectious predispositions to sepsis. A number of questions present themselves in this regard. It is not known how often ARDS precedes other organ failure in sepsis. Further, since aspiration of gastric contents as a cause of ARDS carries a high mortality rate and trauma and drug overdose as causes of ARDS carry lower mortality rates, one wonders if subsequent nosocomial pulmonary infection accounts for the difference in outcome. Agreement on clinical definitions of gastrointestinal, hepatic, and central nervous system failure will be needed to allow this epidemiologic work to proceed. Elucidation of these relationships should aid in our further understanding of the epidemiology of ARDS and help us to target new prophylaxis and treatment modalities more precisely.

References

Ashbaugh, D. G., Bigelow, D. B., Petty, T. L., and Levine, B. E. (1967). Acute respiratory distress in adults. *Lancet,* **2**:319-323.

Bell, R. C., Coalson, J. J., Smith, J. P., Johanson, W. G., Jr. (1983). Multiple system organ failure and infection in adult respiratory distress syndrome. *Ann. Intern. Med.,* **99**:293-298.

Bernard, G. R., Luce, J. M., and Sprung, C. L. (1987). High-dose corticosteroids in patients with the adult respiratory distress syndrome. *N. Engl. J. Med.,* **317**:1565-1570.

Blaisdell, F. W. (1973). Respiratory insufficiency syndrome: Clinical and pathological definition. *J. Trauma,* **13**:195-199.

Bone, R. C., Fisher, C. J., Clemmer, T. P., et al. (1987). A controlled clinical trial of high-dose methylprednisolone in the treatment of severe sepsis and septic shock. *N. Engl. J. Med.,* **317**:653-658.

Buford, T. H., and Burbank, B. (1945). Traumatic wet lung: Observations on certain physiologic fundamentals in thoracic trauma. *J. Thorac. Cardiovasc. Surg.,* **14**:415-425.

Collins, J. A., James, P. M., Bradenberg, C. E., Andersen, R. W., Heisterkamp, C. A., and Simmons, D. L. (1978). The relationship between transfussion and hypoxemia in combat casualties. *Ann. Surg.,* **188**:513-519.

Da Luz, P. L., Shubin, H., Weil, M. H., et al. (1975). Pulmonary edema related to changes in colloid osmotic and pulmonary artery wedge pressure in patients after acute myocardial infarction. *Circulation,* **51**:350-357.

Fagon, J.-Y., Chastre, J., Hance, A. J., Guiguet, M., Trouillet, J.-L., Domart, Y., Pierre, J., and Gibert, C. (1988). Detection of nosocomial lung infection in ventilated patients: Use of a protected specimen brush and quantitative culture techniques in 147 patients. *Am. Rev. Respir. Dis.,* **138**:110-116.

Faling, L. J. (1988a). New advances in diagnosing nosocomial pneumonia in intubated patients. Part I. *Am. Rev. Respir. Dis.,* **137**:253-255.

Faling, L. J. (1988b). Advances in presenting nosocomial pneumonia. Part II. *Am. Rev. Respir. Dis.,* **137**:256-258.

Fein, A., Grossman, R. F., Jones, J. G., Overland, E., Pitts, L., Murray, J. F., and Staub, N. C. (1979). The value of edema fluid protein measurement in patients with pulmonary edema. *Am. J. Med.,* **67**:32-38.

Fowler, A. A., Hamman, R. F., Good, J. T., Benson, K. N., Baird, M., Eberle, D., Petty, T. L., and Hyers, T. M. (1983). Adult respiratory distress syndrome: Risk with common predispositions. *Ann. Intern. Med.,* **98**:593-597.

Fowler, A. A., Hamman, R. F., Zerbe, G. O., Benson, K. N., and Myers, T. M. (1985). Adult respiratory distress syndrome: Prognosis after onset. *Am. Rev. Respir. Dis.,* **132**:472-478.

Fowler, A. A., Fisher, B. J., Hyers, T. M., Bechard, D. E., Centor, R. M., and Webster, R. O. (1987). The adult respiratory distress syndrome: Cell populations and soluble mediators in the airspaces of patients at risk. *Am. Rev. Respir. Dis.,* **136**:1225-1231.

Fry, D. E., Pearlstein, L., Fulton, R. L., et al. (1980). Multiple system organ failure: The role of uncontrolled infection. *Arch. Surg.,* **115**:136-140.

Haupt, H. M., Moore, G. W., and Hutchins, G. M. (1981). The lung in systemic lupus erythematosis. Analysis of the pathologic changes in 120 patients. *Am. J. Med.,* **71**:791-798.

Hyers, T. M., and Fowler, A. A. (1986). Adult respiratory distress syndrome: Causes, morbidity and mortality. *Fed. Proc.,* **45**:25-29.

Johanson, W. G., Jr., Seidenfeld, J. J. , Gomez, P., De Los Santos, R., and Coalson, J. J. (1988a). Bacteriologic diagnosis of nosocomial pneumonia following prolonged mechanical ventilation. *Am. Rev. Respir. Dis.,* **137**:259-264.

Johanson, W. G., Jr., Seidenfeld, J. J., De Los Santos, R., Coalson, J. J., and Gomez, P. (1988b). Prevention of nosocomial pneumonia using topical and parenteral antimicrobial agents. *Am. Rev. Respir. Dis.,* **137**: 265-272.

Knaus, W. A., Draper, E. A., Wagner, D. P., and Zimmerman, J. E. (1985). Prognosis in acute organ system failure. *Ann. Surg.,* **202**:685-693.

Kreuzfelder, E., Joka, T., Keinecke, H.-O., et al. (1988). Adult respiratory distress syndrome as a specific manifestation of a general permeability defect in trauma patients. *Am. Rev. Respir. Dis.,* **137**:95-99.

Luce, J. M., Montgomery, A. B., Marks, J. D., Turner, J., Metz, C. A., and Murray, J. F. (1988). Ineffectiveness of high-dose methylprednisolone in preventing parenchymal lung injury and improving mortality in patients with septic shock. *Am. Rev. Respir. Dis.,* **138**:62-68.

Meakins, J. L., Wicklund, B., Forse, R. A., and McLean, A. P. (1980). The surgical intensive care unit: Current concepts in infection. *Surg. Clin. North Am.,* **60**:117-132.

Montgomery, A. B., Stager, M. A., Carrico, C. J., and Hudson, L. D. (1985). Causes of mortality in patients with the adult respiratory distress syndrome. *Am. Rev. Respir. Dis.,* **132**:485-489.

Murray, J. F. (1975). The adult respiratory distress syndrome (may it rest in peace). *Am. Rev. Respir. Dis.,* **111**:716-718.

Murray, J. F. (1977). Conference report: Mechanisms of acute respiratory failure. *Am. Rev. Respir. Dis.,* **115**:1071-1078.

Pepe, P. E., Potkin, R. T., Reus, D. H., Hudson, L. D., and Carrico, C. J. (1982). Clinical indicators of the adult respiratory distress syndrome. *Am. J. Surg.,* **144**:124-130.

Petty, T. L. (1981). Adult respiratory distress syndrome: Historical perspective and definition. *Semin. Respir. Med.,* **2**:99-103.

Petty, T. L. (1985). Indicators of risk, course, and prognosis in adult respiratory distress syndrome. *Am. Rev. Respir. Dis.,* **132**:471.

Petty, T. L., and Ashbaugh, D. G. (1971). The adult respiratory distress syndrome: Clinical features, factors influencing prognosis, and principles of management. *Chest,* **60**:233-239.

Ribaudo, C. A., and Grace, W. J. (1971). Pulmonary aspiration. *Am. J. Med.,* **50**:510-520.

Rinaldo, J. E. (1986). The prognosis of the adult respiratory distress syndrome. Inappropriate pessimism? *Chest,* **90**:470-471.

Schonfeld, S. A., Ploysongsang, Y., Di Lisio, R., Grissman, J. D., Miller, E., Hammerschmidt, D. E., and Jacob, H. S. (1983). Fat embolism prophylaxis with corticosteroids. *Ann. Intern. Med.,* **99**:438-443.

Seidenfeld, J. J., Pohl, D. F., Bell, R. C., Harris, G. D., Johanson, W. G., Jr. (1986). Incidence, site, and outcome of infections in patients with the adult respiratory distress syndrome. *Am. Rev. Respir. Dis.,* **134**:12-16.

Staub, N. C. (1974). Pulmonary edema. *Physiol. Rev.,* **54**:678-811.

Torres, A., de la Bellacasa, J. P., Rodriguez-Roisin, R., de Anta, M. T. J., and Agusti-Vidal, A. (1988). Diagnostic value of telescoping plugged catheters in mechanically ventilated patients with bacterial pneumonia using the Metras catheter. *Am. Rev. Respir. Dis.,* **138**:117-120.

Veterans Administration Systemic Sepsis Cooperative Study Group (1987). Effect of high-dose glucocorticoid therapy on mortality in patients with clinical signs of systemic sepsis. *N. Engl. J. Med.,* **317**:659-665.

3

Clinical Presentation, Prognostic Factors, and Outcome of ARDS in the European Collaborative Study (1985-1987)

A Preliminary Report

A. ARTIGAS

Hospital de Sabadell
Sabadell
and Universidad Autonoma
Barcelona, Spain

J. R. LE GALL and C. L. CHASTANG

Hôpital Saint Louis
Paris, France

J. CARLET

Hôpital Saint Joseph
Paris, France

L. BLANCH and R. FERNANDEZ

Hospital de Sabadell
Sabadell, Spain

I. Introduction

The adult respiratory distress syndrome (ARDS) is an acute, severe alteration in lung structure and function characterized by hypoxemia, low-compliance lungs with a low functional residual capacity, and diffuse radiographic infiltrates due to increased lung microvascular permeability (Loyd et al., 1984). Since first described in 1967 (Ashbaugh et al., 1987), the syndrome has been associated with a high mortality, and it is disappointing that despite many clinical and laboratory investigations the survival rates have remained virtually unchanged. Patients with the syndrome usually die either from the severity of lung impairment or from common complications. Whether the hypoxemia

*The members of the Coordinator Committee of the European Collaborative ARDS Study are: A. Artigas (principal investigator and chairperson), Barcelona; H. Benzer, Insbruck; J. F. Bernaudin, Paris; J. Carlet, Paris; L. Chastang, Paris; P. Cox, Portland; K. Falke, Berlin; L. Gattinoni, Milano; J. R. Le Gall, Paris; M. Hemmer, Luxembourg; M. Lamy, Liege; J. Qvist, Herlev, and P. M. Suter, Geneva. Other study participants are listed in the Appendix.

of acute respiratory failure is the usual cause of death in patients with ARDS is controversial. However, supportive measures such as mechanical ventilation with positive end-expiratory pressure (PEEP) (Pepe et al., 1984) or extracorporeal membrane oxygenation (Zapol et al., 1979), although technically successful at increasing arterial oxygenation, have had no obvious effect on reducing mortality. This suggests a need to focus on the prevention or treatment of other aspects of this syndrome, such as analysis of the natural history and factors contributing to death in addition to respiratory support measures.

II. Diagnosis of ARDS

The usual definition of ARDS includes only the most severe cases of permeability pulmonary edema. Since the clinical presentation of patients with ARDS has changed little from its original description in 1967, the development of physiologic indices for an accurate definition of the syndrome has been essential for the standardization of "entry criteria" into various clinical studies. These additional features of clinical diagnosis usually include the presence or absence of PEEP ventilation, specific values for the alveolar-arterial oxygen tension gradient (or the arterial alveolar ratio) or calculated right-to-left pulmonary shunt fraction, and measurements of pulmonary compliance. These physiologic criteria are not universally accepted and vary widely among investigators (Table 1). Scoring systems have been described to quantitate the severity of ARDS (Murray et al., 1988).

Following the introduction of bedside pulmonary artery catheterization with the measurement of pulmonary arterial occlusion pressure (PAOP) as a guide to pulmonary capillary and left atrial pressure, it has been possible to quantify the contribution of a raised capillary pressure to the formation of pulmonary edema. Indeed, it is believed essential to measure PAOP in ARDS especially as these patients tend to develop acute pulmonary hypertension and right ventricular dysfunction limiting the value of isolated measurements of central venous pressure. This new invasive technology, although widely applied, has brought with it a number of problems: (1) Although usually reliable, PAOP is occasionally not an accurate measurement of either capillary pressure or left ventricular filling pressure in ARDS, (2) PAOP is rarely related to the prevailing plasma colloid oncotic pressure, and (3) since pulmonary artery catheterization is usually reserved for the most severely ill, a selection bias favoring the entry of severe cases of ARDS into clinical studies has occurred.

Unfortunately, we do not have the means to diagnose ARDS in its early stages. Mild hypocapnia is common in ARDS as well as hypoxemic respiratory failure due to other causes. Furthermore, many patients at high risk of

Table 1 Some Diagnostic Criteria Used to Define Acute Respiratory Failure and ARDS

Investigators and study	Criteria used in diagnosis
Ashbaugh et al. (1967) (original description of ARDS)	Dyspnoea, tachypnea, refractory hypoxemia, reduced pulmonary compliance and bilateral alveolar infiltration on CXR
Pontoppiddan et al. (1985) (MGH scoring system for acute respiratory failure)	Four categories of respiratory failure: 1. *At risk*: one or more risk factors, no/minimal changes on CXR, oxygen by face mask for short periods only 2. *Mild*: minimal diffuse or lobar changes on CXR with or without intubation and CPAP with an F_{IO_2} <0.5 3. *Moderate*: panlobar alveolar infiltrates of one of both lungs of CXR, intubated for more than 24 hr requiring positive airway pressure (CMV, IMV, PEEP, CPAP) with an F_{IO_2} >0.5 4. *Severe*: bilateral panlobar alveolar infiltrates on CXR, intubated requiring CMV and PEEP, Pa_{O_2} <50 mmHg with F_{IO_2} of 1.0 for 8 hr or more, or F_{IO_2} >0.6 for more than 48 hr
Bartlet et al. (1986) (NHI study of acute hypoxic respiratory failure, 1975-1977)	Endotracheal intubation and positive airway pressure for at least 24 hr with an F_{IO_2} >0.50 Five diagnostic categories defined: pneumonitis, capillary leak syndromes (ARDS), high-pressure edema, thromboemboli, and chronic airways obstruction
Zapol et al. (1979) (extracorporeal membrane oxygenation study)	Fast or slow entry criteria: 1. *Fast entry*: Pa_{O_2} <50 mmHg for more than 2 hr with an F_{IO_2} of 1.0 and PEEP >5 cm H_2O 2. *Slow entry*: despite maximal medical therapy for 48 hr, Pa_{O_2} <50 mmHg for more than 12 hr when measured on an F_{IO_2} >0.6 and PEEP >5 cm

Table 1 (*continues*)

Table 1 Continued

Investigators and study	Criteria used in diagnosis
	H_2O with a pulmonary shunt >30% measured on PEEP with and FI_{O_2} of 1.0
Holcroft et al. (1986) (prostaglandin E_1 study)	Patients with ARDS requiring mechanical ventilation with an FI_{O_2} >0.4 and PEEP >5 cm H_2O "not responding to conventional therapy
Upjohn European multicenter trial of prostaglandin E_1 in ARDS	Patients with postoperative ARDS or associated with sepsis or trauma requiring mechanical ventilation, with: an FI_{O_2} >0.5 ± PEEP in two or more determinations at least 2 hr apart in the preceding 24 hr giving a Pa_{O_2} < 75 mmHg or an arterial: alveolar ratio < 0.3 with a pulmonary arterial occlusion pressure < 18 mmHg
European Society of Intensive Care Study of acute respiratory failure	Patients with respiratory distress and a CXR of diffuse bilateral pulmonary infiltrates and severe hypoxemia defined by: Pa_{O_2} < 75 mmHg with an FI_{O_2} > 0.5 for at least 24 hr

CXR, Chest X-ray; Pa_{O_2}, arterial oxygen tension; FI = 2, inspired fraction of oxygen, CMV, continuous mandatory ventilation; IMV, intermittent mandatory ventilation.

developing ARDS develop severe transitory hypoxemia but never progress to the syndrome. Pepe et al. (1982) found that 55% of patients considered at high risk for ARDS who developed "critical hypoxemia" did not progress to ARDS.

The intuitive impression of many clinicians is that most patients in high ARDS risk groups (e.g., posttrauma) who develop pulmonary infiltrates and require mechanical ventilation are now treated more successfully and with a higher survival rate than reported in the majority of published studies (Pepe et al., 1982; Montgomery et al., 1985; Bell et al., 1983a; Fowler et al., 1983). The discrepancy between the present perception of practitioners and the clinical literature suggests that the entry criteria for ARDS into published studies have increasingly selected an atypical population with a high incidence of severe underlying disease(s) or multiple extrapulmonary organ system failure (Rinaldo, 1986).

Two criteria, severe hypoxemia (alveolar/arterial Po_2 ratio < 0.3) and a simultaneous indwelling PA catheter, have increasingly introduced bias into published clinical studies, selecting out a small subset of ARDS patients with an unusually poor prognosis. In order to qualify as having ARDS in many recent published series, poor gas exchange refractory to PEEP, a high FI_{O_2}, and a pulmonary artery catheter needed to be present. Because of increasing awareness of the uncertain risk/benefit ratio for the use of pulmonary artery catheters, different groups treat ARDS patients with PEEP and reduce the FI_{O_2} to a nontoxic level without employing invasive monitoring of the cardiovascular system. If the supportive initial therapy is effective, these patients will not be diagnosed as having ARDS. To better assess the prognosis of acute lung injury, standard criteria for ARDS requiring a low alveolar/arterial Po_2 ratio and a pulmonary arterial catheter may need to be modified. Elimination of measurements obtained with a pulmonary arterial catheter will increase the risk of occasionally including in an ARDS study a patient with unsuspected cardiogenic edema. However, it may be necessary to accept this limitation in order to assess prognosis more accurately in a wider population and evaluate new treatments. The selection of an ARDS group with a high percentage of predictably moribund patients with severe underlying organ failure or irreversible underlying diseases will virtually guarantee that promising drugs undergoing clinical therapeutic trials in ARDS will not be shown to improve outcome. Rinaldo (1986) has recently emphasized this point in 27 patients using a broad clinical criteria for ARDS. Patients with "nonpublishable" ARDS criteria (including young trauma patients without preexisting disease) have a markedly increased ARDS survival rate approximating 70% (Table 2).

To analyze prognostic factors and outcome in ARDS a collaborative European prospective study was carried out by 38 centers from September 1985 to March 1987. Severe hypoxic respiratory failure was defined in 583 patients by the presence of a known risk factor for ARDS, Pa_{O_2} < 75 mmHg

Table 2 Survival Rates for Patients with Different ARDS Criteria

	ARDS		Mortality	
	Number	%	Number	%
A: Nonpublishable	20	74	6	30
B: Publishable	7	26	5	71
Total	27	100	11	40

with $FI_{O_2} > 0.5$ and PEEP 5 cm H_2O, and panlobar infiltration occurring in patients over 15 years of age. Twenty-four hours after admission, mechanical ventilation parameters were fixed (Vt 10 ml/kg, I/E = 1:2, PEEP 5 cm H_2O, $FI_{O_2} = 0.5$) and two groups were identified: *Group A "hypoxemic"* with $Pa_{O_2} > 75$ mmHg and *Group B "Severe ARF"* with hypoxemia ($Pa_{O_2} < 75$ mmHg) and PAOP < 18 mmHG. General medical data and potential prognostic indicator values were collected including illness etiology, previous health status, age, severity of illness (severity indexes and the presence of acute organ system failure), and other physiological variables.

III. Etiology

ARDS occurred in the European Collaborative Study following a variety of overwhelming insults and risk factors (Fig. 1). Some of the nonpulmonary conditions associated with ARDS were shock, sepsis, nonpulmonary trauma, drug overdose, pancreatitis, uremia, eclampsia, central nervous system disease, emboli, burns, and massive transfusion. Pulmonary conditions associated with ARDS include aspiration, lung contusion, infection, radiation, toxic gas inhalation, and near-drowning. Sepsis and trauma were the most common causes of ARDS, the most common cause ranging from one hospital to another depending on local admission policies and clinical specialty practice. In general in medical ICU facilities, bacterial, viral, and aspiration pneumonia patients predominated, whereas such patients accounted for only 28.8% of ARDS admissions to a surgical ICU (Pontoppidan et al., 1985).

Precipitating conditions and specific cause-effect relationships of ARDS often cannot be identified, and the early pathogenetic mechanisms are probably diverse (Rinaldo and Rogers, 1982). The initial insult reaches the lower respiratory tract via the airway or circulation, but regardless of the early pathogenetic mechanisms, the physiologic and morphologic manifestations of ARDS become indistinguishable with time. Clinically, diffuse bilateral pneumonias and contusions both fit the criteria of ARDS, and it is often difficult to distinguish one from the other. Intubated and mechanically ventilated patients usually become colonized with nosocomial bacteria within a few days after admission and can develop a pulmonary superinfection contributing to maintaining or worsening acute lung injury (Montgomery et al., 1985; Bell et al., 1983a; Andrews et al., 1981).

Although no substantial evidence has yet been provided, it is believed that the outcome of ARDS probably depends on the following basic factors: the intensity of the initial acute lung injury; the precipitating cause of ARDS and its response to treatment; and the occurrence of complications and further lung injury. Most deaths in the first days of the syndrome can be attributed to the underlying illness or injury. The majority of late deaths have been

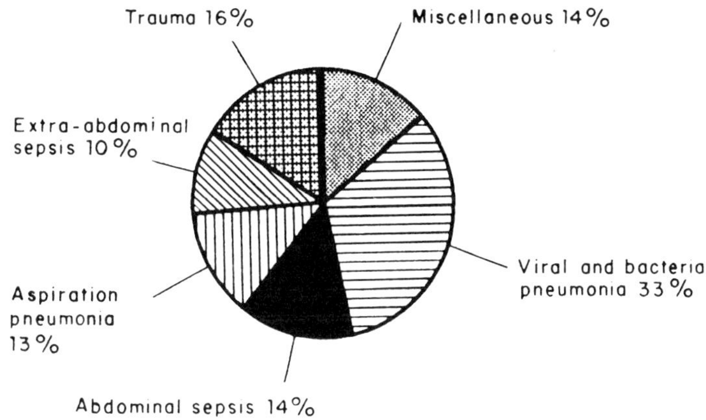

Figure 1 Distribution of etiologies in 583 ARDS patients in the European Collaborative Study. Infectious etiologies (pulmonary and abdominal sources) were the most frequent causes of ARDS.

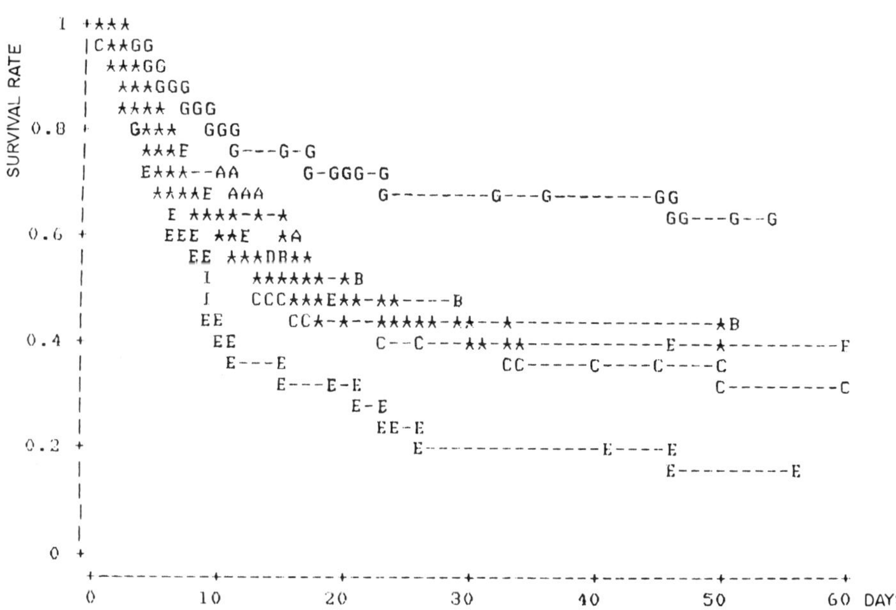

Figure 2 Percent survival of the various etiologies of 583 ARDS patients after 60 days. A, Aspiration; B, extraabdominal infection; C, intraabdominal infection; D, miscellaneous; E, opportunistic pneumonia; F, pneumonia; G, trauma. *$p < 0.0001$.

Table 3 ARDS: Distribution According to Gas Exchange

	No. cases	Survivors	Nonsurvivors	Mortality (%)
Group A Pa_{O_2} > 75 mmHg FI_{O_2} > 0.5 + PEEP 5 cm H_2O	180	111	69	38
Group B Pa_{O_2} < 75 mmHg FI_{O_2} > 0.5 + PEEP 5 cm H_2O	403	126	277	69[a]
Total	583	237	346	59

[a] $p < 0.01$

related to complications, primarily septicemia. Fowler et al. (1983) reported a similar high mortality rate in al ARDS etiologic groups. However, the initial pathogenetic mechanisms differ depending on the precise etiology (septicemia vs. trauma) and the mode of injury (airway vs. circulation). We found the highest mortality rates were due to acute lung injury caused by diffuse infectious processes and pneumonias. ARF following trauma carried an intermediate risk of death, with a lower mortality (38%, $p < 0.0001$) (Fig. 2).

Prior health status is an important prognostic factor in ARDS. Patients with preexisting disease had a higher mortality rate (76%). When ARDS due to an infectious cause developed in an immunocompromised host, the survival rate was very low.

The initial response to treatment (first 24 hr) was useful to distinguish those patients capable of recruiting collapsed alveolar spaces. Patients in group A were associated with a lower mortality rate (Table 3). In this ARDS group we treated predominantly posttraumatic injury patients and other patients without major preexisting diseases.

IV. Mortality and Prognostic Factors

Despite nearly two decades of progress in supportive care for patients with ARDS, recent studies and reviews continue to report a high mortality rate ranging between 41% and 73.8% in patients with ARDS (Pepe et al., 1982; Montgomery et al., 1985; Bell et al., 1983a; Fowler et al., 1983; Fein et al., 1983) and as high as 90% in patients with both sepsis and ARDS; the majority of patients die within 14 days of the onset of the syndrome (Fowler et al., 1983). The mortality rate in the European Study was 59% and lower than the 1976 NHLBI-sponsored Study (see Table 4).

Table 4 Etiologies: Comparison Between American (NHLBI, 1979) and European (1987) Studies

	United States (NHLBI)			Europe		
	NB patients	%	Mortality	NB patients	%	Mortality
Aspiration	93	12.5%	66.6%	65	11.1%	60%
Extra-abdominal infections	—	—	—	45	7.7%	56%
Intra-abdominal infections	94	12.6%	72.4%	97	16.6%	68%
Trauma	55	7.4%	47.2%	109	18.9%	38%
Opportunistic pneumonia	—	—	—	50	8.5%	86%
Interstitial pneumonia	18	2.4	88.9%	—	—	—
Other pneumonia	166	22.4%	68.6%	129	22.1%	61%
Cardiogenic shock	135	18.2%	63.7%	—	—	—
Hypovolemic shock	94	12.6%	68.1%	—	—	—
Miscellaneous	86	11.6%	61.6%	88	15.1%	59%
Total	741	100 %	65.9%	583	100 %	59%

Different authors have recently studied various factors and indicators of poor prognosis in ARDS patients (Montgomery et al., 1985; Fowler et al., 1985; Maunder et al., 1986). The main factors correlating with survival are age and the extent of multisystem organ failure (Artigas and Mancebo, 1987; Mancebo and Artigas, 1987). Eighty-two percent of patients over 70 years of age did not survive (Fig. 3). The mortality rate is directly related to the number of complications and increases to 83% when three or more complications are present (Fig. 4). Patients without complications during their clinical management had a lower mortality rate (38%).

The most frequent complications appearing during the course of ARDS are shock, pulmonary infection, and acute renal failure; all were associated

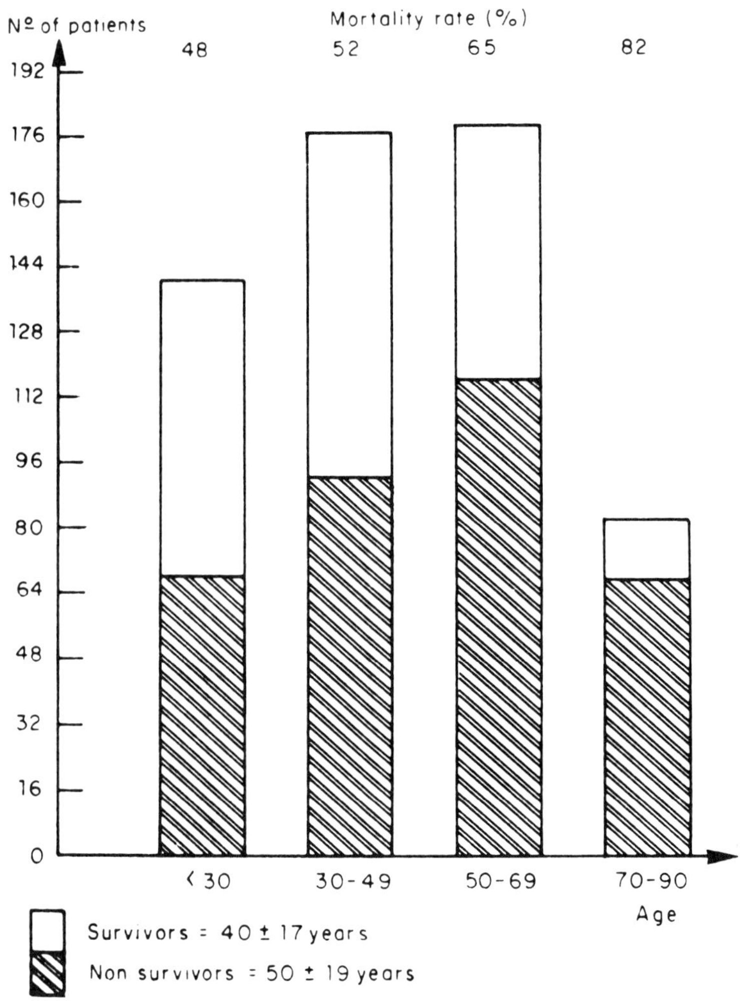

Figure 3 Incidence and survival by age group of 583 patients with ARDS. The average age of survivors was lower than that of nonsurvivors. The majority of patients over 70 years of age died.

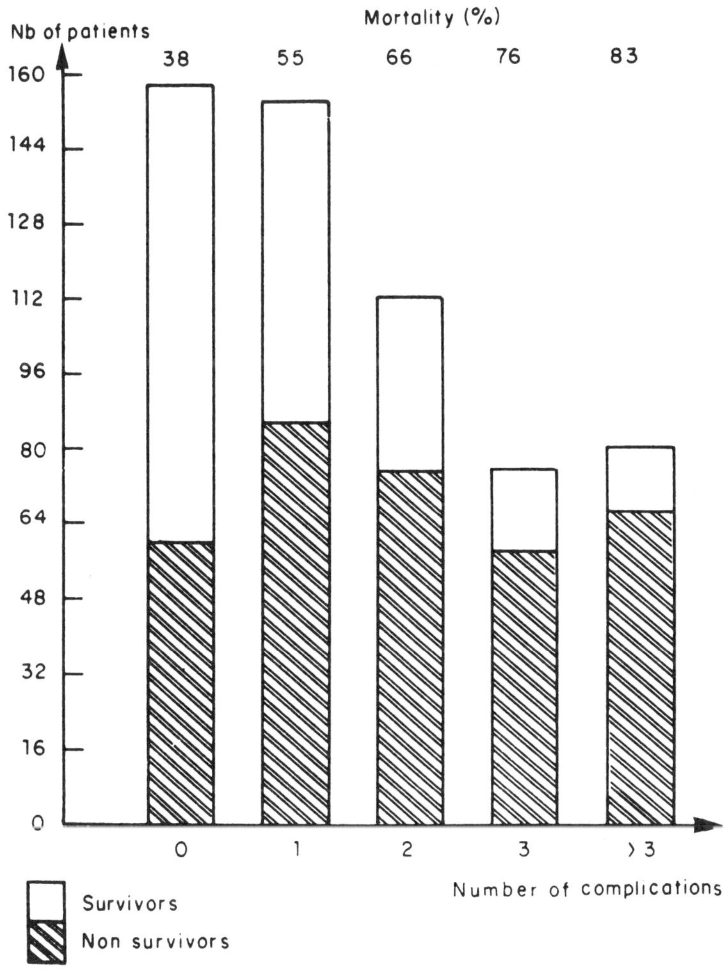

Figure 4 Overall mortality in each group of ARDS patients without complications, with one complication, two complications, and three or more complications appearing during intensive therapy (n = 583 ARDS patients).

with increased mortality. The majority of late deaths are related to the sepsis syndrome, which was present in 73% of ARDS patients (Montgomery et al., 1985; Mancebo and Artigas, 1987); the predominant source of sepsis was the lung. Several investigators have reported that sepsis syndrome, rather than respiratory failure, is the leading cause of death in patients with ARDS

(Pepe et al., 1982; Montgomery et al., 1985; Bell et al., 1983a; Fein et al., 1983; Mancebo and Artigas, 1987; Kaplan et al., 1979).

Linear discriminant analysis has been performed for several physiologic cardiopulmonary variables during the first days of ARDS and correlated with mortality to define prognostic factors. In the NHLBI ARDS study (NHLBI, 1979) no variables or combination of variables was able to determine the survival or death for all groups. However, in the subgroup of ARDS patients with the highest mortality rates, effective respiratory compliance, alveolar-arterial O_2 tension difference ($AaDo_2$), and buffer-base deviation were the best predictors. In another study all patients with an effective compliance below 25 ml/cm H_2O on the first day of study died (Maunder et al., 1986).

Fowler et al. (1985) recently reported four variables were significantly associated with ARDS mortality: presence of less than 10% band forms on the initial peripheral blood smear, persistent acidemia with arterial pH less than 7.40, calculated HCO^-_3 less than 20 mg/dl, and a blood urea nitrogen greater than 65 mg/dl. After eliminating those variables that did not contribute significantly to mortality in the presence of the others, only low band forms, low pH, and low HCO^-_3 were significantly associated with increased mortality.

There was no difference in the initial gas exchange and hemodynamic variables between most groups of ARDS survivors and nonsurvivors, indicating a similar degree of pulmonary deterioration in both groups in the initial phase of ARDS except for the Pa_{O_2}/FI_{O_2} ratio at 10 cm H_2O PEEP (Mancebo and Artigas, 1987; Artigas et al., 1981; Lamy et al., 1976) (Table 5). It is important to evaluate gas-exchange parameters as prognostic factors, relating gas exchange with the response to PEEP and its evolution during the course of ARDS. In one study only survivors decreased Qs/Qt after PEEP was applied (De Latorre et al., 1983). A higher mortality rate was reported by Lamy et al. (1976) in ARDS patients having a "fixed shunt" with severe and irreversible alterations of pulmonary morphology. Oscillations of arterial Po_2 and $AaDo_2$ may indicate the evolution of the ARDS and allow us to make a prognosis. The prognostic value of gas-exchange variables improved at 24 hr with significant differences present between survivors and nonsurvivors in the European Study (Table 6). Consistent $AaDo_2$ values greater than 500 mmHg at FI_{O_2} 1 predicted a fatal outcome and were associated with 100% mortality. A progressive increase of Pa_{CO_2} despite increased ventilatory volume, an increase of VD/VT ratio over 70%, an increase of arterial-end-tidal CO_2 difference, and a persistently high pulmonary vascular resistance are associated with a poor prognosis and with morphologic destruction of the pulmonary circulation (De Latorre et al., 1983).

Biochemical and cellular mediators as early indicators of the severe acute lung injury may predict prognosis in ARDS. In a prospective study

Table 5 Gas Exchange Variables and Hemodynamic Data on Admission (mean ± SD) in Spanish Pilot Study (Mancebo and Artigas, 1987)

	Survivors (n = 11)	Nonsurvivors (n = 24)	p value
F_{IO_2}	0.75 ± 0.18	0.73 ± 0.18	NS
Pa_{O_2} (torr)	86.4 ± 27.2	71.9 ± 32.5	NS
Pa_{CO_2} (torr)	39.1 ± 12.6	37.3 ± 9.7	NS
V_E (liters/min)	13.8 ± 4	13.7 ± 3.3	NS
PEEP (cm H_2O)	8.1 ± 4.6	3.7 ± 3.9	0.025
Qsp/Qt (%)	27 ± 7	32 ± 10	NS
$P(A\text{-}a)_{O_2}$ (Torr)	402.7 ± 120.8	414.7 ± 126.5	NS
MSA (mm Hg)	85.4 ± 13.6	81.7 ± 9.4	NS
HR (beat/min)	109 ± 23.3	121.4 ± 17.6	NS
MPAP (mm Hg)	21.3 ± 4.7	21.3 ± 3.2	NS
WP (mm Hg)	9.6 ± 3	10.2 ± 2.9	NS
Cardiac output (liters/min)	6.9 ± 2.7	5.6 ± 1.3	NS

NS = nonsignificant; V_E = minute ventilation; MSAP = mean systemic arterial pressure; MPAP = mean pulmonary artery pressure; WP = wedge pressure.

Table 6 Comparison of Gas Exchange Between Survivors and Nonsurvivors

	On admission			At 24 hr		
	Surv.	Nonsurv.	p value	Surv.	Nonsurv.	p value
Pa_{O_2}/F_{IO_2} (PEEP = 5 cmH_2O)	110 ± 31	107 ± 30	NS	153 ± 114	100 ± 74	<0.0001
Pa_{O_2}/F_{IO_2} (PEEP = 10 cmH_2O)	145 ± 53	133 ± 51	0.01			
$\Delta Pa_{O_2}/F_{IO_2}$ (PEEP 5 → 10 cmH_2O)	37 ± 46	30 ± 41	NS			
$P(A\text{-}a)_{O_2}/P_{AO_2}$				0.71 ± 0.14	0.85 ± 17	<0.01
Oxygenation index (26)				0.79 ± 0.21	0.90 ± 0.15	<0.0001
Pulmonary failure score (27)				8.96 ± 2.17	9.79 ± 2.25	<0.0001

wherein different mediators were analyzed, antithrombin III, protein C, and alpha-2-macroglobulin demonstrated differences between survivors and nonsurvivors in an early phase of ARDS. Progressive normalization of these measurements occurred with improvement of ARDS (Artigas et al., 1985; Fontcuberta et al., 1986).

V. Severity Scoring Indices

The introduction of standard and accurate methods of scoring the severity of respiratory failure and the disturbances of overall physiology with or without specific and sensitive assays of some mediator(s) predicting the severity of lung injury may make possible the comparison of patient populations and examining the efficiency of therapeutic interventions. However, at present the determination of severity of illness or injury can be given by both specific and general indices.

A. Specific Pulmonary Scoring Indices

Jardin et al. (1982) have proposed an Oxygenation Index calculated from arterial oxygenation which considers the level of FI_{O_2} and PEEP: $AaDO_2/PA_{O_2} + 0.014$ PEEP (cm H_2O). This index has been used from the second day of treatment and thereafter to predict whether the acute lung lesions would subside or develop in severity (Artigas and Mancebo, 1987; Jardin et al., 1982) (Table 7).

Morel et al. (1985) have described a pulmonary failure scoring system, the "Geneva" ARDS Scoring System, using four independent variables, each of which is assigned a score between 0 and 4. A score of 0 corresponds

Table 7 Evolutive Control of Respiratory Severity Index (RSI) and Simplified Acute Physiological Score (SAPS) in 35 ARDS Patients in Spanish Pilot Study (Mancebo and Artigas, 1987)

		Day		
		1	3-5	5
SAPS	Survivors	12.6 ± 4.3	10 ± 3.46	8.78 ± 1.56
	Nonsurvivors	14.3 ± 4.1	15.06 ± 3.46[a]	16.25 ± 5.56[b]
RSI	Survivors	0.8 ± 0.09	0.5 ± 0.11	0.47 ± 0.01
	Nonsurvivors	0.8 ± 0.08	0.7 ± 0.13	0.6 ± 0.014[b]

[a] $p < 0.025$.
[b] $p < 0.001$.

Table 8 Geneva ARDS Scoring System

Score	Chest roentgenogram	$AaDO_2/FI_{O_2}$ (mmHg)[a]	C_{rs} $(ml(cmH_2O)^{-1}$	PAP (mmHg)
0	Normal	<300	>80	<20
1	Moderately increased interstitial marking	300-375	70-80	20-25
2	Markedly increased interstitial marking	375-450	50-70	25-30
3	Patchy air-space consolidation	450-525	30-50	30-35
4	Extensive air-space consolidation	>525	<30	>35

[a]Continuous positive pressure ventilation with continuous positive airway pressure (CPAP) or positive end-expiratory pressure (PEEP) or more than 5 cm H_2O increases this particular score by +1.
$AaDO_2/FI_{O_2}$, alveolar-arterial oxygen tension difference divided by inspired oxygen fraction; C_{rs}, static compliance of the respiratory system; PAP, mean pulmonary arterial pressure.
Source: Morel et al., 1985.

to a normal state, 4 to the most disseased state. By dividing the total number of points scored by the value obtained for each patient (Table 8), they found a significant correlation between the mean score and first-pass lung serotonin uptake. Murray et al. (1988) have described a similar scoring system. The value of some of these indices in a large ARDS population was confirmed in the European Collaborative Study by a close correlation between mortality rates and the first two indices.

B. General Illness Scoring Indices

The APACHE system has been used by Montgomery et al. (1985) for nontrauma patients, while an Injury Severity Score (ISS) has been developed for trauma patients. They prospectively studied 207 patients identified as being at risk for developing ARDS. Forty-seven patients developed ARDS and the remaining 160 provided a comparison control group. In both groups a linear relation was observed between APACHE score and the transformed probability of death. For any given APACHE score, patients with ARDS were more likely to die than those without ARDS. In trauma patients there was a linear relation between the ISS and the transformed probability of death for patients without ARDS, but no relationship was present for patients with ARDS.

Mancebo and Artigas (1987) compared Jardin's oxygenation index with the Simplified Acute Physiologic Score (SAPS) (Le Gall et al., 1983a) in 35 patients with severe ARDS. Dying patients did not demonstrate any improvement in their severity indices during the course of their illness. In contrast, both the SAPS and oxygenation index improved significantly during the clinical course of surviving patients. The European Collaborative Study confirmed a close correlation between mortality rate and SAPS (Table 7).

These studies demonstrate that general indices provide useful prognostic indicators in ARDS because death is often related to extrapulmonary disturbances of organ function. Many researchers now believe that ARDS is not purely acute respiratory disease, but rather reflects a disseminated disorder following or coinciding with a period of respiratory failure and producing widespread tissue damage in the body.

C. Relationship Between Prognostic Factors and Severity Indices

It is important to remember that the various factors influencing the outcome of ARDS are not independent. For instance, previous health status is stat-

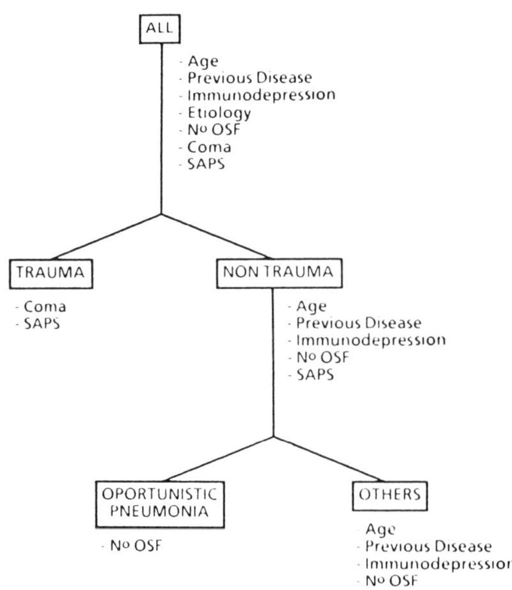

Figure 5 A multivariate analysis of different prognostic factors and physiologic variables separated into two ARDS etiology groups (traumatic vs. nontraumatic ARDS) and the presence of prior immunosuppression.

istically more vital as age increases (Le Gall et al., 1982); severity of illness is more important when previous health status worsens; some diagnoses are more frequent in young or older patients. Diagnosis markedly influences outcome: the SAPS score is correlated with mortality in diagnosis-related groups of patients, but for the same SAPS score the outcome varies according to the primary diagnosis (Le Gall et al., 1983b). The multivariate analysis of the European ARDS Study demonstrated the value of many prognostic factors and physiologic variables in two etiology groups (posttraumatic vs. nontraumatic ARDS), especially the presence or absence of prior immunosuppression (Fig. 5).

VI. Long-Term Recovery

Given the catastrophic degree of acute respiratory failure, the early presence of fibrosis in lung biopsies, the high mortality rate, and the high cost of trying to save these patients, what is the long-term recovery rate for those who do survive? Surprisingly, survivors of ARDS usually lose relatively little pulmonary function and are frequently able to return to their prior activities within 6-12 months after hospital discharge. Thus, the very poor short-term prognosis of ARDS is balanced by the potential for an excellent long-term quality of life in survivors. Studies of 237 ARDS survivors have been reported in 27 articles, and the scatter of the physiologic measurements appears due to differences regarding severity and type of acute lung injury, follow-up times, premorbid pulmonary status including a prior smoking history, presence of nosocomial pneumonia, severity of hypoxemia, barotrauma, and the amount of oxygen received during mechanical ventilation (Alberts et al., 1983; Artigas, 1984; Ingbar and Matthay, 1986; Lakshminarayan and Hudson, 1978). Some of these factors are difficult to assess and many reports do not provide complete information on these various factors that can influence the results of subsequent pulmonary function tests. Table 9 indicates the number of patients and type of information provided in each prior report of ARDS survivors. Most ARDS survivors did not have prior pulmonary function tests since they were previously healthy. Ideally, it would be helpful to know that pre-ARDS pulmonary function was normal before attributing all alterations of lung function to residua of ARDS.

The most common types of physiologic defects reported in survivors of ARDS are a restrictive ventilatory defect, small airways obstruction, airway hyperreactivity, decreased gas exchange with a decrease in DL_{CO}, and hypoxemia with exercise or at rest. The pathology of ARDS reveals edema, congestion, alveolar exudates, hyaline membranes, cellular proliferation, and fibrosis. It is not surprising that in the early phase of recovery, pulmonary function tests commonly reveal a restrictive pattern. Table 10 collates the

Table 9 Data Available in Each Report on ARDS Survivors

	No. of patients	Age	M/F	Clinical status	Roent-genogram	Volume and flow	Airways resistance	Gas exchange Rest	Gas exchange Exercise	Gas exchange Shunt	DL_{CO}
Ashbaugh et al. (1967)	9			*				*			
Interiano et al. (1972)	1	34	1/0		*	*	*	*		*	*
Downs and Olseon (1974)	1	27	0/1	*		*		*	*	*	*
Dine et al. (1974)	1	16	1/0		*	*		*	*		
Llamas (1974)	1	46	1/0	*	*	*		*			*
Yernault et al. (1977)	7	35	1/6	*	*	*	*				*
Glauser and Smith (1975)	1	19	1/0		*	*		*			
Lakshminarayan et al. (1976)	10	42	5/5	*	*	*		*	*	*	*
Klein et al. (1976)	10	22				*	*	*	*	*	
Fallat et al. (1976)	30					*		*	*	*	
Richardson et al. (1976)	2	61	2/0		*	*		*			*
Douglas and Downs (1977)	10	36	8/2	*	*	*		*	*	*	*
Rotman et al. (1977)	6	30	4/2	*	*	*	*	*	*	*	*

Yahav et al. (1978)	15	26	13/2	*	*	*		*	*		*
Leechawengwong et al. (1979)	2	25	2/0	*	*	*	*	*			*
Bachofen and Bachofen (1979)	6	20	5/1	*	*	*		*	*		
Jenkinson and George (1980)	2	25	1/1		*	*					*
Shaw et al. (1981)	2	43	2/0	*	*	*					*
Elliott et al. (1981)	13	30	6/7	*	*	*		*	*		
Xaubet et al. (1981)	9			*	*	*		*	*	*	*
Bell et al. (1983b)	25					*					*
Halevy et al. (1984)	18	39	12/6	*		*		*			
Lakshminarayan and Hudson (1981)	3	28	1/2	*	*	*		*			*
Hudson (1983)	1	42	1/0	*	*	*		*			*
Artigas (1984)	27	40	14/13	*	*	*		*	*	*	*
Buchser et al. (1985)	9	32	7/2		*	*	*	*	*	*	*
Elliott et al. (1985)	16					*					*

M/F = Male/female ratio; DL_{CO} = diffussing capacity for carbon monoxide.
Source: Modified from Alberts et al. (1983).

Table 10 Pulmonary Function Test Results in Survivors of ARDS

	3 months (n = 34)	3-6 months (n = 23)	6 months (n = 105)
Restrictive pattern (TLC < 80%)	11 (32%)	6 (26%)	20 (19%)
Obstructive pattern (normal FEV_1 and FEF_{25-75} < 70%)	4 (12%)	4 (17%)	17 (16%)
Normal	15 (44%)	13 (57%)	68 (65%)
DL_{CO} < 80%	15 (44%)	7 (30%)	22 (21%)

Source: Data compiled from the references listed in Table 9.

reported abnormalities of lung volumes, flow rates, and DL_{CO} at different intervals of recovery time. Approximately one-third of the patients had restrictive airways physiology and half exhibited a decreased DL_{CO} in the first 3 months. With time the restrictive pattern usually resolves and the DL_{CO} rises toward normal. Restrictive ventilatory defects seems to be more common in ARDS patients after thoracic trauma and rib fractures (Hanning et al., 1980). Decreases of expiratory flow rates may occur due to either increased airways resistance or loss of elastic recoil. Most ARDS survivors had no airflow obstruction demonstrated by a decreased forced expiratory volume in 1 sec (FEV_1) and decreased FEV_1/forced vital capacity (FVC) ratio. However, a significant number had reduced midexpiratory flow rates (FEF_{25-75}) often accompanied by increases of RV, RFC, and RV/TLC ratio, with marked (>20%) improvement after administration of a bronchodilator, suggesting air trapping due to reversible small airways changes (Artigas, 1984). Methacholine challenge testing and eucapneic hyperventilation revealed airways hyperreactivity in all cases. Pratt and associates (1979) reported peribronchiolar and alveolar duct inflammation and fibrosis in patients dying from ARDS in the ECMO study, many of whom had received prolonged high levels of oxygen. They suggested that this inflammatory process may be due, at least in part, to oxygen breathing. This hypothesis was not demonstrated in clinical practice; we found no relationship between the duration of mechanical ventilation or the amount of oxygen received and the capacity to normalize the DL_{CO} (Fig. 6). The clinical significance of small airways obstruction and hyperreactive airways is not clear (Simpson et al., 1978). However, it would be logical to employ bronchodilators to treat any clinical symptoms of obstruction.

Most patients have normal resting arterial blood gas tensions, although some ARDS survivors have a diminished Pa_{O_2} and a few have hypoxemia (Pa_{O_2} < 80 mmHg). Are the abnormalities of gas exchange due to chronic

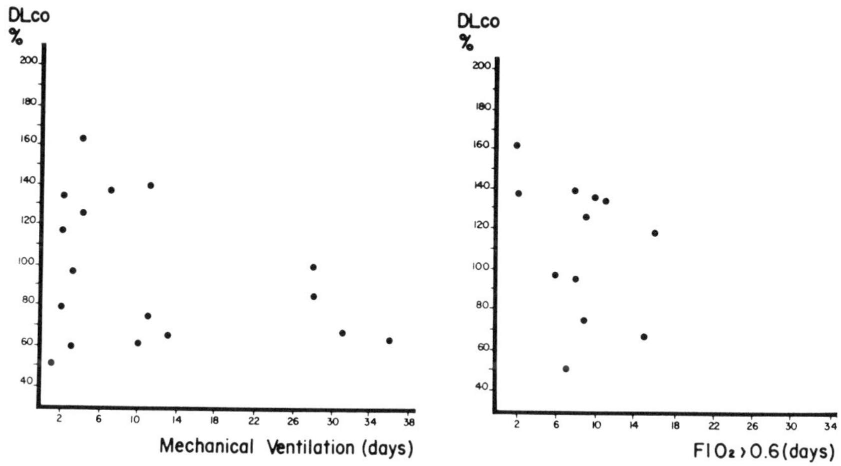

Figure 6 Relationship between the duration of mechanical ventilation or the amount of oxygen received ($FIO_2 > 0.6$ days) during ARDS and the lung diffusing capacity for carbon monoxide (DLco) after one year of recovery of acute episode of lung injury.

vascular obstruction, or due to vascular remodeling during recovery? Elliott et al. (1981) demonstrated in ARDS patients a normally decreasing VD/VT during exercise as a function of CO_2 production rate, suggesting that late chronic vascular obstruction did not account for the decreased DL_{CO} and gas exchange abnormalities. Buchser and co-workers (1985) reported that the diffusing capacity and membrane transfer factor corrected for lung volume were normal, whereas the pulmonary capillary blood volume was significantly decreased to a mean of 49% predicted, suggesting that most of the gas exchange abnormalities are not due to a loss of alveolar gas exchange surface or to diffusion limitation of oxygen transfer, but rather to a decreased or abnormal arrangement of lung capillaries after ARDS.

VII. Summary

In the absence of specific serologic markers, the diagnosis of ARDS remains essentially a form of pattern recognition. As our understanding of ARDS increases and the choice of therapies expands, it is important to identify the prognostic factors and methods of scoring the severity to compare the results of the various different clinical trials reported in the literature. The European Collaborative Study (1985-1987) demonstrated in 583 patients with severe hypoxic respiratory failure that two criteria, severe hypoxemia and pulmonary arterial occluded pressure, have increasingly introduced a selection bias into published clinical studies of ARDS, selecting a small group of patients with an unusually poor prognosis. The prognosis of ARDS is determined by etiology, preexistent disease, age, and other system failure. Because ARDS is not purely a respiratory disease but more a reflection of a disseminated disorder, a general severity of disease classification system is more sensitive to variations in group risk than a comparison of mean values. SAPS and Oxygenation Indexes are useful prognostic variables. The prognostic value of different factors should be correlated to the etiology (posttraumatic vs. nontrauma respiratory failure) and the presence of an immunocompromised host. The majority of ARDS survivors undergo complete recovery of pulmonary function.

Acknowledgments

The authors acknowledge the skillful assistance of Ms. Caroline Newey, Ms. Cuca Ayesta, Ms. Juani Granero, and Mr. Víctor Fuentes in preparing the manuscript. This work was supported by FISS grants #83/909 and 87/909 and by the European Society of Intensive Care Medicine.

VIII. Appendix

The participants of the European Collaborative ARDS Study are: A. Artigas, Barcelona; R. Assmann, Dusseldorf; L. Bossaert, Antwerp; A. Braschi, Pavia; F. Brunet, Paris; J. Carlet, Paris; J. Castañeda, Valladolid; J. M. Caturla, Alicante; J. Cebrián, Valencia; C. L. Chastang, Paris; P. M. Cox, Portland; J. F. Dhainaut, Paris; G. Domenighetti, Locarno; H. Dunkl, Feldkirch; K. Falke, Berlin; Ph. Flandre, Paris; Fumagali, Milan; J. R. Le Gall, Paris; A. Gaspareto, Rome; J. García Pardo, La Coruña; L. Gattinoni, Milan; C. P. Girón, Padova; G. González, Murcia; G. Gritti, Ferrara; T. Hachenberg, Munster; M. Hemmer, Luxembourg; L. Holzapfel, Paris; M. Lamy, Liège; P. Lawin, Munster; F. Lemaire, Paris; J. Mancebo, Barcelona; R. Marcolin, Milan; G. Martinelli, Bologna; J. Motin, Lyon; M. Mutz, Insbruck; F. Nicolas, Nantes; J. Qvist, Herlev; M. Reynaert, Brussels; R. Rodriguez Roisin, Barcelona; J. L. Suennevig, Ulleval; P. M. Suter, Geneva; J. D. Tempe, Strasbourg; A. Tenaillon, Evry; A. Torres, Barcelona; J. Villar, Las Palmas; F. Wattel, Lille; and M. Wendt, Munster.

Pathology Center: Pathology Department, Hôpital Henri Mondor, Paris. J. F. Bernaudin (Chairperson), F. Basset.

Biostatistics and Data Analysis Center: Department of Biostatistics, Hôpital Sant Louis, Paris. C. L. Chastang (Chairperson), Ph. Flandre.

International Advisory Board: G. Johanson, Galveston; W. Knauss, Washington, DC; J. Rinaldo, Nashville; W. Zapol, Boston.

References

Alberts, W. M., Priest, G. R., and Moser, K. M. (1983). The outlook for survivors of ARDS. *Chest,* **84**:272-274.

Andrews, C. P., Coalson, J. J., Smith, J. D., and Johanson, G. (1981). Diagnosis of nosocomial bacterial pneumonia in acute, diffuse lung injury. *Chest,* **80**:254-258.

Artigas, A. (1984). Evaluation pulmonaire des malades survivant a un syndrome de détresse respiratoire aigüe de l'adulte. In *Le syndrome de détresse respiratoire aigüe de l'adulte.* Edited by F. Lemaire. Paris, Masson, pp. 125-136.

Artigas, A., and Mancebo, J. (1987). Etiology and multiple organ system failure as prognostic factors in ARDS. In *Update in Intensive Care and Emergency Medicine.* Edited by J. L. Vincent. Berlin, Springer-Verlag, pp. 163-169.

Artigas, A., Estopa, R., and De Latorre, F. J. (1981). Hemodynamic and gas exchange disorders as prognostic factors in the adult respiratory distress syndrome (abstract). *Crit. Care Med.,* **9**:199.

Artigas, A., Fontcuberta, J., Castella, J., and Rutllant, M. (1985). Coagulation disorders in the adult respiratory distress syndrome. In *Update in Intensive Care and Emergency Medicine.* Edited by J. L. Viccnt. Berlin, Springer Verlag, pp. 84-89.

Ashbaugh, D. G., Bigelow, D. B., Petty, T. L., and Levine, B. E. (1967). Acute respiratory distress in adults. *Lancet,* **2**:319-323.

Bachofen, M., and Bachofen, H. (1979). Der Hilungsverlauf des sheweren "adult respiratory distress syndrome." *Schweiz. Med. Wochenschr.,* **109**:1982-1989.

Bell, R. C., Coalson, J. J., Smith, J. D., and Johanson, W. G. (1983a). Multiple organ system failure and infection in adult respiratory distress syndrome. *Ann. Intern. Med.,* **99**:293-298.

Bell, R. C., Prihoda, T. J., Andrews, C. P., et al. (1983b). Long term pulmonary function in survivors of adult and respiratory distress syndrome and clinical determinants of abnormalities (abstract). *Chest,* **84**:343.

Buchser, E., Leuenberger, P., Chiolero, R., et al. (1985). Reduced pulmonary capillary blood volume as a long term sequel of ARDS. *Chest,* **87**:608-611.

De Latorre, F. J., Estopá, R., and Artigas, A. (1983). Intercambio gaseoso como factor pronóstico en el síndrome de distress respiratorio del adulto. *Med. Intensiva,* **7**:1-6.

Dine, N. L., Myerson, D. A., Myerson, P. J., et al. (1974). Near drowning presenting as the adult respiratory distress syndrome. *Chest,* **65**:347-349.

Douglas, M. E., and Downs, J. B. (1977). Pulmonary function following severe acute respiratory failure and high levels of positive end expiratory pressure. *Chest,* **71**:18-23.

Downs, J. B., and Olsen, G. N. (1974). Pulmonary function following adult respiratory distress syndrome. *Chest,* **65**:92-93.

Elliott, C. G., Morris, A. H., and Cengiz, M. (1981). Pulmonary function and exercise gas exchange in survivors of adult respiratory distress syndrome. *Am. Rev. Respir. Dis.,* **123**:492-495.

Elliott, C. G., Rasmussen, B., Crapo, R. D., et al. (1985). Predictors of pulmonary function abnormalities after adult respiratory distress syndrome (abstract). *Chest,* **88**:638.

Fallat, R. J., Tucker, H. J., and Segovia, L. (1976). Lung function in long term survivors from severe respiratory distress syndrome. *Am. Rev. Respir. Dis.,* **113**:118A.

Fein, A. M., Lippmann, M., Holtzman, H., Eliraz, A., and Goldberg, S. K. (1983). The risk factors, incidence, and prognosis of ARDS following septicemia. *Chest,* **83**:40-42.

Fontcuberta, J., Artigas, A., Sala, N., et al. (1986). Inhibitors of blood coagulation in adult respiratory distress syndrome. *Intens. Care Med.,* **12**:224.

Fowler, A. A., Hamman, R. F., Good, J. T., et al. (1983). Adult respiratory distress syndrome: Risk with common predisposition. *Ann. Intern. Med.,* **98**:593-597.

Fowler, A. A., Hamman, R. F., Zerbe, G. O., Benson, K. N., and Hyers, T. M. (1985). Adult respiratory distress syndrome: Prognosis after onset. *Am. Rev. Respir. Dis.,* **132**:472-478.

Glauser, F. L., and Smith, W. R. (1975). Pulmonary interstitial fibrosis following near drowning and exposure to short term high oxygen concentration. *Chest,* **68**:373-375.

Halvey, A., Sirik, Z., Adam, Y. G., et al. (1984). Longterm evaluation of patients following the adult respiratory distress syndrome. *Respir. Care,* **29**:132-137.

Hanning, C. D., Ledingham, E., and Ledingham, I. McA. (1980). Late respiratory sequelae of blunt chest injury (abstract). *Intens. Care Med.,* **6**:26.

Hudson, L. D. (1983). Prognosis: Immediate and long-term sequelae of acute respiratory failure. *Respir. Care,* **2**:663-671.

Ingbar, D. H., and Matthay, R. A. (1986). Pulmonary sequelae and lung repair in survivors of the adult respiratory distress syndrome. *Crit. Care Clin.,* **2**:629-665.

Interiano, B., Stuard, I. D., and Hyde, R. W. (1972). Acute respiratory distress syndrome in pancreatitis. *Ann. Intern. Med.,* **77**:923-927.

Jardin, F., Prost, J. F., Bazin, M., Desfond, P., Ozier, Y., and Margairez, A. (1982). Modalités évolutives du syndrome de détresse respiratoire aigüe de l'adulte: Valeur pronostique d'un indice de gravité tiré de l'oxygenation artérielle. *Nouv. Press. Med.,* **11**:29-33.

Jenkinson, S. G., and George, R. B. (1980). Serial pulmonary function studies in survivors of near drowning. *Chest,* **77**:777-780.

Kaplan, R. L., Sahn, S. A., and Petty, T. L. (1979). Incidence and outcome of the respiratory distress syndrome in gram-negative sepsis. *Arch. Intern. Med.,* **139**:867-869.

Klein, J. J., Van Haeringen, J. R., and Shurter, H. J. (1976). Pulmonary function after recovery from the adult respiratory distress syndrome. *Chest,* **69**:350-355.

Lakshminarayan, S., and Hudson, L. D. (1978). Pulmonary function following the adult respiratory distress syndrome. *Chest,* **74**:489-490.

Lakshminarayan, S., and Hudson, L. D. (1981). Pulmonary function following adult respiratory distress syndrome. *Semin. Respir. Med.,* **11**: 160-164.

Lakshminarayan, S., Stanfor, R. E., and Petty, T. L. (1976). Prognosis after recovery from adult respiratory distress syndrome. *Am. Rev. Respir. Dis.,* **113**:7-16.

Lamy, M., Fallat, R. J., Koeniger, E., et al. (1976). Pathologic features and mechanisms of hypoxemia in adult respiratory distress syndrome. *Am. Rev. Respir. Dis.,* **114**:267-284.

Leechawengwong, M., Berger, H. W., and Jayamanne, D. S. (1979). Long term serial followup after two episodes of heroin-induced adult respiratory distress syndrome. *Mt. Sinai J. Med.,* **35**:119-121.

Le Gall, J. R., Brun-Buisson, C., Trunet, P., et al. (1982). Influence of age, previous health status and severity of illness on outcome from intensive care. *Crit. Care Med.,* **10**:575-577.

Le Gall, J. R., Loirat, P., and Alperovitch, A. (1983a). Simplified acute physiological score for intensive care patients. *Lancet,* **2**:741.

Le Gall, J. R., Loirat, P., Nicolas, F., et al. (1983b). Utilization d'un indicc de gravité dans huit services de réanimation multidisciplinaire. *Press. Med.,* **12**:1757-1761.

Llamas, R. (1974). Adult respiratory distress syndrome: Report of survival after two episodes. *Chest,* **65**:468-469.

Loyd, J. E., Newman, J. H., and Brigham, K. L. (1984). Permeability pulmonary edema: diagnosis and management. *Arch. Intern. Med.,* **144**: 143-147.

Mancebo, J., and Artigas, A. (1987). A clinical study of the adult respiratory distress syndrome. *Crit. Care Med.,* **15**:243-246.

Maunder, R. J., Shuman, W. P., McHugh, J. W., Marglin, S. I., and Butler, J. (1986). Preservation of normal lung regions in the adult respiratory distress syndrome. Analysis by computed tomography. *JAMA,* **255**: 2463-2465.

Montgomery, B., Stager, M. A., Carrico, C. J., and Hudson, L. D. (1985). Causes of mortality in patients with the adult respiratory distress syndrome. *Am. Rev. Respir. Dis.,* **132**:485-489.

Morel, D., Dargent, F., Bachmann, M., Suter, P. M., and Junot, A. F. (1985). Pulmonary extraction of serotonin and propanolol in patients with ARDS. *Am. Rev. Respir. Dis.,* **132**:479-484.

Murray, J. F., Matthay, M. A., Luce, J. M., and Flick, M. R. (1988). An expanded definition of the adult respiratory distress syndrome. *Am. Rev. Respir. Dis.,* **138**:720-723.

National Heart, Lung and Blood Institute, Division of Lung Diseases (1979). *Extracorporeal Support for Respiratory Insufficiency: A. Collaborative Study.* Bethesda, MD., NIH.

Pepe, P. E., Potkin, R. T., Reus, D. H., Hudson, L. D., and Carrico, C. J. (1982). Clinical predictors of the adult respiratory distress syndrome. *Am. J. Surg.,* **144**:124-130.

Pepe, P. E., Hudson, L. D., and Carrico, C. J. (1984). Early application of positive endexpiratory pressure in patients at risk for the adult respiratory distress syndrome. *N. Engl. J. Med.,* **311**:281-286.

Pontoppidan, H., Hüttemeier, P. C., and Quinn, D. A. (1985). Acute respiratory failure: etiology, demography and outcome. In *Acute Respiratory Failure.* Edited by W. M. Zapol and K. Falke. New York, Marcel Dekker, pp. 1-21.

Pratt, P. C., Volmer, R. T., Shellburne, J. D., et al. (1979). Pulmonary morphology in a multihospital collaborative extracorporeal membrane oxygenation project. I. Light microscopy. *Am. J. Pathol.,* **95**:191-214.

Richardson, J. V., Light, R. W., Baskin, T. L., et al. (1976). Late pulmonary function in survivors of adult respiratory distress syndrome. *South. Med. J.,* **69**:735-737.

Rinaldo, J. E. (1986). The prognosis of the adult respiratory distress syndrome. Inappropriate pessimism? *Chest,* **90**:470-471.

Rinaldo, J. E., and Rogers, R. M. (1982). Adult respiratory distress syndrome: Changing concepts of lung injury and repair. *N. Engl. J. Med.,* **306**:900-909.

Rotman, H. H., Lavelle, R. F., Jr., and Dimcheff, D. G. (1977). Long term physiologic consequences of the adult respiratory distress syndrome. *Chest,* **72**:190-192.

Shaw, R. A., Whitcomb, M. E., and Schonfeld, S. A. (1981). Pulmonary function after adult respiratory distress syndrome associated with Legionnaire's disease pneumonia. *Arch. Intern. Med.,* **141**:741-742.

Simpson, D. L., Goodman, M., and Spector, S. L. (1978). Long term followup and bronchial reactivity testing in survivors of the adult respiratory distress syndrome. *Am. Rev. Respir. Dis.,* **117**:449-454.

Xaubet, A., Naulart, Ll, Estopa, R., Rodriguez Roisin, R., and Agusti Vidal, A. (1981). Evolución clínica, radiológica y funcional respiratoria del síndrome de distres respiratorio del adulto (ARDS). *Med. Clin.* (*Barc.*), **76**:291-295.

Yahav, J., Lieberman, P., and Molho, M. (1978). Pulmonary function following the adult respiratory distress syndrome. *Chest,* **74**:247-250.

Yernault, J. C., Englert, M., and Sergysels, R. (1977). Followup of pulmonary function after "shock lung." *Bull. Eur. Physiopathol. Respir.,* **13**:241-248.

Zapol, W. M., Snider, M. T., Hill, J. D., et al. (1979). Extracorporeal membrane oxygenation in severe acute respiratory failure. A randomized prospective study. *JAMA,* **242**:2193-2196.

4

Tissue Oxygen Delivery and Utilization in Patients with the Adult Respiratory Distress Syndrome

DAVID R. DANTZKER*

The University of Texas Health Science Center at Houston
Houston, Texas

I. Introduction

The adult respiratory distress syndrome (ARDS) was formally named about 20 years ago, although descriptions of non-cardiogenic pulmonary edema preceded this by many years under a number of different appellations (Petty, 1982). The initial reports emphasized the lung injury and resultant hypoxemia, and because of this the therapy that developed was directed toward the correction of these abnormalities. Very soon, it became apparent that advancements in ventilatory therapy and fluid management could effectively reduce the level of intrapulmonary shunting and maintain acceptable pulmonary gas exchange, but the expected improvement in survival was not forthcoming. Although arterial oxygenation could be supported at adequate levels, death resulting from the failure of other organs (Bell et al., 1983; Montgomery et al., 1985) continued to assure mortality rates exceeding 60% (Fowler et al., 1983), which were not very different from those in the initial descriptions.

It is now becoming clearer that in many patients the lung injury seen in ARDS is only one obvious manifestation of a more generalized process in

**Present affiliation*: Long Island Jewish Medical Center, New Hyde Park, New York which multiple organs are involved or at risk. Part of the pathophysiology of this disorder, perhaps better thought of as a syndrome of multiple organ failure, is an abnormality of tissue oxygen transport and utilization (Danek et al., 1980). Thorough reviews of the normal physiologic determinants and control of oxygen delivery and utilization are available. This chapter confines itself to reviewing the normal and abnormal response to an alteration in oxygen transport with regard to tissue oxygen availability and consumption.

Total oxygen delivery, TO_2, is defined as the product of cardiac output, Q, and arterial oxygen content, Ca_{O_2}. Oxygen utilization or consumption, VO_2, is predominantly the oxygen utilized as the terminal electron acceptor for the aerobic generation of adenosine triphosphate (ATP) within the mitochondria via the Krebs tricarboxylic acid cycle (Newsholme and Leech, 1983). ATP is needed to maintain cellular integrity and provide the energy for cell function. This oxygen-dependent reaction in the cytochrome chain has a very high affinity for O_2, and a very low intracellular PO_2 is required to maintain maximum cellular respiration. In preparations of isolated mitochondria, the oxidation of cytochrome c is complete at a PO_2 of 0.5 torr (Jobsis, 1972). Normal healthy individuals can function at a very low Pa_{O_2} (Sutton et al., 1988), and even chronically hypoxemic patients are reasonably well compensated at levels of arterial oxygenation below those found in acutely ill patients dying of apparent hypoxic tissue injury.

A small percentage of VO_2 is utilized for extra-mitochondrial processes, including biosynthesis, degradation, and detoxification of certain substances necessary for cell function. Since the affinity for oxygen is much lower in some of these reactions than for oxidative phosphorylation, it has been suggested that impairment at this level may explain some of the apparent sensitivity to hypoxemia in acutely ill patients (Robin, 1980). Since there is little known about how these reactions may relate to clinical disease, they are not considered further in this review.

II. Normal Response to Reduced TO_2

The normal response of oxygen utilization to a reduction in global oxygen transport is described by a biphasic relationship (Fig. 1) (Cain, 1977; Shibutani et al., 1983). Under normal circumstances, TO_2 is thought to reside on the plateau of the relationship in which oxygen is delivered in excess of the amount required. If TO_2 decreases, VO_2 is maintained by increasing the amount of oxygen extracted from the blood. The extraction ratio (ER = VO_2/TO_2) is represented by the slope of the line from any point on the relationship to the origin. In young, normal subjects at rest, the ER varies from about 20 to 40% (Astrand et al., 1964). To increase the ER, the microvascular bed must

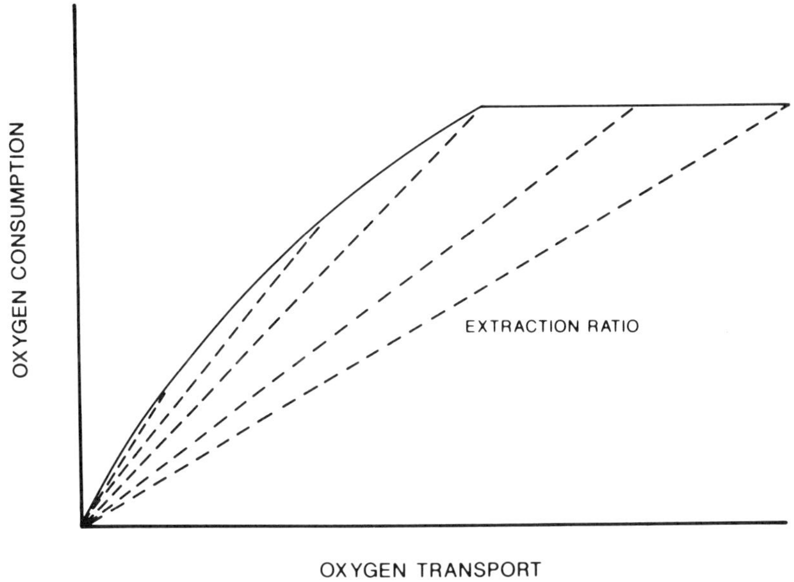

Figure 1 Normal response of oxygen utilization to a reduction in global oxygen transport is described by a biphasic relationship.

be able to augment capillary recruitment and thus provide an optimal milieu for tissue O_2 delivery and diffusion from the capillaries into the tissues. Increased capillarity serves to reduce the distance from the red cell to the mitochondria, improving the transfer of O_2 to the cells at any given capillary PO_2 by improving the diffusion characteristics of the system. The stimulus for vasodilation in response to a falling TO_2 is closely linked to local VO_2, and thus tissue PO_2 or some factor released in response to tissue hypoxia is a likely intermediary (Johnson, 1986).

If TO_2 is reduced beyond the ability of an increase in ER to cope, then VO_2 begins to fall and the individual is now on the linear portion of the relationship in which VO_2 is supply dependent. This critical level of TO_2 (TO_{2crit}) has been determined in animals to be about 8-10 ml O_2/kg body weight/min (Cain, 1977). In one study in anesthetized humans, a similar TO_{2crit} was calculated (Shibutani et al., 1983). In animal studies TO_{2crit} has been found to vary with changes in metabolic rate and the position of the oxyhemoglobin dissociation curve (Warley and Gutierrez, 1988). The ER at TO_{2crit} has been found to vary from 30 to 50% and continues to increase as TO_2 is progressively reduced (Gutierrez et al., 1986).

Once the critical T_{O_2} is reached and V_{O_2} begins to decline below baseline values, energy-dependent cellular demands must be reduced or nonaerobic pathways must be utilized for ATP generation. Some animal species have developed the ability to reduce O_2 requirements below basal levels to compensate for marked reductions in O_2 availability. The exact mechanism of this metabolic downregulation is unclear (Hochachka, 1980).

Anaerobic generation of APT is accomplished through glycolysis or the creatine kinase reaction. When O_2 is not available as the terminal electron acceptor, pyruvate plays this role and is reduced to lactate in the process. This is a much less productive way of utilizing substrate, since each mole of glucose yields only 2 mol of ATP via glycolysis in comparison to the 36 mol of ATP produced during aerobic phosphorylation via the Krebs tricarboxylic acid cycle. An additional drawback to glycolysis as the major source of energy production is the development of lactic acidosis. An alternative to glycolysis, at least in skeletal muscle, heart, and brain, is the production of ATP by the creatine kinase reaction (Piiper et al., 1968). This allows the transfer of a high-energy phosphate bond from the storage compound phosphocreatine (PCr) to ADP to produce ATP:

$$PCr + ADP + H^+ \rightleftharpoons ATP + Cr$$

An additional advantage of this method of ATP generation is that it consumes hydrogen ions and thus limits the metabolic acidosis produced by glycolysis. Although the creatinine kinase reaction constitutes a ready source of energy, its usefulness is limited by the PCr stores.

A major difficulty encountered in studies of the cellular effects of diminished T_{O_2} is the ability to evaluate the effects on tissue bioenergetics. Measurement of total V_{O_2} is likely to be insensitive to the mechanism of change. The development of lactic acidosis, as an index of having exceeded the limits of oxidative phosphorylation, quantitates only the glycolytic contribution to anaerobic energy production and can be influenced by many factors other than the inadequacy of tissue oxygenation. Some tissues, such as the red blood cell, routinely utilize glycolysis for energy production, although their total contribution of lactate is very small. Drugs and chemicals can elevate lactic acid levels (Newsholme and Leech, 1983), as can catecholamine excess, which stimulates glycolysis in excess of the ability of pyruvate to enter the TCA cycle (Greene, 1961). Lactic acid production may also underestimate the significance of tissue hypoxia in situations of marked substrate inadequacy or in the presence of pre-existing metabolic acidosis (Halperin and Fields, 1985).

Nuclear magnetic resonance spectroscopy (MRS) provides a noninvasive method of assessing various biologically important molecules (Gadian, 1982). When tissue is placed in a strong magnetic field and then pulsed by radiofrequency waves, certain isotopic species absorb and then emit some of the energy in the form of a radiofrequency signal. This signal can be characterized and quantitated spectrographically. Phosphorus 31 is the normal stable isotope of phosphorus and forms a part of several molecules important to cellular bioenergetics, including ATP, phosphocreatine, and inorganic phosphate (P_i). Intracellular pH can be measured from the position of the P_i peak, since addition or subtraction of protons shifts its location in the phosphorus spectrum relative to PCr (Moon and Richards, 1973). The ratio of PCr/P_i has been shown to be the equivalent of the cellular phosphate potential (ATP/[ADP][P_i]) and thus the energy charge of the cell (Chance et al., 1985). Phosphate MRS thus has the potential for providing us with a noninvasive measurement of cellular respiration in the intact animal or human.

Other isotopes can be used, the most important of which is ^{1}H or proton MRS. This is used for clinical magnetic resonance imaging (MRI) due to the ubiquitous presence of this isotope in body water. Proton MRS can be used to quantitate many biologically important molecules, such as lactic acid and fatty acids, although there are still insufficient data in living systems to evaluate its potential usefulness.

Utilizing phosphorus MRS, the cellular events during progressive hypoxemia and ischemia were studied in a rabbit hindlimb preparation (Gutierrez et al., 1989). With both perturbations, a fall in To_2 below the critical point was accompanied by a fall in Vo_2, a fall in the PCr/P_i, and a rise in lactate with no change in the ATP concentration. At least in this preparation, therefore, a reduction in To_2 was met by an attempt to maintain energy levels at the baseline level, not by a reduction in ATP requirements. When To_2 was allowed to return to baseline, Vo_2 returned toward baseline in both preparations. In the ischemic preparation, this was accompanied by a resynthesis of PCr and a fall in P_i. By contrast, in the hypoxemic limbs, there was an initial recovery of Vo_2, a failure of PCr synthesis and eventually a fall in ATP concentration, suggesting that unlike the ischemic insult, hypoxemia may have irreversibly damaged the metabolic machinery. Extrapolation of these studies to the intact human may be a bit presumptuous, but they suggest that the fall in Vo_2 that occurs below To_{2crit} is associated with a shift to anaerobic generation of ATP rather than a downregulation of metabolism.

III. To_2-Vo_2 Relationships in ARDS

The biphasic relationship between Vo_2 and To_2 described in animal studies and less well in humans differs from that found in many patients suffering from ARDS. In these patients, Vo_2 has been found to be supply dependent over a very wide range of To_2 (Danek et al., 1980; Gutierrez and Pohil, 1986; Kariman and Burno, 1985), although this is not a universal observation (Annat et al., 1986). In one study, no plateau phase was seen until levels of TO_2 above 21 ml/kg/min (Mohsenifar et al., 1983). Based upon the MRS data discussed above, it would seem reasonable to postulate that over this very wide range of seemingly adequate TO_2 there is inadequate O_2 for aerobic energy production and the tissues turn to alternative strategies for maintaining ATP levels. Quite often, though, no metabolic acidosis is present in these patients despite this obvious pathologic supply dependency. By looking at arterial pH, however, we may be missing evidence of significant tissue acidosis that might be more apparent if we monitored mixed venous PCO_2. As long as minute ventilation increases, no evidence for this increased buffering of metabolic acids would be seen on the arterial side. This situation would be equivalent to the normal arterial pH found during exercise just above the anaerobic threshold at which bicarbonate buffering and alveolar ventilation compensate for the developing lactic acidosis.

Since ARDS is often a manifestation of the syndrome of multiple organ failure, it is tempting to blame this abnormal delivery and supply interaction for the disastrous clinical outcome. In a prospective study of patients admitted to an intensive care unit, those who demonstrated supply dependency had a 70% mortality rate compared to 30% for those without this finding (Gutierrez and Pohil, 1986). A second study found a significantly greater increase in VO_2 subsequent to an increase in TO_2 in patients who died than in those who survived an episode of proven or presumed sepsis (Bihari et al., 1987). The authors interpreted these results as indicating that pathologic supply dependency probably indicated a significant deficit in tissue oxygenation that would eventually result in critical organ failure and death.

How are we to explain this apparent link between TO_2 and VO_2 over such a wide range in patients with ARDS? Perhaps the primary problem is a diffuse cellular defect that interferes with the normal cellular utilization of available oxygen. This type of abnormality of cellular respiration has been previously postulated to exist in patients with sepsis (Harken et al., 1975; Mela et al., 1971). However, it is now generally believed that the ability of the tissues to utilize O_2 in sepsis is normal when adequate amounts are available to the cells (Chandry et al., 1979). There is no evidence to the contrary in patients with ARDS.

An inadequate VO_2 in the face of a seemingly appropriate overall level of O_2 delivery would therefore implicate an abnormality in local O_2 availability, that is, in microvascular blood flow distribution or O_2 diffusion. As already mentioned, tissue blood flow is regulated by local metabolic needs, although the mechanism by which this is accomplished is unknown. Increased regional blood flow improves local TO_2, and increased capillary density enhances the environment for gas diffusion and thus increases the ability to extract O_2. The ability to respond to increasing requirements by increasing blood flow and recruiting additional microvessels varies from organ to organ. For example, during exercise, skeletal muscle can increase blood flow 25 times (Lassen et al., 1976) and increase ER from about 20 to 90% (Astrand et al., 1964) but the heart can only accomplish a 5 times increase in flow and only minimal increase in ER, which is already about 80% at rest.

An inability to autoregulate blood flow to actively metabolizing tissues or the loss of microvessels secondary to occlusion or damage could reasonably be expected to interfere with the ordinary process of matching O_2 needs with availability. The abnormal release of vasoactive substances into the systemic circulation or the failure of diseased lungs to clear these mediators normally could interfere with normal vasoregulation. Hypoxia, inflammation, complement activation, O_2 radical formation, lipid preoxidation, and other events postulated to be occurring as part of the injury process in ARDS could lead to endothelial and vascular smooth muscle cell damage if there is spillover into the systemic circulation. It is not to far-fetched to postulate that this would interfere with the orderly matching of To_2 and Vo_2 by interfering with the regulation of vascular muscle tone, either directly or by disrupting interactions between the endothelium and the smooth muscle. Provisional conformation of this hypothesis is provided from animal studies in which phorbol myristate acetate, administered as a model of acute lung injury, resulted in an increase in the value for To_{2crit} (Mizer et al., 1988). In patients with sepsis, the fall in SVR as a marker of lost autoregulatory ability has been correlated with a reduction in the tissues' ability to extract O_2 (Groenevald et al., 1987). Conversely, a reduction in cardiac output and increase in SVR, suggesting a reversal of the autoregulatory failure, predicted survival in patients with sepsis (Parker et al., 1987).

Microvascular embolization in experimental models also leads to supply dependency over a wider range than normal (Cain, 1984; Ellsworth et al., 1981). These models may mimic the clinical situation in which activation of various inflammatory mediators is postulated to result in endothelial cell injury, granulocyte and platelet agglutination, and capillary occlusion. The resultant loss of capillary cross-sectional area results in an increased diffusion distance from blood to tissue (Tenney, 1974) and a loss of the ability to recruit new capillaries.

An apparent pathologic supply dependency of Vo_2 on To_2 has now been described in patients with chronic disorders, such as chronic obstructive pulmonary disease (Brent et al., 1984) and chronic congestive heart failure (Mohsenifar et al., 1987). In these relatively stable patients, an ongoing inadequacy of oxidative metabolism would appear to be unlikely. This has led to the suggestion that perhaps the observed linear relationship between To_2 and Vo_2 is due to an artifact of the measurements, forced by the presence of a common variable in the calculation of both To_2 and Vo_2. The measurement of TO_2 obviously requires the use of cardiac output and arterial O_2 content measurements. VO_2 can be calculated either directly by volume displacement from a closed system or indirectly by utilizing the principle of conservation of mass:

$$VO_2 = (V_I \times F_{I_{O_2}}) - (V_E \times F_{E_{O_2}}) = Q(Ca_{O_2} - Cv_{O_2})$$

where V_I and V_E are the inspired and expired minute ventilation and Fi_{O_2} and Fe_{O_2} are the inspired and expired fractional concentrations of oxygen. The direct measurement of VO_2 by volume displacement is rarely used because even small leaks in the system will lead to significant error. This is a particular problem in patients on mechanical ventilation. If the patient is in steady state, the amount of oxygen taken up by the lungs equals that taken up by the tissues, and calculations of VO_2 from either the arterial and mixed venous PO_2 and cardiac output or from the inspired and expired gas along with minute ventilation should be the same. In studies in which these two methods have been compared they are usually found to be equal.

In critically ill patients both techniques have significant limitations, with error introduced by the large number of variables that must be accurately measured. Since most clinical studies have used measurements from the blood side, the suggestion has been made that having cardiac output on both the x and y axes artifactually led to the observed relationship. However, this by itself is an unlikely explanation since there are no mathematical constraints forcing this association. Reanalysis of some of the original observations using elegant statistical techniques to account for the influence of common variables did not change the basic conclusions (Moreno et al., 1986).

A more likely problem in the interpretation of the VO_2-TO_2 data reported thus far in the literature is the difficulty of knowing which is the dependent and which is the independent variable (Fig. 2). Reducing TO_2 below TO_{2crit} results in a fall in both TO_2 and VO_2, and in this setting we consider supply to be the independent variable. Normally VO_2 is the independent variable and alterations in O_2 demand are met by rapid changes in TO_2. This has been studied most completely during exercise, when the increase in TO_2 is almost instantaneous with the onset of increased metabolic demands. Many of the clinical studies reported to date have involved a relatively random collection of data. Since O_2 demands as well as delivery are likely to have varied from time to time in these patients, it is difficult to tell which was the dependent and which the independent variable at any given point. If the dependent and independent variables varied from measurement to measurement, it would make it impossible to assess the true presence of pathologic supply dependency in these patients. Clearly, further studies in which carefully controlled interventions are investigated will be necessary to determine the significance of pathologic supply dependency as well as clarify in which disorders it is found.

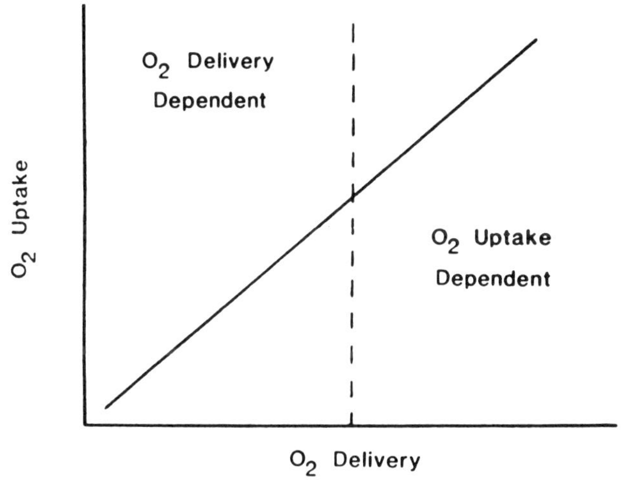

Figure 2 Delivery and uptake of O_2 depicting the difficulty of knowing which is the dependent and which is the independent variable.

References

Annat, G., Viale, J. P., Percival, C., Froment, M., and Motin, J. (1986). Oxygen delivery and uptake in the adult respiratory distress syndrome. *Am. Rev. Respir. Dis.,* **133**:999.

Astrand, P., Cuddy, T. E., Saltin, B., and Stenberg, J. (1964). Cardiac output during submaximal and maximal work. *J. Appl. Physiol.,* **19**:268.

Bell, R. C., Coalson, J. J., Smith, J. D., and Johanson, W. G. (1983). Multiple organ system failure and infection in adult respiratory distress syndrome. *Ann. Intern. Med.,* **99**:293.

Bihari, D., Smithies, M., Gimson, A., et al. (1987). The effects of vasodilation with prostacyclin on oxygen delivery and uptake in critically ill patients. *N. Engl. J. Med.,* **317**:397.

Brent, B. N., Matthay, R. A., Mahler, D. A., Berger, H. J., Zaret, B. L., and Lister, G. (1984). Relationship between oxygen uptake and oxygen transport in stable patients with chronic obstructive pulmonary disease. *Am. Rev. Respir. Dis.,* **129**:682.

Cain, S. M. (1977). Oxygen delivery and uptake in dogs during anemic and hypoxic hypoxia. *J. Appl. Physiol.,* **42**:228.

Cain, S. M. (1984). Supply dependency of oxygen uptake in ARDS: Myth or reality. *Am. J. Med. Sci.,* **288**:119.

Chance, B., Leight, J. S., Clark, B. J., Maris, J., Kant, J., Nioka, S., and Smith, D. (1985). Control of oxidative metabolism and oxygen delivery in human skeletal muscle: A steady-state analysis of the work/energy cost transfer function. *Proc. Natl. Acad. Sci. USA,* **82**:8384.

Chaudry, I. H., Wichterman, K. A., and Bave, A. E. (1979). Effect of sepsis on tissue adenine nucleotide levels. *Surgery,* **85**:205.

Danek, S. J., Lynch, J. P., Weg, J. G., and Dantzker, D. R. (1980). The dependence of oxygen uptake on oxygen delivery in the adult respiratory distress syndrome. *Am. Rev. Respir. Dis.,* **122**:387.

Ellsworth, M. L., Goldfarb, R. D., Alexander, R. S., Bell, D. R., and Powers, S. R. (1981). Microembolization induced oxygen utilization impairment in the canine gracilis muscle. *Adv. Shock Res.,* **5**:89.

Fowler, A. A., Hamman, R. F., Good, J. J., Benson, K. N., Baird, J. M., Eberle, D. J., Petty, T. L., and Hyers, T. M. (1983). Adult respiratory distress syndrome: Risk with common predispositions. *Ann. Intern. Med.,* **98**:593.

Gadian, D.G. (1982). *Nuclear Magnetic Resonance and Its Application to Living Systems.* Oxford, Oxford University Press.

Greene, N. M. (1961). Effect of epinephrine on lactate, pyruvate and excess lactate production in normal human subjects. *J. Lab. Clin. Med.,* **58**:682.

Groeneveld, A. B. J., Kester, A. D. M., Nauta, J. J. P., and Thijs, L. G. (1987). Relation of arterial blood lactate to oxygen delivery and hemodynamic variables in human shock states. *Circ. Shock,* **22**:35.

Gutierrez, G., and Pohil, R. J. (1986). Oxygen consumption is linearly related to O_2 supply in critically ill patients. *J. Crit. Care,* **1**:45.

Gutierrez, G., Warley, A. R., and Dantker, D. R. (1986). Oxygen delivery and utilization in hypothermic dogs. *J. Appl. Physiol.,* **60**:751.

Gutierrez, G., Pohil, R. J., and Narayana, P. (1989). Skeletal muscle O_2 consumption and energy metabolism during hypoxemia. *J. Appl. Physiol.,* **66**:2117-2173.

Halperin, M. L., and Fields, A. (1985). Lactic acidosis: Emphasis on the carbon precursors and buffering of the acid load. *Am. J. Med. Sci.,* **289**:154.

Harken, A. M., Lillo, R. S., and Hufnagel, H. V. (1975). Direct influence of endotoxin on cellular respiration. *Surg. Gynecol. Obstet.,* **140**:858.

Hochachka, P. W. (1980). *Living Without Oxygen.* Cambridge, Mass., Harvard University Press.

Jobsis, F. F. (1972). Oxidative metabolism at low PO_2. *Fed. Proc.,* **31**:1404.

Johnson, P. (1986). Autoregulation of blood flow. *Circ. Res.,* **59**:483.

Kariman, K., and Burns, S. R. (1985). Regulation of tissue oxygen extraction is disturbed in adult respiratory distress syndrome. *Am. Rev. Respir. Dis.,* **132**:109.

Lassen, N. A., Palm, T., and Nielsen, S. L. (1976). Recruitment of muscle capillaries in man. *Bibl. Anat.,* **15**:504.

Mela, L., Bacalzo, L. V., and Miller, L. D. (1971). Defective oxidative metabolism of rat liver mitochondria in hemorrhagic and endotoxin shock. *Am. J. Physiol.,* **220**:571.

Mizer, L. A., Gadek, J. E., and Dorinsky, P. M. (1988). Morphologic alterations in non-pulmonary organs following PMA induced acute lung: Implications for the pathogenesis of multiple organ failure. *Am. Rev. Respir. Dis.,* **137**:A116.

Mohsenifar, Z., Goldbach, P., Tashkin, D. P., and Campisi, D. J. (1983). Relationship between O_2 delivery and O_2 consumption in the adult respiratory distress syndrome. *Chest,* **84**:267.

Mohsenifar, Z., Amin, D., Jasper, A. C., Shah, P. K., and Koerner, S. K. (1987). Dependence of oxygen consumption on oxygen delivery in patients with chronic congestive heart failure. *Chest,* **92**:447.

Montgomery, A. B., Stager, M. A., Carrico, S. C., and Hudson, L. D. (1985). Causes of mortality in patients with the adult respiratory distress syndrome. *Am. Rev. Respir. Dis.,* **132**:485.

Moon, R. G., and Richards, J. H. (1973). Determination of intracellular pH by ^{31}P magnetic resonance. *J. Biol. Chem.,* **248**:7276.

Moreno, L. F., Straton, H. H., Newell, J. C., et al. (1986). Mathematical coupling of data: Correction of a common error for linear calculations. *J. Appl. Physiol.,* **60**:335E.

Newsholme, E. A., and Leech, A. R. (1983). *Biochemistry for the Medical Sciences.* Chichester, John Wiley.

Parker, M. M., Shelhamer, J. H., Natanson, C., et al. (1987). Serial cardiovascular variable in survivors and nonsurvivors of human septic shock: Heart rate as an early predictor of prognosis. *Crit. Care Med.,* **15**:925.

Petty, T. L. (1982). Adult respiratory distress syndrome: Definition and historical perspective. *Clin. Chest Med.,* **3**:3.

Piiper, J., DiPrampero, P. E., and Cerretelli, P. (1968). Oxygen debt and high energy phosphates in gastrocnemius muscle of the dog. *Am. J. Physiol.,* **215**:523.

Robin, E. D. (1980). Of men and mitochondria: Coping with hypoxic dysoxia. *Am. Rev. Respir. Dis.,* **122**:517.

Shibutani, K., Komatsu, T., Kubal, K., Sanchalla, V., Kumar, V., and Bizzari, D. V. (1983). Critical level of oxygen delivery in anesthetized man. *Crit. Care Med.,* **11**:640.

Sutton, J. R., Reeves, J. T., Wagner, P. D., Graes, B. M., Cymerman, A., Malconian, M. K., Rock, P. B., Young, P. M., Walter, S. D., and Houston, C. S. (1988). Operation Everest. II. Oxygen transport during exercise at extreme simulated altitude. *J. Applied. Physiol.,* **64**:1309.

Tenney, S. M. (1974). A theoretical analysis of the relationship between venous blood and mean tissue oxygen pressures. *Respir. Physiol.,* **20**:283.

Warley, A. R., and Gutierrez, G. (1988). Chronic administration of sodium cyanate decreases O_2 extraction ratio in dogs. *J. Appl. Physiol.,* **64**:1584.

5

Bacterial Infection in Adult Respiratory Distress Syndrome

WALDEMAR G. JOHANSON, JR.

University of Texas Medical Branch
Galveston, Texas

I. Introduction

Although the adult respiratory distress syndrome (ARDS) is usually associated with severe respiratory failure, few patients with this syndrome die of uncorrected hypoxemia. Two recent large studies have found that inability to oxygenate the arterial blood was a contributing factor in only 5-15% of deaths among patients with ARDS (Bell et al., 1983; Montgomery et al., 1985). Death during treatment of ARDS is strongly related to the occurrence of impaired function of other, nonpulmonary organs, a process referred to by the term "multiple organ failure" (MOF). Although the organ system may not be "failing" in a conventional sense, for example gastrointestinal bleeding is a common manifestation, MOF has gained acceptance in the absence of a better descriptor. Mortality in ARDS increases progressively with the number of other organs demonstrating impaired function, from 40% for lung failure alone, to 56% with one additional organ, 73% with two, 82% with three, and 100% with four organs "failing" in addition to the lungs (NHLBI, 1979).

Bacterial infection appears to be closely related to the occurrence of MOF. Bell et al. (1983) defined various organ failures by preset criteria and found evidence of such failures in 93% of infected ARDS patients but only 47% of uninfected ARDS patients. Acute renal failure was by far the most common manifestation of other organ involvement, occurring in 55% of infected and 40% of uninfected patients. The sequence of organ failures in relation to ARDS was not clearly defined in that study. Fry et al. (1980) searched for evidence of organ failure by preset criteria in 553 patients who underwent major operative procedures and/or major trauma. Impaired function, "failure" by the criteria chosen, occurred in 145 organ systems in 87 patients with lung, liver, and renal failure occurring with nearly equal frequency; multiple organ failures occurred in 38 patients. Factors that were *not* found to correlate with the development of MOF, once septic patients were removed, included long bone fractures, head injury, oligemic shock, massive fluid therapy, and chest injury. Of 38 patients with MOF, 34 were septic. The sequence of development of MOF was lung, liver, stress gastrointestinal bleeding, and renal; lung failure occurred nearly concomitantly with the recognition of sepsis, whereas renal failure occurred at a mean of 11.6 days following trauma. The sites of infection leading to sepsis were pleuropulmonary in 37%, abdominal in 35%, and miscellaneous sites including urinary tract in 28%. Pulmonary infections accounted for 50% of the septic episodes leading to MOF. Overall 55 patients in this series died. Infection was thought to be the cause of death in 32 (58%), 24 of whom had MOF. The mortality associated with MOF was again noted to increase as the number of organs displaying impaired function increased and was 85% with three organs failing and 100% with four. The authors concluded that bacterial infection is the principal cause of MOF in trauma patients.

Montgomery and colleagues (1985) approached this problem from a somewhat different view but with very similar results. They prospectively identified 207 patients who were judged to be at high risk of developing ARDS, based on earlier observations (Pepe et al., 1982). ARDS did develop in 47, and the remaining patients were used as a control group. Failures of each of eight organ systems were searched for according to preset criteria. In addition, the "sepsis syndrome" was diagnosed in the presence of findings of inflammation and a systemic response (most often hypotension); positive blood cultures were not required. In patients who died, organ dysfunctions and sepsis were categorized as direct, indirect, or contributing factors to the patient's death. A total of 33 (70%) ARDS patients developed the sepsis syndrome. In 13, sepsis preceded ARDS; abdominal sites accounted for 9 of these, and none were pulmonary. In 20 patients, sepsis developed as a complication of ARDS; 15 (75%) of these episodes resulted from pulmonary infections. Positive blood cultures were found in only 7% of patients with the sepsis syndrome from a pulmonary source compared to 41% of patients who were septic from nonpulmonary sites. Only 10% of the control patients developed the sepsis syndrome. Sepsis was the direct or a contributing factor in 72% of deaths among ARDS patients. Only 5 of 32 deaths were due to unresolved respiratory failure, and 4 of these patients were septic at the time of death.

Signs and symptoms of bacterial infection may develop in patients following major surgery or other forms of trauma in the absence of clinically identifiable sites of infection. Meakins et al. (1980) used the term "nonbacteremic clinical sepsis" to refer to patients who appear septic but in whom blood cultures are negative and no site of infection can be recognized with certainty; MOF is commonly present. These investigators found that the syndrome of nonbacteremic clinical sepsis resolved more slowly than that associated with positive blood cultures and a known site of infection but that mortality in the two situations was similar. This concept was pursued in another study in which bacterial infections were categorized at autopsy in 47 patients who died during treatment for ARDS (Table 1). Only 5 patients did not have infections; 9 patients had been noted to be bacteremic prior to death but no definite site had been found clinically. Each of these patients had a localized collection of pus that would have been drained if it had been recognized; 7 were in the abdomen. A total of 10 patients fit the criteria of clinical sepsis. No site of infection had been diagnosed prior to death, although multiple possible sites had been considered in each patient; 8 of these patients had pneumonia as the major site of infection at autopsy. Over 50% of patients

Table 1 Sites of Predominant Infection at Autopsy

	No. clinically diagnosed sites of infection		
	Bacteremic	Clinical sepsis	Known clinical site
Lung	0	8	16
Pleura	1	1	0
Peritoneum	7	0	3
Other	1	1	4
	9	10	23

Source: Adapted from Bell, 1983.

who died with ARDS had pneumonia as the only or major site of infection at autopsy. In the total series of 84 patients, death occurred in 7% of uninfected patients, 39% of patients who were bacteremic from a clinically known site, 71% of patients who had known infections but were not bacteremic, 71% of patients with clinical sepsis, and 100% of patients who were bacteremic from unrecognized sites.

These observations indicate that bacterial infection may play one of several important roles in ARDS. In many studies primary lung infections represent the single most common cause of ARDS if not excluded by the definition of ARDS used (Ashbaugh et al., 1967; NHLBI, 1979; Fowler et al., 1983). ARDS may occur following trauma for any of a variety of reasons, but ARDS developing later than 48 hr after trauma is usually due to sepsis (Walker and Eiseman, 1975). The site of infection, if known, is usually in the abdomen or an infected wound. Bacteremia in the absence of shock or major tissue injury is followed by ARDS in fewer than 5% of cases (Fein et al., 1983; Fowler et al., 1983). In the patient with ARDS, development of a complicating bacterial infection is often manifested by the absence of improvement of lung function over a period of days or the appearance of MOF regardless of the initial etiology of lung injury. These infections are usually in the lungs, although other sites must be searched for with care.

An alternative hypothesis is that the occurrence of MOF as a complication of ARDS is due to bacteria and/or bacterial products released from the gastrointestinal tract. According to this construct, the permeability of the gastrointestinal tract to the large bacterial population contained within it, to endotoxin, or to extracellular products of bacteria is increased, allowing egress of either bacteria or products into the circulation. A presumed corollary to this hypothesis is that the capacity of the reticuloendothelial system (RES) to remove these factors from the circulation is impaired, leading to tissue injury and MOF.

II. Pneumonia as the Source of Sepsis in ARDS

Nosocomial pneumonias occur in 20-40% of intubated, mechanically ventilated patients based on clinical criteria of new fever, infiltrates, leukocytosis, and purulent secretions, and this incidence has not changed over the past 20 years (Johanson et al., 1972; Stevens et al., 1974; Salata et al., 1987). However, autopsy studies have found that up to 72% of patients dying of respiratory failure have pneumonia at the time of death (Coalson, 1982). Obviously, the frequency of nosocomial pneumonia varies with the criteria used for diagnosis as well as with the patient population under study.

We have used the presence of an intense neutrophilic infiltrate centered on airspaces surrounding terminal and respiratory bronchioles to identify bacterial pneumonias (Andrews et al., 1981). In some patients the process is focal, and this geographic localization is readily apparent. In others, the process is more extensive and spreads across many distal lung units; lung tissue necrosis may or may not be present. It is likely, if over 70% of patients who die in respiratory failure have pneumonia by these histologic criteria but only 20-40% of such patients are thought to have pneumonia clinically, that not all histologic pneumonias are clinically significant.

The above-listed clinical criteria for the presence of nosocomial pneumonia may be accurate in many groups of patients, especially in the absence of prior radiographic infiltrates. However, in patients with ARDS and preexisting bilateral infiltrates these criteria have been shown to be inaccurate. Andrews et al. (1981) compared premortem clinical findings with the histology of the lungs at necropsy in ARDS patients who died during ventilatory support. Clinical diagnoses as to the presence or absence of pneumonia were correct in only 70% of patients. Fever, leukocytosis, and pathogenic bacteria in secretions were found in most patients whether pneumonia was present or not, so these criteria had no predictive value. Improvement following antibiotic therapy occurred most often in patients without pneumonia and was therefore of no predictive value. Evaluation of serial chest radiographs also failed to reveal any pattern associated with pneumonia; one-third of dense alveolar infiltrates were due to only pulmonary edema at autopsy.

It is likely that the reported incidence of bacterial pneumonia at necropsy varies with the intensity with which these pathologic findings are sought. In the study of Bell and associates (1983), pneumonias were found in approximately 70% of patients dying with ARDs and 80% of patients who were thought to have clinical sepsis had pneumonia as the only site of infection at necropsy. An average of 12 samples of lung, obtained from all lobes, were examined in that study. In contrast, Marshall et al. (1988) performed autopsies on 20 patients who died following treatment for MOF; although pneumonias were found in perhaps 9 patients, most were thought to be "less serious infections" in the absence of tissue necrosis. These authors found no evidence of "gross infection" in 8 of the 20 patients, and they attributed MOF in these patients to enteric bacteria. Whether small foci of pneumonia may have been overlooked or dismissed cannot be ascertained for certain.

The appearance of the bronchopneumonia lesion requires the presence of about 10^4 bacteria/g lung tissue in both hamsters and nonhuman primates (Johanson et al., 1985). Limited data suggest that a similar number is required in humans (Chastre et al., 1984). The lesion can be readily differentiated from the recruitment of neutrophils that accompanies diffuse alveolar damage by the lack of geographic localization of inflammation in the latter. When experimental bacterial pneumonia is produced in the presence of severe underlying lung damage, such as pulmonary edema due to oxygen toxicity, the intensity of the neutrophil infiltrate may be somewhat reduced but the pattern is not lost. Bacterial inoculation in the presence of a noninfectious lung insult tends to amplify the latter, thereby obscuring the appearance of early pneumonia. Thus, the histologic appearance of bacterial bronchopneumonia appears to be quite specific and if anything tends to underestimate the frequency of this process. For the reasons stated above, however, it is unlikely that all of the histologically evident bronchopneumonia lesions are clinically important but the quantitative relationships between this histologic finding and the clinical course of patients remain unknown.

Nosocomial pneumonias occur with two basic patterns. Early pneumonias, which develop within the first 3 days of hospitalization, are usually caused by organisms that cause community-acquired pneumonias, such as pneumococci and *Hemophilus*. These infections are seen in individuals with acute, sudden illnesses, such as trauma or drug overdoses; presumably the causative organisms were present in the oropharynx at the time of onset of the illness. The second and more common pattern is the development of pneumonia after several days in the hospital, typically around day 7. These infections are most likely to occur in intensive care patients and are predominantly caused by gram-negative bacilli. These organisms are rarely found in the upper respiratory tracts of normal people but are acquired by over 50% of seriously ill patients within a few days in the hospital (Johanson et al., 1972). The mechanisms of colonization of the upper respiratory tract appear to involve increased adherence of gram-negative bacilli to the respiratory epithelial cells of ill patients (Woods et al., 1981), a phenomenon that allows persistence and multiplication of the organisms in the oropharynx. Microaspiration of contaminated oropharyngeal secretions is not prevented by the presence of a cuffed endotracheal tube in the trachea (Cameron et al., 1973). ARDS is accompanied by several factors known to impair the capacity of the lung's antibacterial defenses, including alveolar edema and hypoxia. Thus it is not surprising that many patients with ARDS develop pneumonia. Indeed, it is somewhat surprising that all do not.

When dogs are inoculated endobronchially, bacteria can be recovered within minutes from hilar lymph nodes (Robertson, 1941). This observation indicates that lymphatic removal is at least a contributing component to the dissemination of bacteria to other tissues. Emigration of bacteria from the lungs of hamsters with hyperoxic injury occurs at intrapulmonary concentrations of 10^3 g^{-1} lung tissue (Johanson et al., 1985). Much higher bacterial concentrations are required for demonstration of emigration from the lungs of air-breathing control animals. Although these observations suggest that a much lower threshold for bacterial emigration exists in animals with damaged lungs, other explanations are also possible. One would be that circulating bacteria are removed from the bloodstream more slowly in the presence of lung injury due to concomitant impairment of RES function. In fact, data obtained in hamsters with paraquat-induced lung damage did suggest that prior bacterial infection of the lungs but not paraquat injury led to reduced RES uptake of injected, radiolabeled bacteria (Seidenfeld et al., 1986). A similar impairment of RES function apparently induced by chronic infection has been noted in humans (Bender et al., 1987).

These findings indicate that foci of bronchopneumonia are capable of releasing bacteria, or bacterial products, into the systemic circulation and that necrotizing pulmonary processes are not required for this to occur. Further, bacterial bronchopneumonias are present in most patients following prolonged intubation and mechanical ventilation. The frequency of such pneumonias in seriously ill but nonintubated patients is not known. It is not certain that foci of bronchopneumonia are a sufficient source of bacteria and/or products to initiate the cascade of events leading to MOF or what the quantitative aspects of this relationship might be. However, since clinically unrecognizable pneumonias appear to be a common cause of the syndrome of clinical sepsis, it seems reasonable to believe that MOF might arise from this source as well.

III. The Gastrointestinal Tract as the Source of Sepsis in ARDS

The other prevailing notion to explain clinical sepsis in the absence of definable sites of infection is the release of bacteria or bacterial products from the gastrointestinal tract. This concept is nearly as old as microbiology. Investigators have reasoned that in severe illness bacterial overgrowth might occur in the bowel owing to hypoperistalsis, that bowel permeability to bacterial cells or products might be increased, and/or that the capacity of normal defenses, especially the RES, might be impaired allowing access to the systemic circulation. Evidence exists in support of each of these possibilities.

Serious illnesses are regularly accompanied by disordered bowel motility, and problems with enteral feeding are common among patients in intensive care units. Hypomotility plus the routine administration of agents to reduce gastric acidity have been blamed for colonization of the stomach in critically ill patients. Du Moulin et al. (1982) studied the bacterial flora of the stomach in 60 seriously ill patients. The mean bacterial concentration was 10^8 colony-forming units (CFU)/ml and consisted predominantly of gram-negative bacilli. Bacterial concentrations increased linearly as the pH rose, only rare specimens containing viable gram-negative organisms when the pH was less than 2.0. These authors also found a striking concordance between the flora of the stomach and those of the upper airways, demonstrating both transmission from the stomach to the trachea and from the oropharynx to the stomach on serial cultures in different individuals. Other groups have repeated this study with essentially similar findings (Driks et al., 1987). It appears that stress ulceration prophylaxis with mucosa-protecting agents, such as sucralfate, may be superior to acid neutralization or inhibition because gastric colonization is reduced. However, the observation that sucralfate may have direct antibacterial properties places some doubt on the mechanism of this beneficial change (Tryba and Mantey-Stiers, 1987). The route of gastric colonization remains unclear. Presumably, bacteria proliferating in the hypotonic stomach reflect an overgrowth of the bacteria normally present in small number in the upper gastrointestinal tract, although sequential cultures demonstrating this have not been reported. It remains possible that the gastric flora represent organisms swallowed from the oropharynx. It is probably true that either may occur and that the predominant route may differ from patient to patient.

Evidence in support of altered permeability is less direct. Certainly instances of bacteremia with bowel organisms in the absence of extraluminal sites of infection would tend to support this concept, but it is difficult to be certain that invasive sites of infection were not present. This is particularly true in markedly neutropenic patients in whom the absence of leukocytes makes the formation of pus impossible, thus removing one of the cardinal findings of tissue invasion. However, the finding that nearly 40% of episodes of enterococcal bacteremia in surgical patients occurred in patients with no discernible extraluminal infection is difficult to explain by mechanisms other than increased permeability (Garrison et al., 1982). Neither endotoxin nor intact organisms are present in portal blood in people without bowel or liver disease (van Deventer et al., 1988). Either or both may be present in patients with ulcerating or inflammatory bowel lesions. In animals, alterations in blood flow to the bowel induced by either arterial ligation or portal ligation or the administration of vasoactive substances, such as serotonin, lead to endotoxemia. Systemic endotoxemia is more likely to occur in models in which portal flow is diverted, presumably by avoiding uptake and removal by the liver.

Intraperitoneal administration of endotoxin following prolonged protein deprivation in mice leads to demonstrable translocation of the fecal flora, that is, cultures of mesenteric lymph nodes, liver, and spleen reveal enteric organisms (Deitch et al., 1987). Positive organ cultures occurred rarely in animals that received protein deprivation or endotoxin alone. These findings suggest that the combined insults of protein malnutrition and endotoxin administration increased bowel permeability. Other explanations are also possible. Increased concentrations of bacteria in the bowel might cause translocation without implying increased permeability. Both endotoxin administration and protein malnutrition were associated with increased concentrations of organisms in cecal contents, but neither led to translocation as a single insult, so this mechanism does not explain the observation. It is possible that endotoxin administration impairs RES uptake and killing activity and that the occurrence of positive organ cultures reflects this phenomenon, not increased release of organisms from the bowel. This possibility could not be excluded without additional measurements.

However, these observations do suggest that products of the bowel bacterial flora may be present in the systemic circulation and remote organs of stressed animals in the absence of disease or injury that directly affects the bowel. It is likely that similar events occur in humans, although comparable samples cannot be obtained in humans. However, circulating endotoxin concentrations appear to be directly related to the extent of cutaneous burn injury in humans, for example (Winchurch et al., 1987). In such circumstances, release of endotoxin from the bowel is probably related to alterations in blood flow.

Impairment of the RES as a result of severe illness could contribute to the finding of endotoxin in the blood of these patients. Removal of particulate matter from the blood is accomplished largely by the liver, a function residing primarily in the Kupffer's cells. This process is facilitated by nonspecific serum opsonins, including fibronectin, and specific immunoglobulin opsonins. The rate of removal of particles is dependent on liver blood flow and Kupffer's cell function as well as serum factors. Thus, RES function is difficult to measure in humans, and it is difficult to interpret data in which only some of the above factors have been controlled.

Serum fibronectin concentration falls in patients with sudden, severe injury and clinical improvement has been reported in patients receiving replacement therapy in uncontrolled trials (Scovill et al., 1978). Low fibronectin concentrations have not been found to predict the occurrence of respiratory failure in patients at risk of ARDS in the hands of other investigators (Grossman, 1987), and it seems unlikely that this serum protein will hold the key to RES abnormalities leading to MOF.

New techniques may allow Kupffer's cell function to be assessed more directly. Liver macrophages contain receptors for the complement component C3 and the rate of removal from the blood of particles coated with C3b and iC3b is a function of these cells (Bender et al., 1987). Patients with chronic infections, whether associated with human immunodeficiency virus (HIV) infection or not, demonstrated impaired Kupffer's cell function whereas patients who were HIV positive but without the acquired immunodeficiency syndrome (AIDS) were normal. These findings suggest that RES function may be impaired by bacterial products. Since a major function of the RES is host defense against bacterial infection, such impairment could result in worsening infection, leading to a further decline in RES function, and so forth.

IV. Mechanisms of MOF Related to Sepsis

It is likely that either clinically unrecognized pneumonias or release of bacteria from the gastrointestinal tract, or both, occur in seriously ill patients. The question then becomes how these phenomena might be related, if at all, to the occurrence of MOF. The answer appears to be through one or another of several mediators, which are covered in detail in other chapters and will be only briefly mentioned here. The most likely candidate mediator is tumor necrosis factor (TNF), also known as cachectin. TNF is synthesized and released by macrophages following a priming stimulus. The most potent known priming stimulus is endotoxin (Cybulsky et al., 1988). In fact, many of the long-observed effects of endotoxin infusion in experimental animals and of gram-negative sepsis in humans can now be explained in terms of the effects of TNF or other mediator molecules and are not direct effects of endotoxin. TNF is directly toxic to vascular endothelial cells. In addition, it inhibits the expression of thrombomodulin and induces the production of procoagulant activity (Beutler and Cerami, 1987), all changes that would promote intravascular thrombosis. TNF may increase the production of leukotrienes, platelet-activating factor, and interleukin-1, thereby promoting neutrophil infiltration and the development of systemic signs, such as fever and hypotension. Infusion of recombinant TNF into rats produces ischemic and hemorrhagic inflammatory lesions in the lungs, kidneys, gastrointestinal tract, and pancreas (Tracey et al., 1986). These lesions are similar to those associated with sepsis and MOF in humans dying with ARDS (Coalson, 1986). It is reasonable to postulate that the Kupffer's cells of the liver play a key role in the generation of TNF in patients with ARDS since there is ample evidence that the liver is involved in both subclinical lung infections and in handling bacterial products released from the bowel.

V. Summary

Bacterial infection may *cause* ARDS, as in primary pneumonias or sepsis from nonpulmonary sites.

Infection may *complicate* ARDS, leading to failure of lung function to improve and the occurrence of MOF. Such infections may be clinically apparent or inapparent; in the latter case, bacteria and/or bacterial products are released from foci of bronchopneumonia or the enteric flora.

The systemic effects of bacterial infection are probably caused by host-derived mediators, especially TNF. It is probable that Kupffer's cells in the liver play a key role in this process.

References

Andrews, C. P., Coalson, J. J., Smith, J. D., and Johanson, W. G., Jr. (1981). Diagnosis of nosocomial bacterial pneumonia in acute, diffuse lung injury. *Chest*, **80**:254-258.

Ashbaugh, D. C., Bigelow, D. D., Petty, T. L., and Levine, B. E. (1967). Acute respiratory distress in adults. *Lancet,* **2**:319-323.

Bell, R. C., Coalson, J. J., Smith, J. D., and Johanson, W. G., Jr. (1983). Multiple organ failure and infection in the adult respiratory distress syndrome. *Ann. Intern. Med.,* **99**:293-298.

Bender, B. S., Bohnsack, J. F., Sourlis, S. H., Frank, M. M., and Quinn, T. C. (1987). Demonstration of defective C3-receptor-mediated clearance by the reticuloendothelias system in patients with acquired immunodeficiency syndrome. *J. Clin. Invest.,* **79**:715-720.

Beutler, B., and Cerami, A. (1987). Cachetin: More than a tumor necrosis factor. *N. Engl. J. Med.,* **316**:379-385.

Cameron, J. L., Reynolds, J., and Zuidema, G. D. (1973). Aspiration in patients with tracheostomies. *Surg. Gynecol. Obstet.,* **136**:68-70.

Chastre, J., Viau, F., Brun, P., Pierre, J., Dauge, M., Bouchama, A., Akesbi, A., and Gibert, C. (1984). Prospective evaluation of the protected specimen brush for the diagnosis of pulmonary infections in ventilated patients. *Am. Rev. Respir. Dis.,* **130**:924-929.

Coalson, J. J. (1982). Pathophysiologic features of respiratory distress in the infant and adult. In *Critical Care Medicine: State of the Art,* Vol. 3. Edited by W. C. Shoemaker and W. L. Thompson. Fullerton, CA, Society of Critical Care Medicine, pp. 1-28.

Coalson, J. J. (1986). Pathology of sepsis, septic shock and multiple organ failure. In *New Horizons: Perspectives on Sepsis and Septic Shock.* Edited by W. J. Sibbald and C. L. Sprung. Fullerton, CA, Society of Critical Care Medicine, pp. 27-59.

Cybulsky, M. I., Chan, M. K. W., and Movat, H. Z. (1988). Biology of disease: Acute inflammation and microthrombosis induced by endotoxin, interleukin-1, and tumor necrosis factor and their implication in gram-negative infection. *Lab. Invest.,* **58**:365-378.

Deitch, E. A., Winterton, J., and Berg, R. (1987). The gut as a portal of entry for bacteremia. *Ann. Surg.,* **205**:681-692.

Driks, M. R., Craven, D. E., Celli, B. R., Manning, M., Burke, R. A., Garvin, G. M., Kunches, L. M., Farber, H. W., Wedel, S. A., and McCabe, W. R. (1987). Nosocomial pneumonia in intubated patients given sucralfate as compared with antacids or histamine type 2 blockers. *N. Engl. J. Med.,* **317**:1376-1382.

du Moulin, G. C., Paterson, D. G., Hedley-Whyte, J., and Lisbon, A. (1982). Aspiration of gastric bactria in antacid-treated patients: A frequent cause of postoperative colonisation of the airway. *Lancet,* **1**:242-245.

Fein, A. M., Lippmann, M., Holtzman, H., Eliraz, A., and Goldberg, S. K. (1983). The risk factors, incidence, and prognosis of ARDS following septicemia. *Chest,* **83**:40-42.

Fowler, A. A., Hamman, R. F., Good, J. T., Benson, K. N., Baird, M., Eberle, D. J., Petty, T. L., and Hyers, T. M. (1983). Adult respiratory distress syndrome: Risk with common predispositions. *Ann. Intern. Med.,* **98**:593-597.

Fry, D. E., Pearlstein, L., Fulton, R. L., and Polk, H. C., Jr. (1980). Multiple system organ failure. The role of uncontrolled infection. *Arch. Surg.,* **115**:136-140.

Garrison, R. N., Fry, D. E., Berberick, S., and Polk, H. C., Jr. (1982). Enterococcal bacteremia: Clinical implications and determinants of death. *Ann. Surg.,* **196**:43-47.

Grossman, J. E. (1987). Plasma fibronectin and fibronectin therapy in sepsis and critical illness. *Rev. Infect. Dis.,* **9**:S2420-S430.

Johanson, W. G., Jr., Pierce, A. K., Sanford, J. P., and Thomas, G. D. (1972). Nosocomial respiratory infections with gram-negative bacilli: Significance of colonization of the respiratory tract. *Ann. Intern. Med.,* **77**:701-706.

Johanson, W. G., Jr., Higuchi, J. H., Woods, D. E., Gomez, P., and Coalson J. J. (1985). Dissemination of *Pseudomonas aeruginosa* during lung infection in hamsters. *Am. Rev. Respir. Dis.,* **132**:358-361.

Marshall, J. C., Christou, N. V., Horn, R., and Meakins, J. L. (1988). The microbiology of multiple organ failure: The proximal gastrointestinal tract as an occult reservoir of pathogens. *Arch. Surg.,* **123**:309-315.

Meakins, J. L., Wicklund, B., Forse, R. A., and McLean, A. P. H. (1980). The surgical intensive care unit: Current concepts in infection. *Surg. Clin. North Am.,* **60**:117-132.

Montgomery, A. B., Stager, M. A., Carrico, C. J., and Hudson, L. D. (1985). Causes of mortality in patients with the adult respiratory distress syndrome. *Am. Rev. Respir. Dis.,* **132**:485-489.

National Heart, Lung, and Blood Institute (1979). Extracorporeal support for respiratory insufficiency: collaborative study. U. S. Department of Health, Education, and Welfare, Public Health Service.

Pepe, P. E., Potkin, R. T., Holtman, D., Hudson, L. D., and Carrico, C. J. (1982). Clinical predictors of the adult respiratory distress syndrome. *Am. J. Surg.,* **144**:124-130.

Robertson, O. H. (1941). Phagocytosis of foreign material in the lung. *Physiol. Rev.,* **21**:112-139.

Salata, R., Lederman, M., Shlaes, D., Jacobs, M. R., Eckstein, E., Tweardy, D., Toossi, Z., Chmielewski, R., Marino, J., King, C. H., Graham, R. C., and Ellner, J. J. (1987). Diagnosis of nosocomial pneumonia in intubated, intensive care unit patients. *Am. Rev. Respir. Dis.,* **135**:426-432.

Scovill, W. A., Saba, T. M., Blumenstock, F. A., Bernard, H., and Powers, S. R., Jr. (1978). Opsonic $alpha_2$ surface binding glycoprotein therapy during sepsis. *Ann. Surg.,* **188**:521-529.

Seidenfeld, J. J., Mullins, C. B., III, Fowler, S. R., and Johanson, W. G., Jr. (1986). Bacterial infection and acute lung injury in hamsters. *Am. Rev. Respir. Dis.,* **134**:22-26.

Stevens, R. M., Teres, D., Skillman, J. J., and Finegold, D. S. (1974). Pneumonia in an intensive care unit. *Arch. Intern. Med.,* **134**:106-111.

Tracey, K. J., Beutler, B., Lowry, S. F., Merryweather, J., Wolke, S., Milsark, I. W., Hariri, R. J., Fahey, T. J., III, Zentella, A., Albert, J. D., Shires, G. T., and Cerami, A. (1986). Shock and tissue injury induced by recombinant human cachectin. *Science,* **234**:470-474.

Tryba, M., and Mantey-Stiers, F. (1987). Antibacterial activity of sucralfate in human gastric juice. *Am. J. Med.,* **83**:125-127.

van Deventer, S. J. H., ten Cate, J. W., and Tytgat, G. N. J. (1988). Intestinal endotoxemia. *Gastroenterology,* **94**:825-831.

Walker, L., and Eiseman, B. (1975). The changing pattern of post-traumatic respiratory distress syndrome. *Ann. Surg.,* **181**:693-697.

Winchurch, R. A., Thupari, J. N., and Munster, A. M. (1987). Endotoxemia in burn patients: Levels of circulating endotoxins are related to burn size. *Surgery,* **102**:808-812.

Woods, D. E., Strauss, D. C., Johanson, W. G., Jr., and Bass, J. A. (1981). The role of salivary protease activity in adherence of gram-negative bacilli to mammalian buccal epithelial cells in vivo. *J. Clin. Invest.,* **68**:1435-1440.

6

Prognostic Factors in the Intensive Care Unit with Special Emphasis on Acute Respiratory Failure

WILLIAM A. KNAUS

The George Washington University Medical Center
Washington, D.C.

I. Introduction

The objective of this discussion is to present a model for estimating prognosis from severe acute illness. By using information available at the time patients present for intensive medical care and by following their response to that treatment, we will illustrate our current ability to predict patient outcome. The outcome measure we use is death in the hospital. Hospital mortality does not take into account the quality and length of posthospital survival, but hospital mortality rates can be accurately measured and are a reasonable starting point for this type of analysis.

The model we use assumes that the probability of surviving an acute life-threatening illness is related to four major patient factors:

1. Disease: the acute disease that directly prompted medical treatment

---

The opinions and conclusions are those of the author and do not necessarily represent those of the sponsoring or corroborating institutions.

2. Severity of disease: acute physiologic abnormalities associated with the disease
3. Patient's physiologic reserve: the patient's chronologic age and the presence of severe chronic organ system dysfunction
4. Response to therapy: measured by persistent physiologic abnormalities during the course of treatment

All these factors have been independently shown to correlate with outcome from an acute illness. In this study we illustrate their combined prognostic value for intensive care unit (ICU) acutely ill patients with special emphasis on patients with acute respiratory failure.

II. Source of Patient Information: Validation of APACHE II

The information presented in this study comes from a nationwide effort to validate a severity of disease classification system for acutely ill patients, APACHE II (Knaus et al., 1985a): acute physiology, age, and chronic health evaluation. APACHE II is a simplified form of the original APACHE system (Knaus et al., 1981). The APACHE approach to severity measurement was designed to provide a reliable and objective common method with which clinicians and investigators could measure the severity of disease within most major life-threatening diseases and then use this information to estimate patient prognosis before and during therapy.

The APACHE system was developed using the previously described model. We assumed that the outcome from an acute illness was, in large part, related to the degree of disturbances in the body's major physiologic organ systems and that the risk imposed by these physiologic abnormalities could be estimated on the basis of deviations from normal physiology and on past experience treating acutely ill patients. Thus, the format, design, and weights used in the APACHE II system are not derived from any one group of patients using a data search technique. Rather, they represent general clinical and physiologic principles.

The major part of the APACHE II classification system is an acute physiology score (APS) made up of 12 readily available physiologic determinations. The value of each physiologic measure is given a weight from 0 to 12 depending on its deviation from a predetermined normal range and on its relative importance to patient outcome as decided by an expert multidisciplinary panel of physicians and a review of past experience.

The resulting APS varies from 0 to 45 with a usual range of 0-25. A higher score indicates a greater degree of physiologic derangement and a higher acute risk of death. The APS may be used alone to risk-stratify acutely ill patients at hospital or ICU admission, or it can be measured over time to monitor response to treatment. When used over time, persistent elevations in the APS, despite therapy, represent ongoing physiologic derangement similar to the previously described multiple organ system failure (Bell et al., 1983; Knaus et al., 1985).

To estimate patient prognosis, the APS is combined with additional points or weights provided for a patient's chronologic age and the presence of a severe chronic health problem, both of which reduce a patient's physiologic response to illness, thereby increasing the risk of death. Severe failing health status is defined by one or more positive responses to a series of objective questions regarding chronic organ system dysfunction. For example, for the respiratory system, does the patient have chronic restrictive, obstructive, or pulmonary vascular disease resulting in severe exercise restriction, that is, an inability to climb stairs or perform household duties, or documented chronic hypoxia, hypercapnia, secondary polycythermia, or severe pulmonary hypertension ($\geqslant$ 40 mmHg)?

Points for advanced chronologic age and/or chronic health status are added to those obtained with the acute physiology score to form the full APACHE II classification system. It is a cardinal index number with a theoretical range of 0-71 and an observed range of 0-50. The higher the APACHE II score, the greater is the patient's acute risk of death. The full system is described in Figure 1, and details concerning its origin, development, and design can be found elsewhere (Knaus et al., 1985a).

Both the original APACHE system and the simplified APACHE II have undergone extensive reliability and validity testing. They have been shown to correlate with subsequent hospital mortality rates with patients suffering from a variety of acute diseases and treated in a number of hospitals worldwide (Knaus et al., 1982; Wagner et al., 1984). The overall relationship between APACHE II scores, obtained during the initial 24 hr of ICU treatment, and subsequent hospital mortality rates for 5030 operative and nonoperative ICU admissions was provided in Figure 2.

This ability of the APACHE II score used in combination with the patient's disease to risk or prognostically stratify patients on admission to ICUs by their pretreatment risk of death has made it possible to compare the performance of intensive care among a sample of U.S. hospitals and between a sample of U.S. and French hospitals (Knaus et al., 1982, 1986). The technique of combining information from disease, severity, and physiologic reserve to estimate an individual's risk of death by calculating an anticipated death rate for a group of critically ill patients has been shown to be an improvement over a comparison of the mean values of various patient characteristics as a method of determining the impact of a new treatment on patient

PHYSIOLOGIC VARIABLE	HIGH ABNORMAL RANGE					LOW ABNORMAL RANGE			
	+4	+3	+2	+1	0	+1	+2	+3	+4
TEMPERATURE — rectal (°C)	≥ 41°	39°-40.9°		38.5°-38.9°	36°-38.4°	34°-35.9°	32°-33.9°	30°-31.9°	≤ 29.9°
MEAN ARTERIAL PRESSURE — mm Hg	≥ 160	130-159	110-129		70-109		50-69		≤ 49
HEART RATE (ventricular response)	≥ 180	140-179	110-139		70-109		55-69	40-54	≤ 39
RESPIRATORY RATE — (non-ventilated or ventilated)	≥ 50	35-49		25-34	12-24	10-11	6-9		≤ 5
OXYGENATION: A-aDO$_2$ or PaO$_2$ (mm Hg) a. FiO$_2$ ≥ 0.5 record A-aDO$_2$	≥ 500	350-499	200-349		< 200				
b. FiO$_2$ < 0.5 record only PaO$_2$					PO$_2$ > 70	PO$_2$ 61-70		PO$_2$ 55-60	PO$_2$ < 55
ARTERIAL pH	≥ 7.7	7.6-7.69		7.5-7.59	7.33-7.49		7.25-7.32	7.15-7.24	< 7.15
SERUM SODIUM (mMol/L)	≥ 180	160-179	155-159	150-154	130-149		120-129	111-119	≤ 110
SERUM POTASSIUM (mMol/L)	≥ 7	6-6.9		5.5-5.9	3.5-5.4	3-3.4	2.5-2.9		< 2.5
SERUM CREATININE (mg/100 ml) (Double point score for **acute** renal failure)	≥ 3.5	2-3.4	1.5-1.9		0.6-1.4		< 0.6		
HEMATOCRIT (%)	≥ 60		50-59.9	46-49.9	30-45.9		20-29.9		< 20
WHITE BLOOD COUNT (total/mm3) (in 1,000s)	≥ 40		20-39.9	15-19.9	3-14.9		1-2.9		< 1
GLASGOW COMA SCORE (GCS): Score = 15 minus actual GCS									
[A] Total ACUTE PHYSIOLOGY SCORE (APS): Sum of the 12 individual variable points									
Serum HCO$_3$ (venous-mMol/L) [Not preferred, use if no ABGs]	≥ 52	41-51.9		32-40.9	22-31.9		18-21.9	15-17.9	< 15

[B] AGE POINTS:
Assign points to age as follows:

AGE(yrs)	Points
≤ 44	0
45-54	2
55-64	3
65-74	5
≥ 75	6

[C] CHRONIC HEALTH POINTS
If the patient has a history of severe organ system insufficiency or is immuno-compromised assign points as follows:

a. for nonoperative or emergency postoperative patients — 5 points
or
b. for elective postoperative patients — 2 points

DEFINITIONS
Organ Insufficiency or immuno-compromised state must have been evident **prior** to this hospital admission and conform to the following criteria:

LIVER: Biopsy proven cirrhosis and documented portal hypertension; episodes of past upper GI bleeding attributed to portal hypertension; or prior episodes of hepatic failure/encephalopathy/coma.

CARDIOVASCULAR: New York Heart Association Class IV.

RESPIRATORY: Chronic restrictive, obstructive, or vascular disease resulting in severe exercise restriction, i.e., unable to climb stairs or perform household duties; or documented chronic hypoxia, hypercapnia, secondary polycythemia, severe pulmonary hypertension (>40mmHg), or respirator dependency.

RENAL: Receiving chronic dialysis.

IMMUNO-COMPROMISED: The patient has received therapy that suppresses resistance to infection, e.g., immuno-suppression, chemotherapy, radiation, long term or recent high dose steroids, or has a disease that is sufficiently advanced to suppress resistance to infection, e.g., leukemia, lymphoma, AIDS.

APACHE II SCORE
Sum of [A] + [B] + [C]

[A] APS points ________

[B] Age points ________

[C] Chronic Health points ________

Total APACHE II ________

Figure 1 The APACHE II severity of disease classification system.

outcome (Knaus et al., 1984). As a result, it has been suggested that APACHE II be used to stratify seriously ill gastrointestinal patients by relative risk of death in studies of new surgical and antibiotic treatments (Dellinger et al., 1985).

In of these applications, APACHE and APACHE II have been used to estimate group as opposed to individual death rates. In this study, we will use these same principles to predict outcome for acutely ill patients meeting the criteria for acute respiratory failure (ARF).

A. Data Collection

For each of the 5815 patients in our national validation of APACHE II, we collected information on disease, age, sex, prior health status, and extent of physiologic derangement on admission to the ICU (first day values) and, for physiologic measurements, on all subsequent ICU treatment days. All patients were followed for status at both ICU and hospital discharge. We also recorded whether and when a decision was made to limit, reduce, or end life support as indicated by a DNR (do not resuscitate) decision.

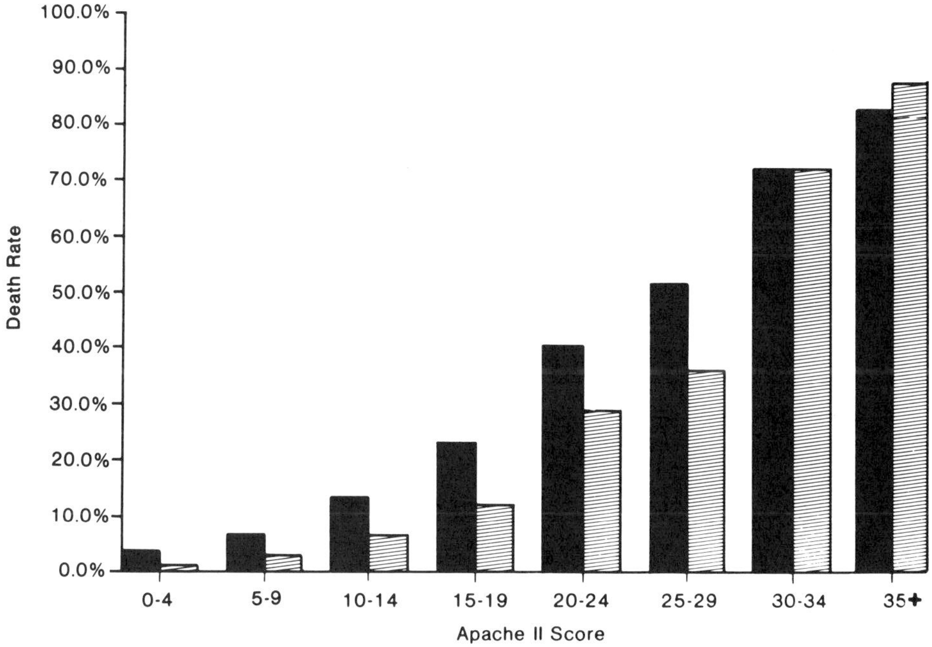

Figure 2 The overall relationship between APACHE II scores and subsequent hospital mortality rates for nonoperative and postoperative patients.

All data were collected on standard forms and sent to a central location for editing, extensive error checking, and analysis. Reported patient outcomes were also independently verified by cross-checking against hospital discharge summaries.

B. Patient Selection for this Study

There were 5815 patients from 13 hospitals in our final APACHE II database. They had a wide variety of acute medical and surgical diagnoses and, with the sole exceptions of burns and acute myocardial infarctions, represent the spectrum of diseases now treated in medical-surgical ICUs. More detailed information on diseases can be found elsewhere (Knaus et al., 1985a).

The 13 hospitals and the intensive care units included in this study are listed in Table 1. Most of the units were mixed medical-surgical, although both dedicated medical and purely surgical units were included. The number of consecutive patients studied per hospital varied from 159 to 500 (Table 1).

Table 1 Hospitals and Intensive Care Units Participating in Study

Hospital	Total number hospital beds	Total number adult ICU beds	Number adult ICU beds studied	Type of ICUs studied
Cooper Medical Center (NJ)	522	14	14	Mixed medical-surgical
Medical College of Georgia (GA)	706	21	6	Medical
George Washington University Medical Center (DC)	450	16	16	Mixed medical-surgical
Johns Hopkins University (MD)	1025	36	7	Medical
Maine Medical Center (ME)	533	32	20	Mixed medical-surgical
University of Maryland Hospital (MD)	729	31	10	Surgical
Massachusetts General Hospital (MA)	1092	90	20	Surgical (two units)
Polyclinic Medical Center (PA)	556	14	6	Mixed medical-surgical
St. Francis Hospital (OK)	802	40	16	Mixed medical-surgical
South Shore Hospital (MA)	280	28	16	Surgical and mixed medical-surgical (two units)
Stanford University Hospital (CA)	633	65	57	Surgical, medical, cardiac surgery (three units)
University of Virginia Medical Center (VA)	683	44	16	Surgical
University of Wisconsin Hospital (WI)	548	36	32	Surgical, medical, mixed medical-surgical (three units)

To concentrate on the acutely ill, we excluded from this study all patients electively admitted to the intensive care unit from the operating room, with the exception of patients with a diagnosis of trauma. From the 2435 total nonoperative patients, we found 224 who were in acute respiratory failure on their third day of ICU treatment and who had a severe degree of hypoxemia ($A\text{-}_aDO_2 \geqslant 350$ mmHg) or hypercapnia ($P_{aCO_2} \geqslant 50$ mmHg). Each was suffering from acute respiratory failure defined as an acute inability to maintain an adequate minute ventilation that was attributed directly to pneumonia or noncardiogenic pulmonary edema. We specifically excluded patients with acute and chronic heart failure and all patients with severe mechanical defects, such as kyphoscoliosis or tracheal stenosis, leading to respiratory failure. Included in this group of acute respiratory failure patients were a number with the adult respiratory distress syndrome (ARDS).

III. Results

The observed hospital death rate for ARF patients was 114 of 224, or 51%. To illustrate the value of the four previously described prognostic factors in this disease group, we first analyzed the influence of the patient's presenting disease. The seven major disease categories present when the patient was admitted to the intensive care unit are listed in Table 2. The nature of the underlying disease strongly influences the prognosis from ARF. Hospital death rates vary from a high of 85% for patients suffering from sepsis to 5% for the 19 patients developing ARF following trauma; only 1 trauma patient died.

Table 2 Initial (First Day) Disease Among 224 Patients Developing Criteria for ARF on Third ICU day

	N	Deceased	%
Sepsis	26	22	85
Gastrointestinal bleeding	10	8	80
Cardiac arrest	11	8	73
Respiratory infection	36	20	56
Respiratory arrest	20	11	55
Pulmonary edema	15	8	54
Trauma	19	1	5

The influence of initial severity of disease on outcome is illustrated in Figure 3, where we have plotted the first day acute physiology score versus hospital outcome for all 224 ARF patients. Hospital mortality rates are low for patients with low initial APS and high for those with initial APS ⩾ 20.

The usefulness of severity information describing the patients' responses to treatment, as measured by the APS over time, is shown in Figure 4. As third day APS increase, implying persistent physiologic imbalances despite ongoing therapy, hospital death rates increase dramatically. By day 3, ARF patients with an APS greater than 20 have very high hospital mortality rates and there is a strong linear relationship between third day APS and hospital mortality rates (Fig. 4).

In Figure 5, we evaluate the relationship between the patient's physiologic reserve status (as measured by their ages) and their observed hospital death rate. The relationship between age and mortality is not as direct as we have seen with severity, but there does appear to be a threshold effect at approximately age 65; thereafter, death rates increase progressively with advancing age.

Finally, we performed a stepwise multivariate logistic regression analysis looking for those factors that are most influential in predicting death in the 224 ARF patients on their third day of ICU care. This analysis, displayed in Table 3, indicates that the most influential single factor is the level of the patient's severity of disease (third day APS) on that day. Next in influence was the patient's age, then whether they met criteria for severe chronic disease

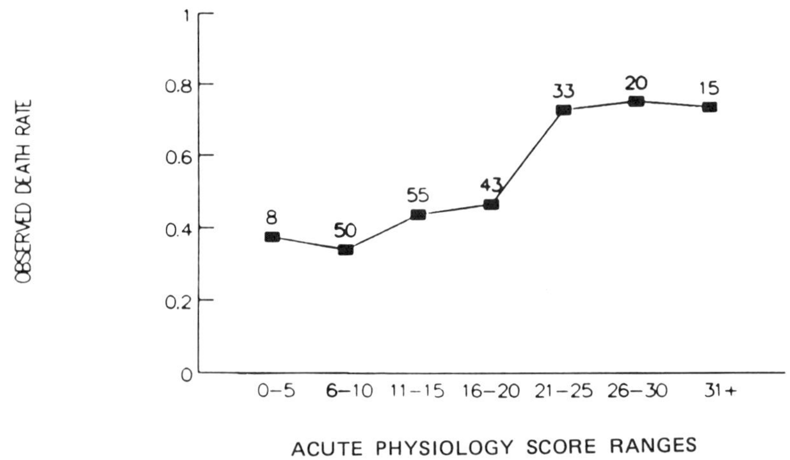

Figure 3 Influence of initial severity of disease (1st day APS) on outcome for 224 ARF patients.

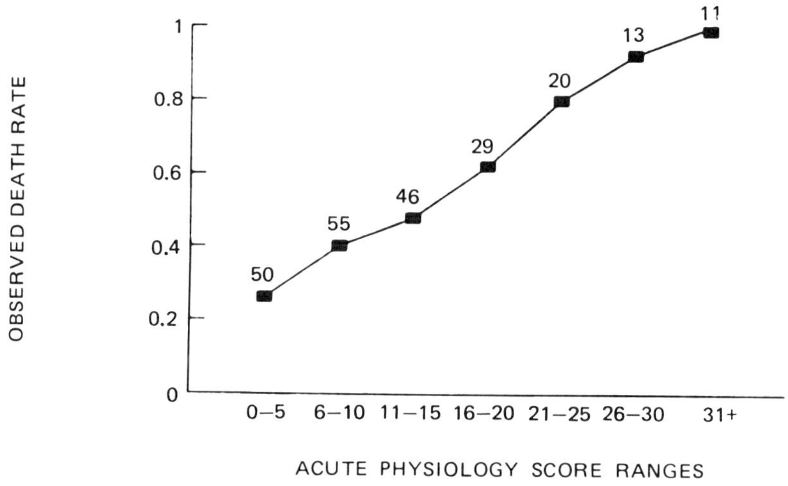

Figure 4 Usefulness of severity information (3rd day APS) describing the patients' responses to treatment.

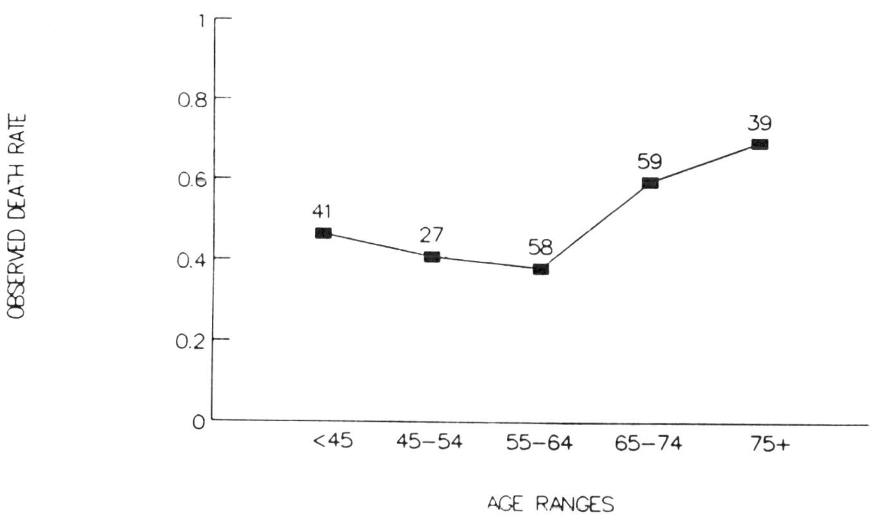

Figure 5 Evaluation of the relationship between patients' ages and mortality rates for 224 ARF patients.

Table 3 Multivariate Analysis of Risk of Death in 224 Patients with Criteria for ARF by Third ICU Day

Significant variables	Chi-square	P
Third day APS	34.8	<0.0001
Age	14.5	<0.0001
Severe chronic disease	9.0	<0.003
Initial disease (sepsis)	4.4	<0.04

according to APACHE II criteria, and, finally, the type of acute disease the patient had on admission to the ICU. For example, sepsis, with the highest death rate, is significant at the $p < 0.04$ level for predicting death.

IV. Discussion

This study has presented a conceptual model for investigating the ability of information availalbe at the time the patient presents for medical care along with that obtained during the course of treatment to predict outcome for patients with acute respiratory failure. We found that prognosis varies by the initial disease process (the seven diseases listed in Table 2) and the severity of that disease, as well as patients' physiologic reserve as determined by their age and chronic health status (Table 3 and Figs. 3, 4, and 5).

These results are encouraging. They suggest there may be an underlying consistent relationship between acute physiologic abnormalities representing severity and an acutely ill patient's risk of death. When information on these physiologic abnormalities is combined with precise descriptions of disease and other patient risk factors, such as age and chronic health status, we have the beginnings of a scientifically valid and reproducible approach to prediction. These new scientific capabilities could improve our ability to document the value of new therapies and improve our use of them.

What are the potential uses of this information? One example was recently provided by gastrointestinal surgeons, who were concerned with the difficulties in interpreting results of treatment studies for acutely ill patients with intra-abdominal infection (Dellinger et al., 1985). Reported mortalities from intra-abdominal infection ranged from 0 to 90%, and no method of relating patient outcome to prior risk existed. This made it impossible to evaluate the incremental value of new or existing treatments. How was it possible to know whether a new antibiotic treatment regimen or a different surgical approach influenced outcome?

To remedy the situation, gastrointestinal surgeons have incorporated the APACHE II system with an anatomic classification of intra-abdominal infections (Dellinger et al., 1985). Their system classifies patients into narrow mortality risk groups (i.e., <10%, 10-20%, >90%, and so on). This stratification allows more precise outcome comparisons by examining patients within each range or by estimating pretreatment death rates. Similar methods could be applied to other diagnoses, such as acute respiratory failure, since the principles used in APACHE II appear to apply to a broad variety of diagnoses, including a major cause of ARF, ARDS (Montgomery et al., 1985). By helping to answer the question of whether the control and treatment groups were similar, risk stratification can improve the precision of clinical research.

In 1982, for example, we published a study comparing the outcome of acutely ill patients treated in French and American ICUs using our original APACHE system (Knaus et al., 1982). For patients with severe gastrointestinal disorders, the French hospital death rate was significantly greater than we predicted on the basis of the U.S. experience. At the time we completed the study, we were uncertain why this variation occurred. It has recently been suggested that some of this variation in outcome was from different indications for surgery in the two countries for patients suffering from acute pancreatitis, one of the common diagnoses in our study (Smadja and Bismuth, 1984).

We are now completing other international comparisons in Australia, Denmark, and New Zealand. We have found that, although the patient selection criteria vary among these countries (in New Zealand, for example, elderly patients and those suffering from chronic diseases are not admitted to ICUs with the same frequency as in the United States), the APACHE II approach to risk stratification appears to work well. Using this system along with information on the patients' disease and major organ system involvement, we were able to compare and contrast the performance of intensive care in these countries (Zimmerman et al., 1988). Using the experience from these studies, we believe we are close to being able to apply these predictive techniques to intensive care units worldwide. Such comparisons would not only help us to determine how important are variations in the coordination of ICU staffs, they could also lead to improvements in our basic understanding of how various patient and medical care factors influence outcome from a severe illness. Until now, isolating various aspects of care has been difficult since so much of the variation in patient outcome has been unaccounted for by traditional methods of prediction or prognostic stratification. Using a combination of disease description and APACHE II scoring, however, it is possible to reduce variation from patient factors so that the influence of other variables may be more apparent.

To accomplish outcome predictions for individual patients, we must first recognize that the factors determining outcome for groups of patients and for individual patients are identical. Scientifically, there is no distinction between the objectives of group versus individual prediction, but there are the possible implications of the findings and the current state of our predictive science. When we speak about individuals, the precision of our predictions must be great and the confidence we have in these estimates must be high. There are two ways to increase confidence: by improving our predictive techniques and by increasing the number of patients studied.

At our current level of understanding, prognostic estimates based on information available prior to treatment enable us to confidently estimate risk in only limited groups of patients regardless of the number studied. We are therefore frequently obligated to treat many patients to determine their response to therapy. Once we have this additional information, however, our estimates of outcome become more accurate.

This is illustrated by the results displayed in Figure 4, where third day APS scores are directly correlated with ARF hospital mortality rates. Evaluating response to treatment using such reproducible physiologic measures is very useful in evaluating an individual patient's ability to respond to future treatment, including mechanical ventilation (Knaus, 1989). This suggests that when physicians are making decisions to limit or reduce therapy for patients who do not respond to therapy, the estimates provided here may represent useful information (McLean et al., 1985). We caution, however, that the prognostic estimates provided in this study are not based on a sufficient number of ARF patients to apply them immediately at the bedside (Hanley and Lippman-Hand, 1983). The trends observed, however, are compatible with previous studies (McLean et al., 1985; Bion et al., 1985), and since the methods used to identify survivors versus nonsurvivors are based on general clinical and physiologic principles, they could be applied to additional ARF patients.

V. Summary

We present a model for relating readily available clinical and physiologic measurements to prognosis from intensive care for acutely ill hospitalized patients in general and for acute respiratory failure patients in particular. Using data from 5815 general intensive care admissions to 13 hospitals, with 224 meeting criteria for acute respiratory failure, this study illustrates the direct relationships among the disease initiating respiratory failure, the acute severity of that disease, and a patient's age and chronic health status to their risk of dying during hospitalization.

The results indicate that all these factors, but especially the severity of disease on the third day of respiratory failure, are very closely related to the patient's subsequent risk of death. Also important in determining outcome were the patient's age, whether they had pre-existing chronic disease, and the exact nature of their admitting disease.

We contend that the increased use of prognostic techniques, many of which have been incorporated in the APACHE severity of disease classification system, can improve the precision of clinical research and will eventually be helpful in individual patient decision-making.

Acknowledgments

Supported by grants from the National Center for Health Services Research, No. HS04857, and the Robert Wood Johnson Foundation, No. 8498.

References

Bell, R. C., Coalson, J. J., Smith, J. D., and Johanson, W. G. (1983). Multiple organ system failure and infection in adult respiratory distress syndrome. *Ann. Intern. Med.,* **99**:293-298.

Bion, J. F., Edlin, S. A., Ramsay, G., McCabe, S., and Ledingham, I. M. (1985). Validation of a prognostic score in critically ill patients undergoing transport. *Br. Med. J.,* **291**:432-434.

Dellinger, E. P., Wertz, M. J., Meakins, J. L., et al. (1985). Surgical stratification system for intra-abdominal infection. *Arch. Surg.,* **120**:21-29.

Hanley, J. A., and Lippman-Hand, A. (1983). If nothing goes wrong, is everything all right? *JAMA,* **249**(13):1743-1745.

Knaus, W. A. (1989). Prognosis with mechanical ventilation: The influence of disease severity of disease, age, and chronic health status on survival from acute illness. *Am. Rev. Respir. Dis.,* **140**:S8-S13.

Knaus, W. A., Zimmerman, J. E., Wagner, D. P., Draper, E. A., and Lawrence, D. (1981). APACHE—acute physiology and chronic health evaluation: A physiologically based classification system. *Crit. Care Med.,* **9**:591-597.

Knaus, W. A., LeGall, J. R., Wagner, D. P., et al. (1982). A comparison of intensive care in the U.S.A. and France. *Lancet,* **2**:642-646.

Knaus, W. A., Wagner, D. P., and Draper, E. A. (1984). The value of measuring severity of disease in clinical research on acutely ill patients. *J. Chron. Dis.,* **37**:455-463.

Knaus, W. A., Draper, E. A., Wagner, D. P., and Zimmerman, J. E. (1985a). APACHE II: A severity of disease classification system. *Crit. Care Med.,* **13**:818-829.

Knaus, W. A., Draper, E. A., Wagner, D. P., and Zimmerman, J. E. (1985b). Prognosis in acute organ-system failure. *Ann. Surg.,* **202**:685-692.

Knaus, W. A., Draper, E. A., Wagner, D. P., and Zimmerman, J. E. (1986). Evaluation of outcome from intensive care in major medical centers. *Ann. Intern. Med.,* **104**:410-418.

McLean, R. F., McIntosh, J. D., Kung, G. Y., et al. (1985). Outcome of respiratory intensive care for the elderly. *Crit. Care Med.,* **13**(8):625-629.

Montgomery, A. B., Stager, M. A., Carrico, C. T., and Hudson, L. D. (1985). Causes of mortality in patients with the adult respiratory distress syndrome. *Am. Rev. Respir. Dis.,* **132**:485-489.

Smadja, C., and Bismuth, H. (1984). Pancreatites aigues necrotiques: Pour une restriction des indications operatures. *Gastroenterol. Clin. Biol.,* **8**:536-540.

Wagner, D. P., Draper, E. A., Campos, R. A., et al. (1985). Initial International use of APACHE: An acute severity of disease measure. *Med. Decision Making,* **4**(3):297-313.

Zimmerman, J. E., Knaus, W. A., Judson, J. A., Havill, J. H., Trubovich, R. V., Draper, E. A., and Wagner, D. P. (1988). Patient selection for intensive care: A comparison of New Zealand and United States hospitals. *Crit. Care Med.,* **16**:318-326.

7

Measurement of Respiratory Elastance and Resistance in Mechanically Ventilated Patients

ANNE M. LORINO and ALAIN HARF

Hôpital Henri Mondor
Créteil, France

I. Introduction

For diagnostic purposes, techniques to measure pulmonary mechanics in spontaneously breathing subjects have been used for a long time in lung function laboratories. These techniques cannot be directly applied to mechanically ventilated patients, and it is only in later years that appropriate methods were developed to investigate respiratory mechanics in such patients. However, if one examines the recent publications, these methods appear to be used in research rather than for clinical management, probably because most of these measurements require long or tedious calculations, which makes them difficult for routine use. Therefore, until now, clinical studies of respiratory mechanics in mechanically ventilated patients with acute respiratory failure have not been widely adopted (Rossi et al., 1985a,b; Bernasconi et al., 1988).

In an intensive care unit, the clinician needs simple and rapid methods to assess respiratory mechanics. For a long time, the maximal inspiratory pressure value displayed on the ventilator has been considered the primary index of the mechanical state of the respiratory system; however, this lumped index does not allow distinction between elastic and resistive parameters.

During the past few years, improved ventilators have provided respiratory elastance and resistance estimates that must, nevertheless, be carefully interpreted. Indeed, the presence of the endotracheal tube, possibly of an intrinsic positive end-expiratory pressure ($PEEP_i$), as well as gas compression in the ventilator tubing when pressure is measured far from the patient, can all lead to inaccuracy in measurements of respiratory mechanics. As a result of the increasing availability of microcomputers, improved methods can be expected to be developed, aiming to provide more accurate on-line assessment of respiratory mechanics.

Respiratory mechanics monitoring in patients with acute respiratory failure would be of great interest clinically to assess the status and progression of lung disease. As emphasized by Bernasconi et al. (1988), routine measurement of respiratory mechanics would allow the clinician to evaluate the efficiency of therapy (e.g., aspiration of bronchial secretions and bronchodilators) and to quantify the degree of inhomogeneity within the lung that plays such an important role in impairing gas exchange in critically ill patients. Furthermore, monitoring of respiratory mechanics could help define the optimal pattern of mechanical ventilation or in carrying out pharmacologic studies.

Each of the many methods proposed to analyze respiratory mechanics in mechanically ventilated patients is based upon an analysis of the relationship between airway pressure, flow, and volume signals, using a rudimentary representation of the respiratory system with a mechanical model. In other words, the interpretation of the parameters derived from each method depends on the model used. Therefore, before reviewing the methods of measuring respiratory mechanics, we will provide a brief preliminary description of the most commonly employed mechanical models. In a general way, despite its complex mechanical behavior, the respiratory system is usually represented by either a single-compartment or a two-compartment model. Each compartment is composed of an elastic element associated with a resistive element, and each element is characterized by a constant elastance or resistance. The mechanical behavior of the respiratory system is then described by the stress-strain equation of the model, wherein stress is the pressure applied P and strain is the corresponding deformation V. In mechanically ventilated patients, P refers to tracheal pressure (with reference to ambient pressure) and V the volume displacement from the resting lung volume, that is, from the elastic equilibrium point corresponding to zero applied pressure. In many cases, the analysis of the respiratory response to a typical strain input (a ramp of applied volume) or stress input (a step of applied pressure) simplifies the measurement of respiratory mechanics. The use of these respiratory responses to assess respiratory elastance and resistance has recently become widespread owing to the recent mechanical improvements in ventilators that allow the simple generation of such inputs at the bedside.

II. Respiratory Models

The mechanical models described below are constant-parameter linear models. They do not include pure viscoelastic components and therefore do not provide a description of the surface tension-induced viscoelastic behavior of the respiratory system. Such "purely viscoelastic" models will be considered later. In a general way, any respiratory model can be represented either by its anatomic configuration (anatomic model) or its mechanical configuration (rheologic model). Although leading to the same equations, these two representations differ in that, in the anatomic configuration, the elements associated in series are subjected to the same strain and those in parallel to the same stress; in the rheologic model the opposite occurs. Therefore a series association of two elements (or components) in the anatomic model corresponds to a parallel association in the rheologic model, and vice versa.

In the following stress-strain equations, $\dot{V}$ and $\dot{P}$ are the first time derivatives of V and P and $\ddot{V}$ is the second time derivative of V.

A. Homogeneous Respiratory Model

The homogeneous respiratory model is the simplest and consists of a single-compartment model (Fig. 1a) corresponding to the rheologic Kelvin model (Fig. 1b).

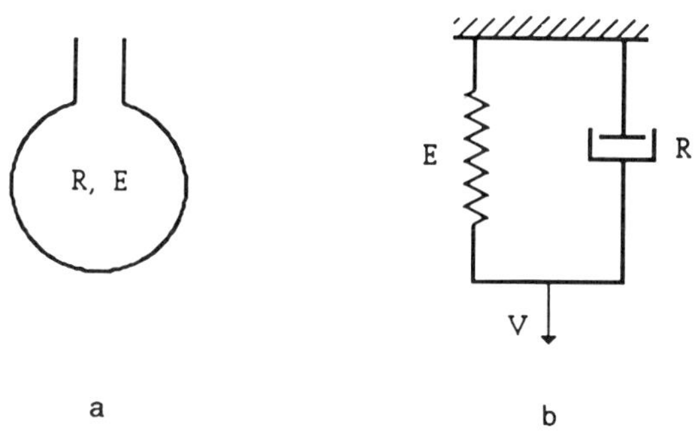

Figure 1 Homogeneous respiratory model composed of a single compartment featuring elastance E and resistance R: (a) anatomic representation and (b) rheologic representation.

Equation of Motion

Total pressure P is the sum of the elastic pressure EV, and the resistive pressure $R\dot{V}$, respectively, derived from each element of the model. Hence,

$$P = EV + R\dot{V} \tag{1}$$

Response to a Ramp of Applied Volume

In response to a ramp of applied volume V = at, that is, in response to a step of flow, $\dot{V}$ = a applied at zero time, P can be expressed as

$$P = Eat + Ra \tag{2}$$

As illustrated in Figure 2a, when t = 0, P exhibits a sudden change equal to the resistive pressure Ra, and then becomes a linear function of time with a slope equal to Ea.

Response to a Step-Applied Pressure

When a step of pressure P = b is applied at zero time, one can express V as

$$V = \frac{b}{E}(1 - e^{-Et/R}) \tag{3}$$

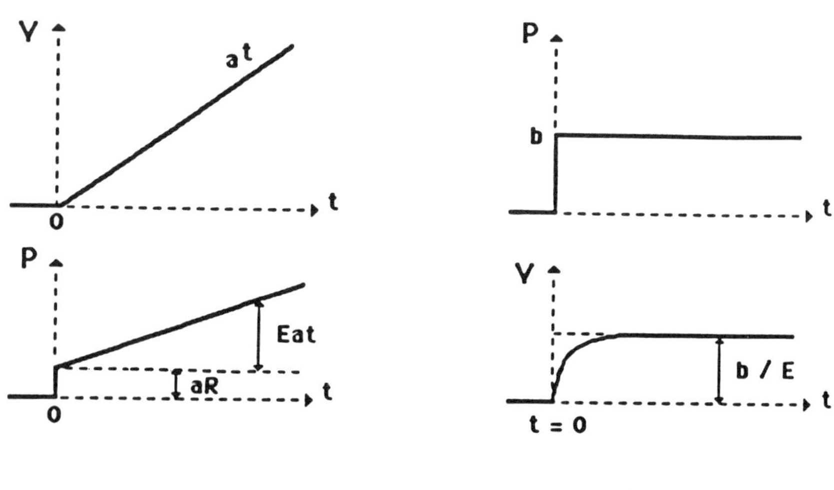

Figure 2 Response of the homogeneous respiratory model to (a) a ramp of applied volume and (b) a step of applied pressure.

Initially, V varies in an exponential manner. Ultimately, the exponential term becomes negligible and P reduces to the constant b/E (Fig. 2b).

B. Homogeneous Thoracopulmonary Model

This model (Fig. 3a) can be easily derived from the preceding one. It is composed of two compartments with pulmonary and chest wall compartments. Both compartments are characterized by their elastance (E_L and E_W, respectively) and their resistance (R_L and R_W, respectively). Figure 3b shows that the behavior of this model is described by the same equations as the homogeneous respiratory model we discussed previously, with $E = E_L + E_W$ and $R = R_L + R_W$.

This model allows the partitioning of the respiratory system into separate lung and chest wall components by measuring pleural (or esophageal) pressure P_{PL}, thereby giving

$$P - P_{PL} = E_L V + R_L \dot{V}$$

$$P_{PL} = E_W V + R_W \dot{V}$$

It should be noted that the last equation applies only to completely relaxed subjects, that is, without activity of their respiratory muscles.

For each compartment, the equation of motion, as well as the response to a ramp of applied volume or a step-applied pressure, is similar to equations obtained for the homogeneous respiratory model.

C. Inhomogeneous Respiratory Model

This model (Fig. 4a) was first proposed by Otis et al. (1956) to describe pulmonary inhomogeneities that can occur in disease and have been recently

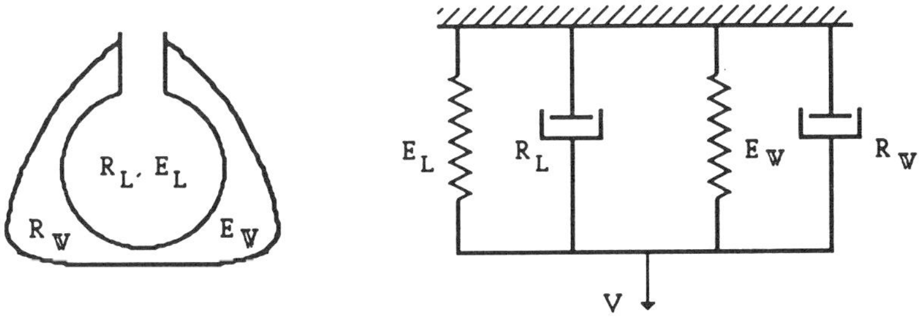

a b

Figure 3 Homogeneous thoracopulmonary model composed of lung (E_L and R_L) and chest wall (E_W and R_W) compartments: (a) anatomic representation and (b) rheologic representation.

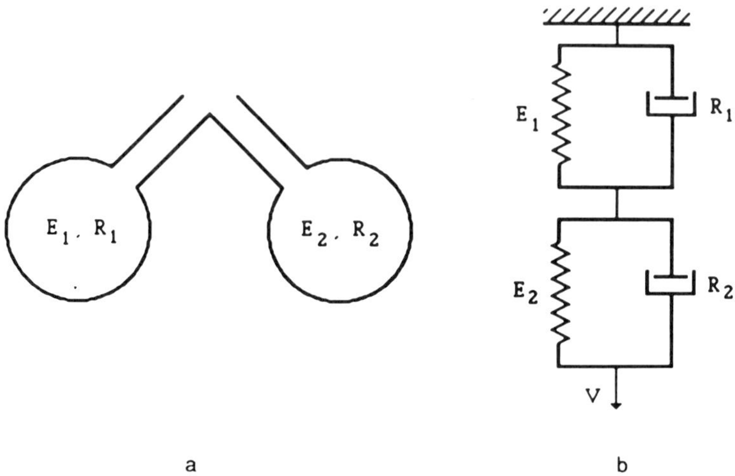

Figure 4 Inhomogeneous respiratory model consisting of two single-compartment models: (a) anatomic representation and (b) rheologic representation.

demonstrated to occur in the adult respiratory distress syndrome (ARDS) (Bernasconi et al., 1988). It consists of two Kelvin models in series (Fig. 4b). Each compartment is characterized by its elastance (E_1 and E_2, respectively) and its resistance (R_1 and R_2, respectively) values.

Equation of Motion

As shown in Figure 4b, the two compartments are subjected to the same stress and the total strain is the sum of that of each compartment. Then, assuming that $(E_2R_1 - E_1R_2)$ is not zero,

$$(E_1 + E_2)P + (R_1 + R_2)\dot{P} = E_1E_2V + (E_2R_1 + E_1R_2)\dot{V} + R_1R_2\ddot{V} \quad (4)$$

Please note that if $E_2R_1 - E_1 R_2$ equals zero, that is, if both compartments are characterized by the same time constant, the equation of motion will reduce to

$$P = \frac{E_1R_2}{R_1 + R_2}V + \frac{R_1R_2}{R_1 + R_2}\dot{V} \quad (5)$$

which is the equation of motion of a homogeneous respiratory model. Therefore, in the following, it is assumed that $E_2R_1 \neq E_1R_2$.

Response to a Ramp of Applied Volume

The response to a ramp of applied volume (V = at) applied at zero time can be obtained by solving the differential equation of motion (4):

$$P = \frac{atE_1E_2}{E_1 + E_2} + a\frac{R_1E_2^2 + R_2E_1^2}{(E_1 + E_2)^2}\left[1 - e^{-t(E_1 + E_2)/(R_1 + R_2)}\right] + a\frac{R_1R_2}{R_1 + R_2}e^{-(E_1 + E_2)t/(R_1 + R_2)} \tag{6}$$

As illustrated by Figure 5a, at time t = 0, when the flow step is applied, P displays a discontinuity corresponding to the resistive pressure generated by the pure resistance:

$$R_{min} = \frac{R_1R_2}{R_1 + R_2} \tag{7}$$

Indeed, R_{min} can be considered the resistance equivalent of the two resistances R_1 and R_2, coupled either in parallel (anatomic model), or in series (rheologic model).

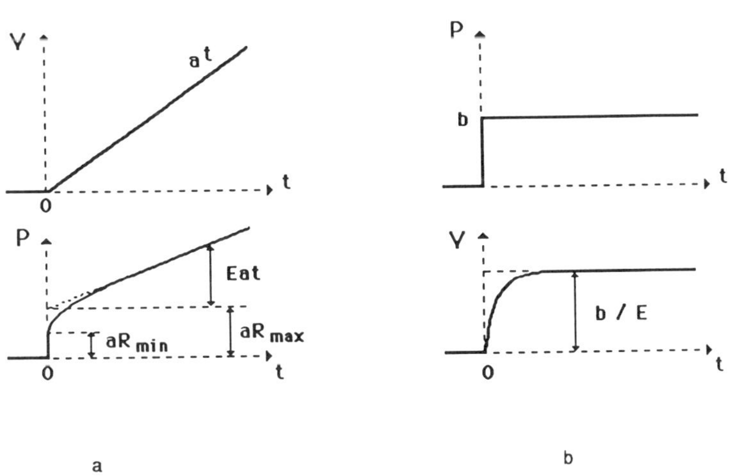

Figure 5 Response of the inhomogeneous respiratory model to (a) a ramp of applied volume and (b) a step of applied pressure. For further explanation, see text.

P varies in an exponential manner, with a time constant equal to $(R_1 + R_2)/(E_1 + E_2)$. Ultimately, when the exponential term becomes negligible, P can be expressed as

$$P = Eat + R_{max}a \tag{8}$$

where $E = E_1E_2/(E_1 + E_2)$ and

$$R_{max} = \frac{R_1E_2^2 + R_2E_1^2}{(E_1 + E_2)^2} \tag{9}$$

Equation (8) demonstrates that, in response to a ramp of applied volume, the inhomogeneous respiratory model behaves like a homogeneous one when a steady state has been reached.

It should be emphasized that the presence of two types of resistance, R_{min} (pure resistance) and R_{max}, which involves pendelluft effects, is due to the presence of inhomogeneities, that is, to the presence of two compartments with unequal time constants, R_1/E_1 and R_2/E_2. In contrast to R_{min}, which can be assessed from the sudden change in pressure occuring after any flow discontinuity, measuring R_{max} requires steady-state conditions, which can only be obtained under constant flow conditions. Furthermore, R_{min} [Eq. 7] does not solely represent airway resistance, since R_1 and R_2, which are the lumped resistances of each of the compartments, include the resistances of all the anatomic structures, that is, airway, lung, and chest wall.

It should also be noted that the mechanical parameters that characterize the inhomogeneous respiratory model (E_1, E_2, R_1, and R_2) cannot be individually determined from the respiratory response to a ramp of applied volume, as was the case for the E and R parameters of the homogeneous model. Only lumped parameters (E, R_{min}, and R_{max}) can be assessed. In a similar manner to our model, a more general inhomogeneous model, consisting of N series Kelvin elements, could be adopted to describe respiratory system behavior (Otis et al., 1956). However, like the two-compartment model, it cannot be characterized completely using a ramp of applied volume: only three lumped parameters can be measured, that is, the equivalent elastance, the instantaneous equivalent resistance, and the resistance involving pendelluft effects.

Response to a Step-Applied Pressure

When a step of pressure P = b is applied at zero time, V can be derived from Equation (4) and expressed as

$$V = \frac{b}{E_1}(1 - e^{-E_1t/R_1}) + \frac{b}{E_2}(1 - e^{-E_2t/R_2}) \tag{10}$$

In response to a step of pressure, V varies as the sum of two exponential terms (Fig. 5b). After a long time, the two exponential terms will have decayed, and P reduces to the constant b/E, wherein $E = E_1E_2/(E_1 + E_2)$. The inhomogeneous respiratory model then behaves like the homogeneous one. Note that both the initial and the steady-state responses to a step-applied pressure are less informative than the response to a ramp of applied volume.

D. Inhomogeneous Thoracopulmonary Model

In the same way as for the homogeneous respiratory model, a thoracopulmonary model can be derived from the inhomogeneous model. One may assume that the chest wall, which is homogeneous, can be represented by a single compartment, whereas the pulmonary model is a two-compartment one (Fig. 6). With such a model, the equation of motion of the pulmonary system can be derived from that of the inhomogeneous respiratory model by replacing P by $P - P_{PL}$ in Equation (4).

In common practice, respiratory mechanics, rather than pulmonary mechanics, are usually assessed because measuring tracheal pressure is far easier than measuring transpulmonary pressure and changes in respiratory mechanics are assumed to represent changes in pulmonary mechanics.

III. Methods for Measuring Respiratory Mechanics

Precautions need to be taken before applying the above-mentioned models of the respiratory system to mechanically ventilated patients. Indeed, in these

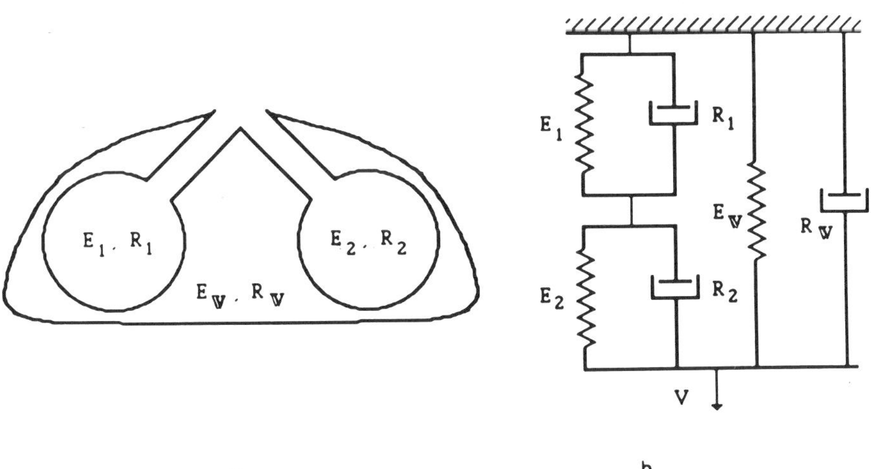

Figure 6 Inhomogeneous thoracopulmonary model consisting of an inhomogeneous pulmonary model associated with a homogeneous thoracic model: (a) anatomic representation and (b) rheologic model.

patients, the presence of an endotracheal tube, as well as the precise conditions of ventilation (e.g., external positive end-expiratory pressure, PEEP, and/or intrinsic positive end-expiratory pressure, $PEEP_i$) need to be taken into account in the equations. In this connection it must be noted that ARDS patients are often mechanically ventilated with PEEP, and that, although low, the $PEEP_i$ values encountered in these patients cannot be disregarded (Bernasconi et al., 1988).

In the prior equations, the deformation was defined as the volume displacement from the resting lung volume corresponding to zero pressure. In the presence of PEEP (external or intrinsic PEEP), the deformation is measured as the volume displacement from a new lung volume level V_0, which corresponds to that PEEP level. Therefore the value of PEEP, that is, the elastic pressure corresponding to the volume V_0, should be subtracted from the measured pressure P (Rossi et al., 1985a). The stable PEEP value is obtained as the static pressure measured at the "endotracheal tube opening" after occluding the expiratory circuit at end-expiratory lung volume.

In mechanically ventilated patients, pressure is generally measured at the proximal extremity of the endotracheal tube and therefore takes into account the resistive pressure drop in the endotracheal tube. The flow resistance of the endotracheal tube R_T has been demonstrated to be flow dependent and is usually represented by Rohrer's equation ($R_T = K_1 + K_2|\dot{V}|$), which is a linear function of flow (Rohrer, 1916). The corresponding resistive pressure $R_T\dot{V}$ can therefore be subtracted from the measured pressure to obtain the actual tracheal pressure, after preliminary determination of K_1 and K_2 in the course of constant flow experiments conducted in isolated tubes (Sullivan et al., 1976). However, since the K_2 value has been reported to differ in isolated tubes and intubated patients (Loring et al., 1979; Chang and Mortola, 1981), direct measurement of tracheal pressure at the distal extremity of the endotracheal tube may be preferable. It must be noted, however, that the frequency response of the endotracheal catheter induces errors in measurement of the pressure signal when rapid changes in airway pressure occur. For example, the assessment of the R_{min} value derived from a sudden change in pressure following a step-applied flow [Eq. (6)] will become uncertain. One method assesses respiratory mechanics directly from pressure measurement at the endotracheal tube opening: the single-breath method, which determines K_2 in situ and requires only the predetermination of K_1.

After pressure has been adequately corrected, we will require a method for determining the respiratory parameters, which need to be suitable for the mechanical model we will use. There are two general methods for measuring respiratory mechanics in mechanically ventilated patients: methods that use the P, $\dot{V}$, and V signals directly derived from mechanical ventilation, and the forced oscillation technique, which requires a strain generator in addition to the ventilator. The main methods, described below, are not presented in chronologic order.

In what follows, respiratory elastance and resistance are respectively referred to as E_{rs} and R_{rs}.

A. Zero Flow and Isovolume Methods

These methods, which are the oldest, are derived from the stress-strain equation of the homogeneous respiratory model [Eq. (1)].

Zero Flow Method

The zero flow method proposed by Von Neergaard and Wirz (1927) measures dynamic elastance by dividing the pressure change between points of zero flow by the tidal volume. After dynamic elastance has been determined, respiratory resistance can be calculated at any given flow as follows: subtraction of elastic pressure from tracheal pressure provides resistive pressure, which is then divided by the corresponding flow to obtain respiratory resistance.

Difficulties in assessing respiratory system elasticity by this method may arise for several reasons. Compared to static elastance, which reflects only the elastic properties of the respiratory system, dynamic elastance takes into account respiratory system inertia (Dosman et al., 1975), as well as possible pendelluft effects due to unequal time constants within the lungs (Otis et al., 1956) and pulmonary stress relaxation induced by surface tension (Mead et al., 1957; Horie and Hildebrandt, 1971). Furthermore, measuring dynamic elastance from only two points of the ventilatory cycle may be very inaccurate if pressure change is rapid near the points of maximal and minimal volume (Marshall, 1965).

Isovolume Method

The isovolume method (Marshall, 1965) evaluates total resistive pressure as the pressure difference measured at two isovolume points, during inspiration and expiration, respectively. This method is based upon two questionable assumptions that dynamic respiratory elastance as well as respiratory flow resistance are the same at an equal lung volume during the inspiratory and expiratory phases.

The zero flow and isovolume methods are based on the assumption that the respiratory system behaves like a homogeneous one-compartment model. Because these methods do not allow the validity of such an assumption to be verified, they may provide erroneous measurements of respiratory mechanics.

B. Constant Inspiratory Flow and Occlusion Methods

These two methods, which both measure inspiratory parameters by analyzing the behavior of the respiratory system at constant inspiratory flow, are presented together. The constant inspiratory flow method can be used with most modern ventilators, which are constant flow generators, in contrast to the occlusion method, which requires ventilators to be supplied with a system allowing occasional closure of the inspiratory and expiratory circuits.

Constant Inspiratory Flow Method

The constant inspiratory flow method was derived by Zin et al. (1983) from the pulse method introduced by Surratt et al. (1980) for measuring respiratory elastance. This method is based on the pressure response of the respiratory system to a ramp of applied volume, that is, to a flow step. Elastance and resistance are determined over the period of inflation corresponding to the steady-state period, that is, while both tracheal pressure and insufflated volume are linear functions of time [Eq. (8)]. Under such steady-state conditions, the linear relationship between the pressure applied by the ventilator and the changes in lung volume allows computation of static elastance and total resistance of the respiratory system; E_{rs} is then estimated as the slope of the linear relationship and R_{rs} as the ratio of the intercept on the pressure axis (resistive pressure) to the constant inspiratory flow (Fig. 7a).

The constant flow method implies that there are no volume-related changes in elastance or resistance. It can therefore be applied even in the presence of unequal time constants within the lungs, provided that a steady state has been reached. Under these conditions, the measured resistance R_{rs} equals R_{max}. This method, which measures inspiratory elastance and resistance, can easily be applied to respiratory mechanics monitoring in the course of mechanical ventilation.

Occlusion Method

The occlusion method was originally introduced to assess static elastance in spontaneously breathing, relaxed subjects (Röhrer, 1916). It was later adapted to respiratory elastance and resistance measurement (Rattenborg, 1956) in patients mechanically ventilated with constant inspiratory flow ventilators and, more recently, improved by Bates et al. (1985). If the respiratory system is suddenly occluded at the airway opening during a steady-state period of constant flow inflation, flow becomes zero and volume constant. The pressure following occlusion is therefore the response of the respiratory system to a step-applied flow [Eq. (6)]. Assuming that airway occlusion is instantaneous, one may determine R_{min} [Eq. (7)] as the ratio of the initial pres-

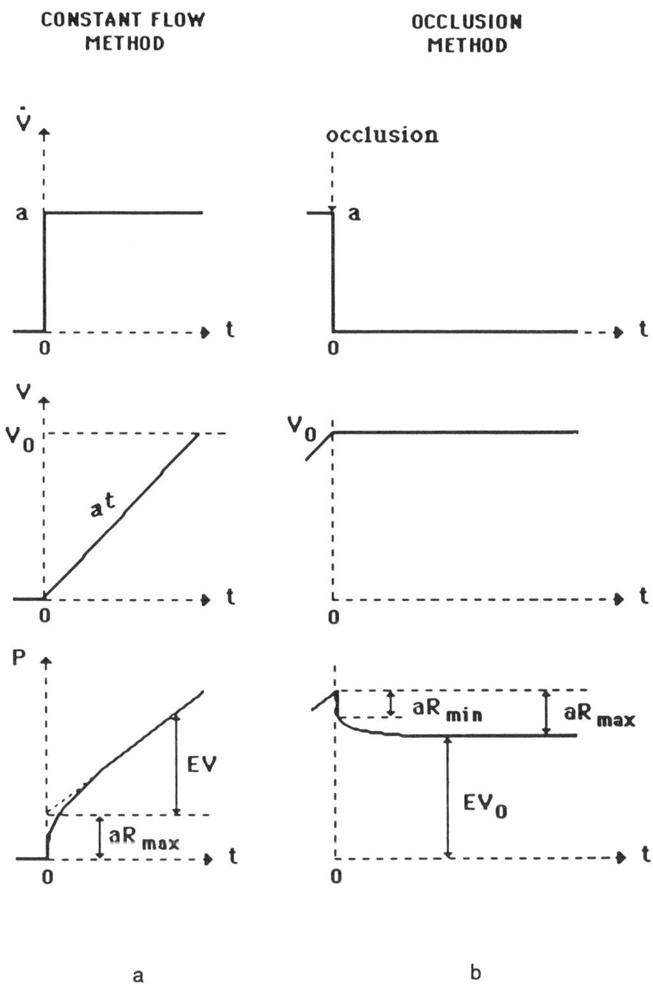

Figure 7 Measurement of respiratory mechanics by (a) the constant inspiratory flow method and (b) the occlusion method. For further explanation, see text.

sure drop immediately following occlusion to the constant preocclusion flow (Fig. 7b). Similarly, when a steady state has been reached, that is, when P has reached a plateau [Eq. (8)], R_{max} can be obtained as the ratio of the total pressure drop to the preocclusion flow and E_{rs} as the ratio of the P plateau value to the insufflated volume (Fig. 7b). This steady state is generally considered achieved within 2 sec following occlusion.

In fact, however, assessment of R_{min} is not so easy. First, measurement of R_{min} relies upon the assumption that a step of flow is applied, that is, that the closure time of the valves can be considered zero. As valves exhibit a finite closure time, R_{min} cannot be readily obtained from the initial pressure drop: during the closure time, V and P are increasing and the pressure signal has to be corrected to obtain the actual value of R_{min} (Bates et al., 1987b). Lastly, valve closure induces oscillations in the pressure signal, which requires appropriate processing of the pressure waveform (Bates et al., 1987a).

Some ventilators now allow automated assessment of total flow resistance, that is, including that of the endotracheal tube, using a technique similar to the occlusion method, provided that a sufficiently long inspiratory pause has been selected: in this case, resistance is obtained as the ratio of the pressure drop during the inspiratory pause to the flow preceding the pause. In such conditions the R_{rs} value, which can be obtained by correcting for endotracheal tube resistance, approximates R_{max} as the inspiratory pause is lengthened.

The occlusion method has recently been used in ARDS patients (Bernasconi et al., 1988). As illustrated by Table 1 (in which respiratory compliance is computed as $C_{rs} = 1/E_{rs}$), these patients exhibit low compliance values, primarily reflecting the loss of ventilated units, and substantially increased R_{max} values that, compared to R_{min} values, demonstrate the presence of time constant inhomogeneities within the lung.

Comparison of Both Methods

The constant flow and the occlusion methods have been compared from theoretical (Bates et al., 1985) and practical (Rossi et al., 1985b) points of view: both methods provide similar values for respiratory elastance and resistance (R_{max}) when tracheal pressure has been corrected for intrinsic PEEP (Rossi et al., 1985a) and when recruitment of new lung units is not present in the early portion of inflation (Rossi et al., 1985b). Indeed, both $PEEP_i$ and lung unit recruitment result in an increased elastic pressure measured by the occlusion method and in an increased resistive pressure measured by the constant flow method, but in contrast to $PEEP_i$, recruitment pressure cannot be assessed.

It should be stressed that both the constant flow and the occlusion methods are based on the response of the respiratory system to step-applied flows of similar amplitude **a**: indeed, $\dot{V}$ rises from zero to **a** for the constant flow method and drops from **a** to zero for the occlusion method. Both methods should therefore be expected to provide similar results (Fig. 7a). Furthermore, if a perfect constant flow ventilator existed (i.e., a ventilator providing a constant flow as soon as the inspiratory phase begins), the constant

Table 1 Respiratory Compliance and Resistance Measured at End-Inspiration[a]

	No.	$PEEP_i$ (cmH_2O)	$C_{st, rs}$ (liter/cmH_2O)	$R_{rs, max}$ (cmH_2O/liter/sec)	$R_{rs, min}$ (cmH_2O/liter/sec)
Group I, COPD	11	5.1 ± 3.2	0.045 ± 0.013	15.8 ± 6.3	8.1 ± 4.3
Group II, ARDS	8	1.3 ± 0.2	0.033 ± 0.007	9.0 ± 4.6	3.7 ± 1.7
Group III, others	10	2.7 ± 1.2	0.044 ± 0.020	7.0 ± 3.3	3.5 ± 2.9

[a]Definition of abbreviations: $PEEP_i$ = "intrinsic" positive end-expiratory pressure; $C_{st, rs}$ = static respiratory compliance; $R_{rs, max}$ and $R_{rs, min}$ = intrinsic maximum and minimum respiratory resistance. Values are mean ± SD. Note that values of $C_{st, rs}$ have been corrected for $PEEP_i$. Mean values of $PEEP_i$ come from three ARDS patients and four patients in Group III.

Adapted from: Bernasconi et al., 1988.

flow method would also allow determination of R_{min}, in the same way as the occlusion method, from the early rise in tracheal pressure following the onset of the inspiratory phase.

The main advantage of the occlusion method for an inhomogeneous respiratory model lies in the determination of two resistances, whose difference, R_{max} - R_{min}, is characteristic of the pendelluft effects due to the inhomogeneities within the lung. It must be remembered however, that if the two compartments to be considered are characterized by similar time constants, that is, when $R_1/E_1 = R_2/E_2$, then the two-compartment model behaves like a one-compartment model [Eq. (5)]. It follows that the notions of R_{min} and R_{max} disappear ($R_{min} = R_{max}$) and the constant flow and occlusion methods are totally equivalent.

C. Single-Breath Method

This method for assessing expiratory respiratory mechanics relies on the response of a homogeneous respiratory model to a stepwise pressure drop [Eq. (3)] performed at end-inflation and to the corresponding V-$\dot{V}$ linear relationship observed for decreasing flows. Two types of analysis of expiratory V-$\dot{V}$ curves have been proposed.

The first, drawn from Brody's observations (1954), was introduced by McIlroy et al. (1963). in conscious relaxed subjects and studied in anesthetized humans by Bergman and Waltemath (1974). It is based upon a comparison of the exponential time constants of Equation (3) obtained in normal conditions and with an added linear external resistance; this method therefore requires several successive passive expirations.

A second type of analysis was introduced by Comroe et al. (1954) and subsequently adapted by Behrakis et al. (1983) to examine the nonlinear V-$\dot{V}$ relationship observed in intubated patients during relaxed expiration: in such patients, the expiratory driving pressure, that is, the elastic recoil pressure, overcomes the nonlinear total resistance of the respiratory system including the endotracheal tube. At the end of the inspiratory phase, airway occlusion is performed, and within 1 or 2 sec, a stable value for tracheal pressure is obtained (Fig. 8a). Immediately afterward, the occlusion is suddenly released, and one may therefore consider that the respiratory system is submitted to a step-applied pressure [Eq. (3)]. During the relaxed expiration that follows, the flow-volume curve is recorded (Fig. 8b). Static respiratory elastance is obtained, as with the occlusion method, by dividing the stable value of tracheal pressure, referenced to the end-expiratory pressure preceding the occlusion, by the insufflated volume V_T. During this relaxed expiration, elastic recoil pressure P_{el}, estimated as $E_{rs}V$, represents the pressure

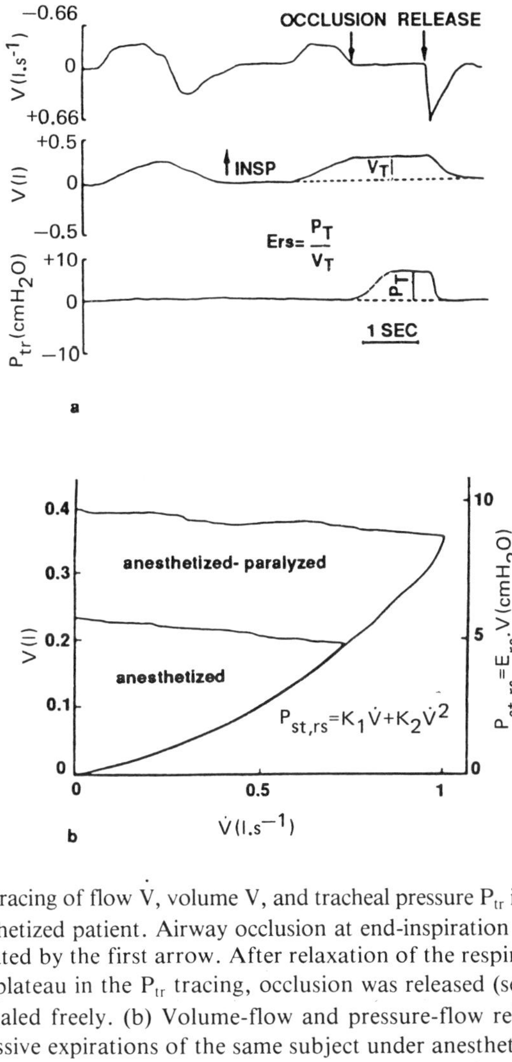

Figure 8 (a) Tracing of flow $\dot{V}$, volume V, and tracheal pressure P_{tr} in a spontaneously breathing anesthetized patient. Airway occlusion at end-inspiration was performed at the point indicated by the first arrow. After relaxation of the respiratory muscles indicated by the plateau in the P_{tr} tracing, occlusion was released (second arrow) and the subject exhaled freely. (b) Volume-flow and pressure-flow relationships corresponding to passive expirations of the same subject under anesthetized and anesthetized-paralyzed conditions. $P_{st,rs}$, elastic recoil pressure. (Reproduced with permission from Behrakis et al., 1983.)

available to overcome the expiratory flow resistance of the total respiratory system (endotracheal tube included), verifying the following equation:

$$P_{el} = (R_{rs} + K_1)\dot{V} + K_2|\dot{V}|\dot{V} \qquad (11)$$

The absence of any inertial term in Equation (11) proves that the respiratory system is represented by the homogeneous respiratory model. Under such conditions, $P_{el}/\dot{V}$ is a linear function of flow, with an intercept equal to $R_{rs} + K_1$ and a slope equal to K_2.

This method, which requires interruption of mechanical ventilation and complete relaxation of respiratory muscles during both occlusion and expiration, appears unsuitable for monitoring respiratory mechanics. Its main advantage is that no assumption of K_2 value is required. The method, however, may not allow one to measure respiratory resistance in ARDS patients since both respiratory elastance and resistance are considered constant over the entire tidal volume in the course of the overall relaxed expiration.

A similar method was recently proposed that does not require interruption of the mechanical ventilation (Benhamou et al., 1987). This method measures dynamic elastance by linear regression analysis of P versus V over the entire ventilatory cycle and then computes respiratory resistance by multiple linear regression of resistive pressure ($P - E_{rs}$ V) versus $\dot{V}$ and $|\dot{V}|\dot{V}$ over the expiratory phase corresponding to decreasing flows. It is therefore subject to criticisms similar to those of the single-breath method regarding inconstant values of respiratory parameters.

D. Interrupter Technique

This consists of one or several brief interruptions (about 100 msec) rapidly performed using a pneumatic valve throughout a relaxed expiration (Fig. 9) and therefore allows assessment of expiratory mechanical parameters. Since two differing analyses of the interrupted passive exhalation have been proposed, two interrupter techniques need to be distinguished.

The first interrupter technique, proposed to measure airway resistance during spontaneous breathing by von Neergaard and Wirz (1927), was extended by Vuilleumier (1944) and employed by Otis and Proctor (1948). It does not rely upon any assumption regarding the respiratory system and can therefore apply to either a homogeneous or an inhomogeneous model. This technique assesses only respiratory resistance, which is obtained by dividing the rapid change in tracheal pressure immediately following the interruption by the flow measured just prior to interruption. This method for R_{rs} measurement, which is comparable to the occlusion method for R_{min} assessment, necessitates similar corrections of the pressure signal to accurately evaluate the instantaneous pressure change (Jackson et al., 1974). Originally, the interrupter technique was believed to measure airway resistance, assuming that tracheal and alveolar pressures equilibrate rapidly upon occlusion. Later it was suggested by several authors (Vuilleumier, 1944; Mead and Whittenberger, 1954; Marshall and DuBois, 1956; Cléments et la., 1959; Peslin and

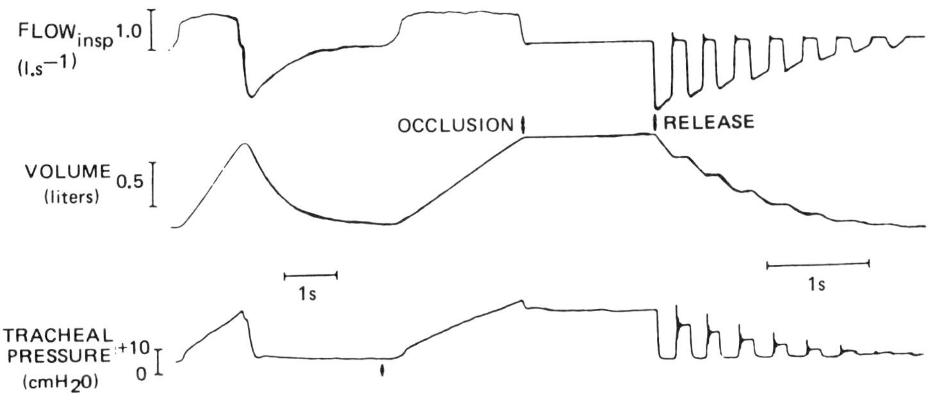

Figure 9 Tracings of flow (top), volume (middle), and tracheal pressure (bottom) in a mechanically ventilated patient. Airway occlusion was performed at end-inspiration (first double arrow) and maintained until a plateau of tracheal pressure occurred. Occlusion was then rapidly released (second double arrow), and a series of interruptions was performed throughout the subsequent passive expiration. During the period of interruption, flow fell promptly to zero and expired volume remained unchanged. After initial oscillations caused by inertial properties, a plateau in tracheal pressure promptly occurred and was consistently observed throughout expiratory interruptions, indicating continued respiratory muscle relaxation. Similarly, the magnitude of flow immediately before and after interruption was not different. (Note change in paper speed indicated by lower arrow.) (Reproduced by permission from Gottfried et al., 1985.)

Andrada, 1967) that this technique measures not only lower airway resistance but also lung tissue and chest wall resistance. Note that, since the occlusion method and this technique measure instantaneous resistances, that is, resistances when pendelluft effects and stress relaxation are excluded, they may be expected to provide similar values for R_{rs} and R_{min}, respectively, when the respiratory system is described by an inhomogeneous respiratory model.

More recently, Gottfried et al. (1985) suggested that another technique of analysis of the pressure signal obtained during an interrupted passive exhalation could assess both respiratory elastance and resistance. Elastance is obtained as the ratio of the end-interruption pressure to the corresponding lung volume, and then elastic pressure P_{el} is analyzed in the same way as with the single-breath method. Indeed, P_{el} is considered the available pressure used, just before the interruption, to overcome the passive expiratory flow resistance of the total respiratory system, including the endotracheal tube [Eq. (11)]. However, since this last relationship is applied only to the expiratory flow immediately preceding the interruption, the nonlinear term of endotracheal tube resistance, K_2, cannot be identified with this analysis, as with the single-breath method. The K_2 parameter must therefore be separately determined. In contrast to the first technique, this second technique, as is the single-breath method, is based upon the assumption of a homogeneous respiratory model and requires complete relaxation of respiratory muscles. One may wonder, however, whether static elastance can be correctly assessed during interruptions far too brief to allow a steady state to be reached, especially in patients with acute respiratory failure (Shephard, 1963) and, consequently, whether respiratory resistance can be derived from the evaluated elastic pressure. Nevertheless, comparative studies of this technique with the single-breath method (Gottfried et al., 1985) showed both methods provide similar resistance values.

It is worth noting that, using any interrupter technique, the accuracy of R_{rs} assessment directly depends on the accuracy in flow measurement. The measurement of flow immediately preceding the interruption is less accurate under dynamic conditions (passive exhalation) than under static conditions (constant flow inflation).

E. Forced Oscillation Technique

Based on the assumption that the total respiratory system behaves linearly, this technique, proposed by DuBois et al. (1956), was widely developed for respiratory mechanics measurement in spontaneously breathing or apneic subjects; its application to ventilated patients remained limited. A random, pseudorandom, or sinusoidal forced flow signal is generated by a special signal generator whose output is amplified and drives loudspeakers. When applied at the airway opening, this forced flow generates a pressure that depends upon respiratory impedance. A Fourier analysis is therefore performed on the pressure and flow signals, and the ratio of the pressure Fourier transform to the flow Fourier transform yields the real and imaginary parts of respiratory impedance Z_{rs} as a function of the frequency f (Fig. 10). The real part of Z_{rs} yields the respiratory resistance, and the imaginary part is equal to the respiratory reactance X_{rs}, which represents both respiratory elastance and inertance ($X_{rs} = 2\pi f I_{rs} - E_{rs}/2\pi f$, where I_{rs} is respiratory inertance). The presence of the inertial term is due to the fact that the inertia of gas, lung, and chest wall can no longer be considered negligible at frequencies higher than 1 Hz. From a theoretical point of view, the extrapolation of the real part of Z_{rs} to zero frequency would equal R_{max} (constant flow); extrapolation to an infinite frequency would equal R_{min} (immediate response to a step-applied flow). Therefore the frequency dependence of the real part of Z_{rs}

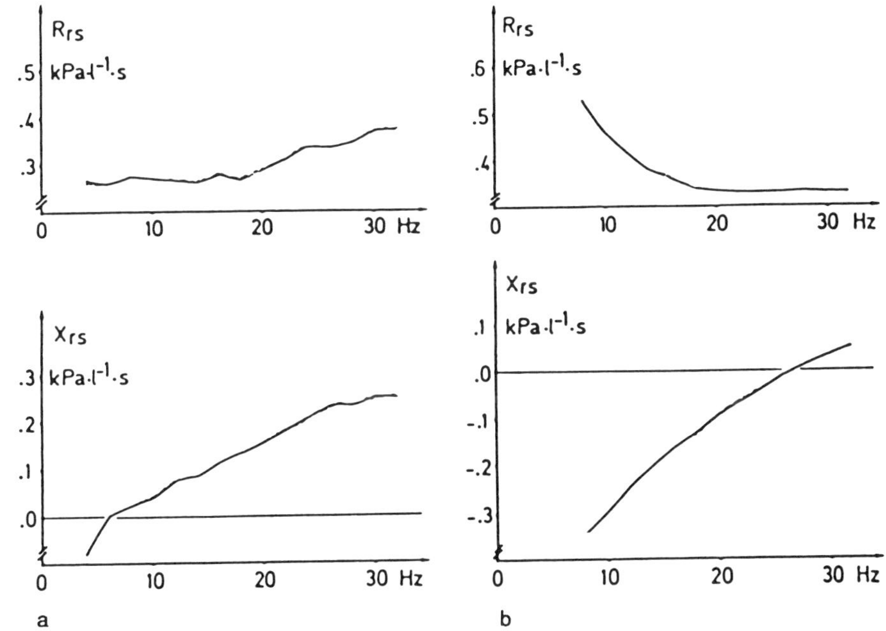

Figure 10 (a) In 10 healthy subjects and (b) in 10 patients with chronic obstructive lung disease, mean values of total respiratory resistance R_{rs} and reactance X_{rs} as a function of frequency. [Adapted with permission from Franken, H., et al., *J. Appl. Physiol.,* **59**:1654-1659 (1985).]

will be marked when the distribution of ventilatory inhomogeneities within the lungs is wide (Grimby et al., 1968; Fredberg and Mead, 1979). When a single frequency is used, respiratory resistance is readily obtained at the input frequency; however, respiratory reactance does not allow computing E_{rs}. Furthermore, when frequencies higher than about 30 Hz are used to explore respiratory system behavior, the simple model characterized by the three lumped parameters (elastance, resistance, and inertance) can no longer be used to describe the frequency dependence of resistance and reactance, which then exhibit maxima and minima.

As the determination of respiratory impedance relies upon the assumption that the respiratory system behaves linearly within the range of forced disturbances, the nonlinear pressure component generated by the flow resistance of the endotracheal tube must be eliminated. If pressure is measured at the endotracheal tube opening, this can be done, provided that measurements are made during a period of apnea by correcting the measured impedance for the apparent series impedance of the endotracheal tube (Tsai et al.,

1977; Fullton et al., 1982). This correction is critical (Delavault et al., 1982). Measurement of tracheal pressure at the distal extremity of the endotracheal tube by means of a retrograde catheter does not allow direct assessment of respiratory impedance: indeed, the measured pressure must be corrected for the transfer function, which includes air compression and heat transfer inside the tube and the kinetic energy losses at the junction between the tube and trachea (Michels et al., 1986; Navajas et al., 1989).

Compared to the other methods described above, the forced oscillation technique is not easily applicable for repeated measurements of respiratory mechanics in mechanically ventilated patients because of the complex apparatus required and the need for time-consuming data processing. Lastly, partitioning of respiratory mechanics into lung and chest wall components requires an appropriate dynamic response of the esophageal balloon at the considered frequencies.

IV. Comparison of the Methods

Several authors have compared respiratory mechanics values obtained by different methods in anesthetized mechanically ventilated patients. Since these comparisons provide an interesting illustration of the theoretical approaches described above, some of them are reported here.

A. Zero Flow, Isovolume, Forced Oscillation, and Passive Exhalation Methods

These four methods were compared by Bergman and Waltemath (1974) in six healthy, anesthetized, and paralyzed artificially ventilated patients. Forced sinusoidal oscillations (amplitude about 50 ml peak to peak and frequency about 3-4 Hz) were applied at a resting end-expiratory lung volume, and data were analyzed according to the method described by Goldman et al. (1970). Measurements were made both with and without an additional external resistance (R = 2.3 cmH_20/liter/sec measured at a flow rate of 0.5 liter/sec). The results obtained for respiratory compliance ($C_{rs} = 1/E_{rs}$) and resistance are summarized in Table 2. Values for R_{rs} were lower when derived from the zero flow or isovolume method, the isovolume method underestimating the value of the additional resistance. As expected, static compliance measured by the passive exhalation method is larger than dynamic compliance measured by the zero flow method.

B. Constant Inspiratory Flow and Occlusion Methods

A comparative study of these two methods has been made by Rossi et al. (1985b) in 11 mechanically ventilated patients with acute respiratory failure,

Table 2 Resistance and Compliance in Anesthetized Subjects[a]

Measurement method	Analytic technique	Compliance (ml BTPS/cmH_2O)		Resistance (cmH_2O/liter/sec)		Measured added resistance
		Control	Added resistance	Control	Added resistance	
Flow-pressure-volume	Neergaard-Wirz	40.9 ± 10.5	40.4 ± 11.3	7.7 ± 1.7	9.9 ± 1.8	2.2 ± 0.8
	Isovolume			6.4 ± 2.0	7.5 ± 2.2	1.1 ± 0.4
Forced oscillation	Forced oscillation			9.0 ± 1.4	11.3 ± 1.9	2.3 ± 0.8
Passive exhalation	Comroe-Nisell-Nims	66.9 ± 14.6	63.8 ± 13.8	10.1 ± 1.9	12.5 ± 2.1	2.4 ± 0.6
	Time constant			10.8 ± 2.2	13.1 ± 2.2	2.3 ± 0.7

[a]Experimental results from six subjects. Values are means ± SD.
Source: From Bergman and Waltemath, 1974.

Table 3 Individual Values of Elastance and Resistance Computed During Inflation and with Occlusion at End-Inspiration[a]

	Inflation		Occlusion		
Subject no.	E_{rs} (cmH_2O/liter)	R_{rs} (cmH_2O/liter/sec)	E_{rs} (cmH_2O/liter)	R_{rs} (cmH_2O/liter/sec)	R_{rs} (min) (cmH_2O/liter/sec)
1	18.7 ± 0.7	4.0 ± 0.8	19.5 ± 1.4	3.5 ± 1.3	2.4 ± 0.5
2	13.1 ± 1.6	5.1 ± 1.5	12.5 ± 1.3	6.0 ± 1.0	2.5 ± 0.8
3	21.0 ± 1.1	4.0 ± 1.6	19.8 ± 0.8	4.5 ± 1.1	1.8 ± 0.7
4	24.3 ± 1.0	12.6 ± 1.7	24.4 ± 0.5	14.9 ± 1.5	4.5 ± 0.9
5	15.4 ± 0.6	10.7 ± 1.3	15.4 ± 0.8	10.7 ± 1.3	6.4 ± 0.7
6	15.4 ± 0.9	6.5 ± 1.7	15.3 ± 0.5	6.5 ± 0.9	2.0 ± 0.4
7	13.1 ± 2.8	13.3 ± 1.6	13.1 ± 1.8	13.9 ± 2.7	9.3 ± 0.8
8	11.7 ± 2.4	34.5 ± 5.3	19.0 ± 1.2	25.7 ± 4.3	15.0 ± 2.2
9	13.2 ± 1.1	8.4 ± 1.6	15.5 ± 0.7	5.5 ± 1.1	3.1 ± 0.6
10	17.2 ± 0.7	9.6 ± 0.8	16.6 ± 0.6	10.4 ± 1.1	6.2 ± 0.4
11	23.9 ± 2.6	18.9 ± 1.9	27.9 ± 1.4	14.6 ± 1.6	7.1 ± 0.7

[a]Values are means ± SD of 10 measurements. E_{rs}, elastance of total respiratory system; R_{rs}, resistance of respiratory system; R_{rs}(min), minimum resistance of respiratory system.
Source: Adapted from Rossi et al., 1985b.

including 1 ARDS (patient 3). All patients were ventilated with PEEP except subjects 8, 9, and 11, who were ventilated with zero end-expiratory pressure (ZEEP). The individual values of elastance and resistance are listed in Table 3. No significant difference was found between the respiratory parameters calculated by both methods in patients on PEEP. However, in patients at ZEEP, a discrepancy was observed and attributed to recruitment of lung units, which is often present at the beginning of inflation in patients with acute respiratory failure.

C. Interrupter and Single-Breath Methods

These two methods were compared by Gottfried et al. (1985) in six patients undergoing general anesthesia for minor surgery. The interrupter method used was that proposed by the authors. The individual values for respiratory elastance and resistance are given in Table 4 and 5, respectively. Results obtained with both methods were not significantly different.

Although providing interesting results, these comparative studies were obtained in healthy subjects whose respiratory system can be represented by a homogeneous model and should not be extended to patients with lung disease. In those patients, different methods based upon the dubious assumption of a homogeneous respiratory system would be expected to provide different results. As a matter of fact, in disease, discrepancies appear between values obtained with the constant flow and occlusion methods (Rossi et al., 1985b).

Table 4 Total Respiratory System Elastance[a]

	Interrupter technique		Single-breath method	
Patient no.	E_{rs} (cmH_2O/liter)	*r*	E_{rs} (cmH_2O/liter)	±SD
1	21.2	0.91	22.9	± 0.7
2	19.8	0.99	18.2	± 1.2
3	21.8	0.99	21.3	± 1.5
4	28.7	0.99	29.4	± 1.0
5	28.0	0.99	31.5	± 1.1
6	33.5	0.98	33.7	± 1.6
Mean ± SD	25.5 ± 5.4		26.2 ± 6.2	

[a]Data obtained from average of eight breaths. Values for interrupter technique obtained by linear regression analysis. Values for single-breath method are means ± SD. E_{rs}, total respiratory system elastance; *r*, correlation coefficient.

Source: Adapted from Gottfried et al., 1985.

Table 5 Total Respiratory System Resistance[a]

	Interrupter technique		Single-breath method	
Patient no.	R_{rs} (cmH_2O/liter/sec)	*r*	R_{rs} (cmH_2O/liter/sec)	*r*
1	1.5	0.95	1.6	0.98
2	1.8	0.99	1.6	0.98
3	1.4	0.99	1.5	0.98
4	3.1	0.99	3.2	0.99
5	2.1	0.95	2.2	0.99
6	1.7	0.95	1.5	0.98
Mean ± SD	1.9 ± 0.6		1.9 ± 0.7	

[a]Data obtained from average of eight breaths. R_{rs}, intrinsic respiratory system resistance; *r*, correlation coefficient.
Adapted from: Gottfried et al., 1985.

V. The Limits of Models and Methods

Accurate assessment of respiratory mechanics depends, above all, upon the adequacy of the model describing the mechanical behavior of the respiratory system and upon the ability of the experimental method to determine the parameters of the model.

A. Respiratory Models

None of the models currently used to describe the mechanical behavior of the respiratory system is satisfactory. Two major criticisms can be formulated, which are presented here.

The Models are Constant Parameter Models

The elastance and resistance parameters that characterize the respiratory models have been taken as constant; that is, an implicit assumption has been made that respiratory elastance and resistance are independent of both deformation and flow rate. This assumption is questionable, especially in ARDS. Indeed, although respiratory parameters have been assumed for a long time, and even verified, to be constant over the volume and flow ranges used for the mechanical ventilation (Rossi et al., 1985b; Gottfried et al., 1985), recent studies conducted in an animal model (Kochi et al., 1988a,b) have proved a volume and flow dependence of pulmonary mechanics. With the forced oscillation technique, in which amplitudes of forced flow and deformation are small, this dependence can be obscured, provided that measurements are made during periods of apnea. With the other methods, taking dependence into account would lead to using nonlinear models with equations of motion that are difficult to solve, even in response to a ramp of applied volume or a step-applied pressure. The advantage of the constant flow and occlusion methods therefore becomes obvious: with these methods, respiratory mechanics can be assessed under precise volume and flow conditions.

The Models Do Not Include Pure Viscoelastic Components

The viscoelasticity of a model may be characterized by the decreased stress (stress relaxation) observed at constant strain, as is the case for the occlusion method. The respiratory system is known to exhibit such behavior (Marshall and Widdicombe, 1960), which can be attributable to the presence of either inhomogeneities (Otis et al., 1956) or pure viscoelastic components, such as pulmonary surfactant (Mead et al., 1957). The stress relaxation induced by inhomogeneities has already been investigated with the occlusion method. Consider now the simplest rheologic viscoelastic model that describes the stress relaxation induced by surface tension in a homogeneous respiratory system (Fig. 11a). Such a model consists of a homogeneous respiratory component (characterized by its own elastance E_1 and resistance R_1), associated with a parallel viscoelastic component (Maxwell model, characterized by its elastance E_2 and its resistance R_2). The equation of motion of this model may be written as

$$E_2P + R_2\dot{P} = E_1E_2V + (E_2R_1 + E_2R_2 + E_1R_2)\dot{V} + R_1R_2\ddot{V} \qquad (12)$$

One may already observe that Equation (12) is roughly comparable to Equation (4). In response to a ramp of applied volume, V = at applied at t = 0, pressure P varies as

$$P = R_1a + R_2a(1 - e^{-E_2t/R_2}) + E_1at \qquad (13)$$

As illustrated by Figure 11b, at time t = 0, P presents a discontinuity corresponding to the resistive pressure generated by the resistance R_1. P then varies in an exponential manner, with a time constant equal to R_2/E_2. Ultimately, the exponential term vanishes, and P can be expressed as

$$P = (R_1 + R_2)a + E_1at \qquad (14)$$

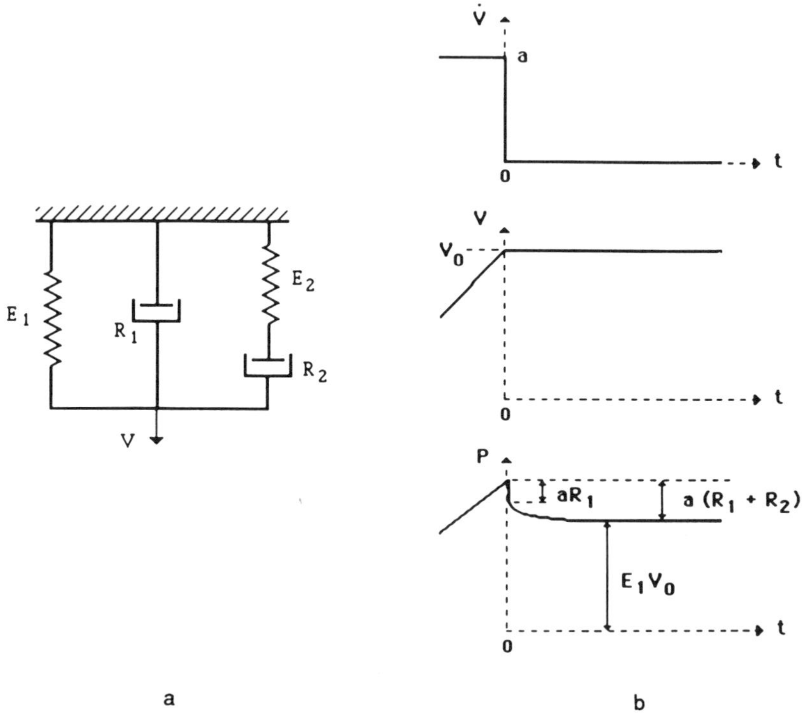

Figure 11 (a) Rheologic representation of a homogeneous respiratory model (E_1, R_1) including a pure viscoelastic component (E_2, R_2). (b) Response of this model to a step of applied flow using the occlusion method. For further explanation, see text.

Comparing Equation (13) to Equation (6) or Figure 11b to Figure 7b, one observes that the response of the homogeneous viscoelastic model of Figure 11a to a step-applied flow is comparable to that of the inhomogeneous model of Figure 4b: similarly, one may define, the "R_{min}" resistance equal to R_1 and the "R_{max}" resistance equal to ($R_1 + R_2$), their difference representing the "viscoelastic resistance" R_2.

Consequently, in the respiratory response to a step-applied flow, the instantaneous resistance R_{min} may be considered to always represent pure respiratory resistance, that is, the resistance in the absence of either inhomogeneities or viscoelastic components. However, the mechanical meaning of R_{max}, depending upon the model selected, appears less clear, and the following question remains unanswered: what does the difference R_{max} -R_{min} actually represent? It is likely that this difference reflects both inhomogeneities within the lung and pure viscoelasticity. To quantify the contribution of each factor, one may represent the respiratory system by a more sophisticated model containing at the same time inhomogeneities and pure viscoelasticity. However, such a representation would only be suitable if each of the parameters of the model could be identified.

B. Methods

Although very sophisticated models can be used to approximate the complex mechanical behavior of the respiratory system, it proves difficult to measure individually the parameters of such models. The major limit to more accurate descriptions of respiratory mechanical behavior using more elaborate models stems from the inability of the methods to measure the key parameters of these models, owing to the few mechanical inputs that can be applied to the respiratory system: only lumped respiratory parameters can be assessed.

VI. Conclusion

It is probably due to methodologic limits that measurements of respiratory mechanics are based on a simplified description of the respiratory system mechanical behavior. Nevertheless, it has become evident that the parameters of such functional descriptions provide useful insights into both the elastic and resistive properties of the respiratory system in mechanically ventilated patients with acute respiratory failure. Among the numerous methods described above, the constant inspiratory flow and the occlusion methods appear most convenient for respiratory mechanics measurement in mechanically ventilated patients. Indeed, both these methods allow simultaneous assessment of respiratory elastance and resistance, do not require special apparatus or interruption of mechanical ventilation, and can apply to whatever respiratory model is chosen. In comparison to the constant flow method, the occlusion method can also quantify the degree of inhomogeneity of time constants within the lung by the difference of R_{max} - R_{min} values, but it must be emphasized that this difference also reflects stress relaxation due to pure viscoelastic components.

Acknowledgments

The authors gratefully acknowledge Dr. Henning Pontopiddan and Dr. Warren Zapol for critical reviewing of the manuscript, and Patrick Muller for helpful advice.

References

Bates, J. H. T., Rossi, A., and Milic-Emili, J. (1985). Analysis of the behavior of the respiratory system with constant inspiratory flow. *J. Appl. Physiol.*, **58**:1840-1848.

Bates, J. H. T., Sly, P. D., and Okubo, S. (1987a). General method for describing and extrapolating monotonic transients and its application to respiratory mechanics. *Med. Biol. Eng. Comput.*, **25**:131-135.

Bates, J. H. T., Hunter, I. W., Sly, P. D., Okubo, S., Filiatrault, S., and Milic-Emili, J. (1987b). Effect of valve closure time on the determination of respiratory resistance by flow interruption. *Med. Biol. Eng. Comput.*, **25**:136-140.

Behrakis, P. K., Higgs, B. D., Baydur, A., Zin, W. A., and Milic-Emili, J. (1983). Respiratory mechanics during halothane anesthesia and anesthesia-paralysis in humans. *J. Appl. Physiol.*, **55**:1085-1092.

Benhamou, D., Lorino, A. M., Lorino, H., Zerah, F., and Harf, A. (1987). Automated measurement of respiratory mechanics in anaesthetized ventilated patients. *Bull. Eur. Physiopathol. Respir.*, **23**:423-428.

Bergman, N. A., and Waltemath, C. L. (1974). A comparison of some methods for measuring total respiratory resistance. *J. Appl. Physiol.*, **36**:131-134.

Bernasconi, M., Ploysongsang, Y., Gottfried, S. B., Milic-Emili, J., and Rossi, A. (1988). Respiratory compliance and resistance in mechanically ventilated patients with acute respiratory failure. *Intensive Care Med.*, **14**: 547-553.

Brody, A. W. (1954). Mechanical compliance and resistance of the lung-thorax calculated from the flow recorded during passive expiration. *Am. J. Physiol.*, **178**:189-196.

Chang, H. K., and Mortola, J. P. (1981). Fluid dynamic factors in tracheal pressure measurement. *J. Appl. Physiol.*, **51**:218-225.

Cléments, J. A., Sharp, J. T., Johnson, R. P., and Elam, J. O. (1959). Estimation of pulmonary resistance by repetitive interruption of airflow. *J. Clin. Invest.*, **38**:1262-1270.

Comroe, J. H., Jr., Nisell, O. I., and Nims, R. G. (1954). A simple method for concurrent measurement of compliance and resistance to breathing in anesthetized animals and man. *J. Appl. Physiol.*, **7**:225-228.

Delavault, E., Saumon, G., and Georges, R. (1982). Nonlinear fluid systems identified by random noise input. *J. Appl. Physiol.*, **53**:1643-1649.

Dosman, J., Bode, J., Antic, R., Martin, R., and Macklem, P. T. (1975). Role of inertia in the measurement of dynamic compliance. *J. Appl. Physiol.*, **38**:64-69.

DuBois, A. B., Brody, A. W., Lewis, D. H., and Burgess, B. F., Jr. (1956). Oscillation mechanics of the lungs and chest wall in man. *J. Appl. Physiol.*, **8**:587-594.

Fredberg, J. J., and Mead, J. (1979). Impedance of intrathoracic airway models during low-frequency periodic flow. *J. Appl. Physiol.*, **47**:347-351.

Fullton, J. M., Hayes, D. A., and Pimmel, R. L. (1982). Pulmonary impedance in dogs measured by forced random noise with a retrograde catheter. *J. Appl. Physiol.*, **52**:725-733.

Goldman, M., Knudson, R. J., Mead, J., Peterson, N., Schwaber, J. R., and Wohl, M. E. (1970). A simplified measurement of respiratory resistance by forced oscillations. *J. Appl. Physiol.*, **28**:113-116.

Gottfried, S. B., Higgs, B. D., Rossi, A., Carli, F., Mengeot, P. M., Calverly, P. M. A., Zocchi, L., and Milic-Emili, J. (1985). Interrupter technique for measurement of respiratory mechanics in anesthetized humans. *J. Appl. Physiol.*, **59**:647-652.

Grimby, G., Takishima, T., Graham, W., Macklem, P., and Mead, J. (1968). Frequency dependence of flow resistance in patients with obstructive lung disease. *J. Clin. Invest.*, **47**:1455-1465.

Horie, T., and Hildebrandt, J. (1971). Dynamic compliance, limit cycles, and static equilibria of excised cat lung. *J. Appl. Physiol.*, **31**:423-430.

Jackson, A. C., Milhorn, H. T., Jr., and Norman, J. R. (1974). A reevaluation of the interrupter technique for airway resistance measurement. *J. Appl. Physiol.*, **36**:264-268.

Kochi, T., Okubo, S., Zin, W. A., and Milic-Emili, J. (1988a). Flow and volume dependence of pulmonary mechanics in anesthetized cats. *J. Appl. Physiol.*, **64**:441-450.

Kochi, T., Okubo, S., Zin, W. A., and Milic-Emili, J. (1988b). Chest wall and respiratory system mechanics in cats: Effects of flow and volume. *J. Appl. Physiol.*, **64**:2636-2646.

Loring, S. H., Eliott, E. A., and Drazen, J. M. (1979). Kinetic energy loss and convective acceleration in respiratory resistance measurements. *Lung*, **156**:33-42.

Marshall, R., and DuBois, A. B. (1956). The measurement of the viscous resistance of the lung tissues in normal man. *Clin. Sci.*, **15**:161-169.

Marshall, R., and Widdicombe, J. G. (1960). Stress relaxation of the human lung. *Clin. Sci.*, **20**:19-31.

Marshall, R. (1965). Objective tests of respiratory mechanics. In *Handbook of Physiology*. Sec. 3, Vol. II. *Respiration*. Fenn, W. O., and Rahn, H., Eds. Washington, D. C., American Physiological Society, Chap. 55, p. 1405.

McIlroy, M. B., Tierney, D. F., and Nadel, J. A. (1963). A new method for measurement of compliance and resistance of lung and thorax. *J. Appl. Physiol.*, **18**:424-427.

Mead, J., and Whittenberger, J. L. (1954). Evaluation of airway interruption technique as a method for measuring pulmonary airflow resistance. *J. Appl. Physiol.*, **6**:408-416.

Mead, J., Whittenberger, J. L., and Radford, E. P., Jr. (1957). Surface tension as a factor in pulmonary volume pressure hysteresis. *J. Appl. Physiol.*, **10**:191-196.

Michels, A., Landser, F. J., Cauberghs, M., and van de Woestijne, K. P. (1986). Measurement of total respiratory impedance via the endotracheal tube; a model study. *Bull. Eur. Physiopathol. Respir.*, **22**:615-620.

Navajas, D., Farre, R., Rotger, M., and Canet, J. (1989). Recording pressure at the distal end of the endotracheal tube to measure respiratory impedance. *Eur. Respir. J.*, **2**:178-184.

Otis, A. B., and Proctor, D. F. (1948). Measurement of alveolar pressure in human subjects. *Am. J. Physiol.*, **152**:106-112.

Otis, A. B., McKerrow, C. B., Bartlett, R. A., Mead, J., McIlroy, M. B., Selverstone, N. J., and Radford, E. P., Jr. (1956). Mechanical factors in distribution of pulmonary ventilation. *J. Appl. Physiol.*, **8**:427-443.

Peslin, R., and Andrada, L. (1967). Facteur pariétal dans la détermination des résistances ventilatoires par interruption du courant gazeux. *Rev. Fr. Etudes Clin. Biol.*, **12**:278-284.

Rattenborg, C. (1956). In *Basic Mechanics of Artificial Ventilation in Management of Life-Threatening Poliomyelitis.* Edited by H. C. A. Lassen. London, Livingstone, chap. 1, p. 23.

Rohrer, F. (1916). Der Zusammenhang der Atemkräfte und ihre Abhängigkeit vom Dehnungszustand der Atemorgane. *Arch. Ges. Physiol.*, **165**:419-444.

Rossi, A., Gottfried, S. B., Zocchi, L., Higgs, B. D., Lennox, S., Calverley, P. M. A., Begin, P., Grassino, A., and Milic-Emili, J. (1985a). Measurement of static compliance of the total respiratory system in patients with acute respiratory failure during mechanical ventilation. *Am. Rev. Respir. Dis.*, **131**:672-677.

Rossi, A., Gottfried, S. B., Higgs, B. D., Zocchi, L., Grassino, A., and Milic-Emili, J. (1985b). Respiratory mechanics in mechanically ventilated patients with respiratory failure. *J. Appl. Physiol.*, **58**:1849-1858.

Shephard, R. J. (1963). Mechanical characteristics of the human airway in relation to use of the interrupter valve. *Clin. Sci.*, **25**:263-280.

Sullivan, M., Paliotta, J., and Saklad, M. (1976). Endotracheal tube as a factor in measurement of respiratory mechanics. *J. Appl. Physiol.*, **41**:590-592.

Suratt, P. M., Owens, D. H., Kilgore, W. T., Harry, R. R., and Hsiao, H. S. (1980). A pulse method of measuring respiratory system compliance. *J. Appl. Physiol.*, **49**:1116-1121.

Tsai, M. J., Pimmel, R. L., Stiff, E. J., Bromberg, P. A., and Hamlin, R. L. (1977). Respiratory parameter estimation using forced oscillatory impedance data. *J. Appl. Physiol.*, **43**:322-330.

von Neergaard, K., and Wirz, K. (1927). Die Messung der Strömungswiderstände in den Atemwegen des Menschen, inbesondere bei Asthma und Emphysem. *Z. Klin. Med.*, **105**:51-82.

Vuilleumier, P. (1944). Über eine Methode zur Messung des intra-alveolären Druckes und der Strömungswiderstände in den Atemwegen des Menschen. *Z. Klin. Med.*, **143**:698-717.

Zin, W. A., Rossi, A., and Milic-Emili, J. (1983). Model analysis of respiratory responses to inspiratory resistive loads. *J. Appl. Physiol.*, **55**:1565-1573.

8

Lung Mechanics in ARDS

Compliance and Pressure-Volume Curves

LAURENT BEYDON and FRANÇOIS LEMAIRE

Hôpital Henri Mondor
Paris Val-de-Marne University
Créteil, France

BJÖRN JONSON

University Hospital
Lund, Sweden

I. Introduction

The existence of lung elastic recoil forces has been described since the nineteenth century (Carson, 1820), but the foundations of modern lung mechanics were laid much later by Rahn et al. (1946) and Fenn (1951), who analyzed the pressure-volume diagram of the respiratory system and its components. Although these concepts were widely used and resulted in great advances in respiratory physiology, they were introduced only recently into intensive care units. In fact, most publications describing lung mechanics during artificial ventilation followed the introduction of positive end-expiratory pressure (PEEP) as a technique to increase arterial oxygen partial pressure in patients ventilated for acute respiratory failure (Ashbaugh et al., 1969). Subsequently, PEEP, as reviewed by Shapiro and co-workers (1984), has been shown to counteract airway closure by increasing alveolar volume and recruiting collapsed airways. Recruitment increases functional residual capacity (FRC) (McIntyre et al., 1969; Kumar et al., 1970) and lung compliance (Falke et al., 1972). Conversely, PEEP may at times depress hemodynamics by reducing cardiac output (Dorinsky and Withcomb, 1983) and reduce perfusion to nonventilated units (Dantzker et al., 1980), leading to vascular derecruitment. Both airways recruitment and vascular derecruitment yield an increased Pa_{O_2} and reduced shunt. Alveolar recruitment appears most desirable, whereas systemic vascular derecruitment is potentially harmful because a reduced cardiac output may decrease systemic perfusion and oxygen delivery (Danek et al., 1980). Pulmonary vascular derecruitment could increase pulmonary vascular injury in ARDS.

II. Titration of PEEP

The complex changes in both ventilatory and hemodynamic parameters that result from the use of PEEP have been the basis for several different attempts to determine an "optimum" level of PEEP.

A positive correlation between the level of PEEP and Pa_{O_2} is a common finding in the adult respiratory distress syndrome (ARDS), but data concerning hemodynamic changes induced by PEEP conflict. Indeed, some authors found no significant depression of cardiac index (CI) or oxygen transport (McIntyre et al., 1969). Other authors have described a marked reduction in these two parameters in proportion to the amount of PEEP. This discrepancy may be explained by the different designs of these studies. Some investigations used only a low level of PEEP; others employed "super-PEEP" (Kirby et al., 1975). Moreover, hemodynamic changes were not consistently prevented by the use of appropriate fluid loading (Walkinshaw and Shoemaker, 1980) or inotropic drugs (Gallagher et al., 1978). Furthermore, comparison between the different studies is hampered because different modes of ventilation, which do not induce the same profiles of intrathoracic pressure, were used. For example, intermittent mandatory ventilation with PEEP (Kirby et al., 1975) or, to an even greater extent, spontaneous ventilation with PEEP (CPAP) (Venus et al., 1979) produces low mean airway pressure and thus preserves venous return. In contrast, controlled ventilation, with its associated higher airway pressures, is likely to induce more marked hemodynamic depression.

In response to these methodologic inconsistences, two ways of titrating PEEP have finally emerged. On the one hand, the "optimal" PEEP was considered that which reduced the shunt to near 15% (Gallagher et al., 1978). This approach often necessitated high levels of PEEP and advocated that any fall in cardiac index receive appropriate treatment, based on hemodynamic monitoring. This method was reported to result in a clear improvement in gas exchange, but the high levels of PEEP achieved, that is, far above 15 cmH_2O, have been proven conclusively to be harmful (Caroll et al., 1988). The risk of barotrauma, pneumothoraces, increased lung water, and epithelial damage, which are the most common side effects of PEEP, must be carefully balanced with the clinical benefit one might gain by reducing shunt (Nelson et al., 1987).

Another trend was initiated as early as 1975 by Suter et al., who reported a biphasic change in static lung compliance C_{ST} during a stepwise increase in the PEEP level. They showed that the level at which C_{ST} peaked corresponded to the point at which oxygen transport was maximal and shunt minimal (Fig. 1). This PEEP threshold, also named "best PEEP," evoked great interest and numerous studies. Since this early publication, lung mechanics have been considered a potentially useful way to titrate PEEP. Even though this approach remained controversial for a long time (Wolff et al., 1982), it was supported by a series of recent publications that gave new clues to validate these early findings. Indeed, lung mechanics and especially pressure-volume loops (P-V loops) appeared to be useful, especially in early stages of ARDS, when alveolar edema and respiratory alterations induce clear-cut modifications in lung mechanics.

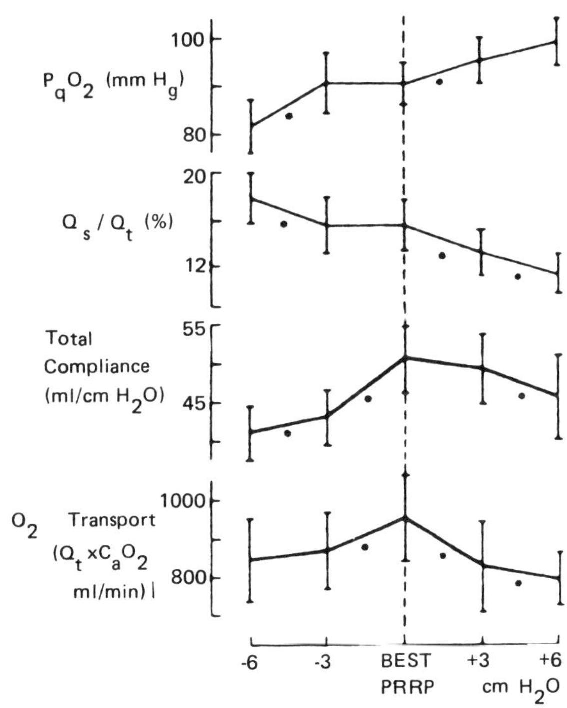

Figure 1 Changes in Pa_{O_2}, shunt (Q_S/Q_T), total compliance, and oxygen transport at values of PEEP higher and lower than an optimum level corresponding to best PEEP. (From Suter et al., 1975.)

In contrast to this "recruitive PEEP" approach, several recent studies restricted the magnitude of PEEP and aimed at determining the lowest PEEP level required to maintain Pa_{O_2} in the normal range with FI_{O_2} remaining below 0.50-0.60. In this "supportive" approach, in which the reduction of shunt is no longer considered a relevant goal (Dobb, 1988), hemodynamic alterations are likely to remain modest and are more easily corrected by the usual therapeutic methods. Nevertheless, such supportive therapy, which supposes a marked response to a low level of PEEP, may fail in severe ARDS and in late stages of ARDS when fibrosis and lung consolidation replace edema. Here, the specific action of PEEP that is, airspace recruitment, is minor.

III. Measurement of the Total Thoracopulmonary Compliance (Static and Dynamic)

We review here different techniques available for bedside assessment of lung mechanics in ARDS. All these techniques are based on the assessment of the pressure response to changes in lung volume of the relaxed respiratory system. Some of them are easily performed by using the ventilator's capabilities, whereas others necessitate special equipment. Because P-V loops are the most complete way to explore not only elastic but also recruitment phenomena and viscoelastic properties of the lung, they are extensively discussed.

To simplify the following descriptions, we first consider only total respiratory system mechanics. Partitioning the total system into lung and chest wall components requires measuring esophageal pressure and is discussed later.

A. Occlusion Methods

Using any type of ventilator, one may easily perform, at the end of a tidal inflation, a manual occlusion followed by a pause, long enough to achieve static conditions (Don and Robson, 1965; Suter et al., 1978). As illustrated in Figure 2, the ratio of the inspired tidal volume (corrected for ventilated compressed volume) to the resulting static pressure corrected for PEEP (external and intrinsic) (Rossi et al., 1985) gives the total static compliance (Jonson et al., 1975) for the corresponding lung volume. Because the pressure-volume relationship of the respiratory system is not linear in the range of vital capacity, the compliance that is measured depends on the amplitude of the tidal volume (Mancebo et al., 1985) and also the end-expiratory lung volume (FRC), that is, on the PEEP level. Thus, C_{ST} as assessed by occlusion at end-inspiration may be used to optimize both tidal volume and PEEP during mechanical ventilation (Suter et al., 1978).

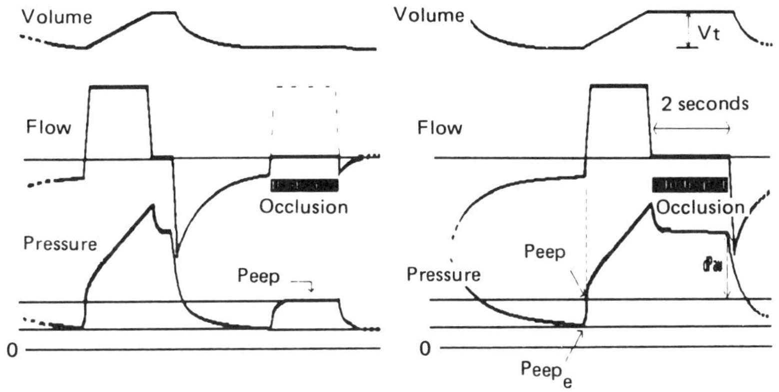

Figure 2 Recordings of volume, flow, and airway pressure during mechanical ventilation. (Left) Measurement of intrinsic PEEP ($PEEP_i$) by an occlusion at the end of expiration. (Right) Static compliance corresponds to the ratio of V_t and dP_{aw}.

B. Effective or Quasi-static Compliance

An alternative to the measurement of C_{ST} by a long pause, in static conditions, is offered by the measurement of the effective compliance (Petty and Ashbaugh, 1971). This method takes advantage of the adjustable post-inspiratory pause built into most ventilators. This pause is routinely used to prolong the duration of inflation and improve gas exchange. Measuring compliance at the end of such a pause reflects the lung mechanics at the preset conditions of ventilation at the moment of measurement. Nevertheless, if this pause is too short to meet static conditions, dynamic parameters will be included in the measurement. Therefore, this quasi-static method must be considered a convenient way to approach lung mechanics without interrupting mechanical ventilation, but it is likely to be less accurate than a "true" static occlusion method. The tidal volume measured value should be corrected for the internal compression volume of the ventilator.

C. Dynamic Compliance

Dynamic compliance is easily obtained during unaltered tidal ventilation (Falke et al., 1972) and corresponds to the ratio of the tidal volume and the pressure difference between two consecutive points of zero flow. Its relevance is limited because it includes both static and dynamic components, that is, flow resistance, inertia, viscoelasticity, and interregional pressure-flow redistributions due to lung inhomogeneities. Thus, the dynamic P-V loops that were primarily used by physiologists to analyze the frequency dependence of lung mechanics and to model hysteresis phenomena are of little interest in clinical applications. Nevertheless, during a constant volume-cycled mechanical ventilation, it may provide a rough approximation of the static and dynamic properties as a whole (Bone, 1976; Thomas et al., 1979).

D. Static Pressure-Volume Loops

All the methods described above, although easy to perform, are somewhat limited in that they provide only the value of compliance during tidal ventilation. In contrast, the P-V loop method gives extensive data on the elastic and viscoelastic components of the respiratory system over a greater range of inflation volume.

Different techniques are available to draw P-V loops, but the super-syringe method is probably the most popular. This method has been widely used in mechanically ventilated patients with acute respiratory failure (Bendixen et al., 1965; Harf et al., 1975; Lemaire et al., 1982a; Matamis et al., 1984; Gattinoni et al., 1986). The experimental device consists of a 2 liter graduated plastic syringe (Janney, 1959) equipped with a pressure transducer and a pneumotachograph or a mechanical system sensing the syringe plunger displacement. Both volume and pressure signals are plotted on an XY recorder. The maneuver is performed as follows. First, the volume history of the lung must be standardized by several large breaths delivered by the ventilator. Then, the syringe is filled with a water-saturated air-oxygen mixture, generally drawn from the ventilator inspiratory limb. The patient is disconnected from the ventilator, and after FRC has been reached, the syringe is connected to the endotracheal tube. The P-V loop is obtained by stepwise 100-200 ml inflations performed until either a pressure of 50 cmH_2O is reached or a plateau of the inspiratory pressure-volume curve is observed, near total lung capacity. This pressure plateau reflects the decrease in compliance in response to lung overdistention. Then, a similar stepwise deflation is performed until pressure returns to atmospheric levels. To ensure static conditions, each volume step is followed by a 2-3 sec pause during which pressure is allowed to stabilize, according to stress adaptation (Sharp et al., 1967; Marshall and Widdicombe, 1960). In these conditions, the P-V loop tracing usually lasts about 60-90 sec. As stated before, this technique requires full relaxation to obviate any muscular participation and ensure static conditions. Moreover, the endotracheal tube must be leakproof because any volume loss during the loop tracing would result in a nonrecoverable drift of the signal.

The resulting P-V curve has a sigmoidal shape. Different distinct points or zones have been described on these loops (Matamis et al., 1984; Gattinoni et al., 1987a), which explore a specific (mechanical) component of the respiratory system in response to the applied deformation, that is, the step changes in volume (Fig. 3):

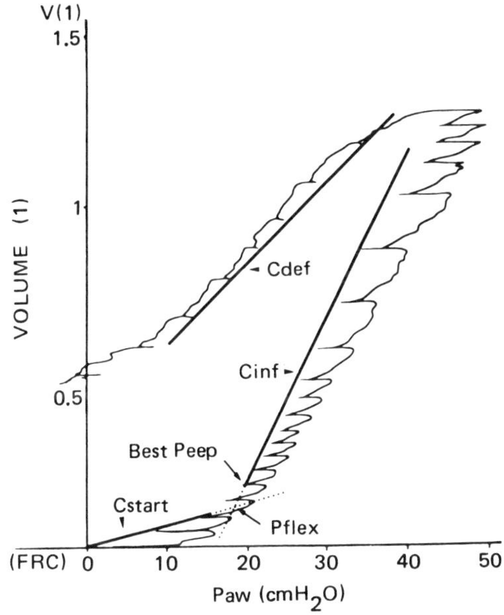

Figure 3 A typical syringe P-V loop with pertinent points illustrated. (From Gattinoni et al., 1987a.)

The compliance, that is, the slope of the P-V curve measured on the first 100-250 ml of inflation (starting compliance, C_{start}), may be different from that seen at volumes ranging from about 250 to 1000 ml (inflation compliance, C_{inf}). The initial poor distensibility of the respiratory system seen at low volume and measured by C_{start} means that a relatively high pressure is needed to reopen closed airways. Indeed, distal airway closure is known to occur at the residual volume (Milic-Emili et al., 1966; Burger and Macklem, 1968; Hughes and Rosenzweig, 1970), especially in dependent lung regions where opening forces, acting on the terminal airways and alveoli, do not counterbalance collapsing forces. In ARDS, airway stability is decreased and occlusion may occur above RFC. Airway collapse contributes to the observed decrease in Pa_{O_2} and to the increase in shunt, physiologic reflections of the pathologic changes occurring in ARDS.

Several phenomena have been proposed to explain the loss of airway stability: possible alteration in surfactant properties (Said et al., 1967; Clements, 1970; Petty et al., 1979) may hinder its ability to lower surface tension at low lung volume and could promote airway closure. Also to be considered is the specific action of the foam resulting from pulmonary edema, producing menisci in the lumen of terminal airways (Faridy and Permutt, 1971; Macklem et al., 1970; Frazer et al., 1979). This liquid accumulation increases the airspace resistance to opening and enhances gas trapping. Similarly, an accumulation of interstitial fluid in the wall of the terminal airspaces could reduce their distensibility and facilitate airway collapse. Lastly, airway closure could result from dynamic compression at the end of expiration (Macklem et al., 1963) if obstructive lung disease is associated with ARDS.

In contrast to C_{start}, C_{inf} represents the optimal elastic behavior one may obtain in response to lung inflation. It quantifies intrinsic respiratory system distensibility when all recruitable aerated zones are open. In normal ventilated patients, C_{inf} ranges from 60 to 100 ml/cmH_2O (Tobin, 1988), but it is notably reduced in ARDS in which values as low as 25 ml/cmH_2O can be measured.

The inflection point P_{flex} is defined as the intersection of C_{start} and C_{inf}. It has been shown on inspiratory (Lemaire et al., 1979) and expiratory P-V curves (Glaister, 1974; Ingram et al., 1974) P_{flex}, when present, may be considered the pressure at which most airspaces are recruited.

Best PEEP corresponds to the pressure at which PEEP must be set to increase the functional residual capacity and maintain airways permanently open. This best PEEP has been described by Gattinoni et al. (1987a) to correspond to the lowest point on the C_{inf} slope.

A third part of the P-V curve can be assessed on the inspiratory limb. It corresponds to the zone where the loop bends, near total lung capacity. This secondary decrease in compliance signals a state of overinflation, which reflects the loss of distensibility displayed by the tissues in response to excessive stretch.

On the expiratory limb, one may identify an extended linear portion, the slope of which corresponds to the deflation compliance (C_{def}) and has the same physiologic significance as C_{inf}. When an inspiratory inflection point is present, an inflection is generally also measured on the expiratory limb. This point means that airway closure phenomena resume near FRC (Demedts et al., 1975; Hida et al., 1979). The terminal part of the expiratory limb is difficult to analyze because of hysteresis. In addition to what was inferred from both the inflation and deflation limbs, the total static compliance may also be determined on the P-V loop. It represents the average elastic properties of the respiratory system and corresponds to the ratio of the total volume insufflated during the P-V maneuver to the corresponding pressure increase. This value must be regarded as imprecise. Indeed, it does not reflect changes in lung distensibility occurring during both inflation and deflation, as assessed by C_{start}, C_{inf}, and C_{def}. Moreover, its value depends on the magnitude of insufflated volume that must be fixed to allow comparison.

Lastly, the area of the P-V loops is not closed. When atmospheric pressure is reached at the end of deflation, the volume recovered in the syringe is always lower than the inflated volume. This reduction in volume is produced by an amount of trapped gas in the lung and by oxygen uptake during the inflation-deflation maneuver. Moreover, the volume of trapped gas has been shown to be higher when inflation is slow and when liquid is accumulating in the airways, resulting in the formation of bubbles or films. Additionally, the respiratory system, owing to viscoelastic properties, displays hysteresis (Mead et al., 1957; Hildebrandt, 1972). Hysteresis, which is represented by the surface area of the loop, means that the total energy supplied during inflation to increase volume is not fully restored during deflation. In the lung, surfactant enhances viscoelasticity. Moreover, in the early stages of ARDS, hysteresis is increased owing to the presence of edema (Cook et al., 1959). Because hysteresis depends upon both the volume and the maximal pressure reached during the P-V maneuver, it can be normalized by the hysteresis ratio (Bachofen and Hildebrandt, 1971). This ratio (HR) is calculated as the quotient of the hysteresis area A and the product of the total change in pressure dP times the total inflated volume V:

$$HR = \frac{A}{dP \times V}$$

E. Constant Flow

To simplify the P-V loop maneuver, another method can replace the cumbersome syringe technique. One may simply use a constant flow to inflate or deflate the lungs. Indeed, if the flow rate is sufficiently small (2 liters/min) near static conditions will be achieved. This constant flow can be achieved by an electric pump or any other calibrated flow generator connected to the endotracheal tube (Suratt et al., 1980; Mankikian et al., 1983; Benito et al., 1985). When overdistension occurs or an airway pressure of 40 cmH_2O is reached at the end of inflation, an expiratory limb is traced by reversing the direction of flow. In this method, the volume increase is a linear function of time and can easily be estimated from the elapsed time. The pressure tracing obtained with the constant flow method has been shown to be identical to that obtained by the syringe technique (Fig. 4).

IV. Recent Concepts of P-V Loops

A. Early and Late ARDS

In accordance with Suter's best PEEP definition, Lemaire et al. (1979) found in 10 of 12 ARDS patients in whom an inspiratory inflection point was present that a dramatic increase in Pa_{O_2} and decrease in shunt occurred when the level of PEEP was increased over P_{flex}. By contrast, when PEEP was set below that threshold, only a slight improvement was seen in oxygenation and

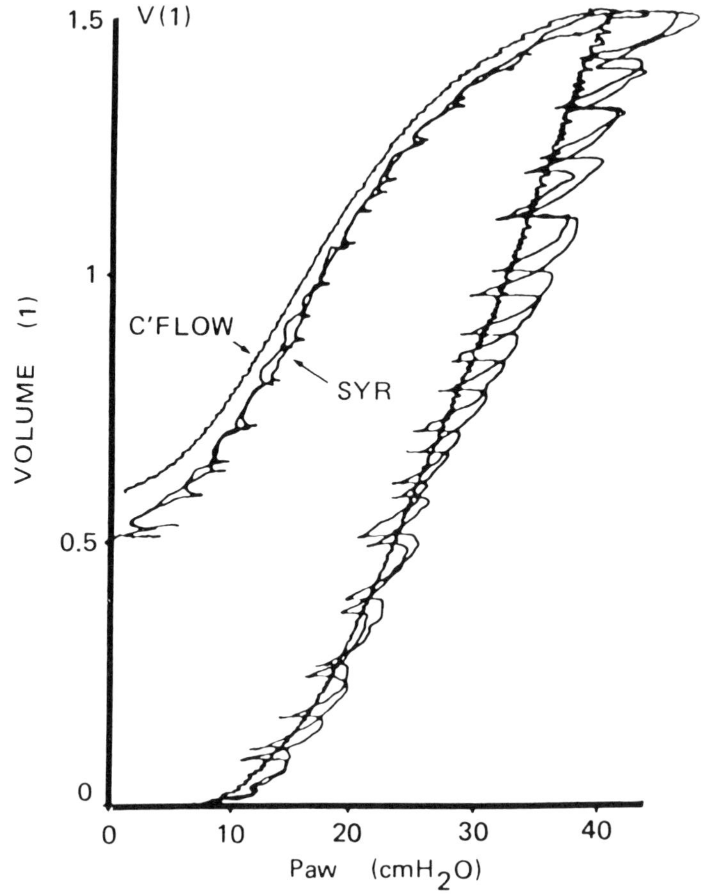

Figure 4 Two consecutive P-V loops with the syringe method (SYR) compared to the constant flow technique (C.FLOW). (From Mankikian et al., 1983.)

shunt. The two patients in whom no inflection was seen did not respond to increasing PEEP up to 32 cmH_2O. Thus, since the paper of Suter et al. (1975) and when an inflection point is present, the best PEEP threshold has become widely used to determine the lowest PEEP level required to optimize oxygenation, maintain a low peak pressure, and limit the risk of barotrauma.

However, some studies challenged these concepts of P_{flex} and best PEEP. Indeed, the inflection point appeared to be inconstant, and even when present, a further improvement in Pa_{O_2} or reduction in shunt could sometimes be achieved at PEEP levels much higher than best PEEP (Tenaillon et al.,

1978). The apparent discrepancies between these different studies were only recently clarified. Holzapfel et al. (1983), comparing early and late stages ARDS (i.e., 2.7 and 31 days after the onset of the lung disease, respectively), found that hysteresis and infection points were only present in the early group on both inspiratory and expiratory limbs. Early ARDS patients improved gas exchange and reduced shunt when PEEP was set above the expiratory P_{flex}. In contrast, in late-stage ARDS patients, in whom fibrosis was likely to have replaced edema, neither an inflection point nor a response to PEEP was observed. This absence of any beneficial effect of PEEP in the late stages of ARDS was similarly emphasized by Klose and Osswald (1981). Matamis et al. (1984) extended these conclusions by finding a correlation between the P-V loop parameters and both clinical and radiologic features (Fig. 5).

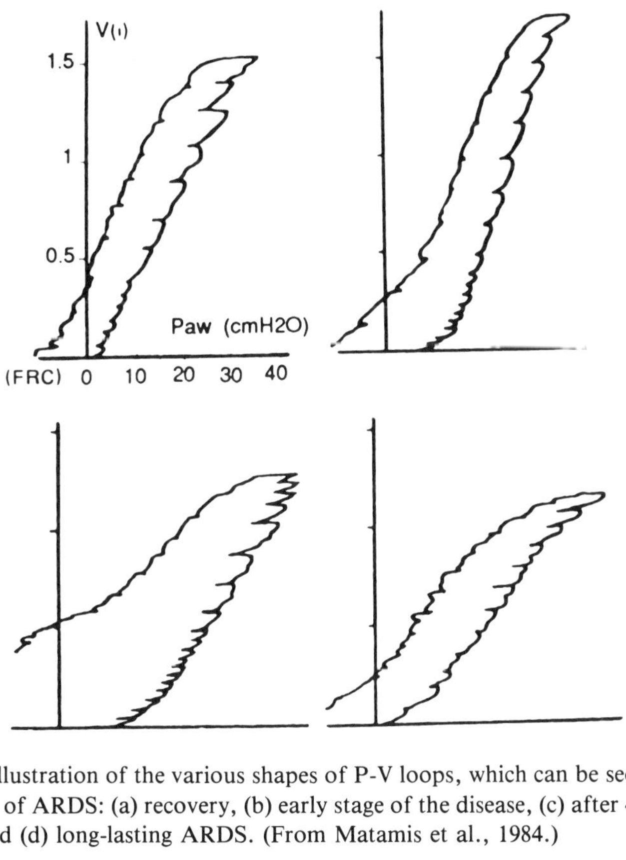

Figure 5 Illustration of the various shapes of P-V loops, which can be seen at different stages of ARDS: (a) recovery, (b) early stage of the disease, (c) after 4 days of evolution and (d) long-lasting ARDS. (From Matamis et al., 1984.)

They showed that the initial stage of the disease was characterized by alveolar opacities on the chest roentgenograms and normal inspiratory and expiratory compliance but increased hysteresis associated with a marked inflection during inflation. Later in the evolution of the disease, the authors noted reduced compliance and hysteresis coincident with interstitial infiltrates replacing the early alveolar opacities. Finally, recovery resulted in normalization of both the compliance and chest x-rays, whereas nonsurvival was associated with a further reduced compliance, persistent interstitial infiltrates, and reduced hysteresis. Thus, hysteresis and the presence of an inflection point were considered characteristic of the early stage of the disease, especially with florid pulmonary edema. At this stage, PEEP is likely to be effective by inducing lung recruitment.

B. Alveolar Recruitment Versus a Cardiac Output Decrease

Brun-Buisson et al. (1987) compared two similar groups of patients with respiratory failure. These two groups differed only by the presence (group I) or the absence (group II) of an inflection on the ascending limb of the P-V curve. All patients were studied at three different levels of PEEP, that is, at a low level, below the value of P_{flex} as measured in group I, at an intermediate PEEP level, just above P_{flex}, and at a high level of PEEP, 5-7 cmH_2O above P_{flex}. In group I patients (presence of inflection), increasing PEEP from the low to the intermediate level resulted in a clearly increased Pa_{O_2} and decreased Q_{VA}/Q_T, but cardiac index did not change. Conversely, a linear relationship was found between changes in Q_{VA}/Q_T and CI when PEEP was further increased to the higher level. In group II patients, this relationship between Q_{VA}/Q_T and CI was seen at all levels of PEEP, without an intermediate state of best PEEP. This study demonstrated that both alveolar recruitment and a decreased cardiac output may have a role in improving Pa_{O_2} during PEEP ventilation. Tracing P-V curves and the recognition of an inflection on the ascending curve may allow prediction of which mechanism will be most prominent.

C. Correlations Between Lung Mechanics and Morphology

Recent progress in understanding lung mechanics during ARDS was provided by Gattinoni et al. (1986, 1987a, 1988) in three complementary studies. They used CT scanning to correlate changes in lung densities with both mechanical and gasometric parameters at different levels of PEEP. This approach confirmed the previous findings insofar as the authors were able to quantify and visualize recruitment by measuring the amount of aerated or nonaerated tissue in ARDS lungs. They found that the densest areas were located in dependent regions, mainly the bases, in contrast to the more aerated nondependent zones. Dense regions were attributed to the presence of atelectasis and edema. The introduction of PEEP increased radiologic lung volume (Fig. 6) and Pa_{O_2} but decreased the amount of lung density. Interestingly, Gattinoni et al. confirmed that the parameters obtained from P-V curves mainly reflect the mechanical behavior of aerated tissues: C_{start} quantitates the amount of the aerated zone at low volume (PEEP of 5 cmH_2O), whereas

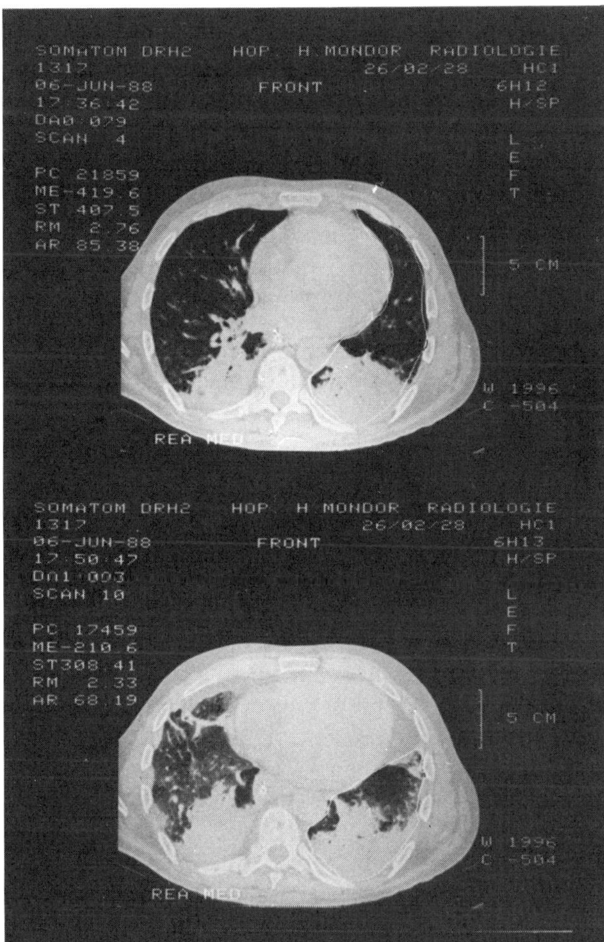

Figure 6 CT scan in ARDS. (Lower) In the absence of PEEP, dependent regions show marked opacities. (Upper) Under PEEP, the radiologic lung volume is increased and the amount of aerated tissue is increased. (By courtesy of A. H. Messadi and N. Vasile, Henri Mondor Hospital.)

the C_{inf}/C_{start} ratio corresponds to the volume recruited by higher PEEP levels. C_{inf} and C_{def} give similar information on the volume of the aerated zone during application of 15 cmH_2O PEEP.

These authors extended their radiographic observations to shunt and cardiac index (CI). They noted a positive correlation between Q_S/Q_T and CI under various levels of PEEP. Moreover, in contrast to parameters of lung mechanics, gasometric changes and especially shunt were directly dependent upon the quantity of nonaerated zones (Fig. 7).

D. Time Dependence

Recruitment by PEEP was investigated by Katz et al. (1981a), who focused on time dependence. To do so, they measured breath-by-breath increases in

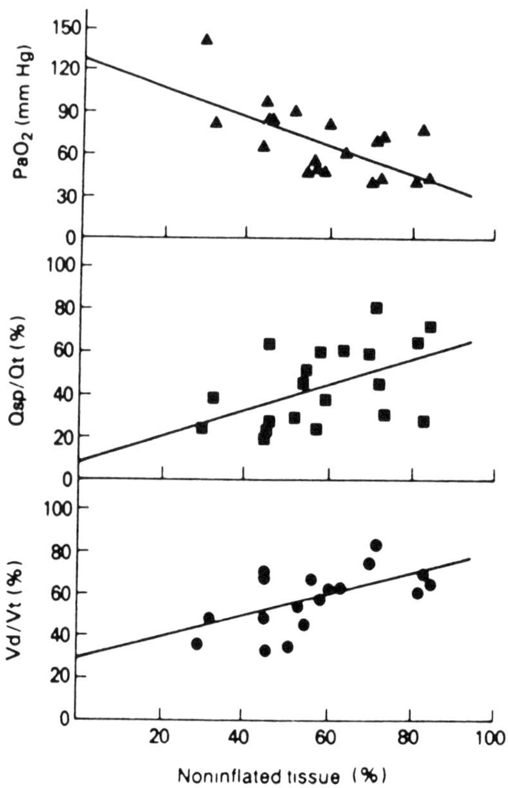

Figure 7 Changes in PA_{O_2}, shunt, and deadspace with the amount of nonaerated tissue measured at a PEEP level of 5 cmH_2O. (From Gattinoni et al., 1988.)

lung volume following the application of 10 cmH_2O PEEP (Fig. 8). They showed that in response to such a constant level of PEEP the volume increase was biphasic. Only 66% of the total increase in lung volume was achieved after the first insufflation following the onset of PEEP. This immediate recruitment was followed by a slow lung volume increase that continued for the next 20 tidal insufflations. This progressive increase in volume verified the earlier findings of Ferris and Pollard (1960) and could be explained by changes in surface tension (Mead et al., 1957; Bachofen and Hildebrandt, 1971) or, more likely, by stress adaptation of the lung in response to PEEP (Sharp et al., 1967). Therefore, the volume change resulting from a given PEEP increment is always greater than the change predicted by the product of that PEEP increment and the compliance measured on the P-V loop.

E. Respiratory System Versus Lung Compliance

Most of the studies dealing with lung mechanics in ARDS examined the total (lung plus chest wall) respiratory compliance, thereby reflecting changes of lung mechanics. Indeed, total compliance represents the summation of elastic forces that mechanical ventilation must overcome. Moreover, changes in the compliance of the respiratory system are assumed to result almost exclusively

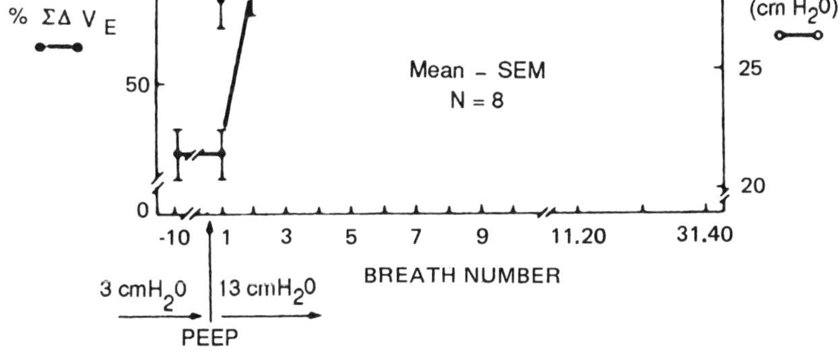

Figure 8 Increase in lung volume and airway plateau pressure during mechanical ventilation, following the change from 3 to 13 cmH_2O of PEEP. Mechanical modifications induced by PEEP take several breaths to be complete. (From Katz et al., 1981a.)

from changes in lung compliance. Although generally true in ARDS (Suter et al., 1978), this may fail in some instances, especially in postoperative situations, when the chest wall is functionally impaired. In this case, the need for a separate measurement of lung and chest wall compliance, instead of total respiratory system compliance, needs to be addressed. This can be done by partitioning total elastic mechanics into lung and chest wall components by measuring eosphageal pressure (Falke et al., 1972; Katz et al., 1981b).

V. Methodologic Limitations

Following this overview of recent reports on P-V loop analysis in ARDS, several methodologic limitations should be pointed out. This method, which is useful to titrate PEEP when an inflection is present, as in early ARDS, is less relevant in the absence of such an inflection. Therefore, in the absence of any sizable recruitment, we recommend that PEEP be adjusted in accordance with other parameters, such as Pa_{O_2}, shunt, and cardiac index. Compliance is nevertheless a useful parameter to examine changes in the elastic properties of the lungs during the course of acute lung disease.

A. Deflation Versus Inflation Compliance

The syringe method to generate the P-V loop allows measurement of both C_{inf} and C_{def}, but these two values generally differ (Lemaire et al., 1982b; Mancebo et al., 1988). C_{def} has been preferred by some authors because it is consistent with the traditional measurement of compliance during expiration as performed in lung function laboratories. Nevertheless, C_{def} is known to depend on the lung volume reached during inflation (Mead and Collier, 1959; Benito et al., 1985), that is, the higher the volume, the higher the compliance. Therefore, this volume must be standardized to allow C_{def} comparisons between different sets of measurements. Additionally, the expiratory inflection point (Salmon et al., 1981) as an indication of closing pressure (Glaister et al., 1973) has greater dependence on hysteresis and volume loss during the maneuver than when measured during inspiration. Consequently, for more accuracy it is preferable to analyze the inflation limb of P-V loops (Lemaire et al., 1979; Gattinoni et al., 1987b).

B. Gas Exchange During the P-V Maneuver

Gattinoni et al. (1987b) provided additional evidence to explain the differences between inspiratory and expiratory compliances. They showed that the ongoing oxygen uptake, no longer balanced by the release of CO_2, which rapidly reaches an equilibrium, could provide a major source of error. The discrepancy is increased not only by increases in humidity and temperature of the inspired gas but also by volume changes due to gas compression. Therefore, the deflation compliance is artificially reduced, and both the hysteresis ratio and area are increased if no corrections are made. In contrast, inspiratory compliance would be less affected because changes in temperature and humidity, on the one hand, and compression, on the other, act in an opposite manner. Dall'Ava-Santucci et al. (1988) have confirmed these limitations of the standard P-V loop method by comparing the compliance values inferred from two different ways of measuring volume change. In the first, true volume changes were measured by external inductive plethysmography, whereas in the second lung volume changes were assessed by the syringe plunger displacement according to the conventional technique. In this way, the errors in volume measurement during the maneuver were assessed and appeared to be more important when the P-V maneuver was prolonged.

Both studies advocate the need for correcting P-V loops, or at least for preferentially analyzing the inspiratory limb after standardization of lung volume history by one or several large volume inflations. Hence, provided these conditions are fulfilled, the loops that are obtained will be highly reproducible.

C. Unilateral Lung Disease

Another limitation of the compliance measurement, whatever the method used, concerns patients with unilateral lung disease (Kvetan et al., 1982). Here, the measured compliance primarily reflects the behavior of the healthy lung and is of little value for assessing the mechanical status of the diseased lung. Similarly, ventilation will be preferentially directed toward the highly compliant, normal lung, thereby increasing ventilation-perfusion inequalities. This problem can be solved by ventilating each lung separately (Glass et al., 1976; Venus et al., 1980) via a double-lumen endobronchial tube with twin ventilators. This technique has also been evaluated in bilateral lung injuries during artificial ventilation in the lateral position (Baehrendtz and Hedenstierna, 1984). When both lungs are independently ventilated, it becomes possible to perform P-V loops and separately titrate PEEP for each lung according to its mechanical variables.

VI. Conclusion

The need to precisely titrate PEEP in daily practice and to limit its potential risks makes the mechanical approach, in particular the P-V curve technique, of great interest when an inflection point is present. In the absence of an inflection point, the usual hemodynamic and gasometric parameters are sufficient and PEEP should be limited to the threshold level required to improve oxygen transport and reduce F_{IO_2} to safe levels (Albert, 1985).

Acknowledgments

The authors would like to thank Professors Henning Pontoppidan and Warren Zapol for reviewing the manuscript.

References

Albert, R. K. (1985). Least PEEP: Primum non nocere. *Chest,* **87**:2-4.

Ashbaugh, D. G., Petty, T. L., Bigelow, D. B., and Harris, T. M. (1969). Continuous positive-pressure breathing (CPPB) in adult respiratory distress syndrome. *J. Thorac. Cardiovasc. Surg.,* **57**:31-41.

Bachofen, H., and Hildebrandt, J. (1971). Area analysis of pressure volume hysteresis in mammalian lungs. *J. Appl. Physiol.,* **30**:493-497.

Baehrendtz, S., and Hedenstierna, G. (1984). Differential ventilation and selective positive end-expiratory pressure: Effects on patients with acute bilateral disease. *Anesthesiology,* **61**:511-517.

Bendixen, H. H., Egbert, L. D., and Hedley Whyte, J. (1965). *Respiratory Care.* St. Louis, C. V. Mosby, p. 50-51.

Benito, S., Lemaire, F., Mankikian, B., and Harf, A. (1985). Total respiratory compliance as a function of lung volume in patients with mechanical ventilation. *Intensive Care Med.,* **11**:76-79.

Bone, R. C. (1976). Diagnosis of cause for acute respiratory distress by pressure-volume curves. *Chest,* **70**:740-745.

Brun-Buisson, C., Abrouk, F., Ben Lakhal, S., and Lemaire, F. (1987). Reduction of venous admixture with PEEP during human ARF. Respective role of alveolar recruitment vs. decrease in blood flow. *Am. Rev. Respir. Dis.* (Suppl.) **135**:A6.

Burger, E. J., and Macklem, P. (1968). Airway closure; demonstration by breathing 100 per cent O_2 at low lung volume and by N_2 washout. *J. Appl. Physiol.,* **25**:139-144.

Caroll, G. C., Tuman, K. J., Braverman, B., Logas, W. G., Wool, N., Goldin, M., and Ivankovich, A. D. (1988). Minimal positive end-expiratory pressure (PEEP) may be "best PEEP." *Chest,* **93**:1020-1025.

Carson, J. (1820). On the elasticity of the lungs. *Philos. Trans. R. Soc. Lond.,* **1**:29-44.

Cléments, J. A. (1970). Pulmonary surfactant. *Am. Rev. Respir. Dis.,* **101**: 984-990.

Cook, C. D., Mead, J., Schreiner, G. L., Frank, N. R., and Craig, J. M. (1959). Pulmonary mechanics during induced edema in anesthetized dogs. *J. Appl. Physiol.,* **14**:177-186.

Dall'Ava-Santucci, J., Armanganidis, A., Brunet, F., Dhainaut, J. F., Chelucci, G. L., Monsallier, J. F., and Lockhart, A. (1988). Causes of error of respiratory pressure-volume curves in paralysed subjects. *J. Appl. Physiol.,* **64**:42-49.

Danek, S. J., Lynch, J. P., Weg, J. G., and Dantzker, D. R. (1980). The dependence of oxygen uptake on oxygen delivery in the adult respiratory distress syndrome. *Am. Rev. Respir. Dis.,* **122**:387-395.

Dantzker, D. R., Lynch, J. P., and Weg, J. A. (1980). Depression of cardiac output is a mechanism of shunt reduction in the therapy of acute respiratory failure. *Chest,* **77**:636-642.

Demedts, M., Clément, J., Stanescu, D. C., and Van De Woestijne, (1975). Inflection point on transpulmonary pressure-volume curves and closing volume. *J. Appl. Physiol.,* **38**:228-235.

Dobb, G. J. (1988). Optimum PEEP: A useful concept? *Crit. Care World,* **5**:114-115.

Don, H. F., and Robson, J. G. (1965). The mechanics of the respiratory system during anesthesia. *Anesthesiology,* **26**:168-172.

Dorindsky, P. M., and Withcomb, M. E. (1983). The effect of PEEP on cardiac output. *Chest,* **84**:210-216.

Falke, K. J., Pontoppidan, H., Kumar, H., Leith, D. E., Geffin, B., and Laver, M. B. (1972). Ventilation with end-expiratory pressure in acute lung disease. *J. Clin. Invest.,* **51**:2315-2323.

Faridy, E. E., and Permutt, S. (1971). Surface forces and airway obstruction. *J. Appl. Physiol.,* **30**:319-321.

Fenn, W. O. (1951). Mechanics of respiration. *Am. J. Med.,* **10**:77-91.

Ferris, B. G., and Pollard, D. S. (1960). Effect of deep and quiet breathing on pulmonary compliance in man. *J. Clin. Invest.,* **39**:143-149.

Frazer, D. G., Stengel, P. W., and Weber, K. C. (1979). Meniscus formation in airways of excised lungs. *Respir. Physiol.,* **36**:121-129.

Gallagher, T. J., Civetta, J. M., and Kirby, R. R. (1978). Terminology update: Optimal PEEP. *Crit. Care Med.,* **6**:323-326.

Gattinoni, L., Mascheroni, D., Torresin, A., Marcolin, R., Fumagalli, R., Vesconi, S., Rossi, G. P., Rossi, F., Baglioni, S., Bassi, F., Nastri, G., and Pesenti, A. (1986). Morphological response to positive end expiratory pressure in acute respiratory failure. Computerized tomography study. *Intensive Care Med.,* **12**:137-142.

Gattinoni, L., Pesenti, A., Avalli, L., Rossi, F., and Bombino, M. (1987a). Pressure-volume curve of total respiratory system in acute respiratory failure. Computed tomographic scan study. *Am. Rev. Respir. Dis.,* **136**: 730-736.

Gattinoni, L., Mascheroni, D., Basilico, E., Foti, Pesenti, A., and Avali, L. (1987b). Volume/pressure curve of total respiratory system in paralyzed patients: Artefacts and correction factors. *Intensive Care Med.,* **13**:19-25.

Gattinoni, L., Pesenti, A., Bombino, M., Baglioni, S., Rivolta, M., Rossi, G., Fumagalli, R., Marcolin, R., Mascheroni, D., and Toresin, A. (1988). Relationships between lung computed tomographic density, gas exchange and PEEP in acute respiratory failure. *Anesthesiology,* **69**:824-832.

Glaister, D. H. (1974). Pressure-volume curves and closing volume. *Scand. Respir. J.* (Suppl.), **85**:209.

Glaister, D. H., Schroter, R. C., Sudlow, M. F., and Milic-Emili, J. (1973). Bulk elastic properties of excised lungs and effects of transpulmonary pressure gradient. *Respir. Physiol.,* **17**:347-364.

Glass, D. D., Tonnensen, A. S., Gabel, J. C., and Arens, J. F. (1976). Therapy of unilateral pulmonary insufficiency with a double lumen endotrachel tube. *Crit. Care Med.,* **4**:323-326.

Harf, A., Lemaire, F., and Lorino, H. (1975). Etude de la mécanique ventilatoire—applications à la ventilation artificielle. *Bull. Eur. Physiopathol. Respir.,* **11**:709-714.

Hida, W., Sasaki, T., Inoue, H., and Takishima, T. (1979). Inflection point of the lung pressure-volume curves using a three-balloon-catheter system. *J. Appl. Physiol.,* **47**:931-937.

Hildebrandt, J. (1972). Models of pressure-volume hysteresis. *Bull. Physiopathol. Respir.,* **8**:337-350.

Holzapfel, L., Robert, D., Perrin, F., Blanc, P. L., Palmier, B., and Guerin, C. (1983). Static pressure-volume curves and effect of positive end-expiratory pressure on gas exchange in adult respiratory distress syndrome. *Crit. Care Med.,* **11**:591-597.

Hughes, J. M. B., and Rosenzweig, D. Y. (1970). Factors affecting trapped gas volume in perfused dogs lungs. *J. Appl. Physiol.,* **29**:332-339.

Ingram, R. H., Jr., O'Cain, C. F., and Fridy, W. W., Jr. (1974). Simultaneous quasi-static lung pressure-volume curves and "closing volume" measurements. *J. Appl. Physiol.,* **36**:135-141.

Janney, C. D. (1959). Super-syringe. *Anesthesiology,* **20**:709-710.

Jonson, B., Nordström, L., Olsson, S. G., and Akerback, D. (1975). Monitoring of ventilation and lung mechanics during automatic ventilation. A new device. *Bull. Physiopathol. Respir.,* **11**:729-743.

Katz, J. A., Ozanne, G. M., Zinn, S. E., and Fairley, H. B. (1981a). Time course and mechanisms of lung-volume increase with PEEP in acute pulmonary failure. *Anesthesiology,* **54**:9-16.

Katz, J. A., Zinn, S. E., Ozanne, G. M., and Fairley, H. B. (1981b). Pulmonary, chest wall, and lung-thorax elastances in acute respiratory failure. *Chest,* **80**:304-311.

Kirby, R. R., Downs, J. B., Civetta, J. M., Modell, J. H., Dannmiller, F. J., Klein, E. F., and Hodges, M. (1975). High level positive end-expiratory pressure (PEEP) in acute respiratory failure. *Chest,* **67**:156-163.

Klose, R., and Osswald, P. M. (1981). Effects of PEEP on pulmonary mechanics and oxygen transport in the late stages of acute pulmonary failure. *Intensive Care,* **7**:165-170.

Kumar, A., Falke, K. J., and Geffin, B. (1970). Continuous positive pressure-ventilation in acute respiratory failure: Effects on hemodynamics and lung function. *N. Engl. J. Med.,* **283**:1430-1436.

Kvetan, V., Carlon, G. C., and Howland, W. S. (1982). Acute pulmonary failure in asymetric lung disease: Approach to management. *Crit. Care Med.,* **10**:114-118.

Lemaire, F., Simoneau, G., Harf, A., Rivara, D., Tesseire, B., Atlan, G., and Rapin, M. (1979). Static pulmonary pressure-volume curve, positive end expiratory pressure and gas exchange in acute respiratory failure. *Am. Rev. Respir. Dis.* (Suppl.), **119**:328.

Lemaire, F., Amamou, M., Rivara, D., Simoneau, G., and Harf, A. (1982a). Static pulmonary pressure-volume curve in acute respiratory failure (abstract). *Am. Rev. Respir. Dis.,* 158.

Lemaire, F., Matamis, D., and Rieuf, P. (1982b). Should compliance of patients in acute respiratory failure be evaluated during inflation or deflation of the lungs? *Am. Rev. Respir. Dis.,* **25**:85.

Macklem, P. T., Fraser, R. G., and Bates, D. V. (1963). Bronchial pressures and dimensions in health and obstructive airway disease. *J. Appl. Physiol.,* **18**:699-707.

Macklem, P. T., Proctor, D. F., and Hogg, J. C. (1970). The stability of peripheral airways. *Respir. Physiol.,* **8**:191-203.

Mancebo, J., Calaf, N., and Benito, S. (1985). Pulmonary compliance measurement in acute respiratory failure. *Crit. Care Med.,* **13**:589-591.

Mancebo, J., Benito, S., Martin, M., and Net, A. (1988). Value of static pulmonary compliance in predicting mortality in patients with acute respiratory failure. *Crit. Care Med.,* **14**:110-114.

Mankikian, B., Lemaire, F., Benito, S., Brun-Buisson, C., Harf, A., Maillot, J. P., and Becker, J. (1983). A new device for measurement of pulmonary pressure-volume curves in patients on mechanical ventilation. *Crit. Care Med.,* **11**:897-901.

Marshall, R., and Widdicombe, J. G. (1960). Stress relaxation of the human lung. *Clin. Sci.,* **20**:19-31.

Matamis, D., Lemaire, F., Harf, A., Brun-Buisson, C., Ansquer, J. C., and Atlan, G. (1984). Total respiratory pressure-volume curves in the adult respiratory distress syndrome. *Chest,* **86**:58-66.

McIntyre, R. W., Laws, A. K., and Ramachandran, P. R. (1969). Positive expiratory pressure plateau: Improved gas exchange during mechanical ventilation. *Can. Anaesthesiol. Soc. J.,* **16**:477-486.

Mead, J., and Collier, C. (1959). Relation of volume history to respiratory mechanics in anesthetized dogs. *J. Appl. Physiol.,* **14**:669-678.

Mead, J., Whittenberger, J. L., and Radford, E. P. (1957). Surface tension as a factor in pulmonary volume-pressure hysteresis. *J. Appl. Physiol.,* **10**:191-196.

Milic-Emili, J., Henderson, J. A. M., Dolovich, M. B., Trop, D., and Kaneko, K. (1966). Regional distribution of inspired gas in the lung. *J. Appl. Physiol.,* **21**:749-759.

Nelson, L. D., Civetta, J. M., and Hudson-Civetta, J. (1987). Titrating positive end-expiratory pressure therapy in patients with early, moderate arterial hypoxemia. *Crit. Care Med.,* **15**:14-19.

Petty, T. L., and Ashbaugh, D. G. (1971). The adult respiratory distress syndrome. Clinical features, factors influencing prognosis and principles of management. *Chest,* **60**:233-239.

Petty, T. L., Silvers, G. W., Paul, G. W., and Stanford, R. E. (1979). Abnormalities in lung elastic properties and surfactant function in adult respiratory distress syndrome. *Chest,* **75**:571-574.

Rahn, H., Otis, A. B., Chadwick, L. E., and Fenn, W. O. (1946). The pressure-volume diagram of the thorax and lung. *Am. J. Phyisol.,* **146**:161-178.

Rossi, A., Gottfried, S. B., Zocchi, L., Higgs, B. D., Lennox, P. M., Calverley, P. M. A., Begin, P., Grassino, A., and Milic-Emili, J. (1985). Measurement of static compliance of the total respiratory system in patients with acute respiratory failure during mechanical ventilation. *Am. Rev. Respir. Dis.,* **131**:672-677.

Said, S. I., Banerjee, C. M., Harlan, W. R., Jr., and Avery, M. E. (1967). Pulmonary edema as a cause of surfactant deficiency. *Jpn. Heart J.,* **8**:742-744.

Salmon, R. B., Primiano, F. P., Saidel, G. M., and Niewoehner, D. E. (1981). Human lung pressure-volume relationships: Alveolar collapse and airway closure. *J. Appl. Physiol.,* **51**:353-362.

Shapiro, B. A., Cane, R. D., and Harrison, R. A. (1984). Positive end-expiratory pressure therapy in adults with special reference to acute lung injury: A review of the literature and suggested clinical correlations. *Crit. Care Med.,* **12**:127-141.

Sharp, J. T., Johnson, F. N., Goldberg, N. B., and Van Lith, P. (1967). Hysteresis and stress adaptation in the human respiratory system. *J. Appl. Physiol.,* **23**:487-497.

Suratt, P. M., Owens, D. H., Kilgore, W. T., Harry, R. R., and Hsiao, H. S. (1980). A pulse method of measuring respiratory system compliance. *J. Appl. Physiol.,* **49**:1116-1121.

Suter, P. M., Fairley, H. B., and Isenberg, M. D. (1975). Optimum end-expiratory airway pressure in patients with acute pulmonary failure. *N. Engl. J. Med.,* **292**:284-289.

Suter, P. M., Fairley, H. B., and Isenberg, M. D. (1978). Effect of tidal volume and positive end-expiratory pressure on compliance during mechanical ventilation. *Chest,* **73**:158-162.

Tenaillon, A., Labrousse, J., Gateau, O., and Lissac, J. (1978). Optimal positive end-expiratory pressure and static lung compliance. *N. Engl. J. Med.,* **299**:774-775.

Thomas, L., Robert, D., and Gerard, M. (1979). Routine use of pressure-volume loops during mechanical ventilation. Determination of optimal combination of flow, tidal volume, and positive end-expiratory pressure. *Chest,* **75**:743-744.

Tobin, M. J. (1988). Respiratory monitoring in intensive care unit. *Am. Rev. Respir. Dis.,* **138**:1625-1642.

Venus, B., Jacobs, H. K., and Lim, L. (1979). Treatment of the adult respiratory distress syndrome with continuous positive airway pressure. *Chest,* **76**:257-261.

Venus, B., Pratap, K. S., and Op'Tholt, T. (1980). Treatment of unilateral insufficiency by selective administration of continuous positive airway pressure through a double lumen tube. *Anesthesiology,* **53**:74-77.

Walkinshaw, M., and Shoemaker, W. C. (1980). Use of volume loading to obtain preferred levels of PEEP. *Crit. Care Med.,* **8**:81-86.

Wolff, G., Langenstein, H., Schwendener, R., and Lischer, P. (1982). Optimal end-expiratory pressure for ventilated patients. *Intensive Care Med.,* **8**:39-48.

9

Minimizing Breathing Effort During Mechanical Ventilation

JOHN J. MARINI

University of Minnesota, Minneapolis
St. Paul Ramsey Medical Center
and Jackson University
St. Paul, Minnesota

I. Introduction

Relief of the breathing work load is a primary objective of mechanical ventilation. By assuming the work burden associated with breathing, mechanical support averts ventilatory failure or arrest. Not only are CO_2 removal and pH homeostasis maintained by mechanical support, but the overtaxed respiratory muscles are given a chance to replenish energy reserves as the primary process that precipitated the crisis is treated. Furthermore, during times of circulatory crisis the nutritive flow commanded by the exercising respiratory muscles can be diverted to other vital organs (Aubier et al., 1981; Viires et al., 1983).

Ideally, the patient would be relieved of excessive burdens during ventilator support but perform enough work to prevent atrophy and build endurance. The multipurpose objective of this discussion is to describe the methods currently available for assessing breathing effort (Table 1), to characterize the magnitude of ventilatory work performed by the machine and patient during mechanical ventilation, and to formulate a strategy for minimizing the breathing work load.

Table 1 Measures of Breathing Effort

Measures of Breathing Effort
Indirect measures
Use of accessory muscles of ventilation
Abnormal breathing patterns
Tachypnea
Paradoxical motion
Ataxic breathing
Respiratory alternans
Direct measures
Oxygen consumption of ventilatory muscles
Electromyography
Integrated signal
Power spectrum
Work of breathing (pressure-volume product)
Force output (pressure-time product)

II. Quantifying Breathing Effort

A. Indirect Measures

The perception of breathing effort is inherently linked to the stress placed on the muscles of the respiratory system relative to their capability to sustain it. The physical examination yields a number of important clues to the status of the power reserve. Such signs as phasic retraction of the intercostal spaces, depression of the substernal notch, vigorous use of the accessory muscles of respiration, asynchrony between the motions of the rib cage and abdomen, ataxic or chaotic breathing, and respiratory alternans all suggest a system poised at the limits of its work performance capability. In recent years there has been an attempt to characterize these abnormalities of breathing motion in a semiquantitative fashion by impedance plethysmography. The maximal compartmental amplitude to tidal volume ratio (MCA/V_T), the percentage of total ventilation provided by rib cage motion, the variability of the rib cage-abdomen excursion ratio, and the phase angle separating excursions of rib cage and abdominal compartments correlate with imposed stress (Tobin et al., 1986). Of these, the MCA/V_T is perhaps the most reliable indicator of system overload. The quantitated dyspnea score (e.g., open-ended modified Borg scale) also correlates well with the level of stress faced by the ventilatory pump in relation to its capacity (Altose, 1986). Although promising, a great deal of additional work remains to be done before the clinical value of these semiquantative indirect measures can be regarded as firmly established.

There is increasing awareness that the central nervous system and the muscles of the respiratory pump form a tightly integrated system. From evidence currently available, it now seems unlikely that the ventilatory control center is programmed to drive the muscles to a non-steady state of energy depletion in pursuit of a ventilatory target. This strategy would eventuate in irreversible cross-bridging of actin and myosin fibers to produce fatal rigor (Roussas and Moxham, 1985). From a survival viewpoint, carbon dioxide retention and respiratory acidosis are more acceptable alternatives. The most reliable measurement of the outflow from the respiratory center available in the clinical setting—the pressure developed in the airway or esophagus 100 msec after a surreptitious airway occlusion (P_{100} or P_1)—appears to have predictive value for the ability of the patient to sustain spontaneous breathing during attempted ventilator discontinuation (Sassoon et al., 1987). This seems consistent with our newer understanding of the interplay between brain and muscle. With this in mind the response of the P_1 to an inhalational challenge of CO_2 would seem to be a particularly attractive way to test the ventilatory reserves (Montgomery et al., 1987). Unfortunately, with the scanty clinical data currently available, it is premature to declare these drive measurements reliable effort indices.

B. Direct Measures

Direct measures of the work performed by the respiratory system include the rate of oxygen consumption by the ventilatory muscles, quantitative electromyography, mechanical (external) work of breathing, and the product of the pressure developed by the inspiratory muscles and the duration of their contraction (the pressure-time index). In theory, each of these, when compared with the maximum levels of which the patient is capable, would provide a reliable effort measure. It must be understood, however, that the interrelationship among them vary greatly with the loads placed on the system, muscular strength, and the efficiency of converting internal energy consumption to external power (Fig. 1).

Ventilation-Related Oxygen Consumption

Precise measurement of the oxygen consumed by the respiratory muscles ($\dot{V}O_{2_R}$) is a difficult task at the bedside. Because $\dot{V}O_{2_R}$ cannot be measured directly, it is usually assessed by measuring total body oxygen consumption before and after a ventilatory stress (e.g., hyperpnea or resistive loading) is imposed or relieved (Bartlett et al., 1958; Cherniack, 1959). Not only is oxygen consumption a difficult measurement to make in the clinical setting, but the respiratory muscles consume only a small fraction of the total body oxygen requirement, especially during machine-supported breathing (Otis, 1964;

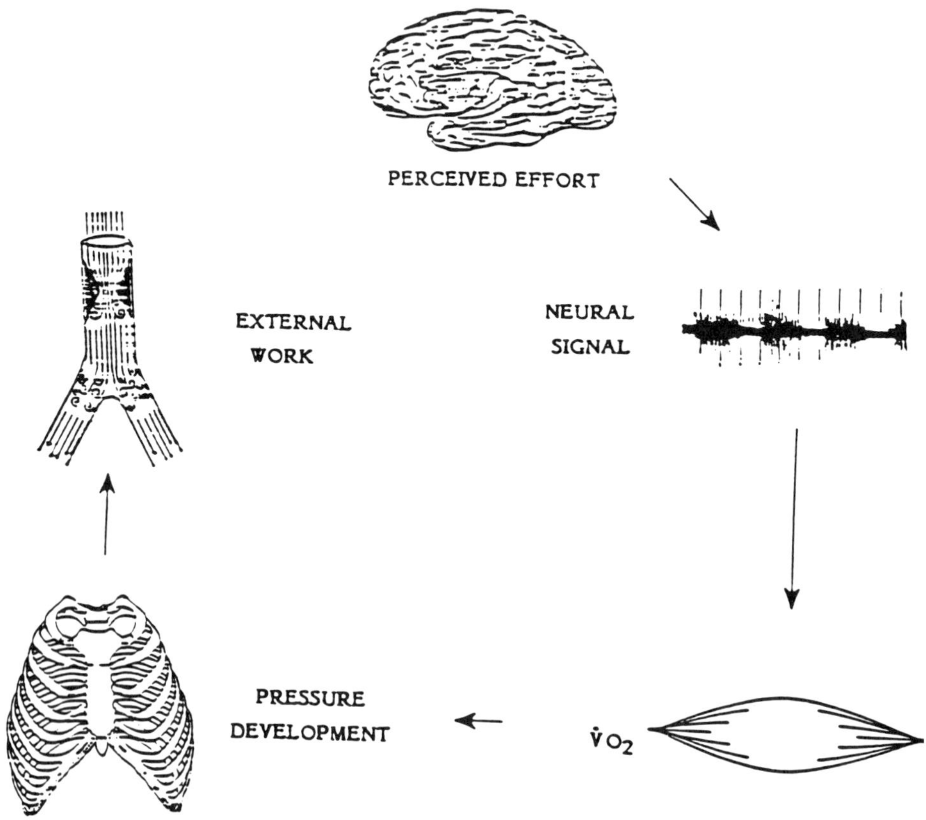

Figure 1 Interrelationships among varied indices of breathing effort. In the progression from perceived effort to mechanical work, reliability deteriorates even as the ease of making precise measurements improves.

Peters, 1969). Furthermore, the poststress increment in oxygen consumption, although attributed in its entirety to the respiratory muscles, is influenced by the activity of nonrespiratory muscle groups. Even within the ventilatory muscle spectrum, simultaneous activation of inspiratory and expiratory muscles can lead to misinterpretation. Finally, by its very nature, the estimation of ventilation-related oxygen consumption requires intervention to accomplish and must be intermittent.

Quantitative Electromyography

Electromyography (EMG), although a step removed from the actual event of respiratory muscle contraction, is a theoretically attractive option, in that the strength of the electromyographic discharge tends to parallel the oxygen consumed by the muscle under observation (Bigland-Ritchie, 1984). Integrated rectified EMG activity parallels the force of muscle contraction relative to force generation capability. Furthermore, the frequency content ("power spectrum") of the EMG shifts under stress to show a disproportionate percentage of low-frequency components (Gross et al., 1979; Loring and Bruce, 1986; Roussos and Moxham, 1985). Electromyography can be conducted on a continuous basis and, therefore, theoretically could serve as a convenient monitor of force output (Fig. 2).

Problems with the clinical application of respiratory electromyography, however, are numerous. By its very nature, the EMG must evaluate only a small subset of the entire array of respiratory muscles. Apart from their discomfort, needle electrodes piercing intercostal or diaphragmatic muscle are highly selective for the impaled fibers and do not necessarily represent the activity of the integrated system. The (transesophageal) diaphragmatic EMG samples its crural component with a catheter lead positioned against the mucosal surface of the esophagus, in close proximity to the diaphragm. However, this semi-invasive technique requires careful electrode placement, and the catheter cannot be left in place indefinitely. Furthermore, the intensity of the signal often varies with cephalocaudal movements of the diaphragm (Grassino et al., 1976). There is controversy as to whether anchoring of the esophageal electrode to the crural region with a gastric balloon is necessary (Loring and Bruce, 1986). Interference of the respiratory EMG signal by nonrespiratory muscle noise (i.e., that of the electrocardiogram) interferes with the quality, accuracy, and selectivity of the integrated EMG.

Skin electrodes at the body surface provide inherently weaker signals that vary with the body habitus of the subject under consideration. Although simple to apply, their respiratory components are almost invariably contaminated by extraneous muscle activity. Perhaps more importantly, there is wide intersubject and (time-dependent) intrasubject variation in signal strength.

Despite all these problems, there has been renewed enthusiasm in the potential use of the EMG applied to the sternocleidomastoid muscle as an indicator of impending system decompensation (Moxham et al., 1980). This easily accessed muscle bundle exhibits increasing activity as the ventilatory pump comes under stress, and its frequency spectrum may yield information suggesting fatigue (Gross et al., 1979; Moxham et al., 1980). Again, however, it is premature to state that such techniques will prove to be of major clinical value.

Force Output and Work of Breathing

In the clinical setting, quantitative assessment of breathing activity can be precisely quantitated by measures of pressure development and work of breath-

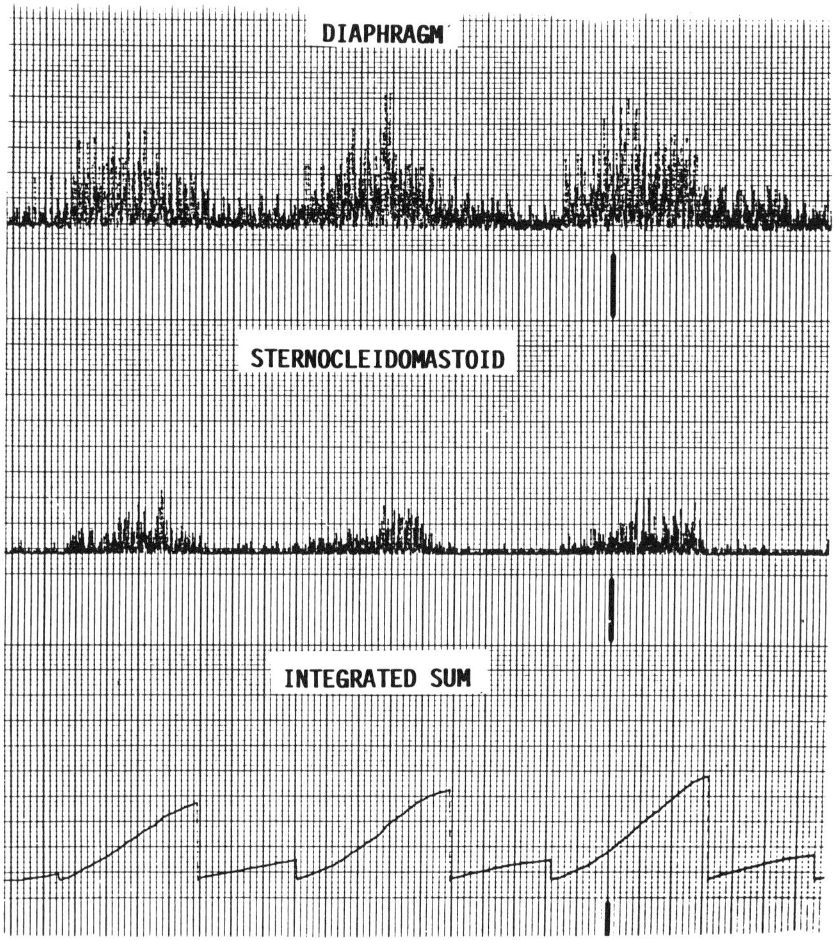

Figure 2 Rectified EMG tracings of diaphragm and sternocleidomastoid and their integrated sum during loaded breathing of a normal subject. These tracings have been filtered free of electrocardiographic artifact. The sum tracing resets with each zero flow point crossing.

ing. Because exhalation is usually driven by energy stored during inspiration, expiratory work is often disregarded in such analyses. When the chest is inflated either by a mechanical ventilator or by the muscles of the patient, alterations occur in the pressure differences between the airway opening and alveolus, between the alveolus and the pleural space, and between the pleural space and the atmosphere. During inflation of a passive subject, a mechanical ventilator applies positive pressure to the airway (Fig. 3). Pressure is dissipated in overcoming flow resistance, with the pressure gradient driving flow the difference between airway pressure (P_{aw}) and alveolar pressure (P_A). Work is also done in expanding the lungs, the relevant forcing pressure change there being $\Delta(P_A - P_{pl})$. Work done in expanding the chest wall is performed by the pressure change developed between the pleural space and atmosphere $[\Delta(P_{pl} - P_{atm})]$.

The work that must be performed by the machine is a pressure-volume product. (To see this more clearly, it is useful to note that from the viewpoint of physics, mechanical work in any system is a force-length product. Because pressure is an expression of force per unit area and volume is an area × length product, pressure volume units are those of force × length, or work.) When a volume change occurs as the *result* of a forcing pressure, the work (W) accomplished is the integral of the product of the relevant forcing pressure (P) and flow ($\dot{V}$) over the time interval of its application t: $W = \int P \dot{V} \, dt$. Pressure-flow integration can be achieved electronically (using a signal integrator) or graphically by planimetry of the area enclosed within the tracing of airway pressure as a function of tidal volume. The area enveloped by the airway pressure-volume tracing during inspiration quantifies all mechanical work done by the machine on the respiratory system in achieving that tidal volume at the selected flow rate. In the clinical setting, a constant flow ventilation mode is commonly used to deliver a specified tidal volume. Under such conditions of constant flow, volume and time are analogs of one another, so

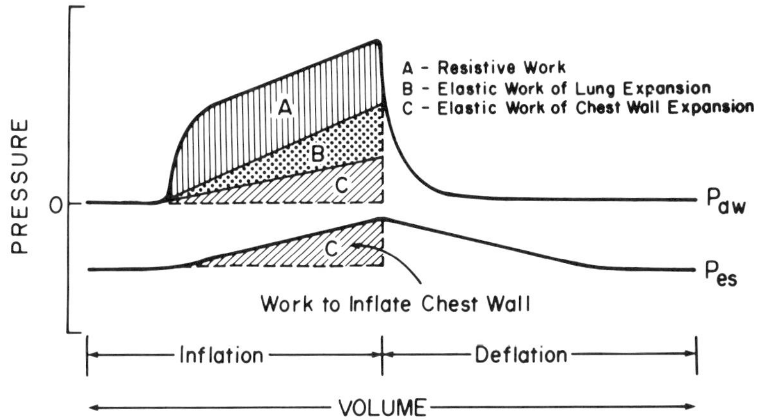

Figure 3 Work to inflate the lung and chest wall during a passive machine cycle delivered with constant flow. Note that the elastic work of chest wall expansion is provided by the ventilator when pleural pressure is greater than atmospheric pressure and by the potential energy stored in the chest wall so long as pleural pressure remains subatmospheric.

that inspiratory pressure-volume and pressure-time plots will subtend similar areas (in terms of equivalent units) during inspiration (Marini et al., 1986b).

Of the total forcing pressure, components are required to drive flow and to expand the lung. When the chest wall is at or above its equilibrium (resting) position at end-exhalation, work must also be performed by the machine in expanding the chest wall. When the chest wall rests below its equilibrium position, however, energy stored as outward-directed elastic tension in the chest wall is recovered during the inspiratory phase to aid the ventilator in achieving expansion. (This work component is usually quite minor.) Thus, the airway pressure profile under passive conditions may slightly underestimate the total work required from all sources to achieve inflation because there is an unquantified component of spring tension from the chest wall adding to the machine's force in expanding the system. Nonetheless, for clinical purposes the work of breathing at the selected tidal volume and flow rate can be quantified acceptably well by the area under the inspiratory airway pressure curve, especially during ventilation in the supine position. Furthermore, the pressure achieved at midcycle is equivalent to the pressure-volume (work) area divided by tidal volume, so that average inspiratory pressure ($\bar{P}$) reflects the work per liter of ventilation (Marini et al., 1986b). At the bedside, central airway pressure can easily be monitored in any ventilated patient using a pressure transducer identical to that used to measure pulmonary arterial pressures, but dedicated to gas pressure measurement. By placing the output of this pressure transducer onto the bedside monitor and/or stripchart recorder, airway pressure can be continuously visualized.

For unchanging resistance and compliance, the inspiratory airway pressure profile described under constant-flow conditions resembles a trapezoid formed by a triangle of elastic pressure and a parallelogram of resistive pressure (Marini et al., 1985a, 1986b). The elastic pressure component appears triangular because the pressure-volume characteristic of the respiratory system is more or less linear throughout the tidal range (Agostoni and Hyatt, 1986). The "resistive" pressure component resembles a parallelogram because, to the extent that inspiratory resistance and flow remain constant, a fixed additional pressure increment is required to overcome nonelastic forces. Assuming a work trapezoid and no dynamic hyperinflation, mean inflation pressure (work per liter) can be estimated at the bedside from the simple measurement of peak dynamic (P_D) and peak static (P_S) pressures: $\bar{P} \simeq P_D - \frac{1}{2}P_S$ (Marini et al., 1986b). For example, if peak dynamic and static pressures were 30 and 20 cmH_2O, respectively, $\bar{P}$ would be $30 - \frac{1}{2}(20) = 20$ cmH_2O and the work per liter of ventilation would be 2.0 J/liter (1 J = 10 $cmH_2O \times 1$ liter). The product of $\bar{P}$ and minute ventilation ($\dot{V}_E$) yields the total work per minute of ventilation. The contour of the work trapezoid can change with alterations in resistance and compliance or with an increase in inspiratory flow rate; the trapezoid becomes more triangular in shape with a reduction in compliance and more rectangular in shape with any increase in flow or resistance in the system (Marini et al., 1986b).

It should be noted that calculations of the work requirement per liter, per breath, or per minute are highly dependent on the pattern of ventilation chosen. $\bar{P}$ can be reduced by lowering tidal volume, and thus, for any specified $\dot{V}_E$ and constant level of resistance, the total work rate per minute is minimized by choosing a small tidal volume—whatever the compliance characteristics of the chest may be. It stands to reason, therefore, that if used unaltered, measurements of work per liter of ventilation made during passive mechanical ventilation do not reflect the work of spontaneous breathing that occurs at different flow rates, flow profiles and tidal volumes.

Work of Spontaneous Breathing

To directly measure the external work of breathing during *spontaneous* breathing cycles, an estimate of pleural pressure must be obtained. This is usually accomplished with an esophageal balloon catheter (Baydur et al., 1982; Loring and Bruce, 1986). Because the lung is a passive structure, the relevant forcing pressure for gas flow and lung expansion remains $\Delta(P_{aw} - P_{pl})$ during spontaneous breathing. The area subtended by a tracing of this pressure against volume from the onset of inspiratory effort to end-inflation quantifies the inspiratory work of breathing across the lung, endotracheal tube, and ventilator circuitry (Fig. 4). The work done across the chest wall cannot be directly measured during spontaneous breathing because the relevant forcing pressure for volume change in the chest wall lies deep within the muscle fibers themselves and is therefore not reflected in the pleural pressure (which is a resultant force of increasingly negative value as inspiration proceeds, oppositely directed and tending to cause chest wall *deflation*). As an estimate for clinical purposes, the area under the esophageal pressure-volume curve described under passive, constant-flow conditions for the appropriate tidal volume is added to the pressure-volume area measured with the esophageal balloon (Otis, 1964; Peters, 1969). Another way of making this adjustment is first to divide tidal volume by the compliance of the passive chest wall to obtain its relaxed end-inflation distending pressure and then to multiply by V_T: chest wall work $\simeq V_T^2/2C$. Whether this additional work increment reflects the actual work of active chest wall expansion (and, more specifically, the work of the respiratory muscles) depends in part on any compliance changes in the chest wall owing to spontaneous muscular contraction and in part on the position from which the chest wall begins expansion. (Stored elastic energy may aid the inspiratory muscles at volumes below the equilibrium position of the chest wall.)

An esophageal balloon is not absolutely mandatory in estimating the work performed during spontaneous breathing. If passive conditions can be

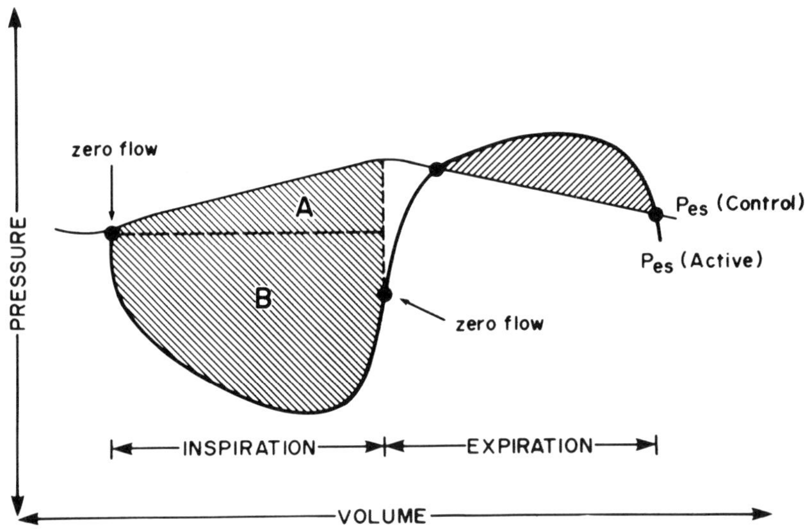

Figure 4 Measurement of inspiratory work (reverse cross-hatching, areas A and B) and expiratory work (cross-hatching) during a vigorous, spontaneous breath. The pressure-volume relationship for the relaxed chest wall (fine line) is made to intersect the active curve (heavy line) at the point corresponding to sharp inspiratory inflection of the simultaneous flow curve. When there is no dynamic hyperinflation (as depicted here), this occurs at the zero flow point. Area A is the work of chest wall inflation. Area B corresponds to work done across the lung and external circuit (From Marini et al., 1988, with permission.)

assured at the tidal volume and inspiratory flow rate that correspond to the spontaneous values, the passive airway pressure curve described during mechanical ventilation closely approximates the actual value computed from esophageal pressure measurements during spontaneous breathing (Marini et al., 1986d). Furthermore, it has recently been shown that the spontaneous work of breathing can also be closely estimated from the peak dynamic and peak static pressure values at normal settings for flow and tidal volume, provided that peak dynamic and peak static pressures are scaled in proportion to their spontaneous counterparts (Truwit et al., 1988). Then, $\bar{P}$ can be approximated as $\simeq$ 0.75 times the modified peak dynamic pressure (Milic-Emili, 1986; Truwit et al., 1988).

Another rough approximation of the mean inflation pressure (work per liter of ventilation) that corresponds to the spontaneously chosen values of flow and tidal volume can be made (assuming constant flow conditions) using a modification of the "equation of motion" (Otis, 1964):

$$P = \dot{V}R + \frac{V}{C} + P_{ex}$$

and

$$\bar{P} = \frac{V_T}{T_I}R + \frac{V_T}{2C} + \text{auto-PEEP}$$

In this calculation, V_T and T_I are tidal volume and inspiratory time, R and C are average values for inspiratory resistance and compliance, and P_{ex}, and auto-PEEP refer to alveolar pressures at end-exhalation. Such estimates of the work of breathing, although artificial in the sense that spontaneous flow is not truly constant, appear to yield acceptable estimates of the work of spontaneous breathing in the clinical setting. The components of the modified equation of motion—tidal volume, inspiratory time, resistance, and compliance—are standard clinical measurements. Auto-PEEP is not. Yet for the clinician, awareness of dynamic hyperinflation and quantification of the resultant auto-PEEP (intrinsic PEEP) is vitally important not only for work estimation, but for reasons related to hemodynamic performance and monitoring of the cardiopulmonary system.

Clinical Importance of Dynamic Hyperinflation

Dynamic hyperinflation occurs when insufficient expiratory time is allocated between tidal breathing cycles to re-establish the equilibrium position (where outward chest wall tension and inward lung recoil counterbalance), relieving net elastic alveolar tension (Bergman, 1972; Kimball et al., 1982). In this setting, flow continues throughout exhalation, with a continual disparity existing between alveolar pressure and pressure monitored in the central airway (Fig. 5). Only when expiratory flow is blocked at end-exhalation will pressures equilibrate between alveolus and central airway long enough to allow auto-PEEP (AP) to be estimated via the standard airway pressure monitor (Pepe and Marini, 1982). When the subject is passive, AP can also be quantified by delaying ventilator cycling to allow complete exhalation of the trapped volume (Tuxen and Lane, 1987). The quotient of this additional expired volume and thoracic compliance approximates the AP value. Another technique estimates AP as the machine pressure required at the onset of passive inflation to counterbalance alveolar pressure and initiate inspiratory flow (Rossi et al., 1985).

To start inspiratory flow, the patient must first put the brakes on exhalation, offsetting positive alveolar pressure with negative inspiratory force. This additional pressure increment adds to the inspiratory tension that must be developed during inspiration, boosting the $\bar{P}$ and total work of breathing. (The offsetting counterpressure is automatically provided by the ventilator

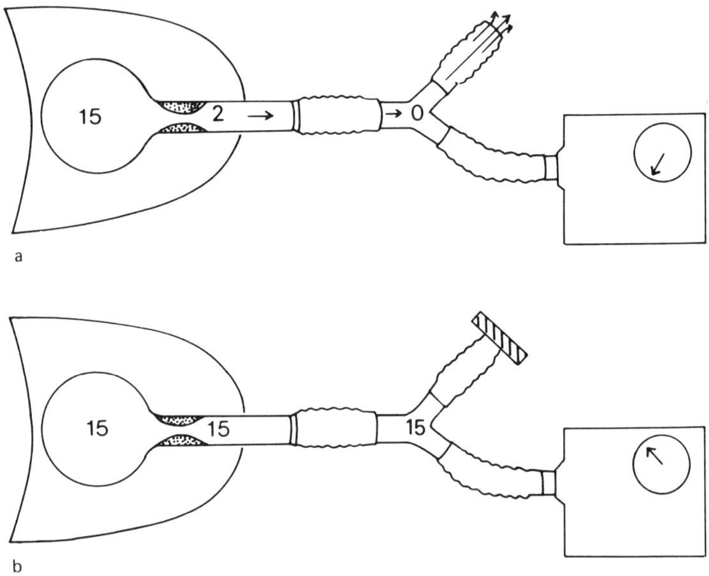

Figure 5 Dynamic hyperinflation and the measurement of auto-PEEP. (a) When expiratory resistance is too great to allow complete decompression of the thorax to the equilibrium position between inflation cycles, positive alveolar pressure and expiratory flow are maintained throughout exhalation. (b) An external manometer downstream from the major site of flow resistance does not record auto-PEEP unless an inspiratory cycle is delayed while expiratory flow is transiently (0.5-1.5 sec) stopped at end exhalation. (From O'Quin, R., and Marini, J. J. (1983). Pulmonary artery occlusion pressure: Clinical physiology, measurement, and interpretation. *Am. Rev. Respir. Dis.,* **128**:319-326, with permission.)

during passive inflation, and therefore the airway pressure tracing obtained under passive conditions includes the AP contribution to $\bar{P}$ and work.) During uninterrupted spontaneous breathing, therefore, the AP level can be estimated using simultaneous tracings of esophageal pressure and flow, provided that P_{es} and flow tracings are in phase. The difference in P_{es} that corresponds to the interval between the first inspiratory deflection of the expiratory flow tracing and the zero flow crossing point corresponds to the AP value.

The hyperinflating effect of auto-PEEP must be taken into account when calculating thoracic compliance (Rossi et al., 1985). Unaccounted for, the apparent pressure needed to achieve a volume will be offset by that amount, falsely lowering the $\Delta V/\Delta P$ (compliance) ratio.

Machine-Assisted Breathing Cycles

When attempting to quantify the patient's work of breathing during triggered or machine-assisted breathing cycles, the "push-pull" nature of the pumping system must be taken into account. The types of patient-initiated assisted breath encountered in the clinical setting are the machine-assisted constant flow, volume-cycled breaths of the assist-control (AMV) or synchronized intermittent mandatory ventilation (SIMV) modes, and the constant-pressure, variable-volume breaths of pressure support ventilation. During the triggered cycles of AMV or SIMV, the patient lowers central airway pressure by 1-2 cmH_2O, signaling the ventilator to activate, to pressurize the airway, and to accomplish the work of breathing (Fig. 6). Conceptually, the patient

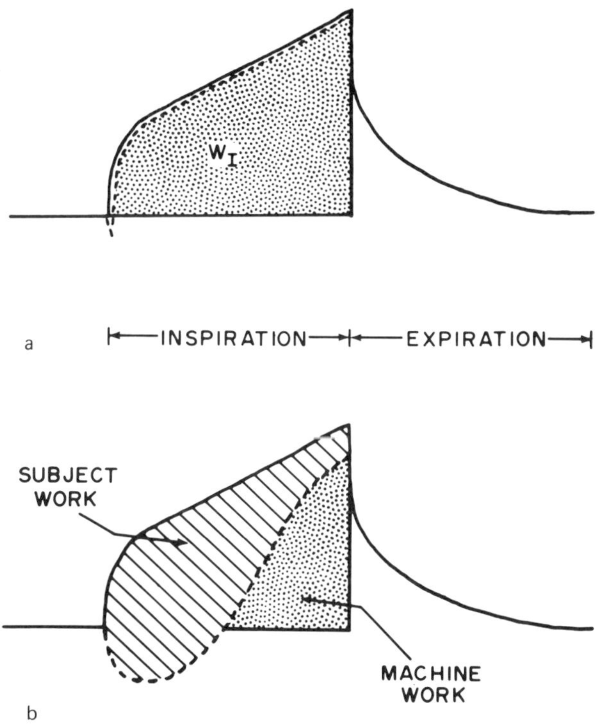

a

b

Figure 6 Calculation of the subject's inspiratory work of breathing during a triggered machine cycle (constant flow) from a plot of airway pressure and volume. (a) Conceptually, the patient would only need to lower airway pressure a small amount before the machine would pressurize to perform the entire inspiratory work of breathing (WI). (b) To the extent that inspiratory effort continues, work is done, quantified by the deficit in machine work between controlled and assisted cycles. (Modified from Marini et al., 1986a, with permission.)

would cease effort after machine activation and would, therefore, do minimal breathing work. The ventilator in turn would do the same amount as during a passive (controlled) cycle. In fact, however, patients do not immediately ease effort with flow onset, and to the extent that the respiratory muscles continue to contract during the machine-aided cycle, the effective "compliance" of the system is improved. The machine therefore needs to perform less work to achieve the same tidal volume and flow. If lung volume and the total work required to inflate the lung-chest wall system remain unchanged (questionable, but not unreasonable assumptions), then any discrepancy in machine work between controlled and triggered machine cycles of identical flow and tidal volume quantifies the work done by the subject during the assisted cycle (Fig. 5) (Marini, 1988b; Marini et al., 1986a). When this irregular pressure-volume area is computed and divided by the volume corresponding to the effort time, the mean inflation pressure provided by the subject ($\bar{P}$) can be quantified. Passive and active curves must be matched at the point of onset of inspiratory effort.

Because all efforts originate in the muscles of the chest wall, the patient's work of breathing can be computed in a similar fashion using esophageal pressure-volume curves recorded under control and assist conditions (Fig. 7). (Marini, 1988a; Marini et al., 1986a). Again, passive and active curves must be matched at the point of onset of inspiratory effort. When there is auto-PEEP, this matching point occurs at the point of inspiratory flow inflection prior to zero flow crossing. Even assuming similar tidal volume and flow settings, such estimations of patient work of breathing will be in error if there are changes in the lung volume or impedance of the chest between the times of recording the "matched" control and assist curves. A change in lung or chest wall compliance between the times at which the control and assisted curves were inscribed will influence the accuracy of both airway and esophageal pressure-based estimates. Unlike the airway pressure, however, the esophageal pressure method is not influenced by changes in airway resistance that occur between the time of assisted and controlled cycle recording. Perhaps, therefore, it is preferable when long periods elapse between the two types of recorded cycle during which such changes can occur (Smith et al., 1988; Truwit and Marini, 1988).

For pressure support cycles, a variant of this technique (employing esophageal pressure) is the only one commonly available to measure subject work (Truwit and Marini, 1988). The esophageal pressure-volume area is quantified in a fashion similar to that for spontaneous cycles. To this is added a triangular work segment that corresponds to the chest wall expansion component, as previously described. (Again, variations in flow profile do not substantially affect the work expended in expanding the chest wall.) Note that, when used alone, airway pressure profiles are of little help in attempt-

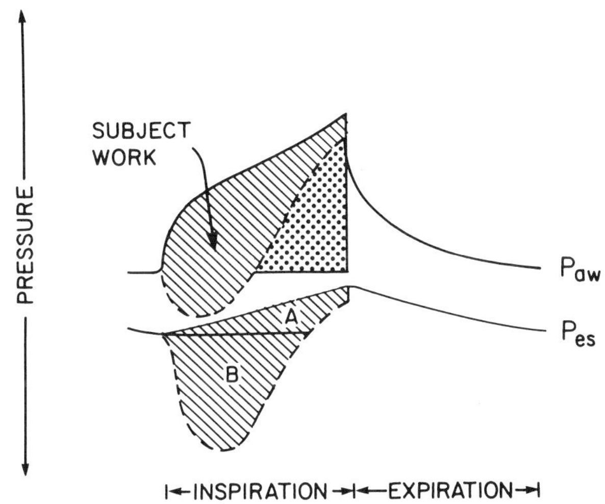

Figure 7 Two methods of computing subject work during machine-assisted cycles from active and passive plots of airway pressure P_{aw} and esophageal pressure P_{es}. Area A represents subject work done across the chest wall, whereas area B represents subject work expended across the lung and external circuit: (——) control; (---) assist. (Modified from Marini, 1988a, with permission.)

ing to assess patient effort during pressure support. For example, if patient effort accelerates flow, the work performed by the machine (the pressure-flow integral) can actually be *greater* during the pressure-supported breath than during the pressure-controlled breath for identical levels of airway pressure and tidal volume. Variations in the flow profile between pressure-controlled and pressure-assisted breaths change the frictional component of work between these types of cycle, violating the "constant work" assumption employed during flow-controlled, volume-cycled breathing (Marini, 1988a; Truwit and Marini, 1988). Recently, a sophisticated computer-aided method utilizing airway pressure and flow information has been described (Kreit et al., 1988), but such methodology requires complex signal processing and extensive clinical validation.

Relation of Work and Pressure Computations to Effort

Absolute measurements of average inflation pressure have limited usefulness in gauging patient effort unless they are viewed against the capability of the subject to generate them. It has long been known that the product of tension and time correlates with the rates of energy usage and oxygen consumption by exercising muscle (Sarnoff et al., 1958). Because the tension of the respiratory muscles cannot be directly measured, pressure—a value that correlates well with global tension for any individual subject—has been widely substituted (Roussos and Macklem, 1977). It should be noted at this point, however, that muscle tension translates only very imprecisely to pressure development, depending on the mechanical advantage of the system. For example, if inspiratory and expiratory muscle tensions were to exactly offset one another, there would be no pressure development in either direction, whatever the oxygen consumption and energy utilization might be. Similarly, if the contracting muscle is ineffectively oriented to develop inspiratory or expiratory pressure, tension does not produce a major change in the measured pressure. For example, when flattened or inverted by hyperinflation, the diaphragm (an inspiratory muscle) is a better generator of expiratory than inspiratory pressure.

One method of normalizing the measured pressure and work values recorded by the techniques just outlined is to relate them to capability using the maximal pressure or maximal pressure-time product that the individual is capable of generating (Bellemare and Grassino, 1982; Roussos and Moxham, 1985). For the diaphragm, this force-time measure is computed as the ratio of average diaphragmatic pressure per tidal breath (P_{dI}) divided by maximum diaphragmatic pressure that can be generated under isometric conditions ($P_{dI_{max}}$), multiplied by the inspiratory time fraction, or duty cycle (T_I/T_{tot}).

Experimentally, it has been found that $P_{dI}/P_{dI_{max}}$ ratios cannot exceed $\simeq 0.5$ at a duty cycle of 0.4 without causing intolerable dyspnea or fatigue either in normal subjects or in patients with chronic obstructive pulmonary disease subjected to breathing loads (Bellemare and Grassino, 1982; Rochester and Arora, 1983; Rochester et al., 1979; Roussos and Macklem, 1977). If T_I/T_{tot} is allowed to change, the highest percentage of the maximum generable force that can be sustained will vary in the opposite direction; whatever the combination of time and pressure, there appears to be a critical pressure-time index of $\simeq 0.2$ that cannot be maintained indefinitely. Although much more data are available for individual muscles (e.g., the diaphragm) than for the integrated respiratory system, it seems reasonable to make such an extrapolation based upon what is currently known.

To compute a pressure-time index for the respiratory system would require knowledge of the relevant $\bar{P}$, P_{max}, T_I, and T_{tot}. The T_I/T_{tot} ratio can be easily measured from a tracing of airflow, or even more simply from a tracing of central airway pressure (Marini, 1988a). The resistance offered by the external circuitry induces sufficient airway pressure fluctuation to generate the timing information of interest around the end-expiratory pressure baseline. Furthermore, $\bar{P}$ can be computed with acceptable accuracy using the techniques already defined. In the clinical setting, then, the major problem in generating the $\bar{P}/P_{max}$ (or pressure-time) index relates to assessment of the maximum inspiratory pressure.

As is widely appreciated, inspiratory P_{max} is influenced by the lung volume at which that inspiratory pressure is generated, especially at lung volumes greater than the equilibrium point (FRC) (Black and Hyatt, 1969). Furthermore, full patient cooperation is necessary to elicit values of pressure close to the maximum values of which the patient is capable. However, the full cooperation of critically ill patients can rarely be guaranteed. Experimentally, high-frequency stimulation of the phrenic nerves can be used to generate near-maximal pressures across the diaphragm. Unfortunately, this technique can be painful and there is no clinical method by which to externally stimulate all inspiratory muscles of the thorax in a coordinated fashion.

At the bedside, maximal pressure is usually recorded by trapping lung volume at FRC and occluding the airway for several breaths while the patient is instructed to forcefully inspire. We have recently shown that inclusion of a one-way valve (selectively allowing expiration) improves the pressures generated and that occlusion must be sustained for at least 20 sec in poorly cooperative subjects before a plateau of negative pressure is reached (Fig. 8) (Marini et al., 1986c). After 20-25 sec, even critically ill, ventilator-dependent

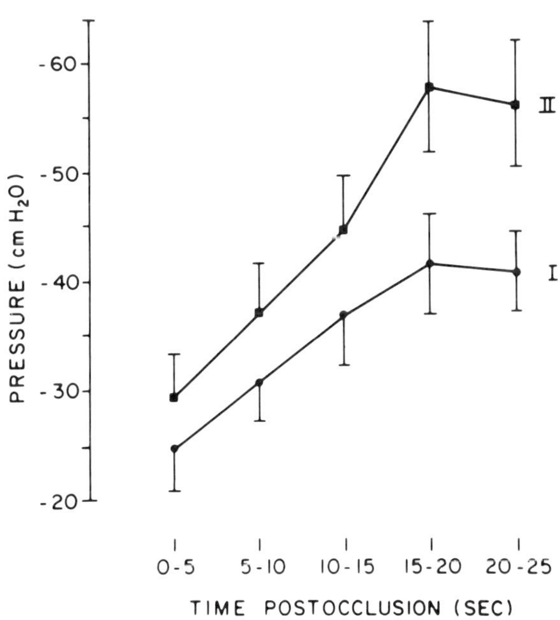

Figure 8 Maximal inspiratory pressures generated during prolonged airway occlusion without (I) and with a one-way expiratory valve inserted into the exhalation line (II). Patients were not coached when making these assessments. (From Marini et al., 1986c, with permission.)

patients usually generate pressures in excess of -40 cmH_2O, casting doubt upon the discriminatory accuracy of currently used weaning criteria for maximum inspiratory pressure (usually suggested to be -25 to -30 cmH_2O) (Sahn et al., 1976). The relationship of the maximum inspiratory pressure spontaneously generated by endogenous breathing efforts during such an airway occlusion maneuver to the maximum voluntary pressure that can be achieved at the same volume is currently unknown (but under investigation). Whether the pressure-time indices developed using such techniques in critically ill patients correspond to those reported in the literature for cooperative subjects hinges largely on the P_{max} measurement and is currently a question widely open to debate.

C. How Much Work Is the Patient Doing During Mechanical Ventilation?

Quantitation of force output or work performance in relation to maximum capability would seem to be crucial information for the physician attempting therapeutic modification of breathing stress. It may or may not be necessary or desirable to minimize the work of breathing during mechanical ventilation, depending on the therapeutic goal. If the objective is to reverse fatigue, then near-total rest of the respiratory system would seem the most effective way to reestablish balance. If the goal is to prevent atrophy, modest exercise might be prescribed. Strength and endurance building would require intermittent high stress and protracted moderate stress, respectively.

In approaching the question of quantifying effort during mechanical ventilation, we recently attempted to characterize breathing effort over the entire spectrum of machine support during critical illness (Marini et al., 1988). For this we selected the mode of synchronized intermittent mandatory ventilation, which juxtaposes natural spontaneous breaths with the machine-aided ("deafterloaded") breaths called for by the patient. By using SIMV we were able to vary the level of support yet compare the work performed by the patient during adjacent spontaneous and machine-aided cycles at fixed levels of chemical drive. Thus, we were also able to assess how well the patient adapts breathing effort to machine assistance within the time span of a single effort. We studied 12 acutely ill patients who were not considered candidates for weaning from mechanical ventilation. The great majority of these patients had acute restrictive illnesses, that is, the adult respiratory distress syndrome (ARDS), pneumonia, and congestive heart failure. We included no patient whose primary problem was obstructive lung disease. In each patient we tested the spectrum of machine support, ranging from fully assisted breathing (100% SIMV, or AMV) to fully spontaneous breathing (0% SIMV). We quantified the work performed by the patient for each type of cycle (spontaneous or machine-assisted) at each level of support.

Breathing frequency increased as average tidal volume fell during SIMV withdrawal. $\dot{V}_E$ remained unchanged. Even during fully assisted breathing, our patients performed considerable work per liter of ventilation, which averaged ≃0.7 J/liter at 100% SIMV (Fig. 9). Thus, the average inspiratory pressure $\bar{P}$ developed by the patient was approximately 7 cmH_2O for each tidal breath. This value corresponded to the expected level of work performed by a healthy subject breathing at a similar minute ventilation (≃ 14 liters/min) (Fleury et al., 1985; Peters, 1969). As SIMV support was withdrawn, there was a progressive and nearly linear increase in $\bar{P}$ over the range of 100-40% SIMV, with leveling off in $\bar{P}$ with further decrements in machine assistance (Fig. 9). Interestingly, at each level of support the pressure developed per spontaneous breath was only about 20% higher than that developed during adjacent machine-aided cycles, and the duration of inspiratory effort was actually longer during machine assistance by a similar percentage. Thus, the pressure-time product per inspiration ($\bar{P} \times T_I$) a correlate of the energy consumed by the contracting respiratory muscles showed no systematic difference between spontaneous and machine-aided cycles at any given level of support. These data suggest that the dyspneic patient does not adapt on a breath-by-breath basis to the "unloading" of the breath by airway pressurization.

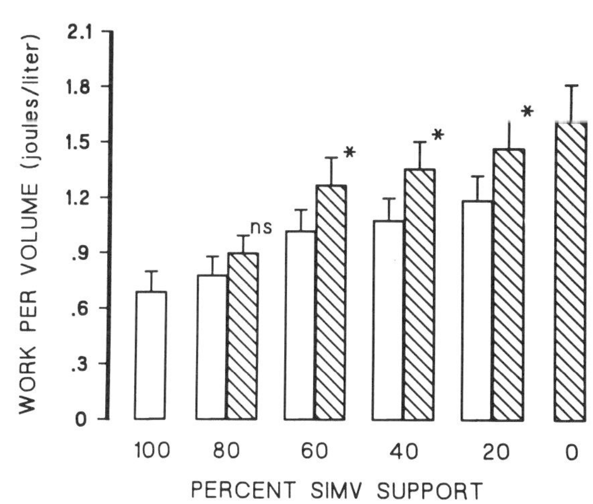

Figure 9 Work per liter of ventilation (mean inflation pressure) during synchronized intermittent mandatory ventilation (SIMV). Significant (*, $p < 0.05$) differences occurred between types of cycle at the lower levels of machine support: (□) assist; (▧) spont. (From Marini et al., 1988, with permission.)

It is instructive to calculate the relative work output of side-by-side spontaneous and machine-assisted breaths. When the work per breath during SIMV was calculated for both types of cycle, the machine-aided cycles were accompanied by *greater* work output per breath than the spontaneous cycles (Fig. 10).Although this finding would seem on the surface to be paradoxical, the results become more understandable when a direct parallel is drawn with the unloading of the heart during congestive failure. As the failing heart is deafterloaded, stroke volume increases at similar systemic pressure, increasing the stroke work of the ventricle (Sagawa, 1978). In other words, for the same contractile effort, work output increases as afterload is reduced. The object lesson is that mechanical measurements of external work do not necessarily reflect patient effort under varying conditions of system loading; the mechanical work output of a system is highly dependent on its loading conditions.

The contraction of the respiratory muscle can be thought of as having isometric and isotonic components. When the system is severely loaded (e.g., by airflow obstruction), there is a large isometric component, in that high tension needs to be developed to maintain slow flow. For the same level of stimulation, flow decreases as pressure increases. Thus, despite enormous effort during exacerbations of chronic obstructive pulmonary disease, measured external mechanical work actually is not a great deal higher than during

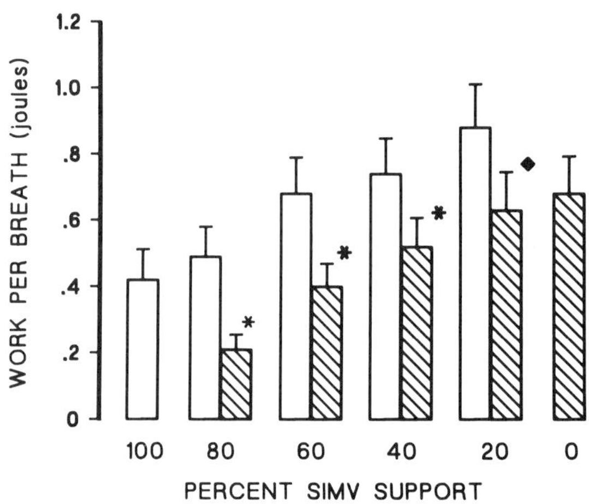

Figure 10 Work per breath during SIMV. Note that work output per breath was significantly greater (*, $p < 0.05$) for machine-assisted cycles at each level: (□) assist; (▨) spont. (From Marini et al., 1988, with permission.)

the efforts of a normal subject breathing at the same minute ventilation—in extreme circumstances it might even be less.

During machine assistance (whether this be during an AMV cycle or a pressure-supported cycle), the work performed by the patient has greatly different pressure-volume characteristics than during an unassisted cycle. During spontaneous breaths high pressures are generated and small volumes are moved, whereas during machine-assisted breaths less pressure is generated but a greater volume change occurs. Such improved length-tension relationships may help to explain (along with modest reductions in the absolute amount of breathing work being done) the marked improvement in dyspnea and sense of well-being that occur during machine assistance (Campbell, 1966).

Although the absolute value of external work itself may be an unreliable indicator of the stress placed on the system, the effort required of the patient is well indexed by the $\bar{P}/P_{max}$ ratio or by the pressure-time index (Grassino and Macklem, 1984). When we computed these effort indices during SIMV (using prolonged one-way valve occlusion to measure P_{max}), our calculated values for $\bar{P}/P_{max}$ and for the PTI index were comfortably below the fatiguing levels reported in the literature only at the 80 and 100% SIMV support levels. Again, our data must be interpreted cautiously, in that we do not know how closely our P_{max} value approximated the true maximum voluntary pressures theoretically available to the patient. Nonetheless, our data suggest that most acutely ill patients who trigger the mechanical ventilator perform substantial amounts of breathing work in relation to their capacity. These levels appear to exceed those needed to prevent atrophy, based on the meager information available in the literature that has addressed this topic (Braun, 1988). We believe it distinctly possible that under conditions of high inflation impedance, muscle weakness, and increased minute ventilation requirement the patient could be pushed to the brink of fatigue, despite receiving substantial ventilatory assistance. Such effort may help to explain why some patients continue to retain carbon dioxide although ventilator supported and fully alert.

D. Minimizing the Work of Breathing During Mechanical Ventilation

The primary interventions available to the physician to reduce the work of breathing during mechanical ventilation are to reduce ventilatory demand to minimize dynamic hyperinflation and to improve the impedance characteristics of the respiratory system (Table 2). The importance of reducing ventilatory demand cannot be overstressed. In critically ill patients, increased CO_2 production may originate from fever, shivering, pain or agitation, trauma, sepsis, or overfeeding or from the workload of breathing itself. Increased

Table 2 Minimizing the Breathing Work Load During Mechanical Ventilation

Reduce ventilatory demand
↓ CO_2 production
↓ Deadspace
↓ Ventilatory drive
Correct metabolic acidosis
Reduce psychogenic stress
Maintain adequate Pa_{O_2}
Consider sedation
Improve respiratory impedance
↓ Airflow resistance
Improve secretion clearance
Reverse bronchospasm
Reduce circuit resistance
↑ Thoracic compliance
Diuresis
PEEP/CPAP
Synchronize machine output to patient demand
Improve breathing efficiency
↓ Auto-PEEP
Appropriate positioning

deadspace fractions are produced by virtually all forms of lung disease, by hypovolemia, by vascular occlusion, and, in certain cases, by the apparatus connecting the endotracheal tube to the Y point of the external circuit. Deadspace fractions as high as 0.7 are not unusual in severe cases of acute respiratory failure. Inappropriate neurogenic or psychogenic stimuli to hyperventilate and the need to compensate for metabolic acidosis can also boost the ventilatory requirement.

Ventilatory demand $\dot{V}_E$ is not only a primary component of the power ($\bar{P} \times \dot{V}_E$) calculation but in itself augments the tidal volume and inspiratory flow rate, thereby increasing the $\bar{P}$ coefficient as well. Furthermore, in patients with obstructive lung disease, $\dot{V}_E$ is a crucial determinant of the auto-PEEP level—a direct contributor to $\bar{P}$ and to the overall work of breathing (Fleury et al., 1985; Marini, 1988a; Milic-Emili, 1986; Truwit and Marini, 1988). In addition, the chest wall expansion that accompanies dynamic hyperinflation foreshortens the skeletal muscle fibers and places the inspiratory muscles at mechanical disadvantage, thereby reducing P_{max} while raising the $\bar{P}/P_{max}$ fraction. Hyperinflation also has obvious detrimental effects on venous return, on the risk of barotrauma, and on the ability to interpret pulmonary arterial occlusion pressure and chest compliance measurements (Pepe and Marini, 1982; Rossi et al., 1985). It must therefore be avoided and its adverse effects compensated.

Reducing Dynamic Hyperinflation

During mechanical ventilation, dynamic hyperinflation can be combated by reducing the minute ventilation requirement, by improving airflow resistance, and by changing the pattern of the breathing cycle. Although taking over the entire work of breathing for the patient would minimize ventilation-related CO_2 production, the negative intrathoracic pressure generated during spontaneous breathing efforts helps to reduce the average intrathoracic pressure and to improve cardiac output. Without question, controlled ventilation can be beneficial when the output demands of the exercising respiratory muscles stress a congested circulation whose output is limited by myocardial failure. However, when preload is a major problem, the benefits of fully controlled ventilation to cardiovascular function are marginal or negative, unless minute ventilation (and auto-PEEP) are reduced sufficiently to lower mean intrathoracic pressure. Thus, for many patients with AP, the assist-control (AMV) mode (rather than controlled mode) may be the best compromise. Of course, other measures should be undertaken simultaneously to reduce the minute ventilation requirement, as already outlined.

Curtailing the inspiratory duty cycle will maximize the time spent in exhalation and thereby help to reduce dynamic hyperinflation, but the benefits are limited and variable. Reductions of T_I require faster inspiratory airflow and increased inspiratory airway pressure. Similarly, adjustments of tidal volume and frequency have little effect so long as $\dot{V}_E$ remains unchanged.

Improving Airflow Resistance

Secretion accumulation, mucosal edema, and bronchospasm contribute greatly to resistance of critically narrowed airways. Bronchodilators, infection control, and maintenance of good bronchial hygiene are crucial adjunctive measures.

Improving Thoracic Compliance

The measures needed to improve lung compliance are largely self-evident: treating infiltrative disease, diuresis, draining air and fluid from the pleural space, decompression of the abdomen, and optimal positioning of the patient. Clearing the fluid from grossly edematous lungs also reduces the ratio of total thoracic volume to the gas volume subcomponent (Scharf and Ingram,

1977), reducing chest wall dimensions and modestly improving muscular efficiency at any specified volume. It is less commonly recognized that the application of positive end-expiratory pressure can improve the compliance characteristics of the lung by recruiting collapsed lung tissue, thereby enlarging the alveolar compartment and improving effective compliance. Once the lung is fully recruited, however, further increases in lung volume tend to reduce effective compliance as the lung and chest wall approach their elastic limits. Again, the attendant hyperinflation disadvantages the respiratory muscles, increasing ventilatory effort.

Improving the Resistance of the Ventilator Circuit

Endotracheal Tube

Assuming that the clinical factors that contribute to chest impedance and to minute ventilation requirement have been addressed, attention should turn to the ventilator circuit itself. It is well known that endotracheal tubes contribute to the total resistance the patient must overcome. Tube resistance, a power function of flow (Gottfried et al., 1985), relates inversely to the fourth power of the radius of the endotracheal tube and directly to its length (Demers et al., 1977). Because of diameter and length considerations, tracheostomy tubes are less resistive than orotracheal tubes, which are in turn less resistive than nasotracheal tubes. Although these concepts are generally well understood, the magnitude of their impact is less commonly appreciated. Secretions, kinking, tip malposition, and other phenomena that occur in situ can dramatically increase the resistance of a fresh tube. In patients with adult respiratory distress syndrome, we have recently found that #8 orotracheal tubes approximately double an already increased level of airflow resistance (Wright et al., 1988). Furthermore, the endotracheal tube resistance is increased in vivo over that measured in vitro prior to insertion. It should be noted that the resistance presented by the endotracheal tube during spontaneous breathing cannot be gauged from the tracing of central airway pressure that in other respects proves so useful. The relevant pressure to gauge the inspiratory resistance of the endotracheal tube during spontaneous breathing is that measured at its carinal tip and referenced to central airway pressure (Marini, 1987). For this purpose, a thin catheter attached to the same type of pressure transducer normally used for pulmonary artery or central airway pressure measurement may be threaded through a large endotracheal tube to record the tracheal pressure deflections. The flatter the inspiratory contour of this pressure tracing, the less resistance is presented by the tube (in combination with the remainder of the inspiratory circuit). The contribution of the tube itself is judged by the difference between the tracheal and external airway pressures. Tube and external circuit resistance assume increasing importance as $\dot{V}E$ increases. Not only does increasing flow $\dot{V}$ raise the pressure increment required, but developing turbulence alters the effective resistance, as reflected by Rohrer's equation:

$$\frac{P_{res}}{\dot{V}} = K_1 + K_2\dot{V}$$

Here P_{res} is the total pressure driving flow $\dot{V}$ and K_1 and K_2 are constants (Rohrer, 1915). Lowering $\dot{V}E$ and replacing a nasal tube with a fresh, large-diameter oral tube or tracheostomy will reduce the upper airway pressure requirement. In certain cases extubation may allow machine withdrawal from a patient who while intubated is otherwise unable to sustain breathing through the circuit.

By augmenting central airway pressure throughout patient-initiated inspiration, pressure support can help compensate for such increases in upper airway resistance (Kacmarek, 1988). Given that the minimal airway resistance offered by a clean, large-diameter endotracheal tube is in the range of 3-5 cmH_2O, it would seem prudent to add 3-5 cmH_2O of pressure support to most patients required to breathe spontaneously through the ventilator's circuitry (Fig. 11).

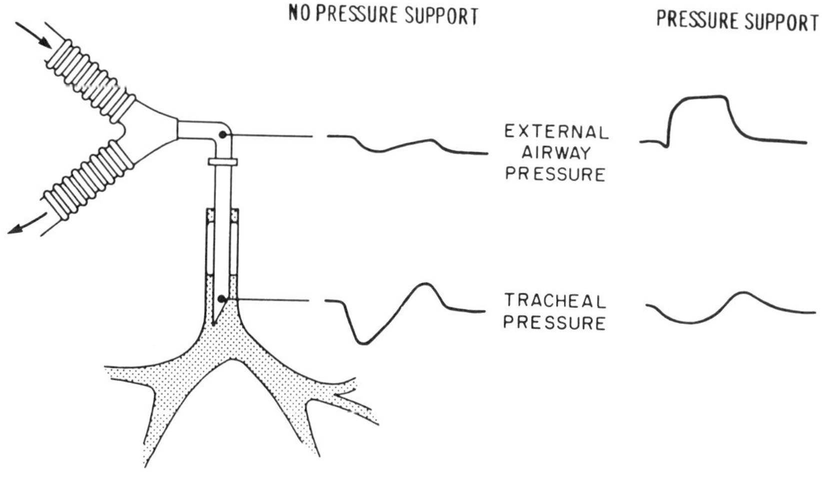

Figure 11 Effect of endotracheal tube resistance on airway and tracheal pressures. The addition of pressure support attenuates the inspiratory effort required, as reflected by the tracheal pressure configuration.

Inspiratory Valve and Connecting Tubing

The inspiratory portion of the ventilator circuit proximal to the endotracheal tube may be of crucial importance to the magnitude of spontaneous inspiratory work. The central (external) airway pressure is an invaluable aid in gauging the work across the inspiratory circuit beyond the endotracheal tube. Whatever the set level of end-expiratory pressure, atmospheric or positive (CPAP), the objective is to maintain the central airway pressure tracing during spontaneous cycles with minimal ripple. Until recently it has generally been believed that continuous flow systems provide conditioned gas flow at minimal energy cost when compared to systems that employ demand valves to meter insiratory gas flow (Gibney et al., 1982). This is not necessarily the case, however. Systems that employ moderate continuous flows, maintaining the set level of end-expiratory pressure against moderately high resistance, are not designed to meet vigorous inspiratory flow demands. Consequently, pressures within the central airway and trachea can fall dramatically during forceful breathing as the patient expends additional energy against friction in the ventilator circuitry. In recent years, systems that employ high baseline flows that can be suddenly augmented by an elastic reservoir or high-pressure source have alleviated many of these problems (Katz et al., 1985; Viale et al., 1985). Some of the newer systems attempt to maintain an unchanging central airway pressure by using flow sensors to regulate the gas flowing in the inspiratory and expiratory limbs, augmenting the machine flow as needed to meet demand. Pressure swings and the clinical importance of differences among systems tend to widen as $\dot{V}_E$ and the inspiratory flow rate increase.

The flow-resistive characteristics of the expiratory side also deserve consideration. Several groups of investigators have demonstrated impressive resistance through standard exhalation valve systems (Banner, 1987; Marini et al., 1985b). Although expiratory valve resistance is usually overcome with energy stored in and released from the elastic components of the respiratory system, additional expiratory muscular effort must be expended when this reserve potential energy is no longer sufficient. The alternative is hyperinflation, with consequent impairment of inspiratory muscle function. Interposition of expiratory resistance also leads to dyspnea during forceful breathing.

Influence of Machine Settings on the Work of Breathing

A number of physician-selectable parameters influence the work done during triggered, volume-controlled machine cycles. In the absence of system leaks, volume control ensures that each breath triggered from the machine provides a breath of the selected size. However, the ventilator's flow profile, mean flow rate, and cycle duration are invariant and stereotyped, failing to correspond to naturally selected patterns. At the ample flow settings usually selected, the machine can usually complete the inflation cycle without vigorous opposition from the patient. However, when there is significant mismatching between the rates of ventilator flow delivery and patient inspiratory demand, when the patient's breathing rhythm is chaotic, or when the tidal volume selected is inappropriate for the patient needs, the potential exists for significant work to be conducted by the patient against the inspiratory circuit of the ventilator. Furthermore, expiratory work must be done against circuit elements when exhalation becomes an active process, as it does during vigorous breathing or when the patient's exhalation cycle precedes the conclusion of flow delivery.

Pressure support ventilation (PSV), a mode of machine assistance in which each triggered cycle is aided by a selected amount of airway pressure, yields control of the cycle length and flow profile to the patient (Banner, 1987). PSV not only reduces the breathing work load in proportion to its set level, but by increasing the volume moved per unit of patient-generated pressure also changes the character and efficiency of the effort (Brochard et al., 1987; MacIntyre, 1986).

The clinician controls a number of parameters that influence the patient's work of breathing during triggered volume-limited machine cycles. In most cases, tidal voluime is set to exceed that spontaneously taken, usually 8-12 ml/kg body weight. Few guidelines exist, however, to indicate the importance of machine triggering sensitivity, inspiratory flow rate, and positive end-expiratory pressure on the patient's work load during triggered cycles. Furthermore, the impact of variations in the patient's endogenous impedance to breathing on the work of machine-aided cycles is not commonly known.

To answer these questions we conducted a series of clinical experiments in normal subjects and in critically ill patients receiving volume-cycled, assist-controlled ventilation. The influence of the flow rate, minute ventilation requirement, and triggering sensitivity were first explored in normal subjects (Kreit et al., 1988). Active work by the subject was assessed in the fashion already described using pressure-volume information inscribed during controlled and assist-control breathing. In that study, we found that CO_2-stimulated hyperpnea sufficient to double the minute ventilation requirement not only increased the overall work of breathing but also increased the work performed per liter of ventilation (i.e., the mean inflation pressure $\bar{P}$). Despite ventilator assistance, our normal subjects performed work at rates that corresponded closely to values predicted for spontaneous breathing at a similar minute ventilation. Although inspiratory flow settings (nominally 80 or 100 liters/min) made no difference to the work performed during baseline levels of minute ventilation ($\simeq 12$ liters/min), the lower flow rate was associated with an increased work rate (higher $\bar{P}$) when these subjects were stimulated to double their ventilation ($\simeq$24 liters/min). Reducing the triggering sensitivity from -2 to -5 cmH_2O/breath increased the active breathing work load at both levels of ventilation.

The influence of minute ventilation, flow rate, and impedance to breathing were then studied in a group of critically ill patients with diverse pulmonary and nonpulmonary problems (Fleury et al., 1985). None of these patients were severely obstructed or had auto-PEEP levels that exceeded 2-3 cmH_2O. As in our normal subjects, stimulation by CO_2 rebreathing markedly increased the patient work rate, expressed as $\bar{P}$. Surprisingly, however, we found no significant influence of peak flow setting (60 and 100 liters/min) on the work performed at either level of $\dot{V}_E$ we tested. Likewise, the resistance and compliance characteristics of the thorax did not influence the measured $\bar{P}$. The reason for the inability of variations in the peak flow setting to influence the work/liter of ventilation was revealed in a comparison of the measured rates of spontaneous inspiratory flow with that provided by the machine. Upon transient disconnection of the mechanical ventilator, 15 of 16 patients demonstrated mean spontaneous inspiratory flow rates less than the lower of the two flow settings we employed (60 liters/min). Only 4 patients exhibited spontaneous peak flow values exceeding 60 liters/min.

The major implications of these studies were that in normal subjects and in patients without obstructive lung disease only ventilatory drive and the inherent strength of the patient determine how much work is performed during a triggered, volume-limited machine cycle, provided that the rates of flow delivered from the machine match or exceed the patient's spontaneous demand. Under these circumstances, the resistance and compliance characteristics of the thorax do not impact on the amount of work the subject performs; that component is met by the powerful pressure-generating potential of the machine. (Indeed, if the patient relaxes immediately after the breath is triggered, the machine performs the entire work of breathing, as suggested by the idealized waveform of Fig. 6.)

Factors that increase the patient's work of breathing during triggered cycles, therefore, are those that influence drive or muscle strength. Apart from the $\dot{V}_E$ commanded by the patient itself, drive can be augmented by reducing the trigger sensitivity, by asynchrony between patient and ventilator cycling rhythms, by inappropriate PEEP settings, by inappropriate tidal volume settings, and, perhaps, by inappropriate peak flow settings and flow profiles. Muscle weakness and supraoptimal PEEP settings impair the patient's ability to perform work. Flow delivery from the machine must be set to exceed the patient's spontaneous demand. If flow delivery falls below the patient's need, the patient not only works against the intrinsic resistance and compliance characteristics of his own thorax but also against the imposed resistance of the endotracheal tube and inspiratory circuit of the machine. Such an event is signaled by an airway pressure tracing that dips substantially below the end-expiratory pressure baseline for a substantial fraction of inspiration. Thus, maintenance of an appropriate flow setting is vital to patient work and comfort. Nonetheless, excessive flows are of no benefit regarding patient work during triggered machine cycles and may actually increase it if they produce discomfort.

Dynamic Hyperinflation, Trigger Sensitivity, and Inadvertent Threshold Loading

As shown by these studies, the triggering sensitivity of the ventilator was an important component of the patient's work of breathing, adversely influencing the level of ventilatory drive (Fleury et al., 1985). It is generally assumed that the triggering sensitivity of the mechanical ventilator is adjusted by the clinician. However, patients who demonstrate dynamic hyperinflation and auto-PEEP have an end-expiratory alveolar pressure that must be counterbalanced before pressure in the central airway can become subatmospheric. No inspiratory flow can begin and the machine will not trigger until the sum of the machine's set trigger sensitivity plus the auto-PEEP level has been overcome by inspiratory effort. In effect, the triggering sensitivity of the machine cycle has been impaired, since a large negative pressure deflection is required to drop central airway pressure even a minimal amount. As a result, some weakened and severely hyperinflated patients fail to trigger the ventilator, despite substantial inspiratory effort relative to their power reserve.

In a recently reported study, we demonstrated that the deliberate addition of low levels of end-expiratory pressure could be beneficial in reducing the work of breathing in patients with measurable auto-PEEP (Smith and Marini, 1988). We studied 10 pharmacologically paralyzed patients with exacerbated chronic obstructive pulmonary disease who exhibited $\geq$5 cmH_2O auto-PEEP during controlled ventilation at a $\dot{V}E$ equivalent to that commanded spontaneously. Some of our patients experienced dramatic reductions in the total work of breathing during AMV when low-level PEEP was added, whereas others showed only modest changes. On average, the work of breathing diminished significantly. During that study we found that PEEP also tended to improve the expiratory flow resistive characteristics at mid- and end-exhalation. Furthermore, the peak (inspiratory) static cycling pressure of the ventilator rose much less than expected when low levels of PEEP (less than the original auto-PEEP) were applied. Once the original auto-PEEP level had been exceeded by added PEEP, there was an approximate 1:1 correspondence between further additions in PEEP and the change in end-inspiratory cycling pressure.

The beneficial effect of PEEP on the work performed by patients with auto-PEEP, we believe, is explicable during this mode of ventilation by an improvement in machine triggering sensitivity (Fig. 12). (After all, no work would be done by the patient if relaxation were to occur immediately after the machine were cycled.) By adding positive end-expiratory pressure downstream of a critical airflow limitation, the effective triggering threshold of the machine can be decreased (Fig. 10). Provided that alveolar pressure at end-exhalation fails to rise in proportion to central airway pressure, the discrepancy between end-expiratory alveolar pressure and central airway pressure is narrowed, improving trigger sensitivity (Smith and Marini, 1988).

It must be emphasized, however, that any such benefit may fundamentally depend on what factors are responsible for generating auto-PEEP. Auto-PEEP can develop for at least three different reasons. Auto-PEEP can arise in subjects with normal mechanics if minute ventilation is so high (greater than 20-25 liters/min) that relaxed equilibrium position cannot be re-established by passive deflation before the onset of the next machine-delivered breath. In this setting, no dynamic airway collapse occurs. The healthy subject then has two options. The first is to dynamically hyperinflate—the option chosen by the patient with chronic obstructive pulmonary disease. Because airway resistance is minimal, end-expiratory alveolar pressure and central airway pressure are not greatly different from one another, and the addition of PEEP would be expected to increase alveolar and central airway pressures by similar amounts, possibly with detrimental effects on hyperinflation, the risk of barotrauma, and inspiratory muscle efficacy.

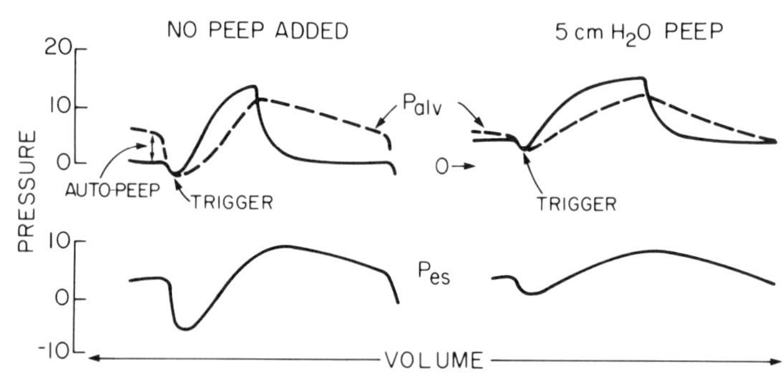

Figure 12 Impact of auto-PEEP on trigger sensitivity and inspiratory effort. To trigger a machine cycle, alveolar pressure PA must fall by the amount of auto-PEEP, plus the set trigger sensitivity. The large dip in esophageal pressure P_{es} reflects this effort. The addition of PEEP downstream from dynamically compressed airways reduces the PA-P_{aw} gradient and attenuates the breathing work load, without a significant increase in end-inspiratory PA.

The second option is to contract the expiratory muscles vigorously to augment expiratory flow. If this action continues throughout exhalation, there may be a component of muscular activity boosting alveolar pressure at end-expiration. Were this the case, the addition of external PEEP might permit storage of (outwardly directed) elastic recoil pressure in the chest wall, provided that a lung volume lower than that dictated by the equilibrium position (corresponding to the applied PEEP level) were achieved. This mechanism enables the expiratory muscles to share the inspiratory work burden. Such a strategy is adapted by some patients during the acute phase of ARDS when PEEP is applied (Coggeshall et al., 1985) and adopted by most normal subjects in the throes of virgorous upright exercise, when expiratory muscle contraction elevates the diaphragm and gravity provides the additional inspiratory pressure boost (Grimby et al., 1968). An increase in expiratory muscle activity, however, does not benefit the patient with critical airflow limitation, in whom auto-PEEP develops at very modest levels of ventilation. In this setting, contraction of expiratory muscles simply enhances dynamic collapse and air trapping, without speeding airflow. Very little, if any, inspiratory boost is achieved.

The airway pressure tracing inscribed during passive inflation at constant flow often gives a clue to the presence of auto-PEEP or to another PEEP-responsive condition—phasic recruitment and derecruitment during the tidal breathing cycle (O'Quin et al., 1985). The airway pressure tracing in both these circumstances is often highly rectangular in shape (Fig. 13) (Blanch et al., 1987; Marini, 1988a; Matamis et al., 1984). As a rule, such a finding should prompt a PEEP trial, as in both instances the patient may benefit from the modest addition of positive end-expiratory pressure.

In closing, it must be re-emphasized that despite the important manipulations of machine circuitry, settings, and pressures just described, perhaps

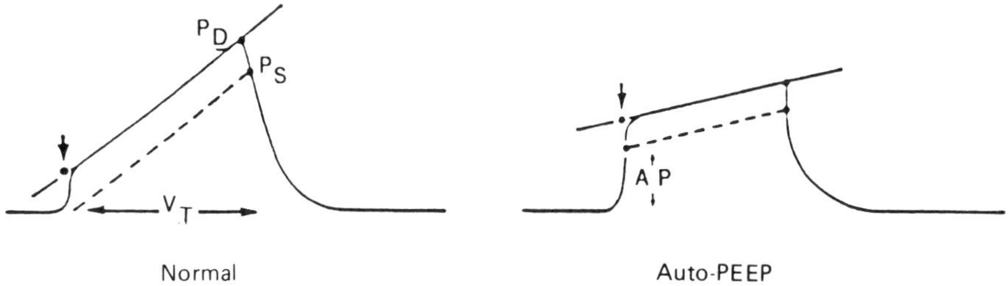

Figure 13 Alteration in the airway pressure profile of a controlled constant flow breath caused by auto-PEEP. The "squared-off" shoulder of pressure at inflation onset represents the sum of resistive pressure losses and the positive airway pressure necessary to counterbalance auto-PEEP.

the single most important factor acting to reduce total work of breathing is to reduce the ventilatory demand.

Acknowledgment

The author is indebted to Brenda F. Plunkett and Lisa Scherer for their skillful assistance in preparation of the typescript.

References

Agostoni, E., and Hyatt, R. E. (1986). Static behavior of the respiratory system. In *Handbook of Physiology*. Edited by A. P. Fishman, P. T. Macklem, and J. Mead. Bethesda, Maryland, American Physiological Society, Chap. 9, pp. 113-130.

Altose, M. D. (1986). Dyspnea. In *Current Pulmonology*, Vol. 7. Edited by D. H. Simmons. Year Book, Chicago. Chap. 7, pp. 199-226.

Aubier, M., Trippenbach, T., and Roussos, C. (1981). Respiratory muscle fatigue during cardiogenic shock. *J. Appl. Physiol.*, **51**:499-508.

Banner, M. J. (1987). Expiratory positive pressure valves: Flow resistance and work of breathing. *Respir. Care,* **32**:431-439.

Bartlett, R. G., Jr., Brubach, H. F., and Specht, H. (1958). Oxygen cost of breathing. *J. Appl. Physiol.*, **12**:413-424.

Baydur, A. Behrakis, K., Zin, W. A., et al. (1982). A simple method for assessing the validity of the esophageal balloon technique. *Am. Rev. Respir. Dis.*, **126**:788-791.

Bellemare, F., and Grassino, A. (1982). Effect of pressure and timing of contraction on human diaphragm fatigue. *J. Appl. Physiol.*, **53**:1190-1195.

Bergman, N. A. (1972). Pulmonary gas trapping during mechanical ventilation at rapid frequencies. *Anesthesiology,* **37**:626-633.

Bigland-Ritchie, B. (1984). Muscle fatigue and the influence of changing neural drive. *Clin. Chest Med.*, **5**:21-34.

Black, L. F., and Hyatt, R. E. (1969). Maximal respiratory pressures. Normal values and relationship to age and sex. *Am. Rev. Respir. Dis.*, **99**: 696-702.

Blanch, L., Fernandez, R., Bernito, S., et al. (1987). Effect of PEEP on the arterial minus end-tidal carbon dioxide gradient. *Chest,* **92**:451-454.

Braun, N. M. T. (1988). Intermittent mechanical ventilation. *Clin. Chest Med.*, **9**:153-162.

Brochard, L., Pluskwa, F., and Lemaire, F. (1987). Improved efficacy of spontaneous breathing with inspiratory support. *Am. Rev. Respir. Dis.*, **136**:411-415.

Campbell, E. J. M. (1966). The relationship of the sensation of breathlessness to the act of breathing. In *Breathlessness*. Edited by J. B. L. Howell and E. J. M. Campbell. Blackwell, Oxford, pp. 55-64.

Cherniack, R. M. (1959). The oxygen consumption and efficiency of the respiratory muscles in health and emphysema. *J. Clin. Invest.*, **38**:494-499.

Coggeshall, J. W., Marini, J. J., and Newman, J. H. (1985). Improved oxygenation after muscle relaxation in the adult respiratory distress syndrome. *Arch. Intern. Med.*, **145**:1718-1720.

Demers, R. R., Sullivan, M. J., and Patiota, J. (1977). The clinical importance of endotracheal tube resistance. *Respir. Care*, **22**:919-921.

Fleury, B., Murciano, C., Talamo, C., et al. (1985). Work of breathing in patients with chronic obstructive pulmonary disease in acute respiratory failure. *Am. Rev. Respir. Dis.*, **131**:822-827.

Gibney, R. T. N., Wilson, R. S., and Pontoppidan, H. (1982). Comparison of work of breathing on high gas flow and demand valve continuous positive airway pressure systems. *Chest*, **82**:692-694.

Gottfried, S. B., Rossi, A., Higgs, B. D., et al. (1985). Noninvasive determination of respiratory system mechanics during mechanical ventilation for acute respiratory failure. *Am. Rev. Respir. Dis.*, **131**:414-420.

Grassino, A., and Macklem, P. T. (1984). Respiratory muscle fatigue and ventilatory failure. *Annu. Rev. Med.*, **35**:625-647.

Grassino, A., Whitelaw, W. A., and Milic-Emili, J. (1976). Influence of lung volume and electrode position on electromyography of the diaphragm. *J. Appl. Physiol.*, **40**:971-975.

Grimby, G., Bunn, J., and Mead, J. (1968). Relative contribution of rib cage and abdomen to ventilation during exercise. *J. Appl. Physiol.*, **24**:159-166.

Gross, D., Grassino, A., Ross, W. R. D., et al. (1979). Electromyogram pattern of diaphragmatic fatigue. *J. Appl. Physiol.*, **46**:1-7.

Kacmarek, R. M. (1988). The role of pressure support ventilation in reducing imposed work of breathing. *Respir. Care*, **33**(2):99-120.

Katz, J. A., Kraemer, R. W., and Gjerde, G. E. (1985). Inspiratory work and airway pressure with continuous positive airway pressure delivery systems. *Chest*, **88**:519-526.

Kimball, W. R., Leith, D. E., and Robins, A. G. (1982). Dynamic hyperinflation and ventilator dependence in chronic obstructive pulmonary disease. *Am. Rev. Respir. Dis.*, **126**:991-995.

Kreit, J. W., Capper, M. W., Pomerleau, C. M., et al. (1988). Work of breathing during pressure support ventilation is not less than the work of breathing during assisted mechanical ventilation. *Am. Rev. Respir. Dis.*, **137**:64.

Loring, S. H., and Bruce, E. W. (1986). Methods for study of the chest wall. In *Handbook of Physiology*. Edited by A. P. Fishman, P. T. Macklem, and J. Mead. Bethesda, Maryland, American Physiological Society. pp. 415-428.

MacIntyre, N. (1986). Respiratory function during pressure support ventilation. *Chest,* **89**:677-683.

Marini, J. J. (1987). The role of the inspiratory circuit in the work of breathing during mechanical ventilation. Respir. Care, **32**(6):419-430.

Marini, J. J. (1988a). Monitoring during mechanical ventilation. *Clin. Chest Med.,* 73-100.

Marini, J. J. (1988b). Work of breathing. In *Current Respiratory Care*. Edited by B. C. Decker. pp. 188-194.

Marini, J. J., Capps, J. S., and Culver, B. H. (1985a). The inspiratory work of breathing during assisted mechanical ventilation. *Chest,* **87**:612-618.

Marini, J. J., Kirk, W., and Culver, B. H. (1985b). Flow resistance of the exhalation valves and PEEP devices used in mechanical ventilation. *Am. Rev. Respir. Dis.,* **131**:850-854.

Marini, J. J., Rodriguez, R. M., and Lamb, V. (1986a). The inspiratory workload of patient-initiated mechanical ventilation. *Am. Rev. Respir. Dis.,* **134**:902-909.

Marini, J. J., Rodriguez, R. M., and Lamb, V. (1986b). Bedside estimation of the inspiratory work of breathing during mechanical ventilation. *Chest,* **89**:56-63.

Marini, J. J., Smith, T. C., and Lamb, V. J. (1986d). Rapid estimation of the inspiratory work of spontaneous breathing (abstract). *Am. Rev. Respir. Dis.,* **133**(4):A120.

Marini, J. J., Smith, T. C., and Lamb, V. (1987c). Estimation of inspiratory muscle strength in mechanically ventilated patients: The measurement of maximal inspiratory pressure. *J. Crit. Care,* **1**:32-38.

Marini, J. J., Smith, T. C., and Lamb, V. J. (1988). External work output and force generation during synchronized intermittent mechanical ventilation. Effect of machine assistance on breathing effort. *Am. Rev. Respir. Dis.,* (September, in press).

Matamis, D., LeMaire, F., Harf, A., et al. (1984). Total respiratory pressure volume curves in the adult respiratory distress syndrome. *Chest,* **86**:58-66.

Milic-Emili, J. (1986). Is weaning an art or a science? *Am. Rev. Respir. Dis.,* **134**:1107-1108.

Montgomery, A. B., Holle, R. H. O., Neagley, S. R., et al. (1987). Prediction of successful ventilator weaning using airway occlusion pressure and hypercapnic challenge. *Chest,* **4**:496-499.

Moxham, J., Wiles, C. M., Newham, D., et al. (1980). Sternomastoid muscle function and fatigue in man. *Clin. Sci. Mol. Med.,* **59**:463-468.

O'Quin, R., Marini, J. J., Culver, B. H., et al. (1985). Transmission of airway pressure to the pleural space during lung edema and chest wall restriction. *J. Appl. Physiol.,* **59**:1171-1177.

Otis, A. B. (1964). The work of breathing. In *Handbook of Physiology,* Sec. 3, Vol. 1. Edited by W. O. Fenn and H. Rahn. Washington, D.C., American Physiological Society, pp. 463-476.

Pepe, P. E., and Marini, J. J. (1982). Occult positive end-expiratory pressure in mechanically ventilated patients with airflow obstruction: The auto-PEEP effect. *Am. Rev. Respir. Dis.,* **126**:166-170.

Peters, R. M. (1969). The energy cost (work) of breathing. *Ann. Thorac. Surg.,* **7**:51-67.

Rochester, D. F., and Arora, N. S. (1983). Respiratory muscle failure. *Med. Clin. North Am.,* **67**:573-597.

Rochester, D. F., Arora, N. S., Braun, N. M. T., et al. (1979). The respiratory muscles in chronic obstructive pulmonary disease (COPD). *Bull. Eur. Physiopathol. Respir.,* **15**:951-975.

Rohrer, F. (1915). Der Stromungswiderstand in den menschlichen Atemwegen. *Pfluegers Arch. Ges. Physiol.,* **162**:225-259.

Rossi, A., Gottfried, S. B., Zocchi, L., et al. (1985). Measurement of static compliance of the total respiratory system in patients with acute respiratory failure during mechanical ventilation. The effect of "intrinsic PEEP." *Am. Rev. Respir. Dis.,* **131**:672-677.

Roussos, C. H., and Macklem, P. T. (1977). Diaphragmatic fatigue in man. *J. Appl. Physiol.,* **43**:189-197.

Roussos, C., and Moxham, J. (1985). Respiratory muscle fatigue. Chapter 27 In *The Thorax.* Edited by C. Roussos and P. T. Macklem. New York, Marcel Dekker, pp. 829-870.

Sagawa, K. (1978). The ventricular pressure-volume diagram revisited. *Circ. Res.,* **43**:677-687.

Sahn, S. A., Lakshminarayan, S., and Petty, T. L. (1976). Weaning from mechanical ventilation. *JAMA,* **235**:2208-2212.

Sarnoff, S. J., Brainwald, E., Welch, G. H., et al. (1958). Hemodynamic determinants of oxygen consumption of the heart, with special reference to the tension time index. *Am. J. Physiol.,* **192**:148-156.

Sassoon, C. S. H., Te, T. T., Mahutte, C. K., et al. (1987). Airway occlusion pressure. An important indicator for successful weaning in patients with chronic obstructive pulmonary disease. *Am. Rev. Respir. Dis.,* **135**:107-113.

Scharf, S. M., and Ingram, R. H., Jr. (1977). Effects of decreasing lung compliance with oleic acid on the cardiovascular response to PEEP. *Am. J. Physiol.,* **233**:H635-641.

Smith, T. C., and Marini, J. J. (1988). Impact of PEEP on lung mechanics and work of breathing in severe airflow obstruction. The effect of PEEP on auto-PEEP. *J. Appl. Physiol.,* (October, in press).

Smith, T. C., Marini, J. J., Taylor, R. F., and Lamb, V. J. (1988). Two measures of the inspiratory work of breathing during triggered machine cycles (AMV). *Am. Rev. Respir. Dis.,* **137**(4, Pt. 2):190.

Tobin, M. J., Perez, W., Guenther, S. M., et al. (1986). The pattern of breathing during successful and unsuccessful trials of weaning from mechanical ventilation. *Am. Rev. Respir. Dis.,* **134**:1111-1118.

Truwit, J. D., and Marini, J. J. (1988). Evaluation of thoracic mechanics in the ventilated patient. Part II. Applied Mechanics. *J. Crit. Care,* **3**(3): 199-213.

Truwit, J. D., Marini, J. J., and Lamb, V. J. (1988). The work of spontaneous breathing can be predicted noninvasively during mechanical ventilation. *Am. Rev. Respir. Dis.,* **137**(4, Pt. 2):216.

Tuxen, D. V., and Lane, S. (1987). The effects of ventilatory pattern on hyperinflation, airway pressures, and circulation in mechanical ventilation of patients with severe air-flow obstruction. *Am. Rev. Respir. Dis.,* **136**:872-879.

Viale, J. P., Annat, G., Bertrand, O., et al. (1985). Additional inspiratory work in intubated patients breathing with continuous positive airway pressure systems. *Anesthesiology,* **63**:536-539.

Viires, N., Sillye, G., Aubier, M., et al. (1983). Regional blood flow distribution in dog during induced hypotension and low cardiac output. *J. Clin. Invest.,* **72**:935-947.

Wright, P., Marini, J. J., and Bernard, G. R. (1988). Increased airway resistance contributes to impaired lung mechanics in the adult respiratory distress syndrome (ARDS). *Am. Rev. Respir. Dis.,* **137**(4, Pt. 2):137.

10

Computed Tomography Scanning in Acute Respiratory Failure

LUCIANO GATTINONI and ANTONIO PESENTI

Università di Milano, Milano
and Ospedale Nuovo S. Gerardo
Monza, Italy

I. Introduction

The adult respiratory distress syndrome (ARDS) is conventionally believed to produce a diffuse involvement of lung parenchyma by inflammatory processes (Ashbaugh et al., 1967). These processes lead to an increased extravascular lung water content and interstitial and intra-alveolar pulmonary edema with a consequently increased radiographic density of the lungs. Computed tomography (CT) can detect such density changes in the lung parenchyma without interference from surrounding structures. In the last several years, the CT scan has been increasingly employed to study ARDS patients despite the logistical difficulty of transporting and positioning critically ill patients. In this chapter we describe our approach to CT scanning of patients with ARDS, emphasizing:

1. The diagnostic value of CT scans compared to conventional x-rays
2. The changing morphologic pattern of ARDS with altered positive end-expiratory pressure (PEEP) and body position

Besides the qualitative or "imaging" value of the CT scan, this technique allows quantitative analysis of lung anatomy, which can be coupled with measurement of lung gas volume. We report in this chapter the correlations between lung anatomy observed by CT scanning and gas transport and hemodynamic measurement changes as a function of PEEP levels and body position in patients with ARDS.

II. Lung Morphology

A. Comparing CT Scans with X-rays

Although both CT scans and conventional radiography employ x-rays to produce images, from the diagnostic point of view their value may dramatically differ. In our experience, in about 10% of patients with ARDS, the CT scan alone (but not the radiograph) revealed a lung abscess or bullae. Moreover, the CT scan can demonstrate localized tension pneumothoraces in either the dorsal or ventral regions of the lung that are not detectable by anteroposterior chest radiography. Figure 1 shows an example of a tension pneumothorax that was only detected with a CT scan.

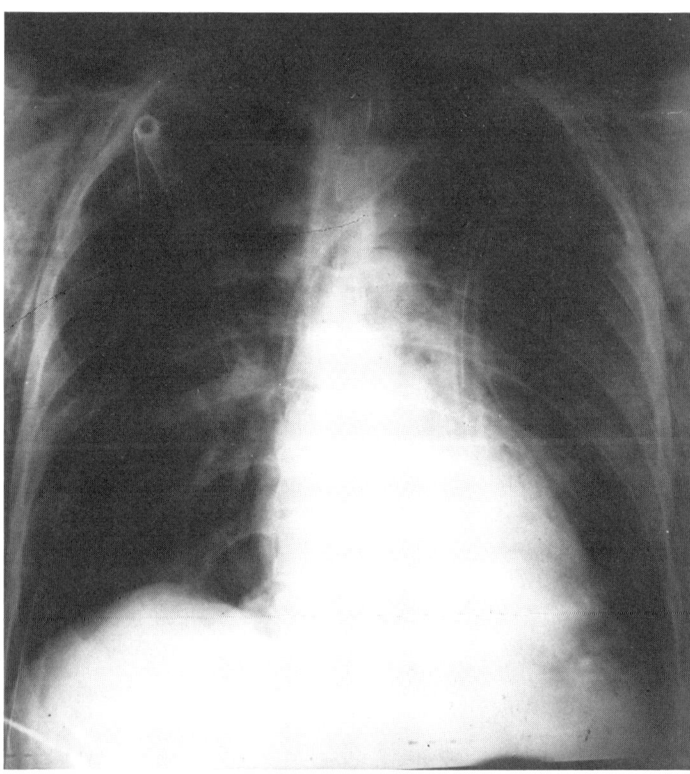

Figure 1 Acute respiratory failure after polytrauma. The CT scan clearly shows an anterior bilateral pneumothorax, not evident in the anteroposterior chest x-ray.

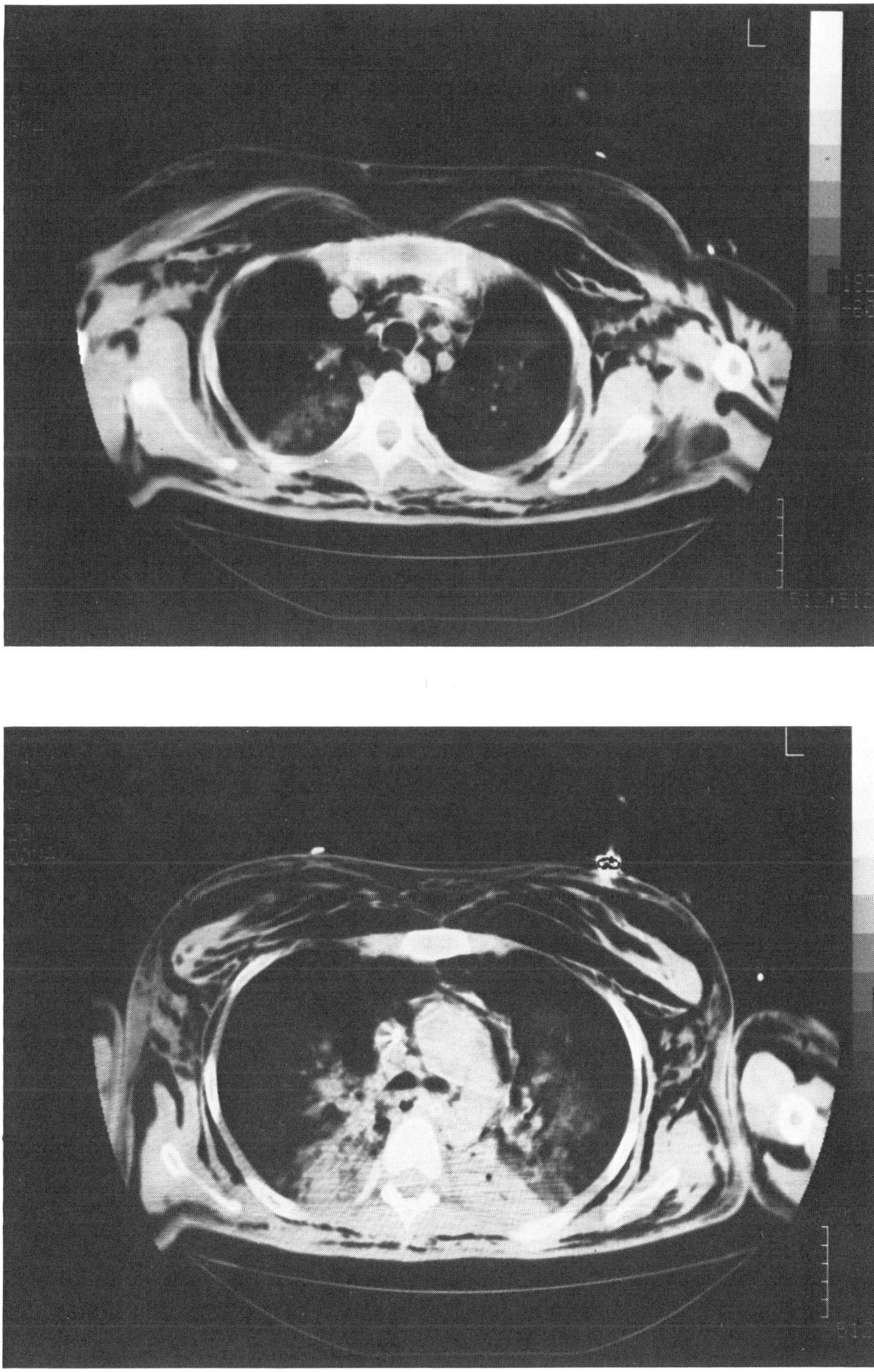

Figure 1 (continued)

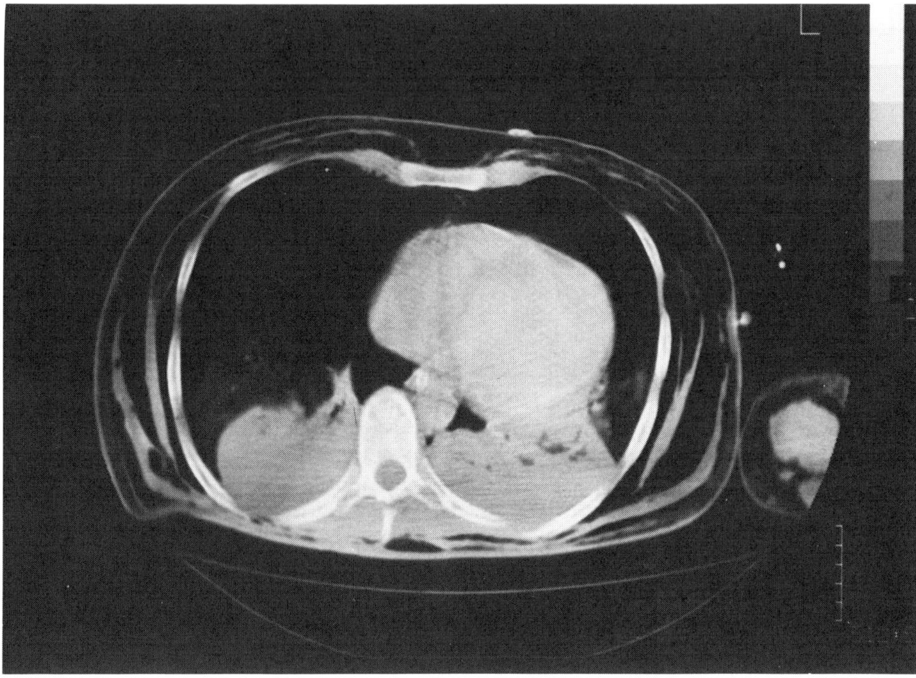

Figure 1 (continued)

When evaluating overall lung edema, we found that the chest radiograph and the CT scan correlated closely when chest X-rays were analyzed by standardized procedures (Gattinoni et al., 1987c), as described by Pistolesi and co-workers (1985) and Halperin and colleagues (1985).

Figure 2 shows the correlation between the chest radiograph and the overall CT scan densities in 17 ARDS patients. We believe a CT scan is indicated for ARDS patients if a tension pneumothorax is clinically suspected that is undetected by the chest radiograph. In these cases, a CT scan may provide an essential tool for diagnosis that may change the patient's clinical course.

B. CT Patterns in ARDS

A major important contribution of the CT scan to our understanding of ARDS has been the visualization of the inhomogeneity of lung parenchymal lesions. Our group (Gattinoni et al., 1986) and others (Maunder et al., 1986; Rommelschein et al., 1983) have shown that the lung densities in ARDS are

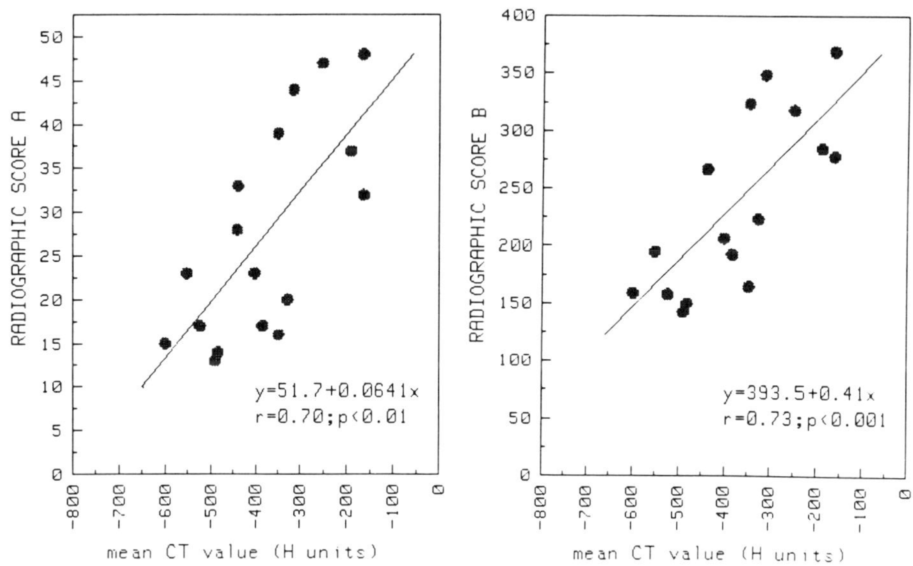

Figure 2 Standardized chest x-ray scoring system of Halperin (A) and Pistolesi (B) versus the CT scan density.

primarily located in dependent regions. This contrasts with the conventional AP chest radiograph, which demonstrates only a diffuse increase of density ("white lungs"). Figure 3 provides a comparison of these two radiographic techniques. The lung inhomogeneity observed by CT scanning poses a question as to the general validity of localized diagnostic lung biopsies, selective bronchopulmonary lavage, and selective or regional angiography. Results from these procedures are likely to be influenced by the region that is sampled. Lung regions can range from a nondependent region with a gas-tissue ratio near normal to a dependent region that is nearly gasless. As we note later, a normal air-tissue ratio does not mean the lung's structure is normal.

C. CT Changes with PEEP

Figure 4 shows two extremes of the changes induced by PEEP. In the upper panel the application of 5-15 cmH_2O PEEP expands previously inflated pulmonary units without evident modification of lung density; the lower panel shows a dramatic response to PEEP with clearing of most of the lung's densities (note in both cases that lung densities, as is common, are located in dependent lung regions).

Figure 4 suggests a morphologic basis may account for the variable gas exchange response to PEEP observed in clinical practice. It is probable that

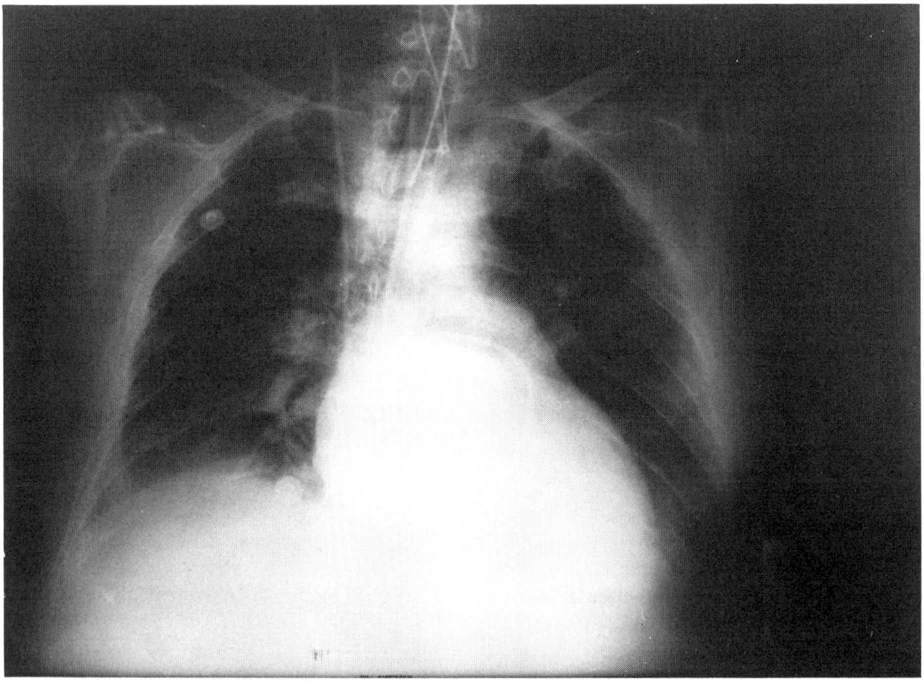

Figure 3 A typical comparison between chest x-ray and CT scan in ARF lung emphasizing the gravity dependency of the densities.

the anatomic composition of the consolidated densities in the upper panel differs from those in the patient scanned in the lower panel (possibly edema or atelectasis).

In general, most ARDS patients show some degree of clearing of lung densities after increasing the level of PEEP, with more consistent clearing at the lung bases and hili and a minor response at the apex (Gattinoni et al., 1986).

D. CT Changes with Altered Body Positioning

After we consistently observed gravity-dependent collapse of dorsal lung regions in supine ARDS patients, we examined the effect of prone positioning to improve gas exchange by better matching of ventilation and perfusion. We hypothesized that a redistribution of blood flow induced by gravity in lung regions with a more normal air-tissue ratio (ventral regions in the supine position) would result in improved oxygenation (Langer et al., 1988).

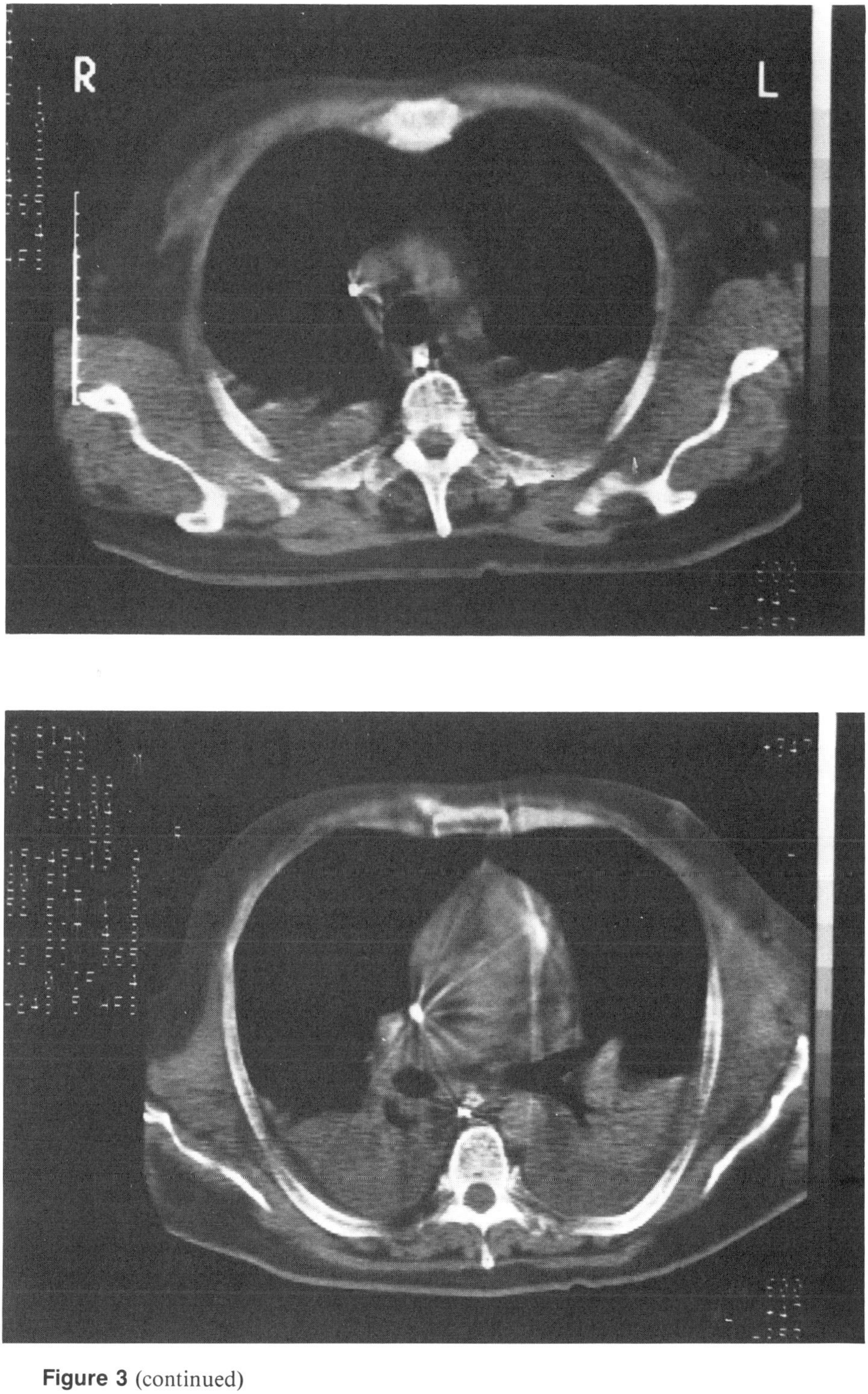

Figure 3 (continued)

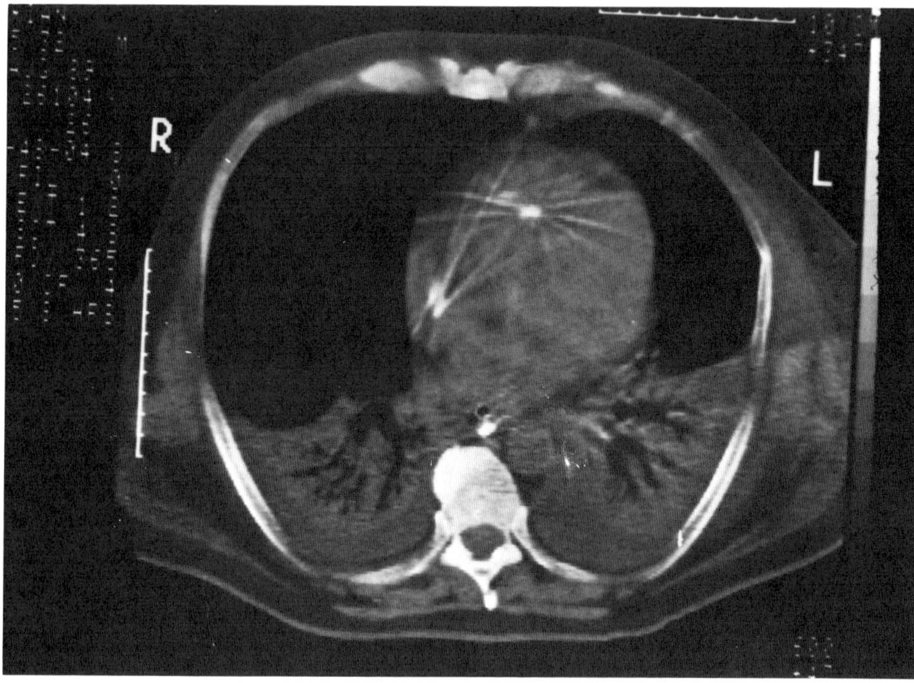

Figure 3 (continued)

The gas exchange response to position changes was quite inconstant, and therefore we studied lung anatomy by CT scanning. Unexpectedly, and almost without exception, we observed a dramatic redistribution of densities when patients were shifted from the supine into the prone position, with "migration" of the high-density lesions from dorsal to ventral regions of the lung, as shown in Figure 5. This anatomic shift occurred independently of gas exchange modifications (Mascheroni et al., 1986).

Figure 4 (a-c) ARF from bacterial pneumonia (patient 1). CT scan of the base at 5, 10, and 15 cmH_2O PEEP. No changes in density and Pa_{O_2} are observed. (a) Pa_{O_2}, 97 mmHg; density, 59%; (b) Pa_{O_2}, 103 mmHg; density, 56%; (c) Pa_{O_2}, 106 mmHg; density, 53%. (d-f) ARF from sepsis (patient 10). CT scan of the base at 5, 10, and 15 cmH_2O. Substantial clearing of the densities is accompanied by an increase in Pa_{O_2}. (d) Pa_{O_2}, 34 mmHg; density, 70%; (e) Pa_{O_2}, 49 mmHg; density, 52%; (f) Pa_{O_2}, 121 mmHg; density, 32%. (From Gattinoni et al., 1986, with permission.)

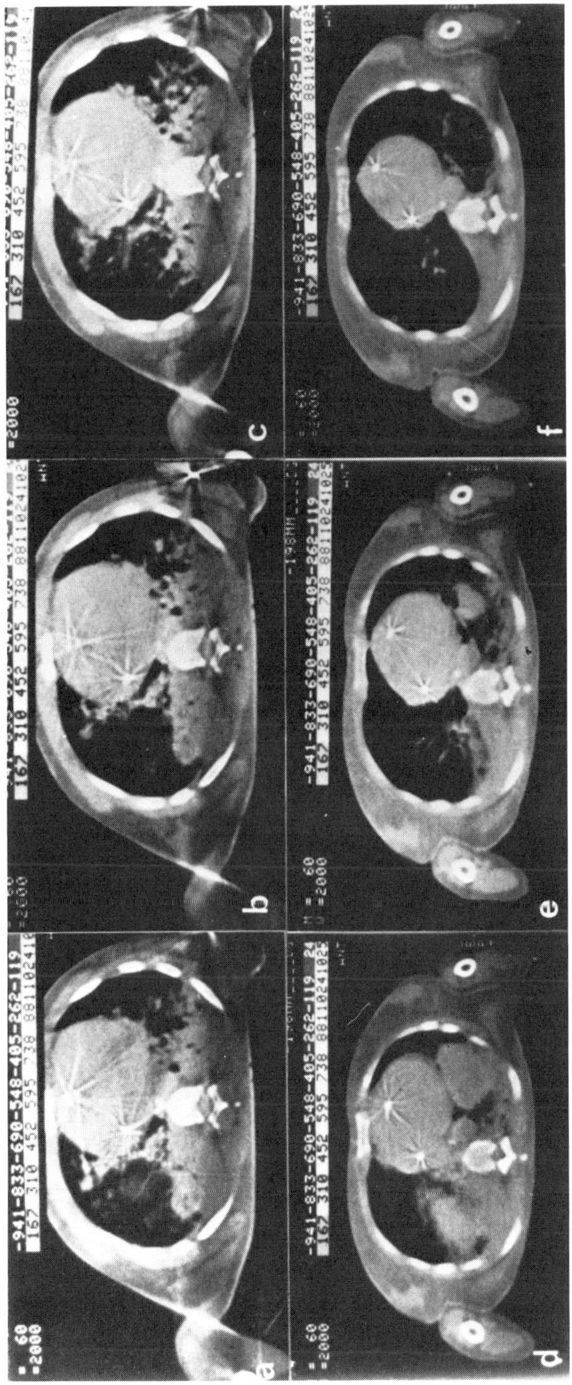

Figure 4

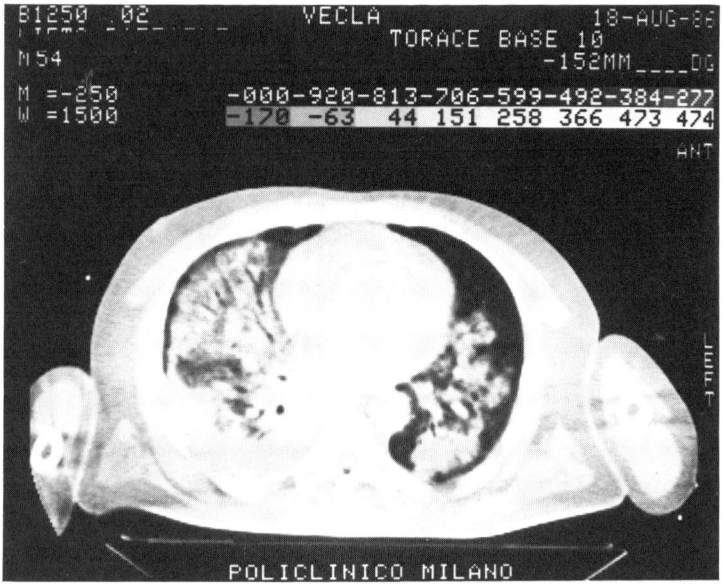

(a)

Figure 5 A typical example of CT scan density redistribution transferring from (a) the supine to (b) the prone positions. (The CT scan in the prone position was taken 10 min after the CT scan in the supine position.)

It is important to emphasize that this dorsal to ventral density redistribution occurs after prone positioning in a very short time (approximately 10 min), the time we required to shift an ARDS patient from supine to prone and obtain a new CT scan.

III. A Quantitative Analysis of CT Scan Images

Our quantitative analysis of the CT scan is based upon a mathematical analysis of the matrix of the CT numbers from which the image is reconstructed and is coupled with a measurement of the lung's gas volume (FRC) (Gattinoni et al., 1988a). The CT number is defined as the difference between the attenuation of the x-ray in a defined volume of the material being studied and the attenuation coefficient of water divided by the attenuation coefficient

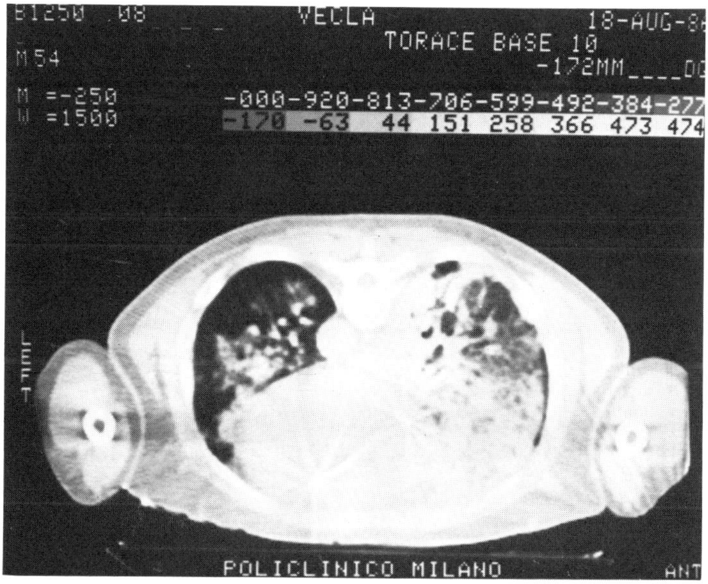

(b)

of water. Each pixel of the image (1.5 × 1.5 × 9 mm) is characterized by a CT number expressed in Hounsfield units (H). Values range over a scale from 0 to −1000 (0 H for water, −1000 H for air). The relationship between the CT number and density (grams per milliliter) is complex, depending upon the incident energy, atomic number of the tissue, and electron mass density, as well as tissue density itself. Under our study conditions (constant incident energy, electron mass, and lung tissue atomic number), variations in CT numbers are mainly related to physical density, that is, the ratio of the volume of gas to the volume of gas plus the volume of tissue (including lung structures, blood, and extracellular lung water). For example, if in a given pixel the CT number is −500 H, the fraction of gas will be 50%; if the CT number is −700 H, the pixel is composed of 70% gas and 30% tissue.

In our ARDS patients we scanned the lung at three levels: apex (1-2 cm above the carina), hilus, and base (1-2 cm above the diaphragm). Each exposure was taken during apnea at the preselected PEEP level, the patient being anesthetized and paralyzed. The transverse area of the thorax was obtained planimetrically. For each lung the boundary was drawn manually along the inside of the ribs and at the edge of the mediastinal organs. The total cross-sectional lung surface area was obtained from the scan of each of the six areas (two apical, two hilar, and two basal) comprising 20,000-40,000 pixels, each defined by a given CT number. A special computer program provided the mean CT number of the total cross-sectional area and the CT number frequency distribution. The CT number frequency distribution was computed relative to 11 equally spaced intervals (from −900 to +100 H in steps of 100 H). After assuming that the total cross-sectional area of the lung is a representative sample of the entire lung, we then computed the average CT number of the lungs [i.e., the average gas/(gas + tissue ratio)] and we also determined the fraction of pixels relative to the total number of pixels, which were included in each compartment (between −900 and −800 H, between −800 and −700 H, and so on).

As the CT number reflects physical density, if the gas volume of the lung (FRC) is measured by an independent technique, such as helium dilution, then by employing the CT number, its frequency distribution, and the measured gas volume, we may estimate the following variables (see Sec. VII for details):

1. Lung weight: the weight, expressed in grams of lung, which includes the weight of lung tissue, intrapulmonary blood, and extravascular lung water. An excess lung weight can be estimated for comparison to the normally expected lung weight for any patient.
2. The weight of normally inflated tissue: we defined this as representing the mass of the lung with a near-normal gas-tissue ratio, that is, between 90% gas-10% tissue and 50% gas-50% tissue. The quantity of normally inflated lung tissue in normal and healthy lungs represents about 80% of the total lung weight.
3. The weight of poorly inflated lung tissue: we defined this as representing the mass of the lung with a gas-tissue ratio between 50% gas—50% tissue, and 10% gas-90% tissue. In the normal lung this accounts for about 15% of the total lung weight.
4. The weight of the noninflated lung tissue: we defined this as representing the mass of lung with a gas-tissue ratio between 10% gas-90% tissue and 0% gas-100% tissue. In the normal lung this accounts for about 5% of total lung weight.
5. Excess lung tissue mass: this represents the percentage increase in lung mass in comparison to the expected normal value for each patient.
6. Recruitment: This is the percentage of lung tissue, relative to the normal lung mass, which by varying the level of PEEP shifts from uninflated or poorly inflated compartments to a compartment with a more normal gas-tissue ratio.

IV. Comparing Physiologic Measurements with CT Scan Anatomy

A. Lung Weight

The lung weight of patients dying from severe ARDS averages 2.5 kg (range 1.75-3.75 kg) (Teplitz, 1976; Zapol et al., 1979). The lung weight we computed from the CT scan in 22 ARDS patients averaged 2.6 + 1.2 kg. The excess lung weight we estimated in patients with acute respiratory failure (ARF) is approximately twice normal (Gattinoni et al., 1988b). It is reasonable to hypothesize that the early lung weight increase is primarily an increase in extravascular lung water (EVLW; i.e., pulmonary edema). Extravascular lung water in severe ARDS has been measured by thermodilution (double-indicator technique) and averaged 14.5 + 4.98 ml/kg body weight, with normal controls at 6.1 + 2.1 ml/kg body weight (Sibbald et al., 1985) accounting for a net increase during ARDS of lung weight by 8.4 ml/kg body weight. This value is much lower than the increase in lung weight we computed by CT scanning during ARDS (21.4 ml/kg body weight). However, it is important to recall that the thermodilution EVLW technique measures extravascular lung water only in perfused lung regions (Effros, 1985) but the CT scan can equally well detect edema in unperfused and underperfused lung regions. The increase in lung weight measured by CT scanning correlates with the mean pulmonary artery pressure, as shown in Figure 6. It is worthwhile emphasizing that a 1 mmHg increase in mean pulmonary artery pressure is associated with a 14% increase from baseline lung weight. These values agree with experimental studies relating the increase in lung weight to an increased pulmonary artery pressure (Ngeow and Mitzner, 1983; Permutt, 1985). We do not know if an increased pulmonary artery pressure causes the increase in lung edema or if lung edema, through vascular compression, causes an increased pulmonary artery pressure. However, the two phenomena seem to be closely associated and are probably of great clinical importance.

B. Lung Anatomy and Compliance

The ARDS lung is generally thought of as stiff and having a decreased compliance (Falke et al., 1972). We have measured the volume-pressure curve (exploring a pressure range from 0 to 40 cmH_2O) and analyzed CT scans taken at 5, 10, and 15 cmH_2O inflation pressure to explore the relationship between lung compliance and variables derived from the CT scan, that is, lung weight and the mass of normally, poorly, and uninflated tissue (Gattinoni et al., 1987b).

The following compliance values, derived from the volume-pressure (V-P) curve of the lung performed by step-by-step inflation during anesthesia and paralysis, were examined (see Fig. 7) (Gattinoni et al., 1987a).

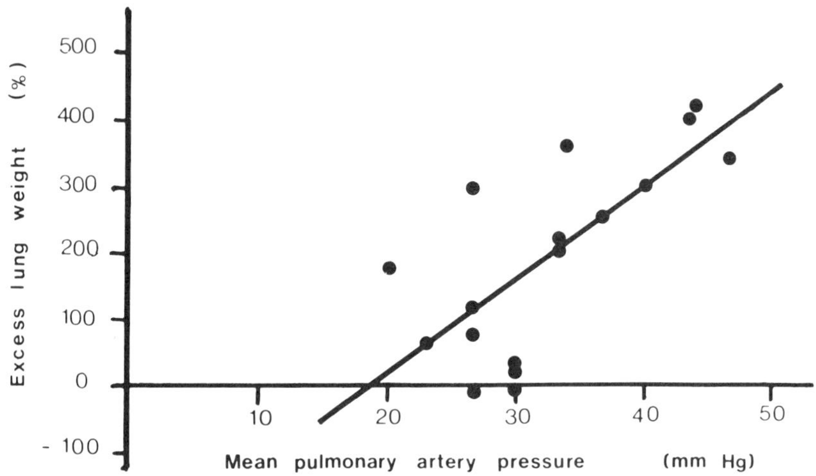

Figure 6 Excess lung weight as a function of mean pulmonary artery pressure (data obtained at 5 cmH_2O PEEP). $r = 0.73$; $P < 0.01$. (From Gattinoni et al., 1986, with permission.)

Starting compliance (C_{start}) is the ratio of the first 100 ml inflation and the corresponding pressure. The C_{start} region examines lung mechanics at a pressure of 3-10 cmH_2O.

Inflation compliance is the slope of the VP curve in its most linear segment.

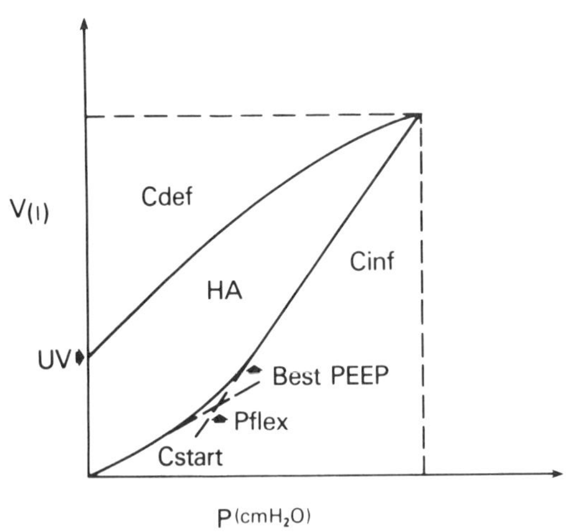

Figure 7 Parameters derived from the pressure-volume curve of the total respiratory system. For explanation, see the text. (From Gattinoni et al., 1987a, with permission.)

Deflation compliance is the slope of the VP curve during deflation in its most linear segment. Both inflation and deflation compliances examine lung behavior at pressures ranging from 5-10 to 40 cmH_2O.

We then sought a mathematical relationship between the starting compliance and the amount of normally, poorly, and uninflated tissue at 5 cmH_2O pressure (the range of pressure explored by C_{start}) and between the inflation and deflation compliances and the same CT scan-derived variables at 15 cmH_2O pressure (i.e., the range of pressures explored by these compliances). It became evident that these differing compliances correlated best with the mass of normally inflated tissue.

Our findings clearly indicate that in the ARDS lung mechanical tests examine the lung regions that contain a near-normal air-tissue ratio but noninflated regions are not "seen" by the V-P curve. Indeed, measurements of lung compliance examine only the mass of lung tissue that remains near "normal" and does not include the mass of lung tissue with edema, atelectasis, or consolidation. Moreover, we demonstrated that the specific compliance in ARDS is normal or higher than normal.

From these studies we conclude that the lungs in ARDS are not uncompliant but rather at low gas volume and that the regions of the lung examined by the V-P curve, that is, the regions with a normal gas-tissue ratio, retain their normal elasticity.

C. Lung Anatomy and Gas Exchange

Since lung compliance reflects the amount of lung tissue with a near-normal gas-tissue ratio (i.e., the gas exchanging regions of the lung), hypoxemia and venous admixture are functions of the mass of uninflated tissue (Gattinoni et al., 1986, 1988b). Employing CT scanning, we cannot discriminate between consolidation, edema, and atelectasis; however, whatever the precise pathology in gasless lung tissue, its mass correlates with shunt-related hypoxemia. Regions of the lung contributing to hypoxemia are likely to be markedly underperfused. The shunt fraction (Q_s/Q_t), in fact, is always less than the computed fraction of uninflated tissue, despite that in normal lungs, blood flow is greater to dependent lung regions, whereas in ARDS there is a greater preponderance of uninflated tissue (for example, 50% uninflated tissue with a 20-25% shunt). Regional hypoperfusion may also account for the discrepancy between excess mass computed by double-indicator techniques and CT scanning. However, we have no direct information on the intrapulmonary distribution of blood flow nor do we understand the mechanisms involved in regional hypoperfusion (e.g., hypoxic vasoconstriction, vascular occlusion, and vascular compression).

V. Alterations in Lung Anatomy and Function with Changing Conditions

A. Effects of PEEP

The precise mechanisms of action of PEEP in ARDS remain controversial. Employing CT scanning, we obtained morphologic evidence of gas recruitment. By quantitative analysis of CT scan images we quantitated anatomic recruitment, independent of hyperinflation, and expressed recruitment as the amount of lung tissue regaining a normal gas-tissue ratio. Figure 8 shows the relationship between anatomic recruitment and the reduction of shunt, suggesting that previously uninflated pulmonary units are perfused and maintain

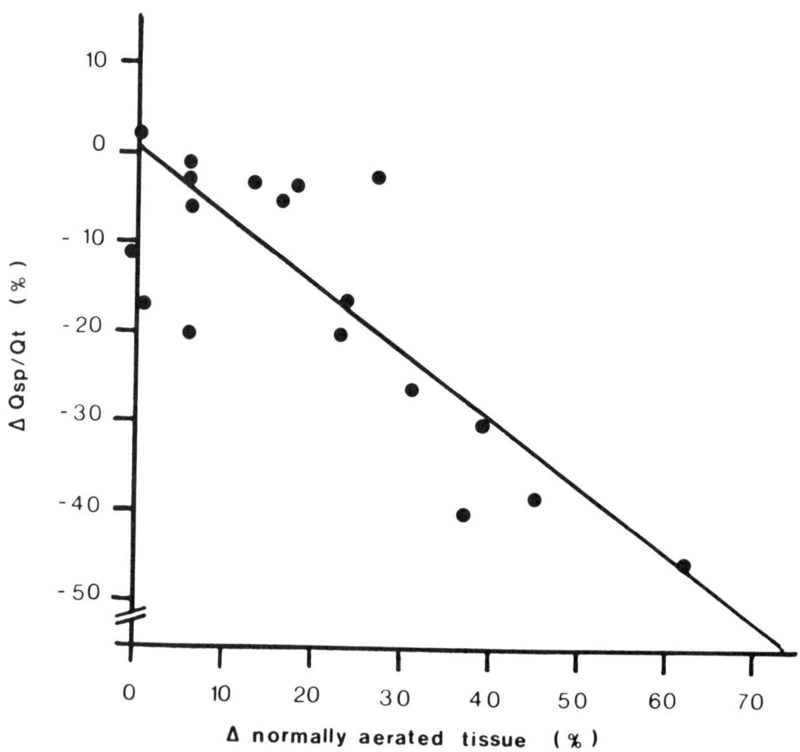

Figure 8 Right-to-left shunt (Q_{sp}/Q_t) changes from 5 cmH_2O PEEP to 15 cmH_2O PEEP (expressed as a percentage change in the Q_{sp}/Q_t values at 5 cmH_2O PEEP) as a function of anatomic gas volume recruitment (data given as a percentage change in normally aerated tissue weight from 5 cmH_2O PEEP to 15 cmH_2O PEEP). $r = 0.78$; $P < 0.01$; $n = 18$. (From Gattinoni et al., 1988b, with permission.)

perfusion when inflated by the action of PEEP (i.e., anatomic gas recruitment parallels functional recruitment). This finding suggests that the main mechanism of action of PEEP consists of recruiting previously uninflated pulmonary units (Gattinoni et al., 1988b).

We may then speculate on the nature of such a recruited unit. It is unlikely that pulmonary units that are consolidated and contain intra-alveolar red cells, fibrin, and fibrosis, for example (as in pneumonia), will reopen, whatever the applied PEEP level. On the other hand, if pulmonary units are filled with edema, it is doubtful that applying PEEP will rapidly clear this edema (the response to PEEP measured in the CT scan is within minutes). Another possibility is that PEEP reopens collapsed units that potentially can be recruited. Collapse of a pulmonary unit may occur for many reasons: surfactant deficiency, gas reabsorption due to occlusion of distal airways, a critical $\dot{V}_A/\dot{Q}$ ratio, or compression by the weight of superimposed pulmonary structures. We investigated this possibility by changing body position.

B. Effects of Prone Body Positioning

As shown in Figure 5, about 10 min after a change in body position from supine to prone, there was a relocation of densities along the gravitational gradient. Dorsal regions decreased in density but ventral regions increased in density. We analyzed this phenomenon quantitatively by dividing the CT scan image, from sternum to vertebra, into fractions of 10% of the total lung height, then derived for each fraction the same anatomic variables we previously computed for the entire lung, that is, weight, excess mass, and the fraction of normal, poorly, and uninflated tissue. Figure 9 shows the changes in density and lung weight from ventral to dorsal in the supine position in normal subjects and ARDS patients. Both the normal lung and the ARDS lung behave similarly, any differences being quantitative, not qualitative. However, we wish to emphasize that during ARDS the weight of overlying structures on the most dependent regions of the lung is approximately 10 cmH_2O, that is, three times the normal compression force. This force may induce the collapse of "healthy" dependent lung units.

By analyzing the excess mass at the different fractions of lung height, from sternum to vertebra (10%, 20%, and so on) we found that excess lung mass was not distributed strictly according to gravity; rather, edema was evenly distributed throughout the lung in the supine and prone positions, as has been reported in experimental models (Hales et al., 1981). Thus two phenomena operate: excess lung mass is not distributed according to the gravity, but densities, which are primary causes of hypoxemia, are gravity dependent. It is possible that compression of airspaces by the weight of overlying structures plays a major role producing the observed pattern.

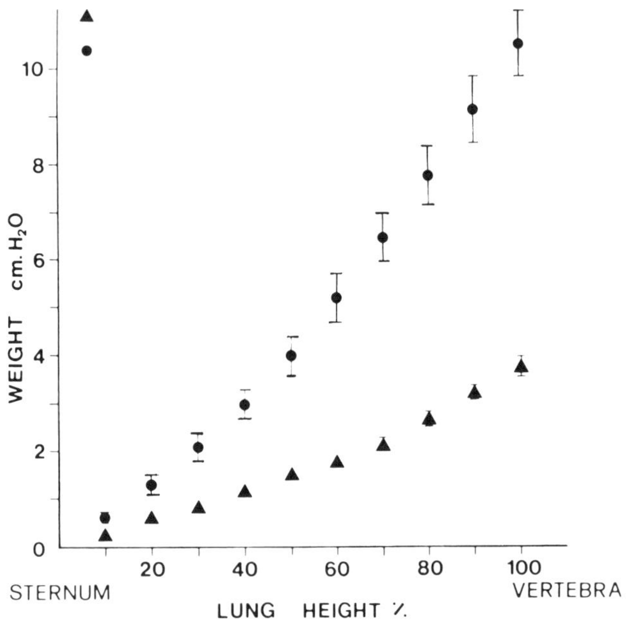

Figure 9 Cumulative lung weight at different lung heights in ARF (n = 10) and normal (n = 7) subjects: (●) ARF; (▲) normal.

We now discuss the mechanisms of density redistribution caused by changes in position. The clearing of the dorsal regions could be due to resorption of alveolar edema; the parallel increase in density in the ventral regions could be attributed to new edema formation. We have discarded this hypothesis because of the brief time in which the phenomenon occurs (10 min). It has been shown in experimental animals that although resorption of saline from alveoli requires several hours, the resorption of protein-rich saline requires days (Staub, 1988). An intrapulmonary shift of interstitial edema from dorsal to ventral regions is also unlikely owing to physical barriers. Moreover, if interstitial edema were free to migrate, we should expect a gravitational distribution of the excess mass in the supine position, a position that was usually maintained for several days before the CT scan. This was not the case for ARDS patients or for patients in whom interstitial edema was due to left heart failure (presumably containing less protein), and edema does not appear to move freely through lung fields (Wollmer et al., 1987).

We cannot exclude a positional shift of intravascular blood volume; however, the absolute changes in densities are far too great to be explained solely by a blood volume shift. In addition, the fractional blood volume is apparently decreased in the most dependent regions of the lung (Wollmer et al., 1984), as is pulmonary blood flow (Bhattacharya et al., 1980; Jones et al., 1976). It is therefore likely that the shifts we observed in lung density from dorsal to ventral with position change are mainly due to alterations in gas distribution, and not to tissue mass distribution.

VI. A Model of the ARDS Lung Derived from CT Scans of the Lung

From the above considerations, we wish to postulate the following evolutionary sequence during ARDS. The first alterations of ARDS are due to endothelial lesions, with increased permeability and the consequent development of interstitial edema. Edema fluid accumulates throughout the lung, independent of gravity. When the excess lung mass reaches a critical value (approximately 100-150% of the original weight), the most dependent regions of the lung collapse owing to the weight of overlying structures, resulting in shunting and hypoxemia. Because of a variety of factors, the cardiac output increases, partly as a response to hypoxemia; consequently, pulmonary hypertension may develop. Of course, many other factors are involved in the development of acute pulmonary hypertension, such as microthrombosis, compression of blood vessels, and hypoxic or other mediator-induced vasoconstriction. Whatever the cause, the increase in pulmonary artery pressure is associated with an increased lung weight. As the lung becomes progressively degassed, the remaining lung mass with a normal gas-tissue ratio decreases and lung compliance decreases. On the other hand, the increased gasless lung mass produces an increased right-to-left shunt with worsening hypoxemia. The therapeutic effects of PEEP on this injured organ are immediate and consist primarily of reopening potentially healthy lung units that were collapsed by the overlying weight, thereby decreasing shunt and hypoxemia.

The lung in ARF may be considered a sponge with an excess mass evenly distributed in all regions. This elastic body is subjected to gravity, and the increased weight causes progressive compression of airspaces and reabsorption and/or compression atelectasis. After turning the patient from supine to prone, dorsal compression atelectasis is relieved and new regions of ventral compression atelectasis rapidly develop. The effects of PEEP and altered positioning may then share a common mechanism, the reopening of weight-induced regional atelectasis. In a preliminary study of 10 patients in whom the PEEP and positioning responses were compared, both responses were highly correlated; that is, the patients showing a greater density redistribution with positioning are the same patients who exhibit greater anatomic recruitment by PEEP.

VII. Appendix: Calculations for Estimating Pulmonary Weight

Our quantitative analysis of the CT scans is based upon two assumptions: that the three slices (apex, hilus, and base) provide a representative sample of the entire lung and that the lung is considered a mixture of gas and tissue (the tissue is analyzed as water density and includes blood, cells, extravascular lung water, and lung structures) (Gattinoni et al., 1988a). The specific weight of the tissue is assumed to be equal to 1 g/cm^3.

A. Actual and Expected Normal Weights

First, the three selected slices are traced manually along the inside margins of the rib cage and mediastinal organs are excluded. Second, the mean CT number of the total cross-sectional area is computed, the total cross-sectional area comprising the sum of the two outlined hemiapical, hemihilar, and hemibasal areas (the CT numbers are 0 H for water, −1000 H for air, and +1000 for bone). Third, the gas volume of the lung is measured by the helium dilution technique. Fourth, the tissue weight of the lung is computed according to the following equation:

$$\text{Total tissue weight} = \frac{G_V(K - CT)}{CT} \tag{1}$$

where G_V is the lung's gas volume measured by helium dilution, K is −1000 H (i.e., the CT number for air minus the CT number for water), and CT is the average CT number of the total cross-sectional area.

The expected normal lung weight is computed according to equation (1), where V_G for normal female subjects is [h(meters) × 1.39] − 0.424 and for normal male subjects is [h(meters) × 5.48] − 7.05 (Ibanez and Rauric, 1990) and CT is −690 H (the mean CT number obtained in normal subjects) (Gattinoni et al., 1988).

B. CT Frequency Distribution

A special computer program generates the CT frequency distribution over 11 compartments (from −1000 H to +100 H, with each compartment spanning 100 H). The weight of normally inflated tissue (compartments between −1000 H and −500 H) is computed as follows:

$$\text{Normally inflated tissue weight} = \frac{L_W}{S_W} + G_V \quad \times f \times \frac{CT}{K} \times Sw \tag{2}$$

where L_W is the total lung weight, S_W is the specific weight of lung tissue, assumed to be 1 g/cm^3, G_V is the total gas volume, f is the fraction of pixels with CT numbers between -1000 H and -500 H, CT is the average CT number of pixels between -1000 H and -500 H, and K equals -1000 H. The amount of poorly inflated lung tissue (CT number between -500 H and -100 H) is computed by the same procedure; the weight of uninflated lung tissue (-100 H to $+100$ H) is computed by subtracting the normally inflated and poorly inflated tissue weights from the total weight of the lung.

C. Recruitment

Alveolar recruitment is computed by subtracting the weight of the normally inflated lung tissue at 5 cmH_2O PEEP from the weight of normally inflated lung tissue at 15 cmH_2O PEEP and then dividing by the expected normal lung weight.

Acknowledgment

Supported in part by grant 87.00750.57 from CNR, Rome, Italy.

References

Ashbaugh, D. G., Bigelow, D. B., Petty, T. I., et al. (1967). Acute respiratory distress in adults. *Lancet,* **2**:319-323.

Bhattacharya, J., Nakahara, K., and Staub, N. C. (1980). Effect of edema on pulmonary blood flow in the isolated perfused dog lung lobe. *J. Appl. Physiol.,* **48**(3):444-449.

Effros, R. M. (1985). Lung water measurements with the mean transit time approach. *J. Appl. Physiol.,* **59**:673-683.

Falke, K. J., Pontoppidan, H., Kumar, A., Leith, D. E., Geffin, B., and Laver, M. B. (1972). Ventilation with end expiratory pressure in acute lung disease. *J. Clin. Invest.,* **51**:2315-2323.

Gattinoni, L., Mascheroni, D., Torresin, A., et al. (1986). Morphological response to positive end-expiratory pressure in acute respiratory failure: Computerized tomography study. *Intensive Care Med.,* **13**:137-142.

Gattinoni, L., Mascheroni, D., Basilico, E., Foti, G., Pesenti, A., and Avalli, L. (1987). Volume/pressure curve of total respir;atory system in paralyzed patients: Artefacts and correction factors. *Intensive Care Med.,* **13**:19-25.

Gattinoni, L., Pesenti, A., Avalli, L., Rossi, F., and Bombino, M. (1987). Pressure volume curve of total respiratory system in acute respiratory failure: Computed tomographic scan study. *Am. Rev. Respir. Dis.,* **136**: 730-736.

Gattinoni, L., Pistolesi, M., Rossi, F., Bombino, M., Bellato, V., and Miniati, M. (1987). Portable x-ray versus CT scan in ARDS (abstract). *Am. Rev. Respir. Dis.,* **135**:A214.

Gattinoni, L., Pesenti, A., Paglioni, S., Vitale, G., Rivolta, M., and Pelosi, P. (1988a). Inflammatory pulmonary edema and positive end-expiratory pressure: Correlations between imaging and physiological studies. *J. Thorac. Imag.,* **3**(3):59-64.

Gattinoni, L., Pesenti, A., Bombino, M., Baglioni, S., Rivolta, M., Rossi, F., Rossi, G. P., Fumagalli, R., Marcolin, R., Mascheroni, D., and Torresin, A. (1988b). Relationships between lung computed tomographic density, gas exchange and PEEP in acute respiratory failure. *Anesthesiology,* **69**:824-832.

Hales, C. A., David, J. K., Ahluwalia, B., Latty, A., Erdmann, J., Javaheri, S., and Kazemi, H. (1981). Regional edema formation in isolated perfused dog lungs. *Circ. Res.,* **48**:121-127.

Halperin, B. D., Feeley, T. W., Mihm, F. G., Chiles, C., Guthaner, D. F., and Blank, N. E. (1985). Evaluation of the portable chest roentgenogram for quantitating extravascular lung water in critically ill adults. *Chest,* **88**:649-652.

Ibanez, J., and Rauric, J. M. (1900). Normal values of functional residual capacity in the sitting and supine position. *Intensive Care Med.,* **8**:173-177.

Jones, T., Jones, H. A., Rhodes, C. G., Buckingham, P. D., and Hughes, J. M. B. (1976). Distribution of extravascular fluid volumes in isolated perfused lungs measured with H_2O. *J. Clin. Invest.,* **57**:706-713.

Langer, M., Mascheroni, D., Marcolin, R., and Gattinoni, L. (1988). The prone position in ARDS patients: A clinical study. *Chest,* **94**:103-107.

Mascheroni, D., Marcolin, R., Fumagalli, R., Gavazzeni, V., Coffano, B., Langer, M., Rossi, G. P., Massa, G., and Gattinoni, L. (1986). Effects of positioning in ARF: CT scan study (abstract). *Intensive Care Med.,* 222.

Maunder, R. J., Shuman, W. P., McHugh, J. W., et al. (1986). Preservation of normal lung regions in the adult respiratory distress syndrome: Analysis by computed tomography. *JAMA,* **25**:2463-2465.

Ngeow, Y. K., and Mitzner, W. (1983). Pulmonary hemodynamics and gas exchange properties during progressive edema. *J. Appl. Physiol.,* **55**:1154-1159.

Permutt, S. (1985). The role of pulmonary arterial pressure in experimentally induced acute lung injury. In *Acute Respiratory Failure.* Edited by W. M. Zapol and K. J. Falke. New York, Marcel Dekker, pp. 227-239.

Pistolesi, M., Miniati, M., Milne, E. N. C., and Giuntini, C. (1985). Chest roentgenogram in pulmonary edema. *Clin. Chest Med.,* **6**:315-344.

Rommelsheim, K., Lakner, K., Westhofen, P., et al. (1983). Das respiratorische distress-syndrome der erwachsenen (ARDS) in computer tomogram. *Anasth. Intensivther. Notfallmed.,* **18**:59-64.

Sibbald, W. J., Short, A. K., Warshawski, F. J., Cunningham, D. G., and Chung, H. (1985). Thermal dye measurements of extravascular lung water in critically ill patients. *Chest,* **87**:585-592.

Staub, N. C. (1988). New concepts about the pathophysiology of pulmonary edema. *J. Thorac. Imag.,* **3**(3):8-14.

Teplitz, C. (1976). The core pathobiology and integrated medical science of acute respiratory insufficiency. *Surg. Clin. North Am.,* **56**:1091-1130.

Wollmer, P., Rhodes, C. G., Deanfiled, J., Rozkovec, A., Allan, R. M., Maseri, A., and Fazio, F. (1987). Regional extravascular density of the lung in patients with acute pulmonary edema. *J. Appl. Physiol.,* **63**(5):1890-1895.

Zapol, W. M., Trelstad, R. L., Coffey, J. W., Trai, I., and Salvador, R. A. (1979). Pulmonary fibrosis in severe acute respiratory failure. *Am. Rev. Respir. Dis.,* **119**:547-554.

11

Cardiorespiratory Interactions

JAMES L. ROBOTHAM

The Johns Hopkins University
Medical Institutions
Baltimore, Maryland

JÜRGEN PETERS

Zentrum fur Anaesthesiologie
Universitat Dusseldorf
Dusseldorf, Federal Republic of Germany

I. Introduction

In a recent review in this series, we outlined many of the factors contributing to ventilation's influence on cardiac output (Robotham and Peters, 1989). In this review, we focus on those mechanical factors that contribute to the net influence of respiration on left ventricular (LV) performance. By this we mean, independently of changes in contractility, how respiration will, by altering preload and afterload, influence the pump performance of the ventricle.

The same principles are shown to apply across the entire spectrum of respiratory modes: (1) spontaneous ventilation with or without airway obstruction; (2) positive or negative pressure mechanical ventilation with or without positive end-expiratory pressure (PEEP); and (3) high-frequency ventilation. These principles should also apply across the entire spectrum of ventricular inotropic states, from normal, to depressed, to absent, that is, cardiac arrest. From this perspective it is apparent that full appreciation of the individual elements or events under one set of conditions (ventilatory mode and cardiac inotropic state) leads to a better understanding of these factors under any other condition.

II. Lung Volume and Intrathoracic Pressure

Changes in lung volume and intrathoracic pressure (ITP) may be either independent or dependent variables. A Mueller maneuver (a fall in intrathoracic pressure with no change in lung volume), a Valsalva maneuver, or chest compression with the airway closed, involves large changes in ITP with no change in lung volume (ignoring small volume changes due to gas compression or decompression). During an inspiratory increase in lung volume, ITP increases with intermittent positive pressure ventilation (IPPV) but decreases with spontaneous ventilation. With the chest widely opened, an increase in lung volume can be associated with no change in ITP. Despite removing the entire rib cage, however, lung inflation can still produce an increase in "local ITP" by direct compression of the heart as the lungs expand. If one places a hand between the heart and lungs as the lungs are inflated, one notes the remarkable degree of force exerted by the expanded lung. (An anesthesiologist who forgets this is rather quickly reminded by a cardiac surgeon.) Thus with the chest closed, stresses applied to the cardiac surface will include both generalized increases in a liquid ITP and a direct contract stress produced by the expanding lungs.

Finally, the increase in abdominal pressure produced by diaphragmatic descent during spontaneous or mechanically produced lung inflation may influence venous return from the abdomen. Ventilatory effects or any mechanical stress applied to the rib cage or abdomen during CPR may affect ITP. Differences in the surrounding compartment pressures influence the gradients for blood flow between them.

III. The Circulatory System

The circulation is by definition a closed circuit. It should therefore not be surprising that attempts to explain or predict all the potential effects of a respiratory perturbation frequently lead to a "circular" argument. At a given instant a substantial number of variables can be altered to affect either total and/or regional blood flow in a specific vascular compartment. As a general principle inherent in a circular system, many of these physiologic mechanisms invoke a "yin-yang" series of events. For example, (1) an increase in blood flow to one compartment through a change in local arterial resistance necessitates a decrease to another; (2) a decrease in intrathoracic pressure increases venous return to the thorax but may decrease arterial outflow; (3) a decrease in LV afterload improves total cardiac output until a fall in coronary perfusion pressure limits myocardial oxygen supply, diminishing the inotropic state of the LV; or (4) an arterial vasodilation increases ventricular output but dilation of the venous capacitance bed reduces venous return.

An important concept derived from the appreciation of these relationships is that, within experimentally obtainable limits, a given respiratory perturbation may have opposite acute and steady-state effects on the circulatory system; for example, a decrease in intrathoracic pressure may transiently decrease LV output but under steady-state conditions increase LV output. From this point of view, an analysis of the influence of respiration on the circulation can either begin by describing the steady state and then deduce the dominant variables or assess the individual variables and deduce their relative importance in different steady-state conditions. It is the latter approach that we have chosen.

Historically, the influence of ventilation on the circulatory system has generally considered the resultant average cardiac output produced by changing a given ventilatory parameter, for example comparing spontaneous and mechanical ventilation, the result of adding PEEP to intermittent positive pressure ventilation (IPPV), or comparison of IPPV and PEEP to high-frequency ventilation. In each case the critically important cardiac output averaged over a minute has been investigated. It was also clear that within all forms of ventilation or cardiopulmonary resuscitation (CPR) there exist cyclically repetitive alterations in the circulatory system that when averaged over time make up the steady-state results. We have found that by using increasingly shorter ventilatory perturbations of the circulatory system, the presence of physiologically distinct events can be definitively determined in a manner impossible with steady-state conditions.

IV. Spontaneous Ventilation and the Left Ventricle

The specific question we shall address, that is, what causes the inspiratory fall in LV stroke volume (LVSV) during spontaneous ventilation?, can serve as a prototype question for understanding cardiorespiratory interactions. The major hypotheses advanced in the literature to explain the inspiratory fall in SV can be divided into two groups: one in which a primary decrease in preload leads by Starling's law to a subsequent decrease in SV; the second in which an increase in afterload or a decrease in contractility leads directly to a decrease in LVSV (Robotham and Peters, 1989). It is obvious that a primary decrease in preload demands a decrease first in the LV end-diastolic volume and then the LV end-systolic volume. An increase in afterload or a decrease in contractility demands first an increase in the LV end-systolic volume and then in the LV end-diastolic volume. Many have used calculated transmural LV pressures, assuming a direct relationship between such pressures and LV volume. However, determination of "true" transmural LV pressure is extremely difficult, requiring simultaneous determination of local intrapericardial pressure over the LV and right ventricular pressure as well as an empirically determined complex weighting ratio (Shabetai, 1988). The most direct approach to solving this problem is to determine changes in LV volume rather than extrapolating a volume change from a potentially misleading pressure measurement.

Advocates of a primary decrease in preload have unequivocally demonstrated in human and animal studies that during either a spontaneous inspiration or a Mueller maneuver the LV free wall to septal diameter acutely decreases and the calculated LV volumes diminish, accounting for the fall in stroke volume (Jardin et al., 1982; Rankin et al., 1982; Robotham et al., 1983; Brinker and Weiss, 1980). Advocates of an increase in LV afterload causing the fall in SV have similarly presented results in both human and animals consistent with increases in LV end-systolic volume (Summer et al., 1979; Buda et al., 1979; Karam et al., 1984). What is perhaps equally important is the appreciation that many studies have a substantial but not statistically significant number of subjects (animals) that qualitatively deviate from the mean results. Using radionuclide techniques in humans during partially obstructed inspiration, Karam et al. (1984) have reported a significant mean increase in the estimated LV end-systolic volume, although a smaller number of individuals decreased their LV end-systolic volume and many exhibited a decrease in LV end-diastolic volume. Using a mechanical device for estimating internal LV circumference in dogs, Wead and Norton (1981) observed early in a Mueller maneuver a presumptive decrease in LV volume but, as the Mueller maneuver was prolonged, an increase in LV volume. Studies using sonomicrometery in dogs have shown an increase in LV volumes during a Mueller maneuver and in the succeeding unobstructed inspiration demonstrated a net decrease in LV volumes (Fig. 1) (Robotham et al., 1983). It is clear that no single mechanism can account for these observations.

Although the majority of studies lead to the conclusion that a diminished preload causes the inspiratory fall in LV stroke volume, other factors are clearly present and may account for the diverse results reported by different groups. Ventricular interdependence or, to some degree, compression of the heart by the inflated lungs (heart-lung interdependence) (Wallis et al., 1983; Guz et al., 1987), that is, increases in either the RV volume or lung volume constraining LV filling, are most commonly believed responsible. Either an increase in afterload and/or a decrease in contractility can explain an increased LV volume with an associated diminished stroke volume.

The phasic change in systemic venous return with respiration should lead to a significant amount of variation in LV output at a normal respiratory rate (Scharf et al., 1980). However, this cannot explain the observed fall in LV stroke volume with the first inspiratory effort after a prolonged apneic period. Accordingly, it becomes necessary to explore the influence of the various potential mechanisms by demonstrating their presence independently of other factors.

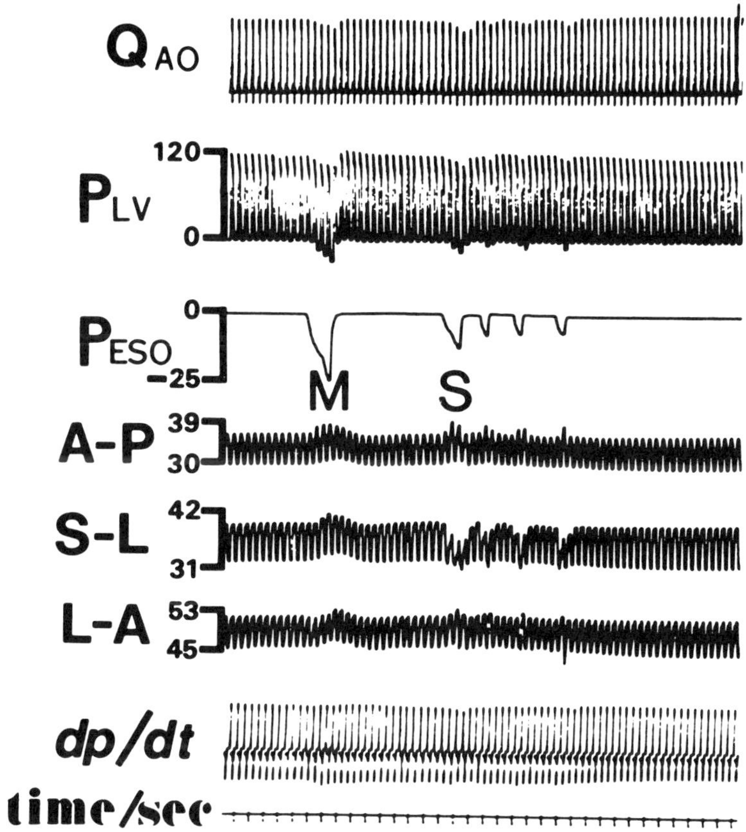

Figure 1 Tracings obtained from a chronically instrumented dog with an implanted ascending aortic flow probe, left ventricular (LV) micromanometer, and endocardial crystals in the anterior-posterior (A-P), septal to free lateral wall (S-L), and long axis (L-A), apex-base dimensions, with an esophageal balloon passed after the dog was anesthetized and endotracheally intubated. The first inspiratory effort is a Mueller maneuver (M) in which a sharp decrease in aortic flow ($\dot{Q}_{AO}$) is noted associated with the fall in LV pressures relative to atmosphere. An increase in heart size both at end-diastole (peak) and end-systole (minimum pen deflection) is noted in all three dimensions, consistent with an acute increase in both LV end-diastolic and end-systolic volumes due to an increased LV afterload. The next inspiratory effort is a large spontaneous sigh (S) in which an even greater fall in aortic flow is noted despite a lesser fall in esophageal pressure (P_{ESO}). The S-L diastolic dimension markedly diminishes, with a small systolic decrease, but both the A-P and L-A dimensions demonstrate increases in end-diastolic and end-systolic dimensions. Similar diastolic and systolic distortions of the left ventricle in the S-L dimension are seen in the following three normal spontaneous tidal breaths. The significant S-L dimension contribution to LV ejection during tidal inspiration is at least partly mediated by heart-lung interdependence. The absence of the fall in S-L dimensions during the Mueller maneuver is consistent with the absence of mechanical compression of the heart. (Reproduced with permission from *Clinics in Chest Medicine,* **4**:173, 1983.)

V. The Cardiac Cycle

The cardiac cycle can be temporally divided into a diastolic period (ventricular filling altering preload) and a systolic period (ventricular ejection altered by afterload and contractility). Within each period, further refinement is possible, such as early diastole with passive filling and late diastole with active (atrial contraction) filling. Similarly, systole can be divided into early isovolumic contraction, ejection, and late isovolumic relaxation periods. If respiration affects ventricular performance, it is reasonable to assume that its influence extends to some or all parts of a cardiac cycle. It is a simplistic but important notion that if ventilation influences only diastole, it could increase or decrease ventricular filling. Assuming a constant preload, if ventilation influenced only systole the resultant stroke volume could increase, decrease, or be unchanged depending on changes in LV afterload and/or contractility. Apparently contradictory results have served as the fuel for the differing schools of thought, each able to marshall data supporting either a predominant diastolic or systolic event. These studies strongly suggest that opposing events are occurring and that a simple explanation is incompatible with the complete picture.

VI. Spontaneous Ventilation: Mitral and Aortic Flows

Our efforts to separate the potential diastolic and systolic influences of respiration on cardiac performance began with studies in anesthetized dogs evaluating blood flow across the mitral valve using an acutely implanted electromagnetic flow probe seated over the mitral valve. Comparison of changes in the integrated mitral and ascending aortic blood flows allows assessment of LV inflow and outflow. This permits an estimate of changes in LV end-diastolic and end-systolic volumes independent of any assumptions about LV shape. Clear respiratory variation was evident in both mitral and ascending aortic integrated flows (Fig. 2). Particularly during the relatively rapid increase in intrathoracic pressure at the beginning of expiration, large increases in mitral flow were usually observed prior to the expected increase in aortic flow. Following vagotomy in the anesthetized dog, respiratory variation in systemic venous is eliminated at the end of the prolonged inspiratory and expiratory periods (Fig. 3). Clear immediate changes were still demonstrable in LV inflow and outflow. However, the cyclic nature of normal spontaneous ventilation and the relatively small changes usually observed between any two cardiac cycles made difficult a clear definition of events at the beginning of an inspiration as due to either primary diastolic or primary systolic events. The relatively rapid increase in ITP at the beginning of expiration was the only portion of the respiratory cycle at which "quasi-square rapid wave" changes in ITP could be observed. For reasons that are not clear, the pento-

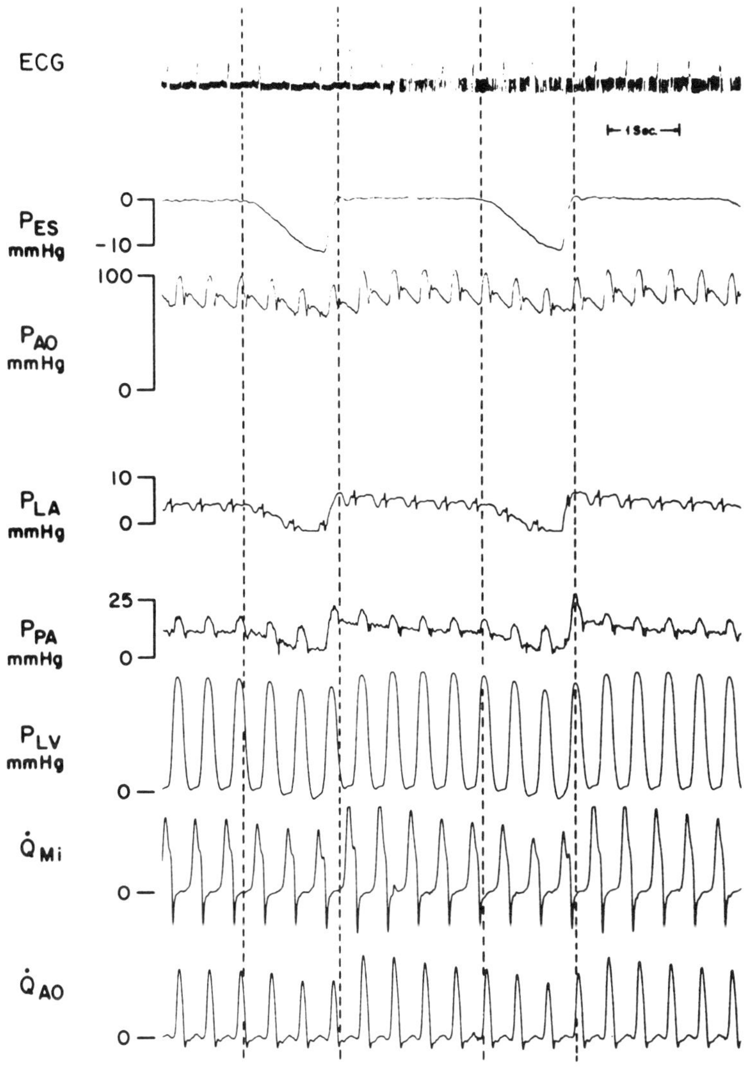

Figure 2 Two consecutive respiratory cycles during partial inspiratory airway obstruction in an anesthetized dog postvagotomy. Vertical dashed lines demarcate the two periods during which esophageal pressure (P_{ES}) is reduced during inspiration. Both integrated mitral ($\dot{Q}_{Mi}$) and ascending aortic ($\dot{Q}_{AO}$) flows diminish during the inspiration and increase with expiration. There is a large inspiratory increase in mitral flow preceding the large increase in aortic flow in both respiratory cycles. Although the rapid increase in eosphageal pressure occurs during systole in the second breath, there is little effect on aortic flow. These two respiratory cycles demonstrate the dominance of mitral flow leading aortic flow during a respiratory cycle. P_{AO}, aortic pressure; P_{LA}, left atrial pressure; P_{PA}, pulmonary artery presure; P_{LV}, left ventricular pressure. (Reprinted with permission from *Anesthesiology,* **69**:522, 1988.)

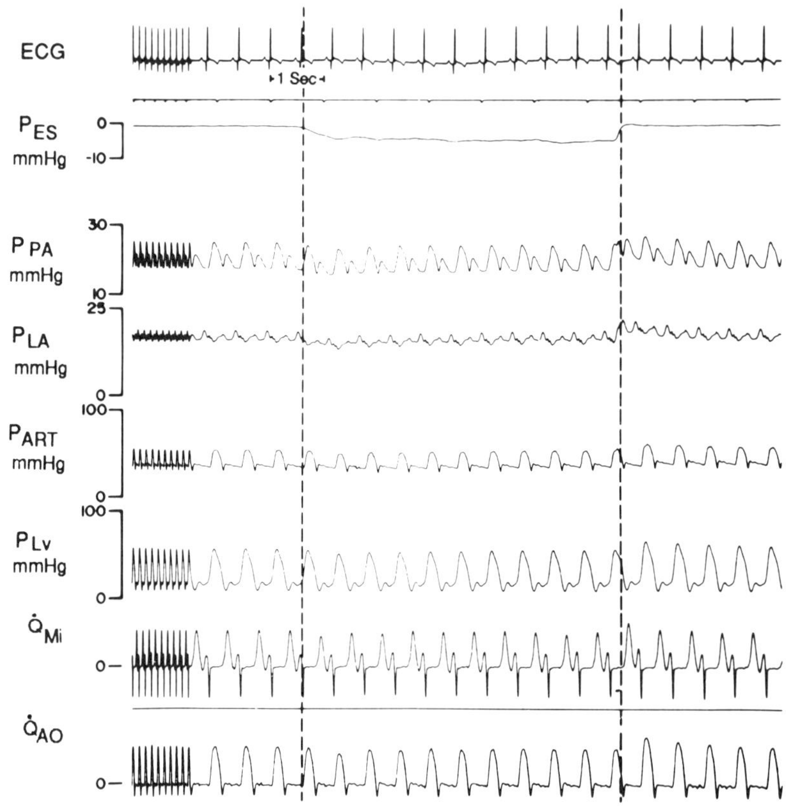

Figure 3 Mueller maneuver in closed chest anesthetized dog following bilateral vagotomy. Abbreviations as in Figure 2. During the prolonged fall in pleural pressure with the Mueller maneuver, defined between the two vertical dashed lines, there are 11 systoles. Aortic flow, as is typical, reaches its minimum during the second beat of the Mueller maneuver and gradually increases to approach but not to exceed the control aortic flows. At the end of the Mueller maneuver, with the rapid increase in esophageal pressure, the aortic flow demonstrates a rebound increase over control values. Mitral flow shows a similar pattern during the Mueller maneuver, with an early decrease and then return toward but not above control diastolic flows. Immediately after the rapid increase in esophageal pressure, marked by the second vertical dashed line, the first event is a large increase in both peak and total mitral flow followed by a large increase in aortic flow. Minimal mitral flow, immediately after the first vertical dashed line, clearly precedes minimal aortic flow, as does the maximal mitral flow immediately after the second vertical dashed line precede maximal aortic flow. Mitral flow demonstrates a clear late atrial component separate from the early passive component. With the initial fall in pleural pressure at the first vertical dashed line, there is a very small decrease in aortic flow prior to any pleural pressure-induced fall in mitral flow. Mitral predominance is demonstrated, but a small systolic effect is suggested. The prolonged expiratory and inspiratory times negate changes in systemic venous return as a consequential influence during the transients occurring immediately following the two vertical lines. (Reproduced with permission from *J. Appl. Physiol.*, **65**:1670, 1988.)

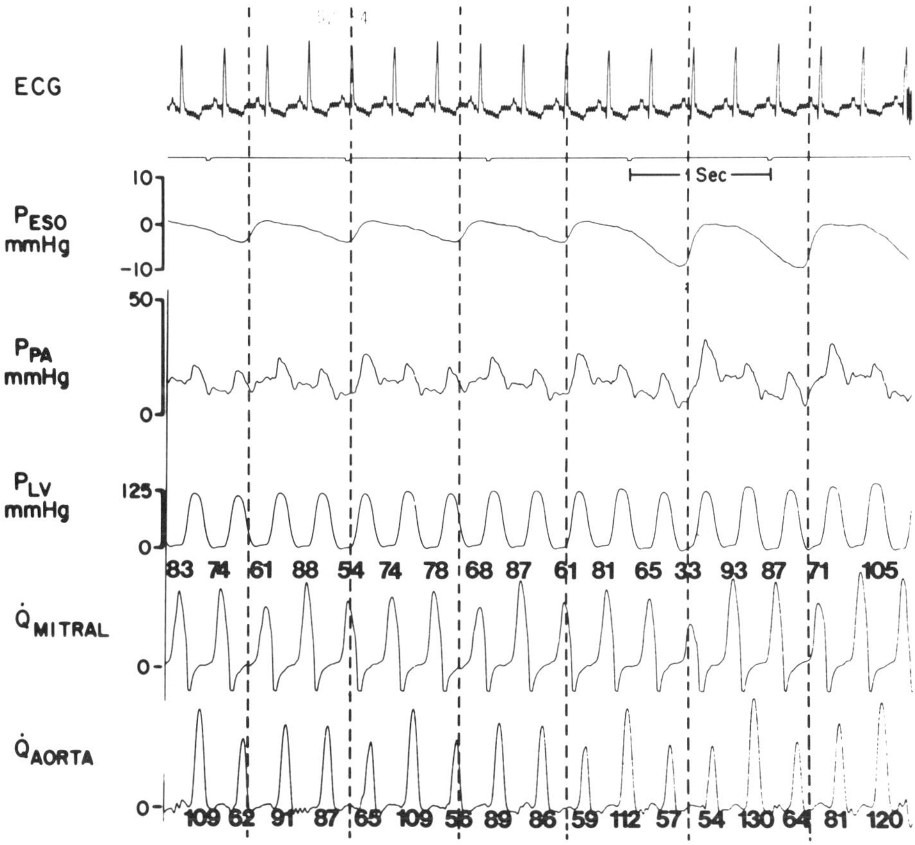

Figure 4 Changes in mitral and aortic flows at a rapid respiratory rate. Tracing obtained during four unobstructed inspiratory efforts followed by two Mueller maneuvers at the far right with large changes in esophageal pressure. Abbreviations as in the previous figures. The numbers above each mitral flow trace and below each aortic flow trace reflect the respective area in arbitrary units. The vertical dashed lines are drawn to coincide with the beginning of the increase in esophageal pressure. The first inspiratory effort demonstrates a large fall in aortic flow (beat 2) independent of the minimal decrease in the immediately preceding mitral flow; that is, end systolic volume has increased. Similarly, in both Mueller maneuvers at the far right, the inspiratory decrease in the aortic stroke volume (beats 12 and 15) cannot be explained by small changes in the preceding mitral inflow volumes. Both Mueller maneuvers suggest an increase in end-systolic volume during the fall in pleural pressure. Conversely, with the rapid increase in pleural pressure at the conclusion of the first Mueller maneuver, there is a large increase in mitral flow (beat 14) preceding the major increase in aortic flow, suggesting an increase in end-diastolic volume with the increase in pleural pressure. (Reproduced with permission from *J. Appl. Physiol.*, **65**: 1673, 1988.)

barbital-anesthetized dog, when not tachypneic, usually begins expiration during diastole. This pattern was noted with or without changes in lung volume during the inspiratory effort, both pre- and postvagotomy. Thus, as illustrated in Figures 2 and 3, an unequivocal increase in diastolic mitral flow and LV filling was demonstrable in every dog studied ($N = 8$) when the expiratory increase in ITP happened to occur during diastole. Under these conditions, a change in LV preload clearly precedes any possible change in LV afterload or contractility as ITP increased. However, because only rarely did the dogs begin expiration during systole, the ability to test statistically whether a systolic event was independently affecting LV output was hampered. Thus unequivocal demonstration of a systolic factor could not be established.

However, recordings obtained during periods of tachypnea in some dogs strongly suggested that separate diastolic and systolic events occur during spontaneous ventilation (see Fig. 4). Under these conditions, rapid fluctuations in intrathoracic pressure occur during various parts of the cardiac cycle. Large changes in mitral flow occurred independently of the preceding systole, during rapid increases and decreases in intrathoracic pressure. As importantly, when ITP fell rapidly during systole, large decreases in the integrated ascending aortic flow can be seen prior to any similarly large decrease in LV filling during the preceding diastolic period.

Review of individual traces in dogs with slow heart rates and, hence, long diastolic periods demonstrated that when the rapid increase in ITP at the beginning of expiration occurred during any part of diastole, an immediate increase in mitral flow was evident. That is, if ITP increased in early diastole, peak mitral flow was augmented, but if the increase in ITP occurred in late diastole, only late diastolic flow was augmented (Fig. 5). These observations

Figure 5 Two consecutive spontaneous unobstructed inspirations with the increase in esophageal pressure (P_{ESO}) demarcated by the vertical dashed line in both breaths. (A) During the fall in esophageal pressure (S_1), both ascending aortic ($\dot{Q}_{AORTA}$) and mitral flow ($\dot{Q}_{MITRAL}$) decrease. The increase in esophageal pressure occurs during diastole, with an obvious increase in mitral flow immediately apparent, the increase in aortic flow following. (B) During the following inspiration (S_2) there is again a decrease in both ascending aortic and mitral flows, but the expiratory increase in esophageal pressure now occurs in late diastole. The increase in area under the mitral flow trace is evident to the right of the vertical line. Ascending aortic flow then exhibits a similar increase. The minimal and maximal mitral flows precede the respective minimal and maximal aortic flows during both respiratory cycles. Diastolic events clearly dominate in determining LV output changes. The elevated left-sided diastolic pressures and low arterial pressure reflect a presumptive degree of LV dysfunction. The ECG demonstrates normal sinus rhythm, arterial pressure (P_{ART}), left atrial pressure (P_{LA}), right atrial pressure (P_{RA}), and left ventricular pressure (P_{LV}), all measured relative to atmosphere. (Reproduced with permission from *Anesthesiology,* **69**:521, 1983.)

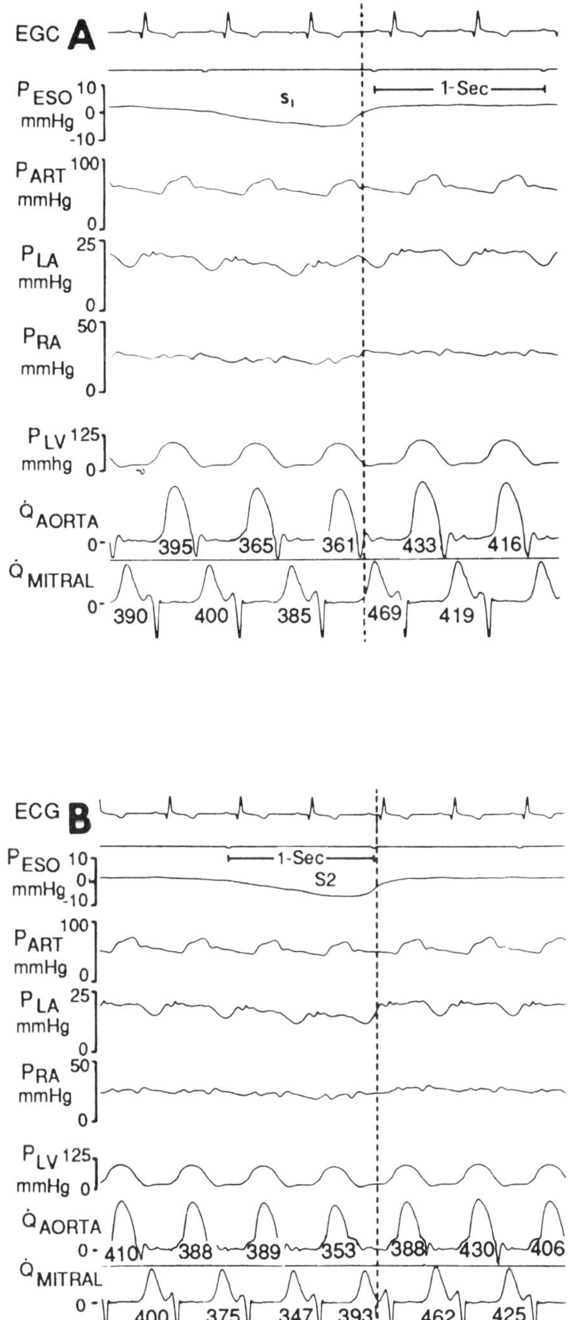
EGC
A
PESO
mmHg
10
0
-10
s1
1-Sec
PART
mmHg
100
0
PLA
mmHg
25
0
PRA
mmHg
50
0
PLV
mmhg
125
0
Q̇AORTA
0
395
365
361
433
416
Q̇MITRAL
0
390
400
385
469
419
ECG
B
PESO
mmHg
10
0
-10
1-Sec
S2
PART
mmHg
100
0
PLA
mmHg
25
0
PRA
mmHg
50
0
PLV
mmHg
125
0
Q̇AORTA
0
410
388
389
353
388
430
406
Q̇MITRAL
0
400
375
347
393
462
425

suggested that mitral flow is exquisitely sensitive to changes in ITP but that a systolic factor, although present, is difficult to consistently demonstrate.

Accordingly, we tested two opposing hypotheses. One hypothesis stated that all respiratory variation in LV volumes is caused by changes in preload during diastole alone; the second hypothesis stated that all respiratory variation is caused only by systolic events, that is, changes in contractility and/or afterload. For the first hypothesis to be accepted, the minimum and maximum values for integrated mitral flow during inspiration and expiration, respectively, should precede the inspiratory minimum and expiratory maximum values for integrated aortic flow. Thus the LV, obeying Starling's law, would vary its output only according to changes in preload. For the second hypothesis to be accepted the inspiratory minimum and expiratory maximum values for integrated aortic flow would precede the respiratory variation in mitral flow. These two hypotheses are mutually exclusive, and as such, if the experimental observations do not conform strictly to one or the other, then neither should be true, that is, both diastolic *and* systolic events interacting to determine the respiratory variation in LV output. We observed that under conditions of unobstructed, partially obstructed, and totally obstructed inspiratory efforts with or without an increase in lung volume, approximately 80% of the time, the minimal and maximal integrated mitral flows preceded the respective minimum and maximal integrated aortic flows. This supports the dominance of preload effects in determining LV output, but systolic mechanisms must also be present since changes in preload did not occur first 100% of the time (Robotham et al., 1988a, b).

The ability of sudden increases in systemic venous return to the right heart to reduce LV compliance, increasing left heart diastolic pressures and diminishing peak and integrated mitral flow, can be demonstrated in the open chest dog (Fig. 6) (Robotham et al., 1988a). Two beats after an increase in systemic venous return and the initial fall in mitral flow, mitral flow increases over baseline, presumably reflecting the increased pulmonary venous return after the initial ventricular interdependence-mediated decrease in mitral flow. This pattern of diminished peak and total mitral flow is exactly that predicted if LV compliance were reduced throughout diastole (see Fig. 7). Once the right heart volume returns to baseline values, the increased systemic venous return, which has been translocated by the RV to the pulmonary vascular bed, raising its intravascular pressure, produces the pressure gradient to immediately increase mitral flow during the subsequent diastole (see Fig. 6). Consistent with pericardially mediated ventricular interdependence being a dominant factor in these relationships, a much smaller reduction in mitral flow is observed when systemic venous return is acutely increased with the pericardium removed (Robotham et al., 1988a).

In contrast, if an increase in LV afterload were the only cause of the inspiratory reduction in LV stroke volume, the initial pattern of change in

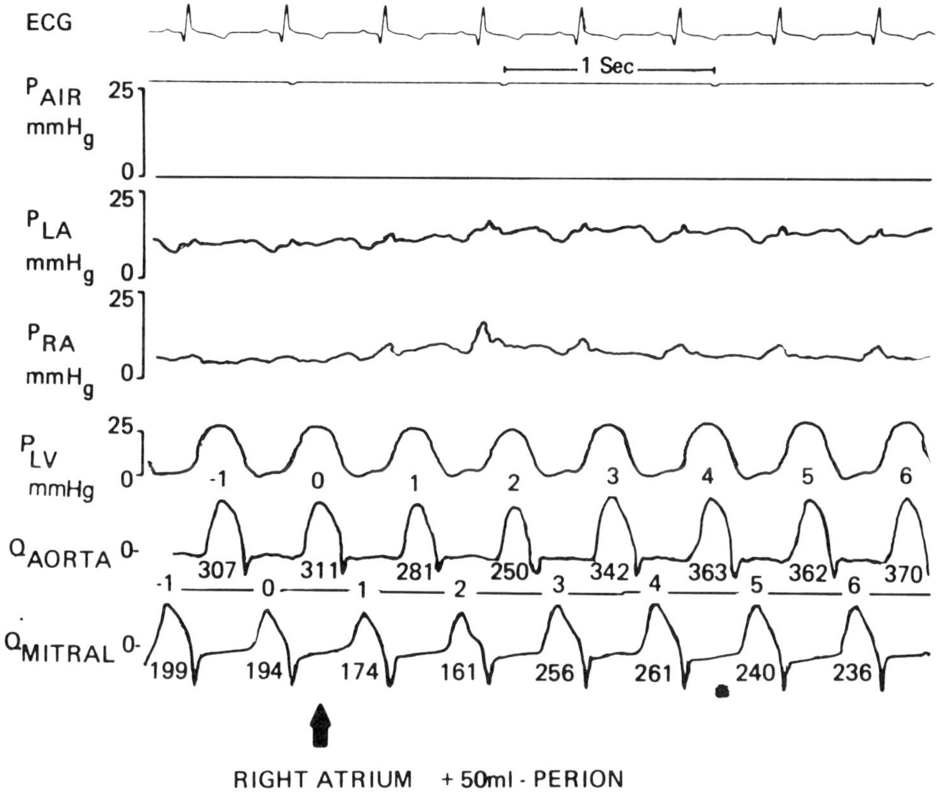

Figure 6 Open chest study during apnea in an anesthetized dog demonstrating the effects of rapid infusion of 50 ml blood into the right atrium with the pericardium on. The rhythm is stable as reflected by the ECG, and airway pressure (P_{AIR}) reflects the apneic state. Left atrial (P_{LA}), right atrial (P_{RA}), and left ventricular (P_{LV}) pressures are measured relative to atmosphere. To facilitate comparisons, the flow traces occurring at the times of the experimental perturbation are designated zero, with sequential negative and positive numbers above each consecutive beat. The areas in arbitrary units under each trace reflect the inflow and outflow volumes. The beginning of the rapid infusion into the right atrium is marked by the thick arrow and is associated with an immediate fall in the next two mitral flow traces ($\dot{Q}_{MITRAL}$), numbered 1 and 2, with a subsequent increase over the control period by the number 3 diastolic period. The aortic flow trace ($\dot{Q}_{AORTA}$) changes follow the mitral, as indicated by the numbered beats. Both right (P_{RA}) and left (P_{LA}) atrial pressures increase during the infusion into the right atrium and are associated with the initial fall and then increase in mitral flow. We interpret this to reflect the right heart first affecting LV filling via interdependence and then increasing LV filling as the increased systemic venous return reaches the left side. A less consistent effect reducing early mitral flow was found when the pericardium was removed. (The bottom two channels are darkened for photographic reproduction.) (Reproduced with permission from *J. Appl. Physiol.*, **65**:1666, 1988.)

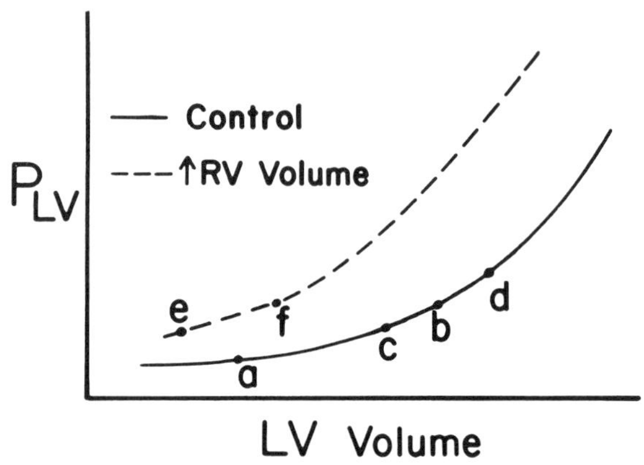

Figure 7 Schematic representation of the diastolic pressure volume relationships at the beginning and end of diastole. Under baseline control conditions, early diastolic pressure and volume at point a moves along the solid line to point b at end-diastole. Assuming steady-state conditions, diastolic filling equals the stroke volume ejected. If an isolated increase in LV afterload is then imposed, LV end-systolic volume moves from point a to point c after a number of beats as a new steady state is approached. The initial beats after the increase in afterload would produce little change in the gradient for peak mitral flow, which occurs early, but as end-diastolic volume moves onto the steep portion of the pressure volume line, late diastolic mitral flow would markedly diminish. Under steady-state conditions of increased afterload, filling would occur from point c to point d, with the gradient for both early and late diastolic filling diminished. In contrast, an acute increase in RV volume changes the LV pressure-volume relationship to the dashed line, which diverges from the control line as the biventricular volume increases. The reduced LV compliance results in diminished initial and end-diastolic volumes with elevated pressures. Thus the gradient for mitral flow is reduced compared to control conditions throughout diastole. Both increasing LV afterload and increasing RV volume via ventricular interdependence diminish LV stroke volume but may have different effects on LV volumes and patterns of mitral flow.

mitral flow should be quite different. Using acute obstruction of the descending thoracic aorta to increase afterload, the first effect must be a decrease in stroke volume producing an increased end-systolic volume. If, as schematically illustrated in Figure 7, this end-systolic volume is located at a point still on the flat portion of the LV diastolic pressure-volume relationship, then one would predict only a minor change in the initial diastolic gradient compared to control and, thus, no change in the early peak mitral flow. Mitral flow later in diastole would decrease. Only after a number of cardiac cycles as a progressive increase in LV end systolic volume occurred due to the increased afterload would the initial gradient for mitral flow diminish and reduce early peak flow. This is exactly what is observed following cross-clamping of the descending thoracic aorta to acutely increase LV afterload (Fig. 8) (Robotham et al., 1988a).

Obviously, if the acute increase in afterload was to be imposed on an LV already on the steep portion of its pressure-volume curve, then even the

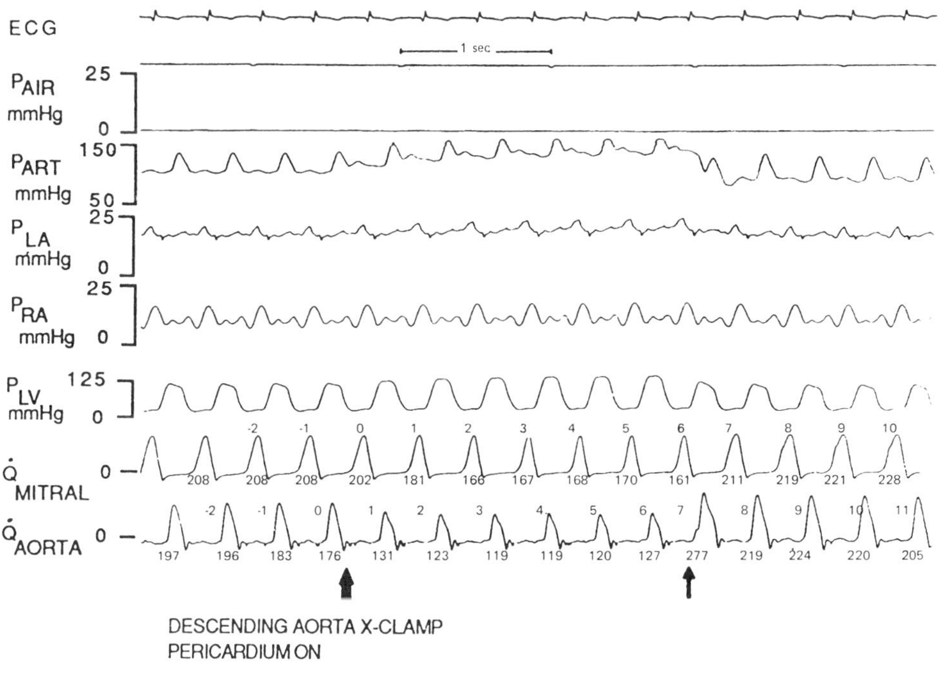

Figure 8 Effects of acute cross-clamping the descending thoracic aorta at approximately the T_8 level in an open chest anesthetized dog preparation. The descending aorta was cross-clamped at the initial thick arrow (beat 0) and the cross-clamp released at the second thin arrow (beat 7). There is an obvious immediate fall in both peak and total aortic flow following the cross-clamp (beat 1), with rebound overshoot in both peak and total flow with the release of cross-clamp (beat 7). Mitral flow demonstrates a lesser percentage fall in total area under the curve as measured in arbitrary units. The most important observation is that aortic flow changes precede mitral changes during definitive changes in LV afterload as indicated by the areas and as measured in arbitrary units under each trace. Similar changes in aortic flow but lesser falls in mitral flow are observed with the pericardium removed during a descending aortic cross-clamp. Neither the mitral flow trace nor the left atrial high-fidelity pressure tracing are consistent with induced mitral valve incompetence. Abbreviations as in the previous figures. P_{ART}, arterial pressure proximal to the aortic clamp. (Reproduced with permission from *J. Appl. Physiol.*, **65**:1668, 1988.)

first cardiac cycle after the increase in afterload could lead to an immediate reduction in both peak and total mitral flow. During spontaneous inspiratory efforts, regardless of the LV end-diastolic pressure, we observed immediate decreases in both peak and integrated mitral flow. Thus, the pattern of change in the mitral flow trace was more compatible with a dominant alteration in preload than in afterload.

VII. Transient Analysis of a Negative ITP

In theory it should be possible to perturb the ventilatory system in an extremely rapid manner such that the separate and independent influences during systole and diastole could be evaluated, for example. Recognition that rapid changes in ITP during spontaneous ventilatory efforts in dogs could produce independent effects on LV filling and emptying (Robotham et al., 1988a, b) led to development of a technique to precisely control ITP within specific periods of a cardiac cycle. The use of electrocardiography (ECG) to trigger bilateral phrenic nerve stimulation permitted an experimental approach to this problem. By appropriately adjusting the delay time after the R wave of the QRS complex, the duration of stimulation, and the frequency of the impulses, a rapid decrease of 15-25 mmHg in ITP can be obtained and confined to either systole or diastole. Further adjustments in the settings permits perturbations confined to early or late diastole.

The approach of analyzing rapid transient changes in lung volume and/or ITP becomes a powerful tool to define separate diastolic and systolic events during respiration since the influence of the RV output in series with the LV is eliminated. By confining the ventilatory perturbation to systole, the influence on the succeeding diastole when ITP has returned to baseline can be evaluated. Similarly, by confining the perturbation to diastole, any influence on the succeeding systole can be evaluated. By confining a perturbation to diastole after the aortic valve has closed, the influence of ventilation on left-sided arterial flow independent of LV function can be evaluated. All this information can then be used to gain maximum insight into a ventilatory perturbation that extends over a complete cardiac cycle.

VIII. Transient Analysis Techniques

A series of studies have been performed in anesthetized dogs, all instrumented acutely to allow ECG-triggered phrenic nerve stimulation and to measure: (1) mitral and ascending aortic flow; (2) LV septal to lateral diameter using sonomicrometery; (3) ascending aortic, descending aortic, and/or carotid flow; or (4) an ascending aortic flow and intrathoracic aortic diameters just distal to the aortic arch.

To minimize the influence of an increase in abdominal pressure during phrenic nerve stimulation affecting either systemic venous return to the right heart or the "regional" LV afterload imposed by increased abdominal pressure (Robotham et al., 1985), Figure 9 demonstrates the influence of phrenic nerve stimulation confined to diastole with the abdomen widely opened and the intestinal contents eviscerated. The airway was unobstructed so that lung volume increased. (*Note*: During a Mueller maneuver with no lung volume change there is only a minimal change in abdominal pressure since diaphragmatic motion is minimal.) When the fall in ITP is confined to diastole, there is an obvious substantial decrease in both the peak mitral flow and the integrated area reflecting LV filling. The subsequent stroke volume when esophageal pressure has returned to baseline is reduced, as expected from Starling's law. The subsequent diastolic and systolic periods demonstrate an increase in both the peak and integrated mitral and aortic flows. The reason for the immediate fall in mitral flow is, in all likelihood, not due to a primary pooling of blood in the pulmonary vascular bed since at end-diastole, when esophageal pressure had returned to baseline, both atrial pressures relative to atmosphere are elevated compared to their previous values during apnea, as is the LV end-diastolic pressure. Thus, for a diminished LV end-diastolic volume, the LV end-diastolic pressure is increased; that is, effective LV diastolic compliance is decreased. Two types of interdependence could account for this, both compatible with the observed increase in right atrial pressure. Heart-lung interdependence in which the expanding lungs compress the heart would reduce the effective compliance of both ventricles, reducing biventricular filling (Wallis et al., 1983). This cannot explain the results when the airway is obstructed completely during the phrenic nerve stimulation, precluding heart-lung interdependence, since the lung volume is constant. The dominant mechanism appears to be ventricular interdependence in which the sudden increase in right ventricular filling (unpublished observation) competes with the LV for space within the intrapericardial sac (Bove and Santamore, 1981). As a result, LV compliance is diminished as the RV volume rapidly increases, thus reducing mitral flow and the subsequent LV stroke volume. Consistent with this, the LV septal to free lateral wall dimension decreases during a transient diastolic negative ITP (Fig. 10). The succeeding diastolic period exhibits a compensatory increase in mitral flow as the blood dammed up during the negative ITP and the increased systemic venous return contribute to LV filling. It takes only 400 msec for an increase in pulmonary arterial inflow to produce an increase in pulmonary venous outflow (Maloney et al., 1968).

The influence of a fall in ITP confined to systole is illustrated in Figure 11, again with the abdomen widely open to minimize the influence of changes in abdominal pressure (Robotham et al., 1985). There is an immediate decrease

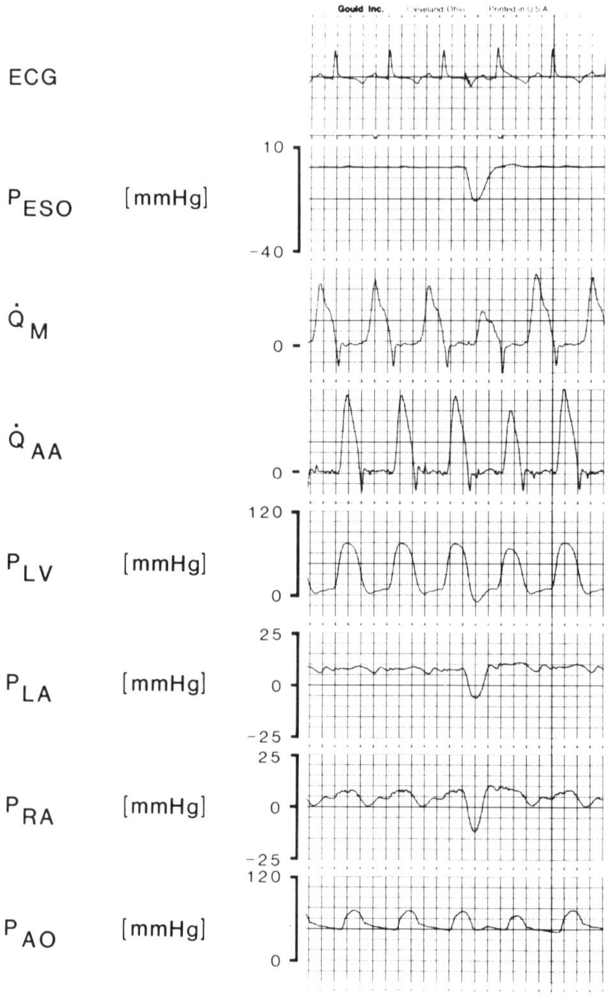

Figure 9 Diastolic phrenic nerve stimulation producing a transient decrease in esophageal pressure (P_{ESO}) confined to diastole in an acutely instrumented anesthetized dog with the abdomen widely opened and the intestinal contents eviscerated to minimize changes in abdominal pressure during the phrenic nerve stimulation. Steady-state mitral ($\dot{Q}_M$) and ascending aortic (Q_{AA}) flows are observed prior to a transient fall in intrathoracic pressure. There is an immediate substantial decrease in peak and total mitral flow. The subsequent LV stroke volume is similarly reduced at a time when intrathoracic pressure has returned to its baseline value such that there could be no effect on LV ejection. The subsequent mitral flow and LV stroke volume demonstrate compensatory increases. Of critical importance, LV end-diastolic pressure (P_{LV}), left atrial pressure (P_{LA}), and right atrial pressure (P_{RA}) are all increased relative to atmosphere at end-diastole when esophageal pressure has returned to baseline values. Since LV inflow has diminished, LV end-diastolic volume is reduced and its pressure increased; thus effective compliance is reduced. The increase in right atrial pressure and pattern of change mitral flow are consistent with ventricular interdependence being responsible for the reduction in LV preload.

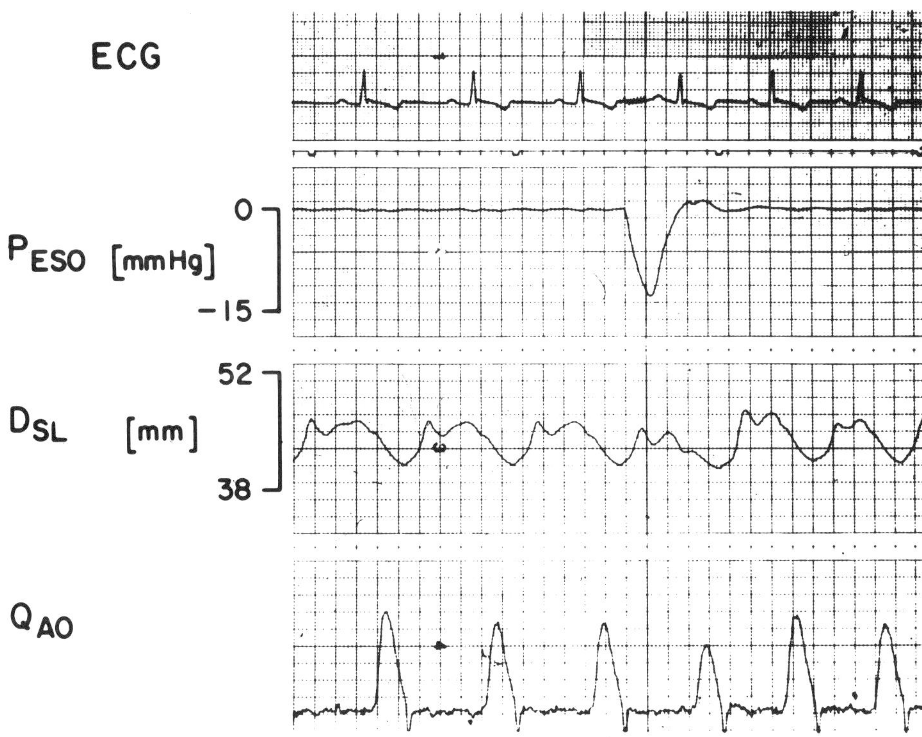

Figure 10 Phrenic nerve stimulation confined to diastole in an acutely instrumented anesthetized dog. During the transient decrease in intrathoracic pressure, the LV septal to free lateral dimension (D_{SL}) is substantially reduced compared to its diastolic dimensions in the preceding control apneic beats. The subsequent ascending aortic flow ($\dot{Q}_{AO}$) is substantially reduced, consistent with the diminished mitral inflow observed in Figure 9. The decrease in the septal to lateral dimension is consistent with ventricular interdependence contributing to the reduction in LV diastolic filling. This pattern was observed whether lung volume was maintained constant or allowed to increase such that heart-lung interdependence alone cannot account for the change.

in the peak and total integrated ascending aortic flow. The decrease is orders of magnitude more than could be ascribed to a possible increase in systolic coronary flow, which is not measured by the aortic flow probe (Schwartz et al., 1982). When an arrythmia did not follow a systolic perturbation in ITP, the subsequent mitral flow was decreased consistent with the presence of an acute increase in the LV end-systolic volume. The fall in LV stroke volume during systolic phrenic nerve stimulation proves that a separate systolic mechanism contributes to the inspiratory fall in LV stroke volume. This means either an acute decrease in contractility or an increase in afterload. Since

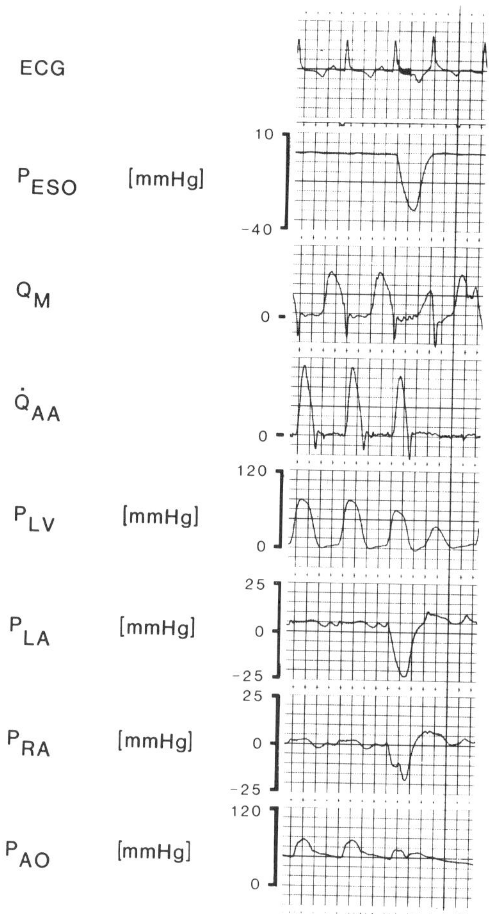

Figure 11 Systolic phrenic nerve stimulation to produce a transient fall in intrathoracic pressure confined to systole in an acutely instrumented anesthetized dog with the abdomen widely opened to minimize changes in abdominal pressure. Following the control apneic period in which steady-state mitral and ascending aortic flows are observed, with the fall in intrathoracic pressure LV stroke volume substantially diminishes compared to control beats with similar end-diastolic volumes. The fall in esophageal pressure is larger than the fall in left ventricular or aortic pressure, all measured relative to atmosphere, and thus the transmural systolic pressures have increased consistent with an increase in afterload. The time course for the decrease in LV output is too rapid for neural reflex arcs.

there are no known reflexes that could mediate such a decrease in contractility within 100 msec, a fall in contractility seems unlikely. However, we have addressed the issue from another perspective by measuring intrathoracic aortic dimensions in the closed chest anesthetized dog during systolic phrenic nerve stimulation. Piezoelectric crystals placed to measure orthagonal diameters using sonomicrometry allow qualitative estimates of the true changes in transmural intrathoracic aortic pressure to be made. The use of the orthogonal diameters, which can then be used to calculate the cross-sectional area of an ellipse, allows us to estimate acute volume changes in the intrathoracic aorta. If anything, an inspiratory effort should increase the length of the intrathoracic aorta. Thus if the cross-sectional area increases, the intrathoracic aortic volume increases. In effect, the aortic dimensions are used to "transduce" the true aortic transmural pressure. Thus, if a primary decrease in contractility accounts for the fall in LV stroke volume, then with less LV output the peak systolic aortic volume should decrease. In contrast, if the primary cause of the fall in LVSV was equivalent to an increased afterload imposed at the junction of the intra- and extrathoracic compartments, then the intrathoracic aortic volume-transmural pressure should increase. Figure 12 illustrates that this is precisely what occurs (Peters et al., 1988b).

Further insight into the influence of a systolic fall in ITP is provided by measuring blood flow at the points of arterial egress from the thorax, that is, in the carotid artery and the descending aorta above the diaphragm (Peters et al., 1988a, b). Adjustment of the timing of the phrenic nerve stimulation to begin in early or midsystole defines two components. The most important factor is a marked reduction in flow into the extrathoracic vascular compartments. Thus, the increased aortic dimensions reflect a diminished volume of blood ejected out of the LV into the aorta as blood leaving the intrathoracic aorta is markedly reduced (Fig. 13). When the phrenic nerve stimulation produces a fall in ITP just as LV pressure begins to rise but before LV ejection begins, a transient retrograde flow can be observed in both the carotid artery and descending thoracic aortic. Thus, another factor contributing to the observed increase in aortic dimensions is movement of blood from the extrathoracic to the intrathoracic arterial compartment. When the decrease in ITP begins after LV ejection has begun, no retrograde flow is seen but the aortic dimensions still increase; that is, retrograde flow is not required to produce the increased aortic dimensions during a fall in ITP confined to systole (Peters et al., 1988b). This implies that the inspiratory reduction in peripheral arterial systolic pressure, commonly referred to as pulsus paradoxus, is produced by not only a reduced LV stroke volume but also by storage of blood in the intrathoracic arterial compartment. The ability to produce brief rapid decreases in ITP during any part of the cardiac cycle allows this principle of independent LV and intrathoracic elastic chambers driven in part by changes

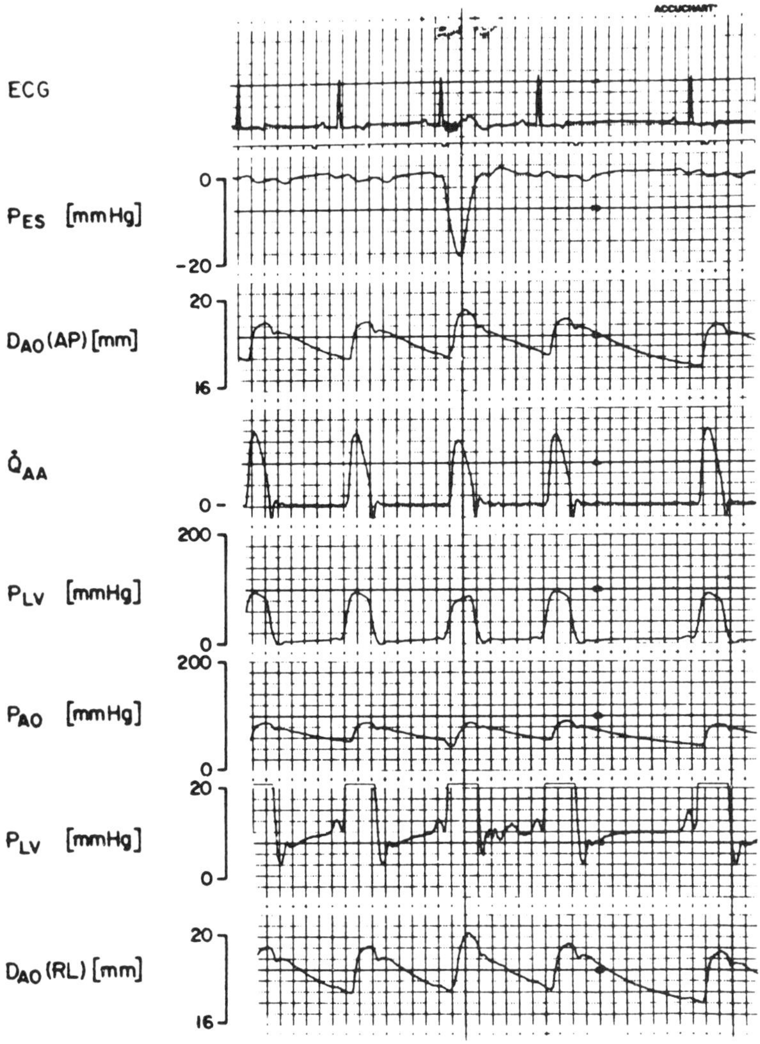

Figure 12 Recording with early systolic phrenic nerve stimulation (PNS) and the airway obstructed in an anesthetized dog. The decrease in esophageal pressure (P_{ES}) causes an increase in systolic anteroposterior intrathoracic aortic diameter [D_{AO}(AP)] but a fall in left ventricular stroke volume derived from the ascending aortic blood flow ($\dot{Q}_{AA}$). Both systolic left ventriuclar (P_{LV}) and aortic pressure (P_{AO}) fall relative to atmospheric pressure. Neither the LV end-diastolic pressure (recorded with a fluid-filled catheter) immediately before PNS nor R-R interval change compared with the preceding cardiac cycle. Congruent with the increase in systolic D_{AO}(AP), right-to-left aortic diameter [D_{AO}(RL)] also increases. The decrease in LV stroke volume associated with increased D_{AO} is compatible with an increased LV afterload. The same qualitative changes are observed when lung volume is allowed to increase with the fall in esophageal pressure, such that a decrease of intrathoracic pressure alone with or without a change in lung volume is sufficient to explain the fall in Q_{AA} and LV stroke volume and the increase in D_{AO}. (Reproduced with permission from *J. Appl. Physiol.*, **64**:1520, 1988.)

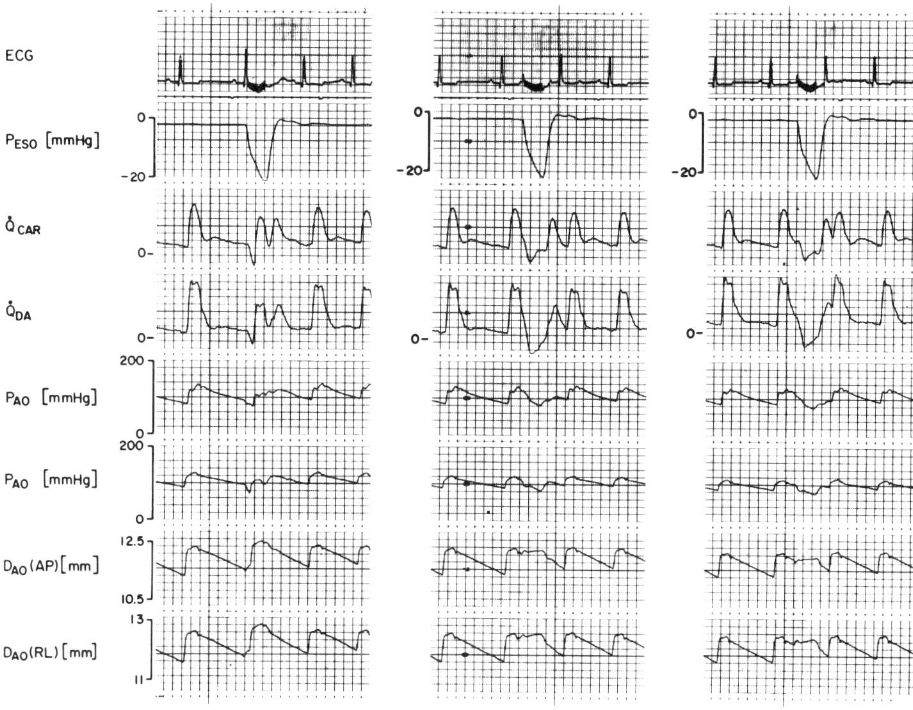

Figure 13 Effects of negative intrathoracic pressure on carotid ($\dot{Q}_{car}$) and descending aortic blood flow ($\dot{Q}_{DA}$) as the decrease in intrathoracic pressure is "walked" through the cardiac cycle (airway obstructed, paper speed 50 mm/sec). Transient retrograde flow from the extrathoracic into the intrathoracic arterial compartment is observed in both arteries during phrenic nerve stimulation (PNS) beginning during isovolumic systole (left) as well as during diastole (middle and right), along with an increase in both anteroposterior (AP) and right-to-left (RL) aortic diameters (D_{AO}). Note that negative flow in both vessels returns toward zero baseline even before peak negative esophageal pressure (P_{es}) is reached, presumably because continuous extrathoracic drainage of blood into the peripheral arterial circulation tends to re-establish pressure gradients that favor blood flow from intrathoracic to extrathoracic arterial compartment. With the rapid increase in intrathoracic pressure in late diastole after PNS, there is a bolus antegrade flow in both vessels as the aorta discharges its retained volume into the extrathoracic compartments independently of LV ejection. (Reproduced with permission from *J. Appl. Physiol.*, **64**:1512, 1988.)

in ITP to be demonstrated in Figure 13 by a series of negative ITP pulses "marched through" the cardiac cycle. The changes in ITP contribute to blood being stored or released from the intrathoracic aorta. It is even possible to dissociate changes in LV output from the changes in blood flow to the extrathoracic compartment.

These results contribute to an understanding of the physiologic events when a negative ITP is prolonged to more normal periods of time. When a negative ITP occurs during diastole, the normal diastolic runoff to the periphery is impeded and may in the extreme be reversed, that is, retrograde arterial flow. The transmural pressure of the intrathoracic aorta is unequivocally increased. This is accomplished by changing the hydrostatic gradient between the intra- and extrathoracic compartments. Thus, as the ITP is progressively lowered, blood flow is first reduced, then stopped, and finally reversed. Since the LV exists within the thorax in continuity with the intrathoracic aorta, an increase in the transmural aortic pressure reflects an increased afterload to LV ejection. This is an important distinction since many at first perceive the increased aortic dimensions associated with a fall in pressure relative to atmosphere as "vasodilation" that would reduce the LV afterload. The latter would be true only if the LV existed in an extrathoracic compartment. This is precisely what occurs in patients with an artificial heart (Robotham, unpublished observation). However, if the LV experiences a similar fall in surrounding pressure as does the aorta, then the increased intrathoracic aortic volume reflects the increased impedance to blood leaving the thorax in the same way an isolated increase in the hydrostatic pressure of the extrathoracic aorta would cause the intrathoracic aorta to increase in size. If a fall in ITP begins in diastole, mitral inflow diminishes and reduces preload and the normal diastolic aortic flow runoff is impeded, that is, increasing the intrathoracic aortic transmural pressure. The ensuing systole with the negative ITP still present then reflects the combined influences of a decreased preload and increased afterload (see Fig. 14), that is, a marked diminution in LV stroke volume.

It is also clear that as this continues for an increasing number of cardiac cycles, (1) the increased systemic venous return will lead to a gradual increase in LV stroke volume despite an increase in LV afterload; (2) the increased afterload will tend to preserve the end-diastolic volume by increasing the end-systolic volume; and (3) an increased, decreased, or absent net change in LV volumes can occur during a fall in ITP. Thus, in the light of our results, it is not surprising that conflicting and confusing results have been published. Each group of studies reflects the balance of systolic and diastolic influences on LV volumes. It is not until the opposing factors are clearly understood within a single cardiac cycle that the discussions generated by such apparently discordant results can be easily reconciled.

IX. Positive Pressure Ventilation and Cardiopulmonary Resuscitation

Pinsky and his colleagues have used a positive pressure ventilator gated to the ECG to produce positive pressure transients in ITP and lung volume

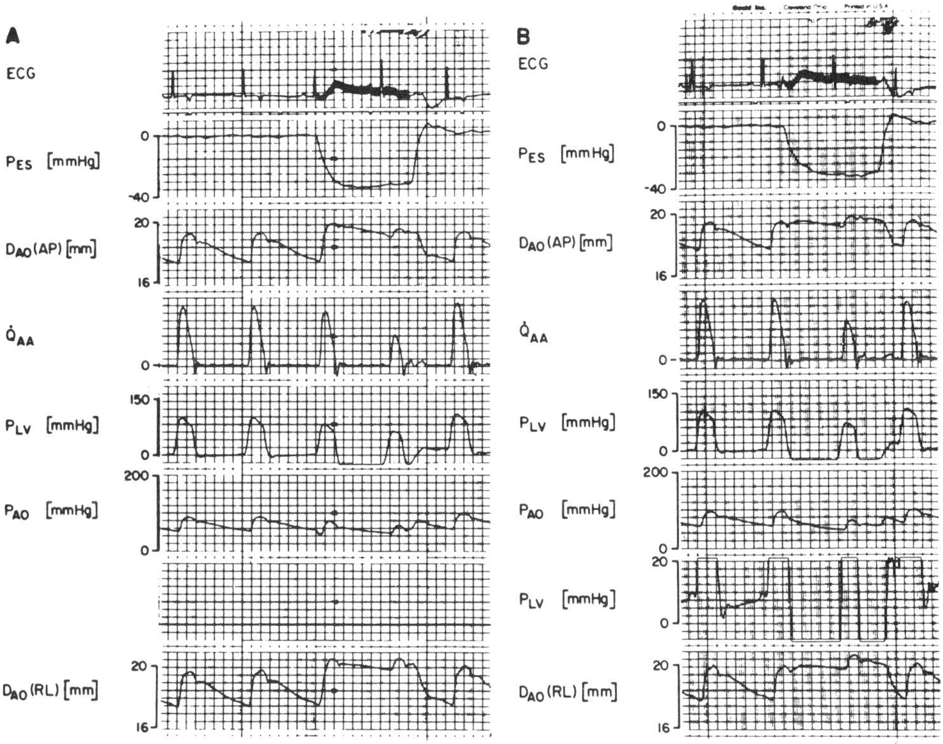

Figure 14 Effects of a decrease in intrathoracic pressure with electrocardiogram (ECG)-triggered phrenic nerve stimulation beginning in either systole (a) or diastole (b) and extending into the ensuing cardiac cycle (airway obstructed, paper speed 50 mm/sec). (a) With esophageal pressure (P_{ES}) beginning to decrease in systole and consistent with an increased afterload imposed on the left ventricle, ascending aortic flow ($\dot{Q}_{AA}$) immediately decreases but the intrathoracic aortic diameter (D_{AO}) increases in both anteroposterior (AP) and right-to-left (RL) dimensions. Left ventricular (P_{LV}) and aortic pressures (P_{AO}) decrease relative to atmospheric pressure. The ensuing ejection takes place into a markedly distended aorta and is associated with a pronounced fall in LV stroke volume. (b) With the decrease in P_{ES} beginning in diastole, D_{AO} shows a minimal decrease consistent with a reduced diastolic runoff and increased aortic transmural pressure as LV preload is presumptively limited via ventricular interdependence. The ensuing ejection thus occurs with a reduced LV preload and increased afterload combining to reduce LV stroke volume. (Reproduced with permission from *J. Appl. Physiol.*, **64**:1524, 1988.)

(Pinsky et al., 1986). They have focused on maximizing the steady-state cardiac output while we have focused on the individual mechanisms that contribute to the mean steady-state results. Fessler et al. (1988) have recently published studies on the effects of positive pressure in an isolated heart-lung system. Both groups find that LV output is enhanced when a positive ITP occurs in systole. This has little influence on diastolic filling, which is predominantly early in diastole. Thus, the effective afterload for blood to move from the intrathoracic to the extrathoracic aorta is reduced when the ITP remains elevated during systole, reducing LV work. If the ITP falls rapidly during early systole, this abolishes the intra- to extrathoracic compartment gradient. However, to the extent that the intrathoracic aorta has been emptied during the previous diastole, analogous to systolic deflation of an intra-aortic balloon assist device, the LV work is reduced as it ejects into a relatively empty, low-pressure intrathoracic aorta. From this perspective, positive pressure pulses should enhance total cardiac output and reduce LV work under conditions of LV failure. A diastolic positive ITP producing a diminution in venous return will reduce LV preload and hence the radius of curvature will decrease and wall thickness increase. This would reduce systolic LV wall stress. If as systole commences the ITP surrounding both the LV and the intrathoracic aorta is still elevated, the gradient to pump blood to the extrathoracic (not the intrathoracic) compartments is reduced. (*Note*: If the abdominal pressure increases to the same extent as ITP rises, no benefit is gained with regard to diminishing the "regional afterload" imposed by the arterial supply to the abdomen; Robotham et al., 1985.) If the ITP falls as systole begins, LV ejection proceeds into an empty intrathoracic aorta. A lowered ITP simultaneously enhances systemic venous return to the intrathoracic compartment. This perception of gated cardiac cycle-specific positive pressure ventilation is completely consistent with studies of the influence of negative intrathoracic pressure on LV performance. To understand the cardiorespiratory interactions during one form of ventilation is to understand such interactions in any other form of ventilation.

The physiologic principles examined in our studies of spontaneous ventilation are equally applicable to understanding events during CPR. An increase in ITP during asystole will effectively promote egress of blood from both the LV and intrathoracic aorta into the extrathoracic compartments, which do not experience an equivalent increase in the surrounding pressure. During CPR, if the mitral valve is open, an increase in ITP would also promote flow out of the pulmonary vascular bed toward the extrathoracic beds. If abdominal pressure were to increase an amount equal to ITP during either an IPPV inspiration or CPR compression, then no gradient between these two compartments would be produced. An increase in ITP would then tend to empty the intrathoracic aorta toward the head. However, any increase in

ITP will reduce systemic venous return. Thus, just as complex results from a negative ITP can be predicted based on the duration and timing of the ITP fluctuation, the same potential for a net decrease, increase, or absent net change exists with a positive ITP regardless of the inotropic status of the LV.

X. Conclusion

Analysis of cardiorespiratory interactions during transient perturbations of ITP offers the ability to separate independent systolic and diastolic factors that determine the net changes in ventricular volumes and stroke volume. Using a negative ITP as the paradigm, a diastolic event, which is most likely ventricular interdependence, reduces LV preload and LV stroke volume. During systole a negative ITP produce an effective increase in LV afterload that will both decrease LV stroke volume and tend to increase steady-state LV preload. The influence of changes in ITP on the intrathoracic aorta may affect both LV performance and the net movement of blood to the extrathoracic compartment. Finally, a negative ITP will increase systemic venous return, which by increasing LV preload may overcome the adverse effects of ventricular interdependence and increased afterload on LV stroke volume. These findings resolve many conflicting issues with regard to cardiorespiratory interactions during spontaneous ventilation and describe principles that are equally applicable to the analysis of cardiorespiratory interactions during spontaneous ventilation, mechanical ventilation, and cardiopulmonary resuscitation.

Acknowledgments

The authors wish to express their sincere thanks to Ms. Trudy Campbell for her excellent secretarial assistance. Supported by NIH R01-HL39138-02.

References

Bove, A. A., and Santamore, W. P. (1981). Ventricular interdependence. *Prog. Cardiovasc. Dis.,* **23**:365-388.

Brinker, J. A., and Weiss, J. L. (1980). Leftward septal displacement during right ventricular loading in man. *Circulation,* **61**:623-633.

Buda, A. J., Pinsky, M. R., and Ingels, Jr., N. B. (1979). Effect of intrathoracic pressure on left ventricular performance. *N. Engl. J. Med.,* **301**:453-459.

Fessler, H. E., Brower, R. G., Wise, R. A., and Permutt, S. (1988). Mechanism of reduced LV afterload by systolic and diastolic positive pleural pressure. *J. Appl. Physiol.,* **65**:1244-1250.

Guz, A., Innes, J. A., and Murphy, K. (1987). Respiratory modulation of left ventricular stroke volume in man measured using pulsed doppler ultrasound. *J. Physiol.* (*Lond.*), **393**:499-512.

Jardin, F., Farcot, J. C., Boisante, L., Prost, J. F., Gueret, P., and Bourdarias, J. P. (1982). Mechanism of paradoxic pulse in bronchial asthma. *Circulation,* **66**:887-894.

Karam, M., Wise, R. A., Natarjan, J. K., Permutt, S., and Wagner, H. W. (1984). Mechanism of decreased left ventricular stroke volume during inspiration in man. *Circulation,* **69**:866-873.

Maloney, J. E., Bergel, D. H., and Glazier, J. B. (1968). Transmission of pulsatile blood pressure and flow through the isolated lung. *Circ. Res.,* **23**:11-24.

Peters, J., Kindred, M. K., and Robotham, J. L. (1988a). Transient analysis of cardiopulmonary interactions. I. Diastolic events. *J. Appl. Physiol.,* **64**:1506-1517.

Peters, J., Kindred, M. K., and Robotham, J. L. (1988b). Transient analysis of cardiopulmonary interactions. II. Systolic events. *J. Appl. Physiol.,* **64**:1518-1526.

Pinsky, M. R., Matuschak, G. M., Bernardi, L., and Klain, M. (1986). Hemodynamic effects of cardiac cycle-specific increases in intrathoracic pressure. *J. Appl. Physiol.,* **60**:604-612.

Rankin, J. S., Olsen, C. O., Arentzen, C. E., Tyson, G. S., Maier, G., Smith, P. K., Hammon, J. W., Jr., Davis, J. W., McHale, P. A., Anderson, R. W., and Sabiston, D. C., Jr. (1982). The effects of airway pressure on cardiac function in intact dogs and man. *Circulation,* **66**:108-120.

Robotham, J. L., and Peters, J. (1989). Mechanical effects of intrathoracic pressure on ventricular performance. In *Heart/Lung Interactions.* Edited by S. Scharf and S. Cassidy. New York, Marcel Dekker, pp. 251-283.

Robotham, J. L., Badke, F. R., Kindred, M. K., and Beaton, M. K. (1983). Regional left ventricular performance during normal and obstructed spontaneous respiration. *J. Appl. Physiol.,* **55**:569-577.

Robotham, J. L., Wise, R. A., and Bromberger-Barnea, B. (1985). Effects of changes in abdominal pressure on left ventricular performance and regional blood flow. *Crit. Care Med.,* **13**:803-809.

Robotham, J. L., Stuart, R. S., Doherty, K., Borkon, A. M., and Baumgartner, W. (1988a). Effects of changes in left ventricular loading and pleural pressure on mitral flow. *J. Appl. Physiol.,* **65**:1662-1675.

Robotham, J. L., Stuart, R. S., Doherty, K., Borkon, A. M., and Baumgartner, W. (1988b). Mitral and aortic flows during spontaneous respiration in dogs. *Anesthesiology,* **69**:516-526.

Scharf, S. M., Brown, R., and Saunders, N. (1980). Hemodynamic effects of positive pressure inflation. *J. Appl. Physiol.,* **49**:124-131.

Schwartz, G. G., McHale, P. A., and Greenfield, J. C. (1982). Hyperemic response of the coronary circulation to brief diastolic occlusion in the conscious dog. *Circ. Res.,* **50**:28-37.

Shabetai, R. (1988). Pericardial and cardiac pressures. *Circulation,* **77**:1-5.

Summer, W. R., Permutt, S., and Sagawa, K. (1979). Effects of spontaneous respiration on canine left ventricular function. *Circ. Res.,* **45**:719-728.

Wallis, T., Robotham, J. L., Compean, R., and Kindred, M. K. (1983). Mechanical heart-lung interaction with PEEP. *J. Appl. Physiol.,* **54**: 1039-1047.

Wead, W. B., and Norton, J. F. (1981). Effects of intrapleural pressure changes on canine left ventricular function. *J. Appl. Physiol.,* **50**:1027-1035.

12

Cardiovascular Function During Acute Respiratory Failure

WILLIAM E. HURFORD

Harvard Medical School and
Massachusetts General Hospital
Boston, Massachusetts

JEAN-LOUIS TEBOUL

INSERM U 296
Université Paris XII
Hôpital Henri Mondor
Créteil, France

I. Introduction

Patients with acute respiratory failure (ARF) continue to die at an alarming rate. From 1978 to 1987, the overall mortality for ARF in the Respiratory/Surgical Intensive Care Unit of the Massachusetts General Hospital was 41%. Mortality was 86% for patients with severe adult respiratory distress syndrome (ARDS) but only approximately 10% of the deaths resulted directly from hypoxemia (Pa_{O_2} < 50 mmHg). Instead, patients usually died with intractable circulatory failure characterized by a normal cardiac output in the days before death, a low peripheral vascular resistance, and multiple organ failure. Reports from other centers parallel our own (Bartlett et al., 1986; Montgomery et al., 1985).

Undoubtedly, multiple mechanisms are responsible for the circulatory failure that occurs during ARF. This chapter focuses upon the cadiovascular changes accompanying the acute pulmonary artery hypertension measured during severe ARDS. The role of hemodynamic changes secondary to sepsis is discussed. We also examine hemodynamic changes occurring due to the use and discontinuation of mechanical ventilation with positive end-expiratory pressure.

II. Assessing Cardiac Function During ARDS

A. Transmural Pressure

Critical to the study of the cardiovascular changes occurring during ARF is an understanding of transmural pressure since the heart fills and ejects, not as a function of intracavitary pressure, but rather as a function of transmural pressure. For in vitro heart preparations, transmural pressure is simply the intracardiac pressure referenced to atmospheric pressure. The intact patient, however, is more complex, for the heart is exposed to constantly changing pleural pressure and is physically compressed by the lungs. Transmural pressure is then equal to intracavitary pressure minus pericardial or pleural pressure. Changes in pleural pressure in turn are dependent upon changes of lung volume and the compliance of the chest wall.

To complicate matters further, transmural pressure has been measured differently by various investigators, producing at times very different and often conflicting conclusions. Esophageal pressure, used by many investigators as a reference for transmural pressure, may not always reflect juxtacardiac pressure since lung expansion rotates the heart anteriorly and lifts it off the posterior mediastinum and esophagus (Marini et al., 1982). In addition, the lungs may directly compress the heart, increasing juxtacardiac pressure more than pleural pressure (Marini et al., 1981a; Culver et al., 1981; Wise et al., 1981). Careful studies by Marini and his coworkers (1982) and Craven and Wood (1981) have shown that juxtacardiac pressure is best estimated by directly measuring lateral pericardial pressure or by measuring esophageal pressure with the subject in a lateral or prone position.

In the critically ill patient, however, the measurement of juxtacardiac pressure is complicated and often impractical. One must then rely upon the measurement of central venous pressure or pulmonary capillary wedge pressure referenced to ambient pressure. Lozman and co-workers (1974) have noted a poor correlation between the pulmonary capillary wedge pressure (PCWP) and left ventricular end-diastolic pressure (LVEDP) in patients ventilated with PEEP after cardiac surgery. The correlation between these two measurements may be improved by following several guidelines. To minimize the effects of varying intrathoracic pressure throughout the respiratory cycle, measurements are best made at end-expiration (O'Quin and Marini, 1983; Luce, 1984). Some authors have advocated that intravascular pressure measurements be made after the patient is taken off PEEP ventilation (Powers and Dutton, 1975; LaBrousse et al., 1976). It may be more prudent, however, to continue mechanical ventilation with PEEP during the measurements. In this way, steady-state values are obtained rather than values influenced by increased venous return occurring when PEEP is removed (Zarins et al., 1977; Qvist et al., 1975). In addition, the temporary deterioration in gas exchange that may accompany the removal of PEEP may be avoided (DeCampo and Civetta, 1979; Luterman et al., 1978).

In normal patients, the distal end of the pulmonary artery catheter must be properly positioned if the PCWP is to accurately reflect left atrial pressure. Since pulmonary microvessels collapse when alveolar pressure exceeds pulmonary capillary pressure, PCWP can reflect left atrial pressure only if pulmonary venous pressure exceeds airway pressure (O'Quin and Marini, 1983). This condition is equivalent to zone 3 described by West and colleagues (1964). If the catheter terminates in a portion of the lung described by zone 1 or 2 conditions, in which airway pressure is greater than pulmonary arterial or pulmonary venous pressure, respectively, then the wedge pressure reflects airway pressure rather than left atrial pressure. The result is a falsely elevated PCWP measurement.

The probability of the catheter tip residing in a zone 3 region during PCWP measurements can be increased by measuring PCWP with the patient in a recumbent position and by ensuring with a lateral chest radiograph that the distal end of the catheter terminates at or below the level of the left atrium (O'Quin and Marini, 1983; Luce, 1984; Tooker et al., 1978).

Fortunately, the distal end of the pulmonary artery catheter usually resides in a zone 3 region, since the flow-directed catheter tends to be directed toward dependent, high-flow regions of the lung (Kronberg et al., 1979). This was confirmed by Teboul and co-workers (1988), who used lateral supine chest radiographs to examine 150 critically ill patients with indwelling Swan-Ganz catheters. In their study, the pulmonary artery catheter terminated at or below the level of the left atrium in 147 of 150 patients.

In ARDS patients, PCWP measurements correlate closely with simultaneous measurements of LVEDP despite the application of PEEP levels up to 20 cmH_2O (Figs. 1 and 2) (Teboul et al., 1989). This high degree of correlation may be secondary to the predominance of zone 3 conditions during ARDS. Increased pulmonary anatomic shunt during ARDS may effectively shield microvessels from increased alveolar pressure. In addition, the transmission of alveolar pressure to the pulmonary microvasculature may be reduced secondary to decreased microvascular and lung compliance.

B. Ventricular Volume

To avoid the pitfalls of assessing transmural pressure in critically ill patients, more direct assessments of ventricular volume and function have been developed. The most commonly used techniques are two-dimensional echocardiography, radionuclide angiocardiography, and thermodilution.

Two-dimensional echocardiography can provide dynamic images of both the right and left ventricles. Ultrasonic imaging is entirely noninvasive and can provide repeatable indices of ventricular size and contractility. Jardin

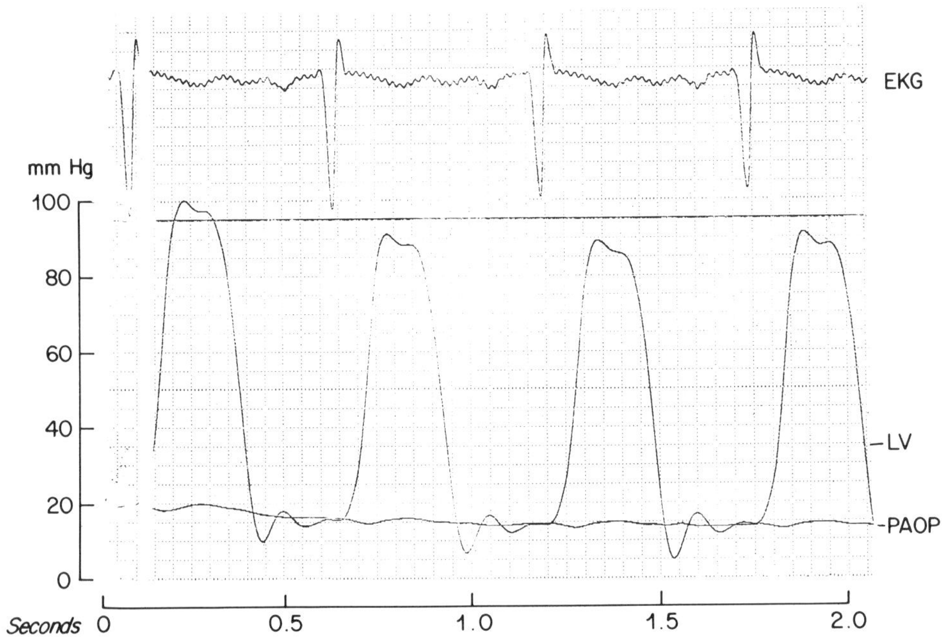

Figure 1 A high-speed recording of pulmonary artery occlusion pressure (PAOP), LV pressure, and EKG in an ARDS patient mechanically ventilated with 20 cmH_2O PEEP. A close correspondence of LVEDP and PAOP is shown. (Reprinted from Teboul et al., 1989.)

and coworkers (1981, 1985, 1987) have reported indices of ventricular volume and function in a large number of critically ill patients during both spontaneous and mechanical ventilation. The number and quality of sonographic views that may be obtained in the mechanically ventilated, critically ill patient are limited. Jardin et al. obtained a subcostal four-chamber view to image the ventricles along the long axis of the heart. Since only a single axis was scanned to measure ventricular volume and function, the assumption must be made that changes in ventricular dimension along the long axis accurately reflect changes in the other planes. This may not be the case under all conditions. Two-dimensional transesophageal echocardiography may provide additional views in the mechanically ventilated patient.

Radionuclide angiocardiography using autologous erythrocytes labeled with ^{99m}Tc-pyrophosphate has been used to assess right and left ventricular function in several studies of critically ill patients (Sibbald et al., 1986; Dhainaut et al., 1986; Hurford et al., 1986). Both "first-pass" and gated equilibrium blood pool angiocardiograms can be performed (Pitt and Strauss, 1977).

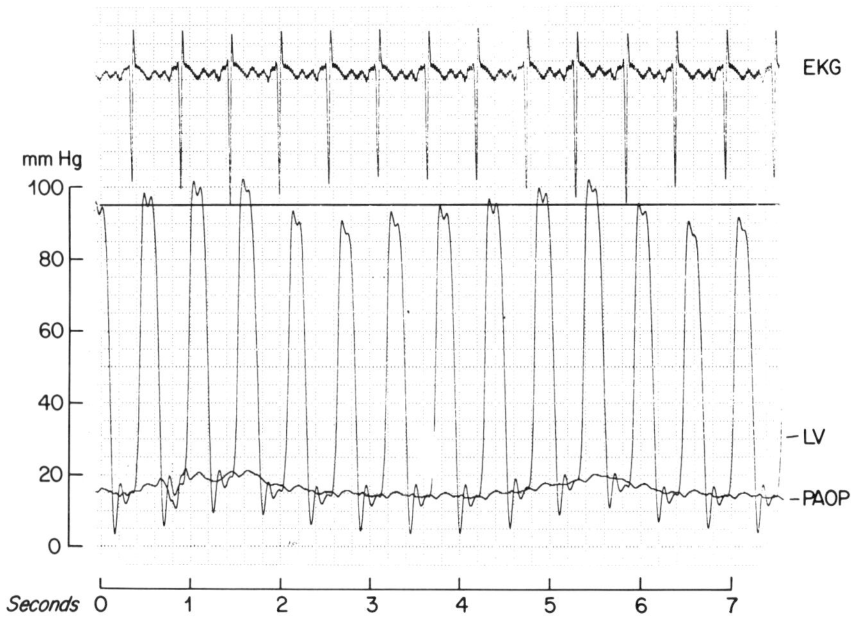

Figure 2 A slow-speed recording of pulmonary artery occlusion pressure (PAOP), LV pressure, and EKG in a second ARDS patient mechanically ventilated with 20 cmH_2O PEEP. Note the correspondence of LV pressure and PAOP. This correspondence was maintained during periods of peak mechanical lung inflation. (Reprinted from Teboul et al., 1989.)

In a first-pass study, sequential images are acquired as a bolus of the radionuclide mixes within the central circulation and passes through the heart. Time-activity curves for a region of interest positioned over the ventricle are produced by a computer, and the ejection fraction is calculated by dividing the difference between end-diastolic and end-systolic activity within the region of interest (stroke counts) by the activity in the ventricle at end-diastole. This technique requires no assumptions concerning the shape of the ventricle or pattern of contraction. The first-pass technique minimizes the inclusion of atrial activity within the ventricular region of interest since activity within the atrium peaks prior to the accumulation of radioactivity within the ventricle. Multiple first-pass studies in a single patient are difficult to obtain because of the accumulation of background activity and the hazards of exceeding safe radiation limits. First-pass techniques using ultrashort half-life isotopes, such as iridium 191m (Rajagopalan et al., 1982) or krypton 81m (Nienaber et al., 1985), could circumvent these problems, but these isotopes are rarely available.

Equilibrium multiple-gated blood pool angiocardiography is available in many hospitals and can be performed with a mobile gamma camera at the patient's bedside. With this technique, sequential images are acquired and gated to the R wave of the electrocardiogram. The ejection fraction is calculated in an analogous fashion to the first-pass scan. The major problem with using equilibrium angiocardiography is that right ventricular function is difficult to assess accurately. Geometric separation of overlapping right atrial and ventricular activity can be difficult. The technique may therefore systematically underestimate the RV ejection fraction. This error may be minimized by carefully positioning the gamma camera to maximize the apparent separation of cardiac chambers and by calculating the ejection fraction from separately defined systolic and diastolic regions of interest. Using this technique in normal subjects and in patients with coronary artery disease, Maddahi et al. (1979) found a close correlation between RV ejection fraction calculated by multiple-gated equilibrium and first-pass techniques.

Thermodilution techniques have been developed to clinically assess right ventricular function. In current applications of this technique, a bolus of iced saline is injected into the right atrium and mixes within the right ventricle. The reduction in temperature in pulmonary artery blood is then measured with a rapid-response thermistor mounted on a pulmonary artery catheter (Kay et al., 1983). The downslope of the thermal washout curve, as detected by the pulmonary artery thermistor, follows an exponential decay interrupted by a series of diastolic plateaus. Each successive increase in blood temperature in the pulmonary artery represents an RV ejection of progressively warmer blood as the bolus of cold indicator in the RV is diluted with warm inflowing blood and subsequently ejected from the right ventricle. Calculation of the ratio between the temperature increases of two successive diastolic plateaus yields an estimate of the residual fraction (RF), that is, the fraction of blood remaining in the ventricle. The ejection fraction (EF) is calculated as $EF = 1 - RF$. Recently, computer algorithms have been developed that determine the best fitting curve to the exponential washout using least-squares regression (Vincent et al., 1986; Dhainaut et al., 1987). This method simplifies the tedious and sometimes difficult task of manually identifying each diastolic plateau.

Values derived by the thermodilution technique compare acceptably with indices of RV volume and function obtained by two-dimensional echocardiography and radionuclide angiocardiography. Systematic errors induced by damping of the response time of the catheter-mounted thermistor and errors induced by arrhythmias, injection technique, and tricuspid regurgitation limit the accuracy of the method (Hurford and Zapol, 1988).

III. Effect of Acute Pulmonary Artery Hypertension

Severe ARDS is associated with the development of acute pulmonary artery hypertension believed due to vasoconstriction, compression, and destruction of pulmonary vessels, as well as intravascular thrombosis (Zapol and Snider, 1977; Tomashefski et al., 1983). The increased RV afterload may alter RV performance and limit cardiac output. Figure 3 plots the cardiac index and pulmonary vascular resistance of 19 patients with moderate or severe ARDS who were studied with a combination of invasive monitoring and gated blood pool scans using ^{99m}Tc-labeled red cells. In these patients, cardiac index was

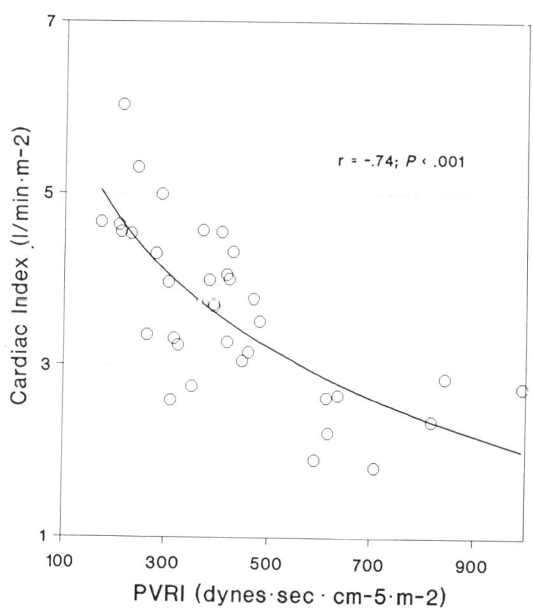

Figure 3 Cardiac index and pulmonary vascular resistance (PVRI) determined in 19 patients with moderate or severe ARF. Patients were studied with a combination of invasive monitoring and gated blood pool scans using ^{99m}Tc-labeled red cells at various times during their illness. Cardiac index was reduced when the pulmonary vascular resistance was elevated.

reduced, sometimes quite severely, when the pulmonary vascular resistance was markedly elevated. In cases of a marked increase in pulmonary vascular resistance, right ventricular ejection fraction was reduced (Fig. 4) and right ventricular end-systolic and end-diastolic volume index (Fig. 5) increased. Sibbald and co-workers (1986) have reported similar correlations.

In the view of Guyton and colleagues (1954), the dilation of the RV and the decreased RV ejection fraction measured during acute pulmonary arterial hypertension may reflect compensatory mechanisms to maintain stroke volume rather than ischemia or myocardial dysfunction. Right ventricular ischemia may occur at very high pulmonary artery pressures or during systemic hypotension (Vlahakes et al., 1981). In canine models of moderate acute pulmonary artery hypertension (mean pulmonary artery pressure less than 50 mmHg), right ventricular myocardial blood flow is increased as long as systemic blood pressure is maintained (Gold and Bache, 1982; Hurford et al., 1987a). Diastolic compliance may be reduced by alterations in septal position and motion as the right ventricle dilates (Jardin et al., 1981; Hurford

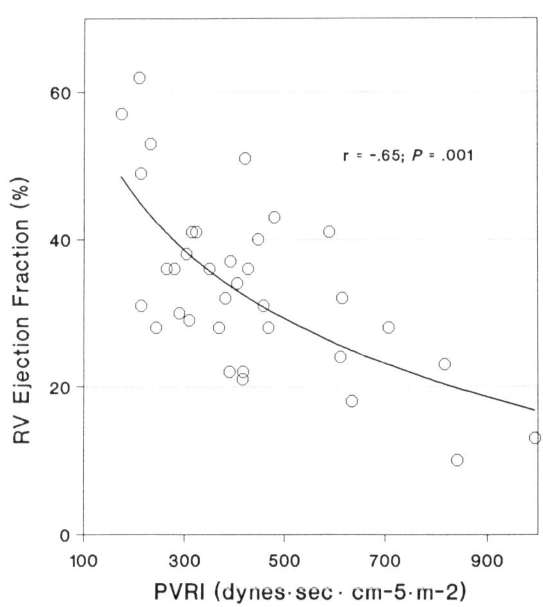

Figure 4 Right ventricular ejection fraction and pulmonary vascular resistance (PVRI) in the ARF patients described in Figure 3. Right ventricular ejection fraction was determined from equilibrium angiocardiograms using ^{99m}Tc-labeled red cells. Right ventricular ejection fraction was reduced in patients with increased PVRI.

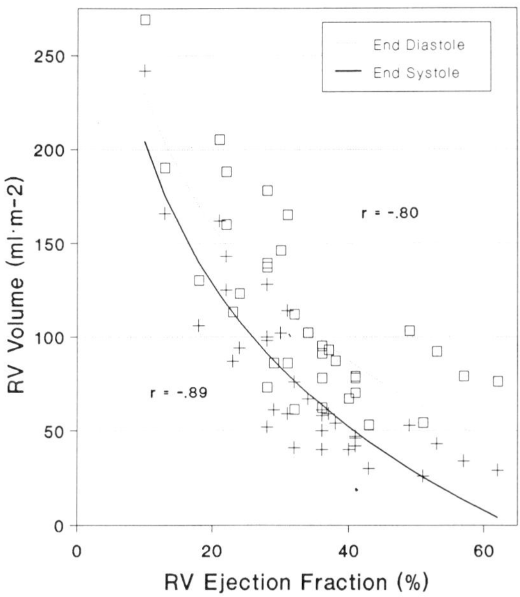

Figure 5 Right ventricular volume and ejection fraction in the ARF patients described in Figure 3. Right ventricular ejection fraction was determined from equilibrium angiocardiograms using ^{99m}Tc-labeled red cells. Right ventricular end-diastolic volume (squares) was estimated by dividing the thermodilution-derived stroke volume by the RV ejection fraction calculated from a simultaneously acquired equilibrium radionuclide angiocardiogram. Right ventricular end-systolic volume (crosses) was calculated by subtracting the stroke volume from the end-diastolic volume. Right ventricular volume was increased in patients who had a decreased RV ejection fraction.

et al., 1987a). Left ventricular compliance may also be restricted by the surrounding pericardium if the RV is excessively dilated (Bove and Santamore, 1981; Weber et al., 1981).

Left ventricular contractility appears unaffected by acute pulmonary injury. During experimental lung injury induced by infusing glass beads into the pulmonary circulation of dogs, Calvin and co-workers (1986) demonstrated that the relationship between LV stroke work and end-diastolic size was unchanged following pulmonary microvascular injury. In their study, changes in stroke volume following pulmonary injury appeared secondary to changes in end-diastolic volume. Similarly, Qvist et al. (1988) reported that the decrease in stroke volume observed after infusing thrombin into the pulmonary vasculature of dogs was due to decreased LV diastolic compliance

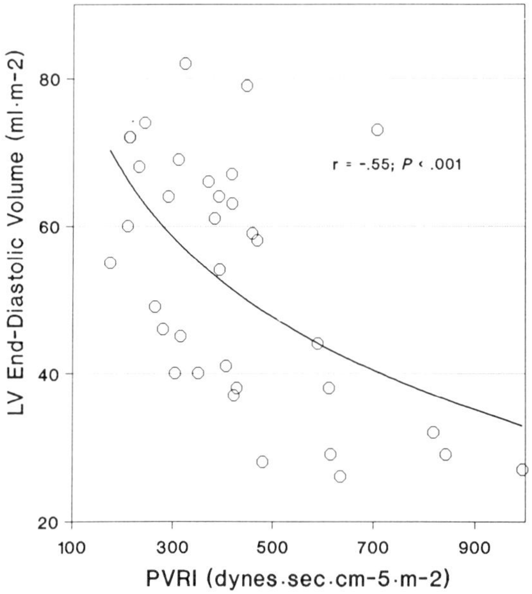

Figure 6 Left ventricular end-diastolic volume and pulmonary vascular resistance (PVRI) in the ARF patients described in Figure 3. Left ventricular end-diastolic volume was estimated by dividing the thermodilution-derived stroke volume by the LV ejection fraction calculated from a simultaneously acquired equilibrium radionuclide angiocardiogram. Left ventricular end-diastolic volume was reduced in patients who had an elevated PVRI.

rather than decreased systolic performance. In the ARDS patients we studied, left ventricular ejection fraction was unaffected by the level of pulmonary artery pressure. Left ventricular end-diastolic volume was decreased in these patients (Fig. 6). The decrease was proportional to the degree of pulmonary hypertension and may be due to either decreased RV output or decreased diastolic compliance secondary to an enlarged right ventricle. Current human studies have not demonstrated conclusively which mechanism, if any, is predominant during severe ARDS.

IV. Effect of Sepsis

Sepsis or septicemia accompanies approximately 25% of ARDS cases at the Massachusetts General Hospital. The clinical course of such patients is often complicated by a normal or increased cardiac output, a low peripheral vascular resistance, and multiple organ failure (Montgomery et al., 1985; Hyers and Fowler, 1986; Bell et al., 1986). Experimental models in which endotoxin or whole bacteria are infused into laboratory animals or human volunteers mimic these derangements and are characterized by myocardial depression, systemic hypotension, increased pulmonary artery pressure, and complement and coagulation cascade activation with thrombocytopenia and leukopenia (Suffredini et al., 1987; Parker and Adams, 1985). The similarity between the clinical and biologic manifestations of sepsis in humans and those induced experimentally by gram-negative endotoxin infusion strongly supports the role of endotoxin as a triggering factor for the cardiovascular consequences of sepsis.

An understanding of the cardiovascular effects of endotoxin and its secondary mediators is crucial to developing successful therapies and improving survival in ARDS. The death rate is much higher in ARDS patients with multiple organ dysfunction. Likely causes of multisystem failure in these patients is that systemic perfusion is either relatively inadequate (secondary to myocardial dysfunction) or inappropriately distributed to the periphery (possibly secondary to decreased systemic vascular resistance, arteriovenous shunting, and/or local vasoconstriction) (Siegel et al., 1967; Parker and Adams, 1985; Parker et al., 1984; Bihari et al., 1987). Increased blood flow to respiratory muscles secondary to increased work of breathing during sepsis may contribute to the hypoperfusion of other organs (Hussain and Roussos, 1985). Despite the presence of an apparently adequate systemic blood flow, blood pressure, and arterial oxygen tension, inadequate tissue oxygenation may occur due to microembolic phenomenon or the inappropriate and uncontrolled release of the mediators of acute inflammation into the microcirculation (Movat et al., 1987). A defect in tissue oxygen uptake has recently been demonstrated in ARDS patients (Bihari et al., 1987). A similar defect, increased lactate flux from the canine hindlimb, has been demonstrated after the infusion of the monokine tumor necrosis factor α (TNF-α) (Tracey et al., 1987b). These metabolic derangements may be amenable to treatment by the infusion of vasoactive mediators. Prostacyclin infusion for 30 min has been shown to increase oxygen delivery and uptake in ARDS patients who subsequently died with multiple organ failure (Bihari et al., 1987). A 7 day infusion of a related compound, prostaglandin E_1, improved survival and reduced the development of multiple organ failure in patients with ARDS (Holcroft et al., 1986).

Experimental and clinical evidence suggests that reversible myocardial depression and decreased left ventricular compliance occur during the first several days of sepsis (Parker et al., 1984; Parker and Adams, 1985; Parrillo et al., 1985; Natanson et al., 1986). Decreased LV compliance and contractility would increase pulmonary capillary wedge pressure, which is already moderately elevated (usually 15-20 mmHg) in many ARDS patients. This in turn would contribute to increased pulmonary microvascular pressure and pulmonary edema formation in the face of increased microvascular permeability.

The cause of cardiac dysfunction during sepsis is unclear. The decreased myocardial contractility does not appear to be associated with global myocardial ischemia. In a study of seven patients with septic shock (mean arterial blood pressure less than 60 mmHg), Cunnion and co-workers (1986) found preservation of coronary blood flow and no evidence of myocardial lactate production. Of the seven patients, four had a transient decrease in LV ejection fraction to below 45%. These decreases were not correlated with changes in coronary blood flow, myocardial lactate metabolism, or myocardial oxygen utilization.

Circulating mediators may directly depress myocardial contractility. Parrillo and co-workers (1985) isolated a low-molecular-weight compound from the sera of septic patients that decreased the contractility of myocytes in primary culture. In addition, Michelassi et al. (1982, 1983) demonstrated that leukotrienes C_4 and D_4, which may be liberated during some types of acute lung injury, were potent coronary vasoconstrictors and produced a myocardial depressant effect independent of their reduction of coronary blood flow, since blocking the decrease in coronary blood flow by a leukotriene receptor antagonist did not prevent the depression of myocardial contractility. Additional myocardial depressant factors probably exist in sepsis. Tracey and co-workers (1987b) found that TNF-α infusion was associated with a hypodynamic state despite very high levels of circulating catecholamines and suggested that cardiac function was reduced either directly by TNF-α or through the activity of other, uncharacterized factors released after TNF-α infusion.

Antagonism of the effects of endotoxin by (1) administration of antibodies directed against lipopolysaccharide (LPS) core components, (2) inhibition of mediator production, or (3) through use of blockers of receptor binding represent promising methods of defining the importance of the various mediators and treating the cardiovascular sequelae of sepsis. Antibodies to *Escherichia coli* J5 LPS have been developed, and their administration has increased the survival time of septic patients in two prospective, randomized trials (Ziegler et al., 1982; Baumgartner et al., 1985). As a proximal mediator of the pathophysiologic consequences of endotoxemia, TNF-α is a prime target for immunologic blockade during experimental sepsis. Preliminary experiments suggest that the administration of anti-TNF-α antibodies may improve survival and organ function during sepsis. When mice were passively immunized with a polyclonal rabbit antiserum to TNF-α, they were protected from the lethal effects of LPS produced by *E. coli* (Beutler et al., 1985). Similarly, protection against shock, organ failure, and death was conferred upon three anesthetized baboons by passive immunization against TNF-α performed 2 hr prior to a lethal intravenous infusion of *E. coli* (Tracey et al., 1987a).

The administration of cyclooxygenase inhibitors would be expected to block those effects of endotoxin and TNF-α that are mediated through the actions of prostacyclin, thromboxane A_2, or other eicosanoids. The administration of indomethacin has been reported to ameliorate pulmonary and circulatory dysfunction in patients with gram-negative sepsis (Short et al., 1981). In addition, Kettelhut and co-workers (1987) have shown that indomethacin or ibuprofen administered intravenously to rats prior to an intravenous injection of TNF-α blocked the adverse physiologic effects of the monokine and reduced its lethality by 70%.

V. Positive-Pressure Ventilation and PEEP

Positive end-expiratory pressure (PEEP) improves oxygenation by increasing alveolar pressure and lung volume. The increased airway pressure is in turn transmitted to the pleura, heart, and great vessels. PEEP influences cardiovascular performance in several ways, including limiting peripheral venous return, increasing right ventricular afterload, decreasing left ventricular diastolic compliance, and decreasing left ventricular afterload. The subject has been reviewed extensively by many authors (Luce, 1984; Robotham, 1981; Robotham and Scharf, 1983; Eaton et al., 1983; Goldberg and Rabson, 1981; Laver et al., 1979; Pick et al., 1982; Cassidy and Mitchell, 1981; Dorinsky and Whitcomb, 1983).

A. Right Ventricular Preload

Initial studies of the hemodynamic effects of PEEP concentrated upon its effects on cardiac output and peripheral venous return. Cournand et al. (1948) demonstrated that PEEP decreased human cardiac output. Cournand measured both right ventricular and pleural pressure and found that the decrease in cardiac output was directly related to the decrease in transmural right ventricular pressure. In 1957, Braunwald and co-workers reported that positive-pressure breathing decreased cardiac output and central blood volume. They were able to reverse these effects by infusing metaraminol, which increased peripheral venous pressure, arteriolar tone, and myocardial contractility. Qvist and co-workers (1975) examined the effects of PEEP on central hemodynamics. Studying anesthetized beagles, they found that cardiac output and transmural pressures decreased in response to the application of 12 cm PEEP. The hemodynamic measurements returned to normal after the infusion of 25 ml/kg of autologous blood. The investigators concluded that PEEP decreased cardiac output at least in part by decreasing transmural filling pressures and reducing venous return. Multiple studies in humans (Jardin et al., 1981; Prewitt et al., 1981; Calvin et al., 1981; Viquerat et al., 1983; Dhainaut et al., 1986; Potkin et al., 1987) and in other animals (Prewitt and Wood, 1979; Fewell et al., 1980a, b; Haynes et al., 1980) have confirmed these findings.

B. Right Ventricular Afterload

Positive pressure ventilation may also act to increase right ventricular afterload. Afterload, defined from in vitro muscle fiber experiments, is the tension that develops in a muscle fiber after the onset of contraction. When considering the intact heart, it is nearly impossible to define afterload precisely. Most investigators accept that ventricular afterload is related to the wall tension developed during systole. According to the law of Laplace, tension is directly proportional to intracavitary pressure and chamber size. In turn, these factors are directly related to outflow resistance or, in the case of the right ventricle, pulmonary vascular resistance.

High levels of PEEP increase alveolar pressure and may compress pulmonary microvessels. When alveolar pressure exceeds pulmonary microvascular pressure, outflow pressure becomes limited by alveolar pressure rather than left atrial pressure. As a consequence, pulmonary vascular resistance rises and transpulmonary blood flow decreases (Roos et al., 1961; Rankin et al., 1982). Support for this concept was provided by the laboratory studies of Glazier and colleagues (1969), who showed that increasing airway pressure reduced pulmonary capillary width and pulmonary capillary red cell density, and also by Thorvaldson's group (1985), who showed that increasing PEEP progressively reduced pulmonary blood volume. In addition, Henning (1986) demonstrated that pulmonary vascular resistance increased and stroke volume decreased when anesthetized dogs were exposed to 20 cmH_2O PEEP. The stroke volume remained depressed despite restoration of the right ventricular end-diastolic volume by volume infusion, suggesting that right ventricular afterload was increased by PEEP. Although Henning did not measure left atrial pressure in his experiments, it is likely that the large increase in pleural pressure produced by 20 cmH_2O PEEP would have exceeded left atrial pressure. The resulting rise in pulmonary vascular resistance would in turn increase right ventricular afterload and limit the systolic function of the right ventricle.

Biondi and co-workers (1988), using thermodilution measurements of RV ejection fraction and volume, studied the effects of increasing PEEP on RV function in patients with acute respiratory failure or recovering from surgery. They found that increasing PEEP above 15 cmH_2O increased pulmonary vascular resistance and decreased RV ejection fraction and volume.

This finding is consistent with an increase in pulmonary vascular resistance due to lung inflation by high levels of PEEP. With the application of 5 cmH_2O PEEP in their study, however, pulmonary vascular resistance and RV ejection fraction were unchanged but RV end-diastolic volume was reduced, consistent with decreased RV filling.

Studies by Schulman and associates (1988) suggest that the effect of PEEP on right ventricular function may vary depending upon the patient's pre-existing RV function. In their study, patients with an RV ejection fraction (EF) of 30% or less had a decreased RV ejection fraction and an increased RV volume in response to increasing PEEP. Patients with an RV EF greater than 30% had no change of RV volume despite increasing PEEP to 20 cmH_2O.

C. Left Ventricular Preload

Several mechanisms may limit left ventricular filling during mechanical ventilation with PEEP. First, since right ventricular output is reduced, less volume is available to fill the left ventricle. In addition, left ventricular diastolic compliance appears to be reduced during PEEP. That is, for a given transmural LV diastolic pressure, LV volume is decreased during ventilation with PEEP.

Jardin et al. (1981), studying the application of PEEP in patients with ARDS, suggested that lung inflation would increase RV loading and restrain left ventricular performance via a leftward shift of the interventricular septum. Such a shift may be reflected by an increased radius of curvature of the interventricular septum as measured by two-dimensional echocardiography. In the patients they studied, the septal radius of curvature increased only at PEEP levels of 20 cmH_2O or greater. Lower levels of PEEP were associated with a decreased LV volume without a change in septal curvature, suggesting decreased LV filling.

Lung inflation plays an important role in transmitting positive pressure to the heart. This point has been controversial in the past. Manny and coworkers (1978) reported that the hemodynamic effects of PEEP persisted and in fact were exacerbated when the entire chest walls of their experimental animals were removed. It was assumed that complete chest wall excision would have eliminated any direct effects of increased pleural pressure upon the heart and great vessels. Subsequently, Marini, Culver, and Butler (Marini et al., 1981a, b; Culver et al., 1981) published a series of articles demonstrating that PEEP increased pericardial pressure even when pleural pressure was zero after excision of the chest wall. Also, Fewell and co-workers (1980b) showed that physically holding the lungs away from the heart eliminated the decrease in cardiac output and ventricular end-diastolic volume caused by increased expiratory pressure.

The hemodynamic effects of PEEP depend in part upon lung and chest wall compliance (Wallis et al., 1983). Both compliances may be affected by acute or chronic lung injury. The effects of different types of lung injury on the cardiovascular effects of PEEP, however, have not been studied extensively. Pulmonary edema produced by infusing oleic acid in dogs, for example, has no significant modifying effect on the transmission of PEEP to the pleural space (Henning, 1986). Similar results were reported by Scharf and Ingram (1977), who reported that oleic acid infusion decreased both lung and chest wall compliance equally. Since lung and chest wall expansion were restricted to the same degree, the presence of pulmonary edema secondary to oleic acid had no net effect on the transmission of airway pressure to the pleural space.

In patients with ARDS, however, lung compliance is markedly reduced but chest wall compliance remains relatively normal (Suter, 1985). Lung volume in these patients may change only minimally with PEEP, resulting in little change in transmitted pressure. As a result, the hemodynamic effects of PEEP may be relatively small in patients with ARDS (Hurford et al., 1986 and 1987b). Patients with highly compliant lungs may respond differently to PEEP. Mechanically ventilated patients with chronic obstructive lung disease may have inadequate time for exhalation, resulting in air trapping, hyperexpansion of their lungs, and an elevated functional residual capacity (FRC) (Pepe and Marini, 1982; Kimball et al., 1982). Pleural pressures can be quite high in such patients, even at low levels of PEEP. Although extensive hemodynamic studies have not been performed in such patients, it is possible that lung hyperinflation by positive end-expiratory pressure could produce exaggerated hemodynamic effects.

D. Myocardial Contractility

It has been difficult to separate the cardiovascular effects of alterations in pleural pressure and lung volume from changes in myocardial contractility. Depending upon the pressure used by investigators to reference transmural pressure—atmospheric, pleural, esophageal, or pericardial pressure—ventricular function curves showing either depression (Scharf et al., 1977; Manny et al., 1978; Cassidy et al., 1978; Prewitt and Wood, 1979) or preservation (Qvist et al., 1975; Scharf et al., 1979; Fewell et al., 1980a; Robotham et al., 1980; Haynes et al., 1980; Calvin et al., 1981; Wise et al., 1981; Prewitt et al., 1981; Marini et al., 1981a, b) of ventricular contractility have been constructed. When transmural pressures are referenced to true juxtacardiac pressure or esophageal pressure measured with the subject in the lateral or prone position, no change in myocardial contractility occurs during ventilation with PEEP (Wise et al., 1981).

Other indices of contractility have been studied by Fewell and his co-workers (1980a). In dogs ventilated with either zero end-expiratory pressure or 12 cmH_2O PEEP, they found no significant difference in right or left ventricular dP/dt or ejection time. Further, measurements of regional myocardial blood flow showed no change with the application of 12 cmH_2O PEEP.

E. Left Ventricular Afterload

Changes in left ventricular afterload may occur during positive-pressure breathing. Afterload alterations may be especially great when the changes in intrapleural pressure are large or when cardiac function is compromised.

Permutt and co-workers have suggested that transmural left ventricular pressure more accurately reflects left ventricular afterload than does systolic aortic pressure (Robotham and Scharf, 1983). This hypothesis would explain the hemodynamic effects seen in humans during rapid changes in intrapleural pressure.

Buda and co-workers (1979) examined eight patients who had metal myocardial markers implanted during cardiac transplant or coronary bypass surgery. Each patient was studied during spontaneous breathing and during inspiration against a closed glottis to -60 cmH_2O (a Mueller maneuver). They found that negative intrathoracic pressure increased left ventricular volume and decreased left ventricular ejection fraction despite lowering systemic blood pressure. The transmural LV pressure increased during the Mueller maneuver. These changes are consistent with an increased LV afterload induced by decreasing intrathoracic pressure.

It is attractive to hypothesize that the opposite situation may also occur: increasing positive end-expiratory pressure may act to decrease LV afterload and actually improve left ventricular function in some patients. This hypothesis was tested by Mathru and his colleagues (1982) in 16 patients with an LVEDP > 16 mmHg who had undergone coronary bypass surgery. Patients were taken from controlled ventilation to an equivalent level of intermittent mandatory ventilation (IMV) and then 5 cmH_2O PEEP was added to the IMV. Mean airway pressure levels decreased when the patients were placed on IMV and then returned to their previous level when PEEP was added. In this group of patients, cardiac output and stroke volume fell when airway pressure was decreased. The decreased cardiac output occurred despite a concomitant reduction in arterial blood pressure. Increasing airway pressure with PEEP restored the cardiac output.

Two factors may be responsible for these changes. First, placing the patients on IMV decreased pleural pressure and may have suddenly increased left ventricular afterload, fostering LV dysfunction. Second, the sudden decrease in intrathoracic pressure may have rapidly increased venous return.

The increase in left ventricular pressure in turn would have increased left ventricular volume and wall stress. Increasing airway pressure with PEEP may reverse these effects. Further evidence for this effect has been provided by Pinsky and co-workers, who have documented increased cardiac output when intrathoracic pressure is increased both in dogs with cardiac failure (Pinsky et al., 1983) and in patients with severe shock (Pinsky and Summer, 1983).

F. Heart Rate

Most clinical studies have found that heart rate changes little when positive-pressure ventilation with PEEP is instituted (Viquerat et al., 1983; Prewitt et al., 1981; Mathru et al., 1982; Jardin et al., 1981; Dhainaut et al., 1986). Calvin and co-workers (1981), on the other hand, found that heart rate decreased slightly with the application of 14 cmH_2O PEEP. Cassidy et al. (1979a) found a slightly increased heart rate when normal volunteers were exposed to positive-pressure ventilation with 10 cm PEEP. Laboratory studies of positive end-expiratory pressure have documented both increased (Stinnett, 1981) and decreased (Cassidy et al., 1979b) heart rate. These variable changes may be secondary to hyperinflation and reflex stimulation of pulmonary stretch receptors, which causes tachycardia and hypertension, and C fiber receptors, which causes bradycardia and hypotension (Coleridge et al., 1965). Both effects may be abolished by vagotomy. Increased vagal activity caused by lung inflation may also be offset by increased sympathetic activity from aortic and carotid baroreceptors (Stinnett, 1981; Cassidy et al., 1979b). Anesthetics or concurrent drug therapy may alter the balance of sympathetic and parasympathetic tone.

VI. Cardiovascular Function During Weaning from Mechanical Ventilation

Many patients who survive an episode of ARF have difficulty weaning from mechanical ventilation (MV). The Massachusetts General Hospital has a daily census of approximately 12 such patients who do not require further intensive care therapy but remain dependent upon MV. Commonly, their course has been complicated by advanced age and pre-existing pulmonary and/or cardiac disease.

Recent studies suggest that cardiac dysfunction during weaning can play a major role in preventing successful weaning of patients whose pulmonary and respiratory muscle function appears adequate to sustain spontaneous ventilation (SV). Lemaire and colleagues (1988) prospectively studied the hemodynamics, respiratory mechanics, and ventricular volumes of 15 patients whose inspiratory force, vital capacity, tidal volume, and minute ventilation met generally accepted criteria for successful weaning but who nevertheless were unable to wean from mechanical ventilation. The most important finding in these patients was that mean transmural LV filling pressure, as gauged by PCWP or LVEDP, rose from 7.5 ± 5 to 24.5 ± 13 mmHg (mean ± SD) during spontaneous ventilation (Figs. 7 and 8). Furthermore, both LV and RV volumes measured by radionuclear angiocardiography were increased. Worsening of wall motion abnormalities during spontaneous ventilation was demonstrated in 3 patients with LV wall motion abnormalities during mechanical ventilation. After 10 min of spontaneous ventilation esophageal pressure was reduced, but cardiac index, heart rate, and central venous, pulmonary artery, and systemic blood pressure were increased.

Following the initial study, patients were given a diuretic (furosemide, 80 mg/day). A total of nine patients were able to wean successfully on this

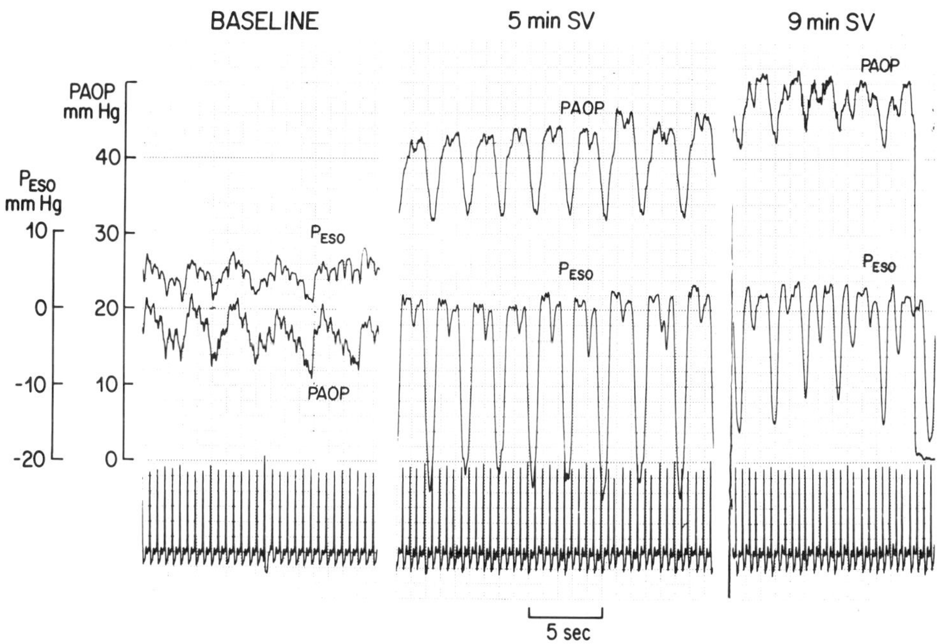

Figure 7 Weaning from mechanical ventilation (baseline) to spontaneous ventilation (SV) of a COPD patient recovering from acute cardiopulmonary decompensation. There is a progressive increase in pulmonary artery occlusion pressure (PAOP) from 14 mmHg (baseline) to 50 mmHg (9 min SV). The esophageal pressure is reduced during SV, with marked negative inspiratory excursions. (Reprinted from Lemaire et al., 1988.)

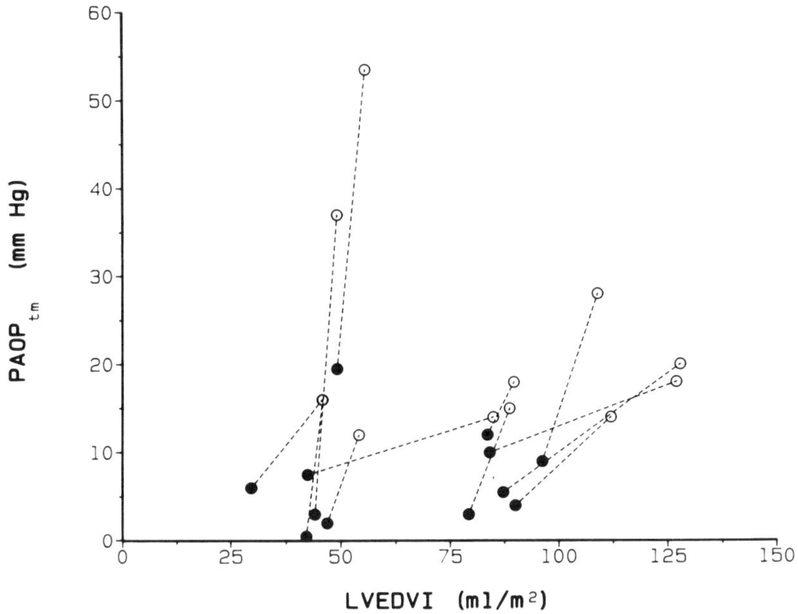

Figure 8 Changes in transmural pulmonary artery occlusion pressure ($PAOP_{tm}$) and left ventricular end-diastolic volume index (LVEDVI) during the transfer from mechanical ventilation (MV) to spontaneous ventilation (SV) in 12 chronic obstructive pulmonary disease (COPD) patients recovering from acute respiratory failure: (●) MV; (○) SV. (Reprinted from Lemaire et al., 1988.)

regimen, and eight were restudied about 1 week after the initial study. During the second study, LV filling pressure remained unchanged at 9 ± 3 mmHg during spontaneous ventilation.

A high incidence of organic heart disease in patients unable to wean after recovery from ARF was noted in the study. Of the six patients who remained dependent upon mechanical ventilation, five died in the hospital. Of these five three underwent autopsy and each demonstrated extensive coronary atherosclerosis.

The increases in central venous pressure (CVP), LVEDP, and PCWP associated with these weaning episodes suggest that LV volume overload may occur secondary to a redistribution of blood volume from peripheral to cardiopulmonary compartments (Permutt, 1988). Additionally, reduced intrathoracic pressure during SV can increase LV afterload (Buda et al., 1979; Scharf et al., 1981; Robotham, 1981; Mathru et al., 1982). It is possible that these hemodynamic stresses produced by spontaneous, as opposed to positive-pressure, ventilation could result in altered myocardial perfusion and LV dysfunction.

To evaluate the possibility that myocardial ischemia may occur when ventilator-dependent patients breathe spontaneously, Hurford and co-workers (1988b) performed a study using thallium 201 myocardial scintigraphy to determine the occurrence of myocardial perfusion inhomogeneities during the weaning of 15 ventilator-dependent patients (9 women and 6 men, aged 71 $\pm$ 7 years). The patients had been mechanically ventilated for 9-68 days. These patients had a spontaneous respiratory rate of 32 $\pm$ 8 bpm (mean $\pm$ SD), a spontaneous tidal volume of 280 $\pm$ 140 ml, a maximal inspiratory force of -24 ± 6 cmH_2O, stable or improving acute pulmonary disease as evidenced by serial chest radiographs and arterial blood gas tensions, and were able to spontaneously breathe comfortably for at least 10 min. A total of 14 patients were studied with thallium 201 myocardial scintigraphy during both mechanical ventilation (IMV) and, on a separate day to minimize background activity, after at least 10 min of spontaneous breathing via a T piece (SV). The remaining patient was studied while on SV only. During SV, 8 of 15 patients had areas of decreased myocardial thallium uptake with redistribution of the label on delayed images, indicating decreased myocardial perfusion during SV. Of the 14 patients, 5 had an increased LV cavity size during SV. The change from IMV to SV was accompanied by an increased heart rate, diastolic and mean arterial pressure, and spontaneous minute ventilation and decreased pH_a. Further, preliminary outcome data suggested that the patients with positive thallium scans during SV were hospitalized longer than those with negative scans (86 $\pm$ 47 versus 39 $\pm$ 12 days).

These studies suggest that abruptly shifting mechanical ventilator-dependent patients to SV can be associated with increased central venous pressure, increased LV preload and afterload, and alterations in myocardial perfusion. These changes may result in cardiac dysfunction and provide the reason that many patients with borderline pulmonary function and respiratory mechanics, especially those with coexisting coronary artery disease, cannot wean from mechanical ventilation.

VII. Summary

Pulmonary hypertension associated with the development of severe ARDS decreases cardiac output by increasing right ventricular afterload. Right ventricular ejection fraction decreases and RV volume increases as the pulmonary artery pressure is increased. Left ventricular contractility appears unaffected. Stroke volume may be decreased as a consequence of decreased RV output or decreased LV diastolic compliance secondary to an enlarged right ventricle, as well as to changes in the shape and motion of the interventricular septum.

Concurrent sepsis may confound the cardiovascular management of patients with acute respiratory failure. Multiple organ failure secondary to either inadequate or inappropriately distributed peripheral perfusion increases mortality. Reversible myocardial depression may occur early during sepsis. Myocardial depression may be due to the release of circulating myocardial depressant factors.

Supporting patients with positive-pressure ventilation and PEEP decreases venous return by raising intrapleural pressure. At high levels of PEEP, when alveolar pressure exceeds pulmonary capillary pressure, pulmonary vascular resistance increases, in turn increasing right ventricular afterload. PEEP limits left ventricular filling by decreasing right ventricular output, by hyperinflating the lungs and physically compressing the heart, and, at high levels of PEEP, by shifting the interventricular septum toward the LV free wall. PEEP may improve the systolic function of the left ventricle by reducing left ventricular afterload. Myocardial contractility per se does not appear to be affected by PEEP.

In patients with concurrent pulmonary and/or cardiac disease, the discontinuation of positive-pressure ventilation may be associated with signs and symptoms of cardiac dysfunction and myocardial ischemia. Limiting the increase in LV filling pressure during SV through the use of diuretics and vasodilators may aid the process of weaning such patients from mechanical ventilation.

References

Bartlett, R. H., Morris, A. H., Fairley, H. B., Hirsh, R., O'Connor, N., and Pontoppidan, H. (1986). A prospective study of acute hypoxic respiratory failure. *Chest,* **89**:684-689.

Baumgartner, J.-D., McCutchan, J. A., van Melle, G., Vogt, M., Luethy, R., Glauser, M. P., Ziegler, E. J., Klauber, M. R., Muehlen, E., Chiolero, R., and Geroulanos, S. (1985). Prevention of gram negative shock and death in surgical patients by antibody to endotoxin core glycolipid. *Lancet,* **2**1:59-63.

Bell, R. C., Coalson, J. J., Smith, J. D., and Johanson, W. G., Jr. (1986). Incidence, site, and outcome of infections in patients with the adult respiratory distress syndrome. *Am. Rev. Respir. Dis.,* **134**:12-16.

Beutler, B., Milsark, I. W., and Cerami, A. C. (1985). Passive immunization against cachectin/tumor necrosis factor protects mice from lethal effect of endotoxin. *Science,* **229**:869-871.

Bihari, D., Smithies, M., Gimson, A., and Tinker, J. (1987). The effects of vasodilation with prostacyclin on oxygen delivery and uptake in critically ill patients. *N. Engl. J. Med.,* **317**:397-403.

Biondi, J. W., Schulman, D. S., Soufer, R., Matthay, R. A., Hines, R. L., Kay, H. R., and Barash, P. G. (1988). The effect of incremental positive end-expiratory pressure on right ventricular hemodynamics and ejection fraction. *Anesth. Analg.* (Cleve), **67**:144-151.

Bove, A. A., and Santamore, W. P. (1981). Ventricular interdependence. *Prog. Cardiovasc. Dis.,* **23**:365-388.

Braunwald, E., Binion, J. T., Morgan, W. L., Jr., and Sarnoff, S. J. (1957). Alterations in central blood volume and cardiac output induced by positive pressure breathing and counteracted by metaraminol (Aramine). *Circ. Res.,* **5**:670-675.

Buda, A. J., Pinsky, M. R., Ingels, N. B., Daughters, G. T., II, Stinson, E. B., and Alderman, E. L. (1979). Effect of intrathoracic pressure on left ventricular performance. *N. Engl. J. Med.,* **301**:453-459.

Calvin, J. E., Driedger, A. A., and Sibbald, W. J. (1981). Positive end-expiratory pressure (PEEP) does not depress left ventricular function in patients with pulmonary edema. *Am. Rev. Respir. Dis.,* **124**:121-128.

Calvin, J. E., Baer, R. W., and Glantz, S. A. (1986). Pulmonary injury depresses cardiac systolic function through Starling mechanism. *Am. J. Physiol.,* **251**:H722-H733.

Cassidy, S. S., and Mitchell, J. H. (1981). Effects of positive pressure breathing on right and left ventricular preload and afterload. *Fed. Proc.,* **40**: 2178-2181.

Cassidy, S. S., Robertson, C. H., Pierce, A. K., and Johnson, R. L., Jr. (1978). Cardiovascular effects of positive end-expiratory pressure in dogs. *J. Appl. Physiol.,* **44**:743-750.

Cassidy, S. S., Eschenbacher, W. L., Robertson, C. H., Jr., Nixon, J. V., Blomqvist, G., and Johnson, R. L., Jr. (1979a). Cardiovascular effects of positive-pressure ventilation in normal subjects. *J. Appl. Physiol.,* **47**:453-461.

Cassidy, S. S., Eschenbacher, W. L., and Johnson, R. L., Jr. (1979b). Reflex cardiovascular depression during unilateral lung hyperinflation in the dog. *J. Clin. Invest.,* **64**:620-626.

Coleridge, H. M., Coleridge, J. C. G., and Luck, J. C. (1965). Pulmonary afferent fibres of small diameter stimulated by capsaicin and by hyperinflation of the lungs. *J. Physiol.* (*Lond.*), **179**:248-262.

Cournand, A., Motley, H. L., Werko, L., and Richards, D. W., Jr. (1948). Physiological studies of the effects of intermittent positive breathing on cardiac output in man. *Am. J. Physiol.,* **152**:162-174.

Craven, K. D., and Wood, L. D. H. (1981). Extrapericardial and esophageal pressures with positive end-expiratory pressure in dogs. *J. Appl. Physiol.,* **51**:798-805.

Culver, B. H., Marini, J. J., and Butler, J. (1981). Lung volume and pleural pressure effects on ventricular function. *J. Appl. Physiol.,* **50**:630-635.

Cunnion, R. E., Schaer, G. L., Parker, M. M., Natanson, C., and Parrillo, J. E. (1986). The coronary circulation in human septic shock. *Circulation,* **73**:637-644.

DeCampo, T., and Civetta, J. M. (1979). The effect of short-term discontinuation of high level PEEP in patients with acute respiratory failure. *Crit. Care Med.,* **7**:47-49.

Dhainaut, J.-F., Devaux, J. Y., Monsallier, J. F., Brunet, F., Villemant, D., and Huyghebaert, M.-F. (1986). Mechanisms of decreased left ventricular preload during continuous positive pressure ventilation in ARDS. *Chest,* **90**:74-80.

Dhainaut, J.-F., Brunet, F., Monsallier, J. F., Villemant, D., Devaux, J. Y., Konno, M., DeGournay, J. M., Armaganidis, A., Iotti, G., Huyghebaert, M.-F., and Lanore, J. J. (1987). Bedside evaluation of right ventricular performance using a rapid computerized thermodilution method. *Crit. Care Med.,* **15**:148-152.

Dorinsky, P. M., and Whitcomb, M. E. (1983). The effect of PEEP on cardiac output. *Chest,* **84**:210-216.

Eaton, R. J., Taxman, R. M., and Avioli, L. V. (1983). Cardiovascular evaluation of patients treated with PEEP. *Arch. Intern. Med.,* **143**:1958-1961.

Fewell, J. E., Abendschein, D. R., Carlson, C. J., Murray, J. F., and Rapaport, E. (1980a). Continuous positive-pressure ventilation decreases right and left ventricular end-diastolic volumes in the dog. *Circ. Res.,* **46**:125-132.

Fewell, J. E., Abendschein, D. R., Carlson, C. J., Rapaport, E., and Murray, J. F. (1980b). Mechanism of decreased right and left ventricular end-diastolic volumes during continuous positive-pressure ventilation in dogs. *Circ. Res.,* **47**:467-472.

Glazier, J. B., Hughes, J. M. B., Maloney, J. E., and West, J. B. (1969). Measurements of capillary dimensions and blood volume in rapidly frozen lungs. *J. Appl. Physiol.,* **26**:65-76.

Gold, F. L., and Bache, R. J. (1982). Transmural right ventricular blood flow during acute pulmonary artery hypertension in the sedated dog. *Circ. Res.,* **51**:196-204.

Goldberg, H. S., and Rabson, J. (1981). Control of cardiac output by systemic vessels: Circulatory adjustments to acute and chronic respiratory failure and the effect of therapeutic interventions. *Am. J. Cardiol.,* **47**:696-702.

Guyton, A. C., Lindsey, A. W., and Gilluly, J. J. (1954). The limits of right ventricular compensation following acute increases in pulmonary circulatory resistance. *Circ. Res.,* **2**:326-332.

Haynes, J. B., Carson, S. D., Whitney, W. P., Zerbe, G. O., Hyers, T. M., and Steele, P. (1980). Positive end-expiratory pressure shifts left ventricular diastolic pressure-area curves. *J. Appl. Physiol.,* **48**:670-676.

Henning, R. J. (1986). Effects of positive end-expiratory pressure on the right ventricle. *J. Appl. Physiol.,* **61**:819-826.

Holcroft, J. W., Vassary, M. J., and Weber, C. J. (1986). Prostaglandin E_1 and survival in patients with the adult respiratory distress syndrome: A prospective trial. *Ann. Surg.,* **203**:371-378.

Hurford, W. E., and Zapol, W. M. (1988). The right ventricle and critical illness: A review of anatomy, physiology, and clinical evaluation of its function. *Intensive Care Med.,* **14**:448-457.

Hurford, W., Barlai-Kovach, M., Lynch, K., Zapol, W. M., Strauss, H. W., and Lowenstein, E. (1986). Effect of the adult respiratory distress syndrome (ARDS) and PEEP in biventricular function (abstract). *Am. Rev. Respir. Dis.,* **133**:A304.

Hurford, W. E., Barlai-Kovach, M., Strauss, H. W., Zapol, W. M., and Lowenstein, E. (1987a). Canine biventricular performance during acute progressive pulmonary microembolization: Regional myocardial perfusion and fatty acid uptake. *J. Crit. Care.,* **2**:270-281.

Hurford, W. E., Lynch, K., Strauss, H. W., and Zapol, W. M. (1987b). The effect of positive end-expiratory pressure on the pulmonary blood volume of patients with ARDS (abstract). *Am. Rev. Respir. Dis.,* **135**: A6.

Hurford, W. E., Lynch, K., Keech, F., Wilson, D., Strauss, H. W., Lowenstein, E., and Zapol, W. M. (1988b). Thallium-201 myocardial perfusion defects appear during the weaning of mechanical ventilator-dependent patients (abstract). *Am. Rev. Respir. Dis.,* **137**:293.

Hussain, S. N. A., and Roussos, C. (1985). Distribution of respiratory muscle and organ blood flow during endotoxic shock in dogs. *J. Appl. Physiol.,* **59**:1802-1808.

Hyers, T. M., and Fowler, A. A. (1986). Adult respiratory distress syndrome: Causes, morbidity, and mortality. *Fed. Proc.,* **45**:25-29.

Jardin, F., Farcot, J.-C., Boisante, L., Curien, N., Margairaz, A., and Bourdarias, J.-P. (1981). Influence of positive end-expiratory pressure on left ventricular performance. *N. Engl. J. Med.,* **304**:387-392.

Jardin, F., Gueret, P., Dubourg, O., Farcot, J.-C., Margairaz, A., and Bourdarias, J.-P. (1985). Right ventricular volumes by thermodilution in the adult respiratory distress syndrome: A comparative study using two-dimensional echocardiography as a reference method. *Chest,* **88**: 34-39.

Jardin, F., Dubourg, O., Margairaz, A., and Bourdarias, J.-P. (1987). Inspiratory impairment in right ventricular performance during acute asthma. *Chest,* **92**:789-795.

Kay, H. R., Afshari, M., Barash, P., Webler, W., Iskandrian, A., Bemis, C., Hakki, A.-H., and Mundth, E. D. (1983). Measurement of ejection fraction by thermal dilution techniques. *J. Surg. Res.,* **34**:377-346.

Kettelhut, I. C., Fiers, W., and Goldberg, A. L. (1987). The toxic effects of tumor necrosis factor in vivo and their prevention by cyclooxygenase inhibitors. *Proc. Natl. Acad. Sci. USA,* **84**:4273-4277.

Kimball, W. R., Leith, D. E., and Robins, A. G. (1982). Dynamic hyperinflation and ventilator dependence in chronic obstructive pulmonary disease. *Am. Rev. Respir. Dis.,* **126**:991-995.

Kronberg, G. M., Quan, S. F., Schlobohm, R. M., Lindauer, J. M., and Goodman, P. C. (1979). Anatomic location of the tips of pulmonary artery catheters in supine patients. *Anesthesiology,* **51**:467-469.

LaBrousse, J., Tenaillon, A., Massabie, P., Simonneay, G., and Lissac, J. (1976). Artificial ventilation and pulmonary capillary wedge pressure in acute respiratory failure. *Lancet,* **1**:974.

Laver, M. B., Strauss, H. W., and Pohost, G. M. (1979). Right and left ventricular geometry: Adjustments during acute respiratory failure. *Crit. Care Med.,* **7**:509-519.

Lemaire, F., Teboul, J.-L., Cenotti, L., Giotto, G., Abrouk, F., Steg, G., Macquin-Mavier, I., and Zapol, W. M. (1988). Acute left ventricular dysfunction during unsuccessful weaning from mechanical ventilation. *Anesthesiology,* **69**:171-179.

Lozman, J., Powers, S. R., Jr., Older, T., Dutton, R. E., Roy, R. J., English, M., Marco, D., and Eckert, C. (1974). Correlation of pulmonary wedge and left atrial pressures: A study in the patient receiving positive end expiratory pressure ventilation. *Arch. Surg.,* **109**:270-277.

Luce, J. M. (1984). The cardiovascular effects of mechanical ventilation and positive end-expiratory pressure. *JAMA,* **252**:807-811.

Luterman, A., Horovitz, J. H., Carrico, C. J., Canizaro, P. C., Heimbach, D., and Colocousis, J. (1978). Withdrawal from positive end-expiratory pressure. *Surgery,* **83**:328-332.

Maddahi, J., Berman, D. S., Matsuoka, D. T., Waxman, A. D., Stankus, K. E., Forrester, J. S., and Swan, H. J. C. (1979). A new technique for assessing right ventricular ejection fraction using rapid multiple-gated equilibrium cardiac blood pool scintigraphy. *Circulation,* **60**:581-589.

Manny, J., Patten, M. T., Liebman, P. R., and Hechtman, H. B. (1978). The association of lung distention, PEEP and biventricular failure. *Ann. Surg.,* **187**:151-157.

Marini, J. J., Culver, B. H., and Butler, J. (1981a). Effect of positive end-expiratory pressure on canine ventricular function curves. *J. Appl. Physiol.,* **51**:1367-1374.

Marini, J. J., Culver, B. H., and Butler, J. (1981b). Mechanical effect of lung distention with positive pressure on cardiac function. *Am. Rev. Respir. Dis.,* **124**:382-386.

Marini, J. J., O'Quin, R., Culver, B. H., and Butler, J. (1982). Estimation of transmural cardiac pressures during ventilation with PEEP. *J. Appl. Physiol.,* **53**:384-391.

Mathru, M., Rao, T. L. K., El-Etr, A. A., and Pifarre, R. (1982). Hemodynamic response to changes in ventilatory patterns in patients with normal and poor left ventricular reserve. *Crit. Care Med.,* **10**:423-426.

Michelassi, F., Landa, L., Hill, R. D., Lowenstein, E., Watkins, W. D., Petkau, A. J., and Zapol, W. M. (1982). Leukotriene D_4: A potent coronary artery vasoconstrictor associated with impaired ventricular contraction. *Science,* **217**:841-843.

Michelassi, F., Castorena, G., Hill, R. D., Lowenstein, E., Watkins, W. D., Petkau, A. J., and Zapol, W. M. (1983). Effects of leukotrienes B_4 and C_4 on coronary circulation and myocardial contractility. *Surgery,* **94**: 267-275.

Montgomery, A. S., Stager, M. A., Carrico, C. J., and Hudson, L. D. (1985). Causes of mortality in patients with the adult respiratory distress syndrome. *Am. Rev. Respir. Dis.,* **132**:485-489.

Movat, H. Z., Cybulsky, M. I., Colditz, I. G., Chan, M. K. W., and Dinarello, C. A. (1987). Acute inflammation in gram-negative infection: Endotoxin, interleukin 1, tumor necrosis factor, and neutrophils. *Fed. Proc.,* **46**:97-104.

Natanson, C., Fink, M. P., Ballantyne, H. K., MacVittie, T. J., Conklin, J. J., and Parrillo, J. E. (1986). Gram-negative bacteremia produces both severe systolic and diastolic cardiac dysfunction in a canine model that simulates human septic shock. *J. Clin. Invest.,* **78**:259-270.

Nienaber, C. A., Spielmann, R. P., Wasmus, G., Mathey, D. G., Montz, R., and Bleifeld, W. H. (1985). Clinical use of ultrashort-lived radionuclide Krypton-81m for noninvasive analysis of right ventricular performance in normal subjects and patients with right ventricular dysfunction. *J. Am. Coll. Cardiol.,* **5**:687-698.

O'Quin, R., and Marini, J. J. (1983). Pulmonary artery occlusion pressure: Clinical physiology, measurement, and interpretation. *Am. Rev. Respir. Dis.,* **128**:319-326.

Parker, J. L., and Adams, H. R. (1985). Development of myocardial dysfunction in endotoxin shock. *Am. J. Physiol.,* **248**:H818-H826.

Parker, M. M., Shelhamer, J. H., Bacharach, S. L., Green, M. V., Natanson, C., Frederick, T. M., Damske, B. A., and Parrillo, J. E. (1984). Profound but reversible myocardial depression in patients with septic shock. *Ann. Intern. Med.,* **100**:483-490.

Parrillo, J. E., Burch, C., Shelhamer, J. H., Parker, M. M., Natanson, C., and Schuette, W. (1985). A circulating myocardial depressant substance in humans with septic shock. *J. Clin. Invest.,* **76**:1539-1553.

Pepe, P. E., and Marini, J. J. (1982). Occult positive end-expiratory pressure in mechanically ventilated patients with airflow obstruction. *Am. Rev. Respir. Dis.,* **126**:166-170.

Permutt, S. (1988). Circulatory effects of weaning from mechanical ventilation: The importance of transdiaphragmatic pressure. *Anesthesiology,* **69**:157-160.

Pick, R. A., Handler, J. B., Murata, G. H., and Friedman, A. S. (1982). The cardiovascular effects of positive end-expiratory pressure. *Chest,* **82**:345-350.

Pinsky, M. R., and Summer, W. R. (1983). Cardiac augmentation by phasic high intrathoracic pressure support in man. *Chest,* **84**:370-375.

Pinsky, M. R., Summer, W. R., Wise, R. A., Permutt, S., and Bromberger-Barnea, B. (1983). Augmentation of cardiac function by elevation of intrathoracic pressure. *J. Appl. Physiol.,* **54**:950-955.

Pitt, B., and Strauss, H. W. (1977). Evaluation of ventricular function by radioisotopic technics. *N. Engl. J. Med.,* **296**:1097-1099.

Potkin, R. T., Hudson, L. D., Weaver, L. J., and Trobaugh, G. (1987). Effect of positive end-expiratory pressure on right and left ventricular function in patients with the adult respiratory distress syndrome. *Am. Rev. Respir. Dis.,* **135**:307-311.

Powers, S. R., Jr., and Dutton, R. E. (1975). Correlation of positive end-expiratory pressure with cardiac performance. *Crit. Care Med.,* **3**:64-68.

Prewitt, R. M., and Wood, L. D. H. (1979). Effect of positive end-expiratory pressure on ventricular function in dogs. *Am. J. Physiol.,* **236**: H534-H544.

Prewitt, R. M., Oppenheimer, L., Sutherland, J. B., and Wood, L. D. H. (1981). Effect of positive end-expiratory pressure on left ventricular mechanics in patients with hypoxemic respiratory failure. *Anesthesiology,* **55**:409-415.

Qvist, J., Pontoppidan, H., Wilson, R. S., Lowenstein, E., and Laver, M. B. (1975). Hemodynamic responses to mechanical ventilation with PEEP: The effect of hypervolemia. *Anesthesiology,* **42**:45-55.

Qvist, J., Mygind, T., Crottogini, A., Jordening, H., Mogensen, T., Dorph, S., and Laver, M. B. (1988). Cardiovascular adjustments to pulmonary vascular injury in dogs. *Anesthesiology,* **68**:341-349.

Rajagopalan, B., Cheng, C., Strauss, H. W., Treves, S., Quinn, D., and Zapol, W. M. (1982). Cardiopulmonary interactions in patients with ARDS: Studies of right ventricular function using first pass nuclear angiography with iridium 191m (abstract). *Am. Rev. Respir. Dis.,* **125**:77.

Rankin, J. S., Olsen, C. O., Arentzen, C. E., Tyson, G. S., Maier, G., Smith, P. K., Hammon, J. W., Jr., Davis, J. W., McHale, P. A., Anderson,

R. W., and Sabiston, D. C. (1982). The effects of airway pressure on cardiac function in intact dogs and man. *Circulation,* **66**:108-120.

Robotham, J. L. (1981). Cardiovascular disturbances in chronic respiratory insufficiency. *Am. J. Cardiol.,* **47**:941-949.

Robotham, J. L., and Scharf, S. M. (1983). Effects of positive and negative pressure ventilation on cardiac performance. *Clin. Chest Med.,* **4**:161-187.

Robotham, J. L., Lixfield, W., Holland, L., MacGregor, D., Bromberger-Barnea, B., Permutt, S., and Rabson, J. L. (1980). The effects of positive end-expiratory pressure on right and left ventricular performance. *Am. Rev. Respir. Dis.,* **121**:677-683.

Roos, A., Thomas, L. J., Nagel, E. L., and Prommas, D. C. (1961). Pulmonary vascular resistance as determined by lung inflation and vascular pressures. *J. Appl. Physiol.,* **16**:77-84.

Scharf, S. M., and Ingram, R. H., Jr. (1977). Effects of decreasing lung compliance with oleic acid on the cardiovascular response to PEEP. *Am. J. Physiol.,* **233**:H625-H641.

Scharf, S. M., Caldini, P., and Ingram, R. H., Jr. (1977). Cardiovascular effects of increasing airway pressure in the dog. *Am. J. Physiol.,* **232**: H35-H43.

Scharf, S. M., Brown, R., Saunders, N., Green, L. H., and Ingram, R. H., Jr. (1979). Changes in canine left ventricular size and configuration with positive end-expiratory pressure. *Circ. Res.,* **44**:672-678.

Scharf, A. M., Bianco, J. A., Tow, D. E., and Brown, R. (1981). The effects of large negative intrathoracic pressure on left ventricular function in patients with coronary artery disease. *Circulation,* **63**:871-874.

Schulman, D. S., Biondi, J. W., Matthay, R. A., Barash, P. G., Zaret, B. L., and Soufer, R. (1988). Effect of positive end-expiratory pressure on right ventricular performance: Importance of baseline right ventricular function. *Am. J. Med.,* **84**:57-67.

Short, B. L., Gardiner, M., Walker, R. I., Jones, S. R., and Fletcher, J. R. (1981). Indomethacin improves survival in gram-negative sepsis. *Adv. Shock Res.,* **6**:27-36.

Sibbald, W. J., Driedger, A. A., Cunningham, D. G., and Cheung, H. (1986). Right and left ventricular performance in acute hypoxemic respiratory failure. *Crit. Care Med.,* **14**:852-857.

Siegel, J. H., Greenspan, M., and Del Guercio, L. R. (1967). Abnormal vascular tone, defective oxygen transport and myocardial failure in human septic shock. *Ann. Surg.,* **165**:504-517.

Stinnett, H. O. (1981). Altered cardiovascular reflex responses during positive pressure breathing. *Fed. Proc.,* **40**:2182-2187.

Suffredini, A. F., Parker, M. M., Brenner, M., Schlesinger, T., and Parrillo, J. E. (1987). Endotoxin administration produces abnormal cardiovascular responses in normal humans. *Clin. Res.,* **35**:386A.

Suter, P. M. (1985). Assessment of respiratory mechanics in ARDS. In *Acute Respiratory Failure.* Edited by W. M. Zapol and K. J. Falke. New York, Marcel Dekker, pp. 507-519.

Teboul, J.-L., Besbes, M., Axler, O., Brun-Buisson, C., Andrivet, P., Rekik, N., and Lemaire, F. (1988). A bedside index for determination of zone III condition of pulmonary artery (PA) catheter tips during mechanical ventilation (MV) (abstract). *Am. Rev. Respir. Dis.,* **137**:139.

Teboul, J.-L., Zapol, W. M., Brun-Buisson, C., Abrouk, F., Rauss, A., and Lemaire, F. (1989). A comparison of pulmonary artery occlusion pressure and left ventricular end-diastolic pressure during ARDS. *Anesthesiology,* **70**:261-266.

Thorvaldson, J., Ilebekk, A., and Kiil, F. (1985). Determinants of pulmonary blood volume. Effects of acute changes in airway pressure. *Acta Physiol. Scand.,* **125**:471-479.

Tomashefski, J. F., Jr., Davies, P., Boggis, C., Greene, R., Zapol, W. M., and Reid, L. (1983). The pulmonary vascular lesions of the adult respiratory distress syndrome. *Am. J. Pathol.,* **112**:112-126.

Tooker, J., Huseby, J., and Butler, J. (1978). The effect of Swan-Ganz catheter height on the wedge pressure-left atrial pressure relationship in edema during positive-pressure ventilation. *Am. Rev. Respir. Dis.,* **117**:721-725.

Tracey, K. J., Fong, Y., Hesse, D. G., Manogue, K. R., Lee, A. T., Kuo, G. C., Lowry, S. F., and Cerami, A. (1987a). Anti-cachectin/TNF monoclonal antibodies prevent septic shock during lethal bacteremia. *Nature,* **330**:662-664.

Tracey, K. J., Lowry, S. F., Fahey, T. J., III, Albert, J. D., Fong, Y., Hesse, D., Beutler, B., Manogue, K. R., Calvano, S., Wei, H., Cerami, A., and Shires, G. T. (1987b). Cachectin/tumor necrosis factor induces lethal shock and stress hormone responses in the dog. *Surg. Gynecol. Obstet.,* **164**:415-422.

Vincent, J.-L., Thirion, M., Brimioulle, S., Lejeune, P., and Kahn, R. J. (1986). Thermodilution measurement of right ventricular ejection fraction with a modified pulmonary artery catheter. *Intensive Care Med.,* **12**:33-38.

Viquerat, C. E., Righetti, A., and Suter, P. M. (1983). Biventricular volumes and function in patients with adult respiratory distress syndrome ventilated with PEEP. *Chest,* **83**:509-514.

Vlahakes, G. J., Turley, K., and Hoffman, J. I. E. (1981). The pathophysiology of failure in acute right ventricular hypertension: Hemodynamic and biochemical correlations. *Circulation,* **63**:87-95.

Wallis, T. W., Robotham, J. L., Compean, R., and Kindred, M. K. (1983). Mechanical heart-lung interaction with positive end-expiratory pressure. *J. Appl. Physiol.,* **54**:1039-1047.

Weber, K. T., Janicki, J. S., Shroff, S., and Fishman, A. P. (1981). Contractile mechanics and interaction of the right and left ventricles. *Am. J. Cardiol.,* **47**:686-695.

West, J. B., Dollery, C. T., and Naimark, A. (1964). Distribution of blood flow in isolated lung; relation to vascular and alveolar pressure. *J. Appl. Physiol.,* **19**:713-724.

Wise, R. A., Robotham, J. L., Bromberger-Barnea, B., and Permutt, S. (1981). Effect of PEEP on left ventricular function in right-heart-bypassed dogs. *J. Appl. Physiol.,* **51**:541-546.

Zapol, W. M., and Snider, M. T. (1977). Pulmonary hypertension in severe acute respiratory failure. *N. Engl. J. Med.,* **296**:476-480.

Zarins, C., Virgilio, R., Smith, D., and Peters, R. (1977). The effect of vascular volume on positive end-expiratory pressure-induced cardiac output depression and wedge left atrial pressure discrepancy. *J. Surg. Res.,* **23**:348-60.

Ziegler, E. J., McCutchan, A., Fierer, J., Glauser, M. P., Sadoff, J. C., Douglas, H., and Braude, A. I. (1982). Treatment of gram negative bacteremia and shock with human antiserum to a mutant *Escherichia coli. N. Engl. J. Med.,* **307**:1225-1230.

13

Corticosteroids in Adult Respiratory Distress Syndrome

KENNETH L. BRIGHAM

Center for Lung Research
Vanderbilt University School of Medicine
Nashville, Tennessee

I. Introduction

Of the several pharmacologic agents that may reasonably be expected to prevent or alter the course of acute diffuse lung injury, corticosteroids have the longest history. Clinical use of these drugs in patients with the adult respiratory distress syndrome (ARDS) was originally largely empirical. As more information about the pathogenesis and pathophysiology of ARDS emerged, the rationale seemed more sound. The focus of many investigations on neutrophil activation and generation of lipid mediators as crucial events in the pathogenesis of the syndrome suggested that corticosteroids may be effective, if not in reversing the process, at least in preventing it.

For a very long period of time, steroids were used as therapy for ARDS without benefit of controlled clinical trials to establish efficacy. Based mostly on anecdotal impressions, clinicians tended to divide themselves into pro and anti steroid groups, each position maintained with equal passion and each position equally indefensible. Clinical trials were late in coming because of strong clinical impressions and because, as research progressed, the science seemed to validate those impressions.

Although the final answer may not yet be in for every subset of patients with ARDS, at least the general question of efficacy has been addressed with appropriate studies. Discussion of the topic provides an opportunity for interesting insights into some of the processes by which new therapies can or cannot be developed.

II. Actions of Corticosteroids That May Be Beneficial in ARDS

Corticosteroids are "anti-inflammatory" drugs; the classification preceded knowledge of specific actions of the drugs or mechanisms by which inflammation was inhibited. Since ARDS was presumed to result from diffuse injury to the lungs and since acute tissue injury can result from or cause an acute inflammatory response, or both, a general rationale for corticosteroids as therapy for ARDS was obvious even when the syndrome was first recognized (Ashbaugh et al., 1967; Petty and Ashbaugh, 1977).

A popular hypothesis explaining acute diffuse lung injury holds that activation of neutrophils is an early and central event in the process (Brigham, 1987). Neurophils then adhere in the lung microcirculation and generate aggressive oxygen species and proteases that injure the endothelium (and other lung cells). Several lines of evidence support this notion. Activated neutrophils can injure lung endothelial cells in culture (Repine et al., 1982). Several animal models of diffuse lung injury appear to depend on the presence of neutrophils, at least for the full expression of the injury (Heflin and Brigham, 1981; Flick et al., 1981). Neutrophils accumulate in the lungs and the airspaces of patients with ARDS, and the severity of the neutrophilic alveolitis may correlate with the severity of the lung injury. There is evidence in both whole-animal and organ preparations and in cell culture studies that oxidant mechanisms are important in injury resulting from a variety of stimuli (Fantone and Ward, 1982; Brigham, 1986). Neutrophil proteases, especially neutrophil elastase, are released in the lungs of humans with ARDS and can be identified in bronchoalveolar lavage fluid.

At least in vitro, high concentrations of corticosteroids inhibit some responses of neutrophils to activating stimuli. For example, corticosteroids can inhibit neutrophil aggregation in response to complement exposure (Hammerschmidt et al., 1979). It has also been reported that corticosteroids can inhibit neutrophil superoxide generation and other activation responses (Nelson and Ruhmann-Wennhold, 1978; MacGregor et al., 1974).

Among the several humoral mediators that may participate in the pathophysiologic alterations in ARDS, eicosanoids, biologically active metabolites of arachidonic acid, have assumed prominence. Figure 1 and Table 1 illustrate how eicosanoids are generated and list the effects of some eicosanoids on lung

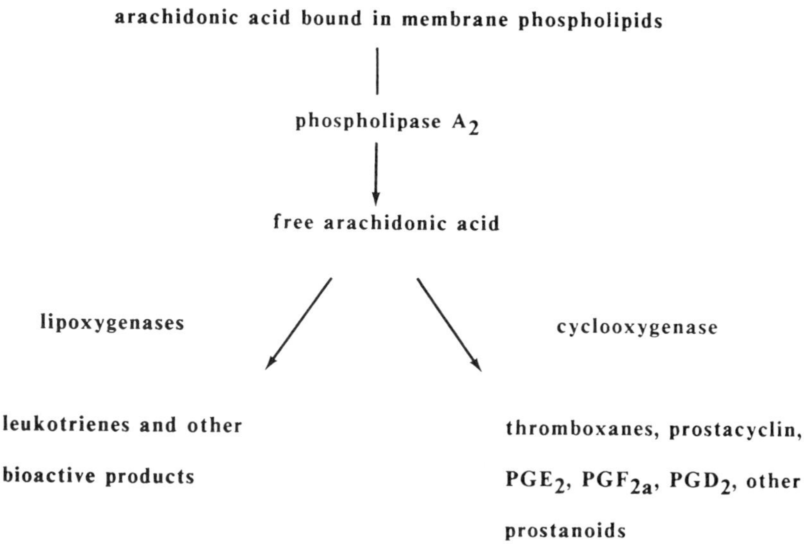

Figure 1 A simplified scheme of eicosanoid generation.

function. Many of the 40-odd cell types present in the lungs possess the necessary metabolic machinery to generate cyclooxygenase and lipoxygenase products of arachidonic acid. Such products are generated when arachidonic acid is liberated from membrane phospholipids. That process involves activation of the enzyme phospholipase A_2, and corticosteroids can inhibit this step in the process and thus have the potential for preventing generation of all eicosanoids in response to an injurious stimulus.

Since several eicosanoids can have deleterious effects on the lungs (Table 1) and since interventions that injure the lungs cause increased generation

Table 1 Effects of Some Eicosanoids on the Lungs

Eicosanoid	Effect
Thromboxane A_2	Vasoconstriction, bronchoconstriction
Prostacyclin	Vasodilation
PGE_2	Vasoconstriction (mild)
$PGF_{2\alpha}$	Vasoconstriction, bronchoconstriction
Leukotriene D_4	Bronchoconstriction, vasoconstriction
Leukotriene C_4	Same as LTD_4 but less potent

of both cyclooxygenase and lipoxygenase products of arachidonic acid (Brigham et al., 1986), inhibition of the eicosanoid response to injury may have a beneficial effect. However, it should be mentioned that at least part of the eicosanoid response may be homeostatic. Particularly prostaglandin E_2 and prostacyclin have some anti-inflammatory effects. Prostacyclin is also a potent pulmonary vasodilator, and infusion of prostaglandin E_2 can moderate the pathologic response to some interventions in experimental animals (Brigham et al., 1988). It is therefore possible that inhibition of production of all eicosanoids could have both beneficial and deleterious effects on the response.

Cells other than neutrophils and mediators other than eicosanoids may also participate in the pathogenesis of acute lung injury. For example, lymphocytes sequester in the lungs following endotoxin infusion in a sheep preparation (Meyrick and Brigham, 1983). In fact, the numbers of lymphocytes sequestering in the lung microcirculation in that model are similar to the numbers of neutrophils, and the lymphocytes appear activated by electron microscopy. In some models of lung injury, alveolar macrophages are activated to release substances that are chemotactic for neutrophils (Duke et al., 1989), and production of aggressive oxygen species by alveolar macrophages has been suggested as a mechanism of lung injury. Activated monocytes are also seen in ultrastructural studies of the sheep lung response to endotoxemia (Meyrick and Brigham, 1983). Tumor necrosis factor (TNF), a product of monocytes and macrophages, is released in response to bacterial endotoxin exposure, and it has been shown recently that infusion of TNF into animals can reproduce many of the pathophysiologic effects of endotoxin infusion (Johnson et al., 1988). Other cytokines, especially interleukin-2, a lymphocyte product, can alter lung function when administered exogenously (King et al., 1987). Corticosteroids may have a beneficial effect on acute lung injury by preventing the release of injurious cytokines (Rinehart et al., 1974).

III. Evidence of Efficacy of Corticosteroids in Animal and Organ Models

High doses of corticosteroids have been shown clearly to alter responses of the lungs to some injurious stimuli in laboratory preparations. We have studied the effects of steroids on the responses of the lungs to endotoxemia in chronically instrumented unanesthetized sheep (Brigham et al., 1981).

Infusion of gram-negative bacteria or their endotoxins into sheep causes a series of responses, many of which resemble ARDS (Brigham et al., 1983). If sufficient doses of endotoxin are given, the animals develop severe pulmonary edema and respiratory failure, a response pathophysiologically indistinguishable from ARDS in humans (Esbenshade et al., 1982).

If sheep are treated with high intravenous doses of methylprednisolone prior to infusing endotoxin, the response is attenuated (Begley et al., 1984). The increase in flow of protein-rich lung lymph, indicating increased lung microvascular permeability, which occurs several hours after endotoxin infusion, is diminished in steroid-treated animals (Fig. 2). Pretreatment with steroids also prevents sequestration of neutrophils in the lungs as assessed by light microscopy (Fig. 3).

However, even very high doses of corticosteroids do not completely prevent the endotoxin response. As shown in Figure 4, endotoxin-induced pulmonary hypertension still occurs in steroid-treated animals (Begley et al., 1984). Other studies indicated that the early-phase endotoxin-induced pulmonary hypertension is mediated by vasoconstrictor prostanoids, probably thromboxanes (Snapper and Brigham, 1985), and one would have expected that corticosteroids would prevent this effect. Some of the differences between the in vitro and in vivo effects of steroids are discussed in Section IV.

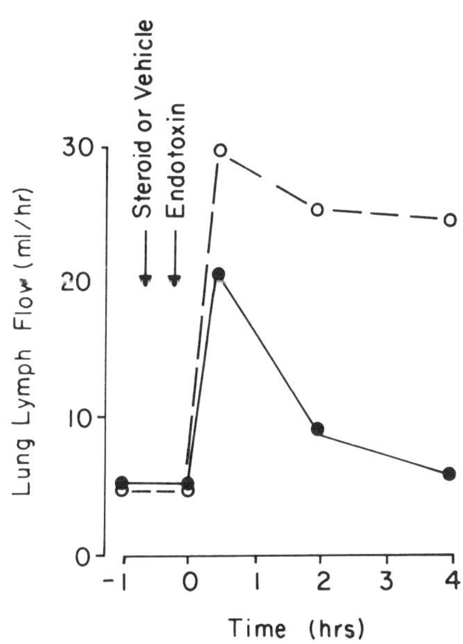

Figure 2 Lung lymph flow in sheep given endotoxin in the presence and absence of high doses of methylprednisolone. The late phase of high flow of protein-rich lung lymph indicative of increased microvascular permeability is attenuated in the steroid-treated animals: (O-O) vehicle; (●-●) steroid. (Redrawn and printed with permission from Begley et al., 1984.)

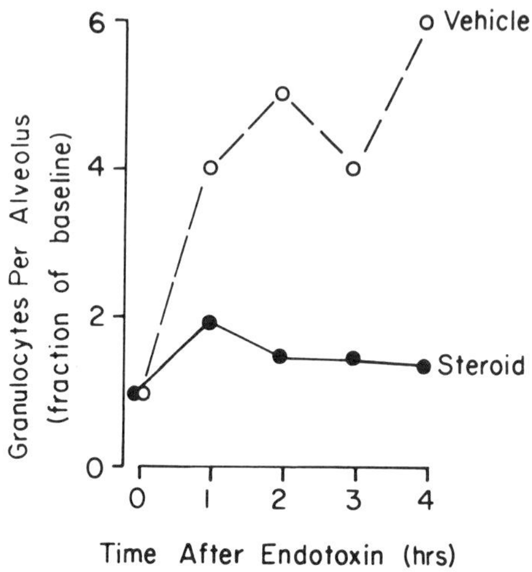

Figure 3 Numbers of neutrophils in light microscopic sections of lungs from sheep given endotoxin in the absence or presence of high doses of methyl prednisolone. Corticosteroids prevented the sequestration of neutrophils in the lungs following endotoxin infusion: (○-○) vehicle; (●-●) steroid. (Redrawn and printed with permission from Begley et al., 1984.)

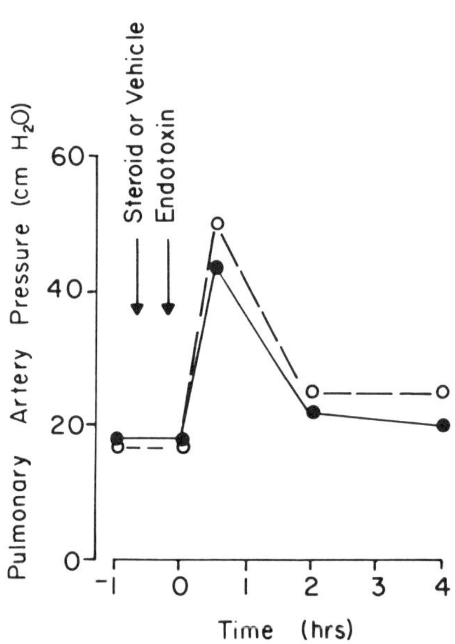

Figure 4 Effects of high doses of methyl prednisolone on the pulmonary artery pressure response to endotoxin infusion in unanesthetized sheep. Steroid therapy did not prevent the early pulmonary hypertension caused by endotoxin: (○-○) vehicle; (●-●) steroid. (Redrawn and printed with permission from Begley et al., 1984.)

High doses of corticosteroids do not prevent some forms of lung injury in animal models, even though the injury is associated with an acute inflammatory response. Unanesthetized sheep made to breathe pure oxygen for several days develop severe lung injury, increased vascular permeability, pulmonary edema, and respiratory failure (Newman et al., 1983). As shown in Figure 5, this oxygen-induced toxic response is associated with increased numbers of neutrophils in the lungs. Activation of inflammatory mechanisms is also indicated by the appearance of neutrophil chemotactic activity in lung lymph as the toxic response progresses.

However, treatment of the animals with high doses of corticosteroids does not prevent pulmonary oxygen toxicity (Newman et al., 1986). As shown in Figure 5, neutrophils still accumulated in the lungs of steroid-treated animals. Figure 6 illustrates the lung lymph response in animals breathing pure oxygen with and without steroid treatment. As illustrated in Figure 7, steroid treatment also did not affect the deterioration in gas exchange as oxygen toxicity developed. Pulmonary edema also occurred to an equal degree in animals whether or not they were treated with steroids (Fig. 8). It is not yet completely clear what role the inflammatory response plays in pulmonary oxygen toxicity. It is possible that the response is not important in the pathogenesis of the injury but is a response to direct oxidant injury. It is also possible

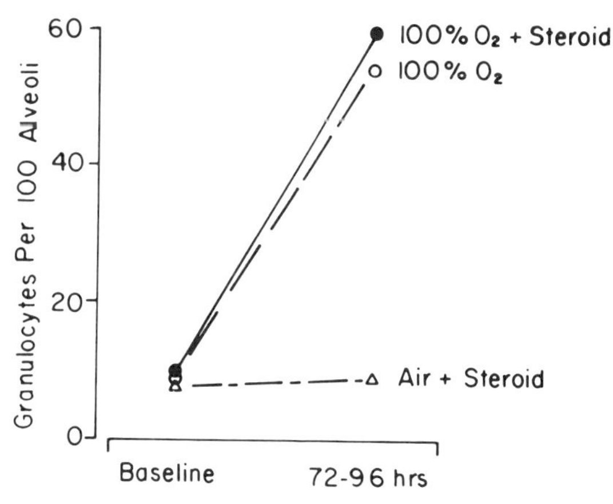

Figure 5 Numbers of neutrophils in light microscopic sections of lung tissue taken from sheep at baseline and after 72-96 hr of breathing pure oxygen with or without treatment with methylprednisolone. Neutrophils accumulate in the lungs with oxygen toxicity, and steroid treatment does not prevent this response. (Redrawn and printed with permission from Newman et al., 1986.)

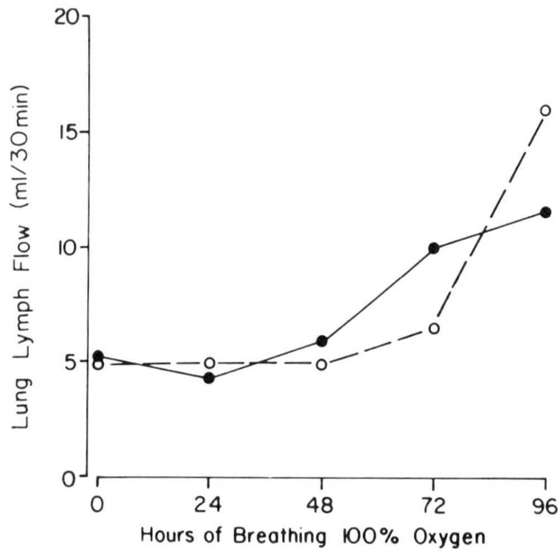

Figure 6 Lung lymph flow in sheep breathing pure oxygen with or without steroid treatment. Steroid treatment did not alter the large increase in lung lymph flow caused by oxygen toxicity: (○-○) oxygen alone; (●-●) oxygen plus steroid. (Redrawn and printed with permission from Newman et al., 1986.)

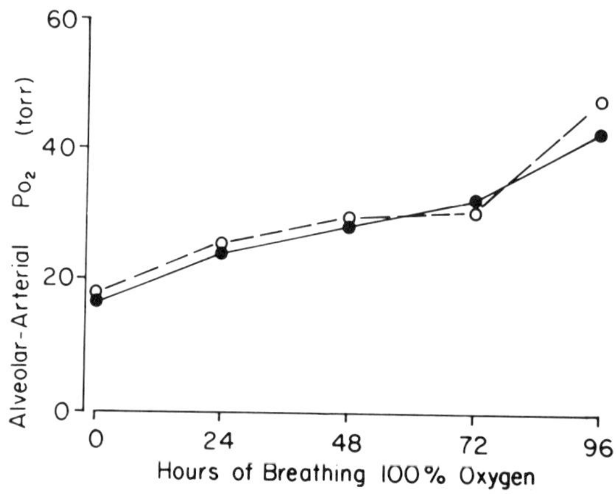

Figure 7 Alveolar to arterial oxygen partial pressure in sheep breathing pure oxygen with or without steroid treatment. Steroid treatment did not affect the deterioration of oxygenation as oxygen toxicity developed: (○-○) oxygen alone; (●-●) oxygen plus steroids. (Redrawn and printed with permission from Newman et al., 1986.)

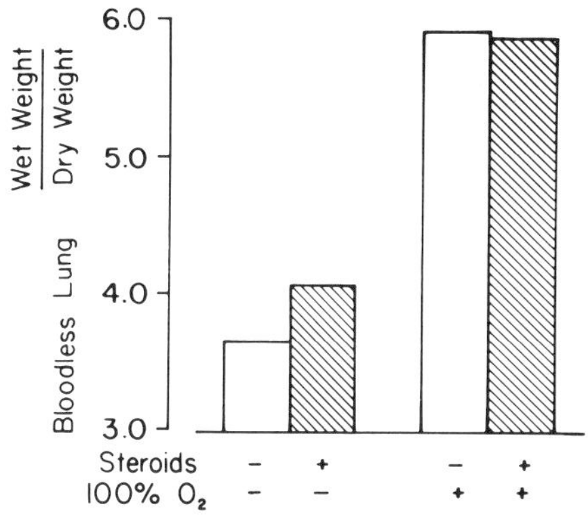

Figure 8 Postmortem wet-dry weight ratio of bloodless lungs from sheep breathing either air or pure oxygen for 72-96 hr with and without steroid therapy. Steroid treatment did not affect the development of pulmonary edema in oxygen-breathing animals. (Drawn from data from Newman et al., 1986, and printed with permission.)

that even high doses of corticosteroids do not adequately suppress the inflammatory response. This is discussed further in the next section.

IV. In Vitro Versus In Vivo Effects of Corticosteroids

Much of the rationale for the use of corticosteroids in acute lung injury is based on the implicit assumption that these agents have the same effects when administered to intact animals (including humans) as they have in preparations in vitro. This assumption is false. That in vitro and in vivo effects may be different should not be surprising in view of the complexity of responses in the whole animal.

For example, corticosteroids inhibit many neutrophil functions in vitro, but altered leukocyte trafficking in response to inflammatory stimuli may not necessarily be prevented even by very high doses of the drugs in intact animals. For example, peripheral blood leukocyte counts decrease dramatically in sheep over the course of the response to intravenous infusion of endotoxin, and treatment of the animals with corticosteroids does not prevent this response (Begley et al., 1984). Steroids did not prevent the disappearance of neutrophils from the blood, but the drugs did alter the leukocytes' destination. As shown in Figure 3, steroid-treated animals did not accumulate neutrophils in their lungs following endotoxemia (Begley et al., 1984). The leukocytes must have sequestered in other organs.

Table 2 Granulocyte Aggregation in Response to Zymosan-Activated Plasma

Granulocytes	Hank's	Normal plasma	Steroid plasma
Control	42 ± 4	42 ± 5	46 ± 5
Steroid	52 ± 2	49 ± 4	50 ± 5

Source: Reprinted with permission for Newman et al. (1986).

In humans with ARDS, high-dose corticosteroid treatment usually means 30 mg/kg of methyl prednisolone every 6 hr. This is a very high steroid dose compared to physiologic concentrations, and the dose is largely empirical. However, even this high dose of corticosteroids may not have the same effects on leukocyte function seen in preparations in vitro. Table 2 shows the aggregation response of neutrophils isolated from normal and steroid-treated sheep in the presence of plasma from normal and steroid-treated sheep. All the responses were identical (Newman et al., 1986). Table 3 shows similar values for phorbol ester-stimulated superoxide production by granulocytes from normal and steroid-treated sheep. Again, no differences could be detected (Newman et al., 1986). Steroid treatment of the animal did not affect neutrophil behavior, and plasma from steroid-treated sheep did not affect responses of neutrophils from either normal or steroid-treated animals. The in vitro and in vivo effects of steroids on neutrophil function may be very different.

Even pharmacologic doses of corticosteroids may not have the same effects on eicosanoid generation as predicted from in vitro studies (Lewis and Piper, 1975). We measured lung lymph concentrations of thromboxane and prostacyclin metabolites and concentrations of the lipoxygenase product, 12-hydroxyeicosatetraenoic acid (12-HETE) following endotoxin infusion into unanesthetized sheep with and without treatment with high doses of methylprednisolone given prior to endotoxin infusion (Ogletree et al., 1986).

Table 3 Superoxide Production by Sheep Granulocytes (nmol O_2^- per 10^6 cells)

Granulocytes	*n*	Hank's	Control plasma	Steroid plasma
Control	5	21.8 ± 3.4	2.3 ± 0.6	—
Steroid	6	29.2 ± 7.3	—	3.2 ± 0.5

Source: Reprinted with permission from Newman et al. (1986).

Figures 9 and 10 show the time course of lung lymph eicosanoid concentrations in the steroid-treated and control experiments. Steroid treatment diminished the release of prostacyclin metabolite into lung lymph and also, markedly, the release of 12-HETE after endotoxin infusion. However, substantial increases in thromboxane metabolite occurred after endotoxin infusion, even in the presence of high concentrations of corticosteroids. More specific cyclo-

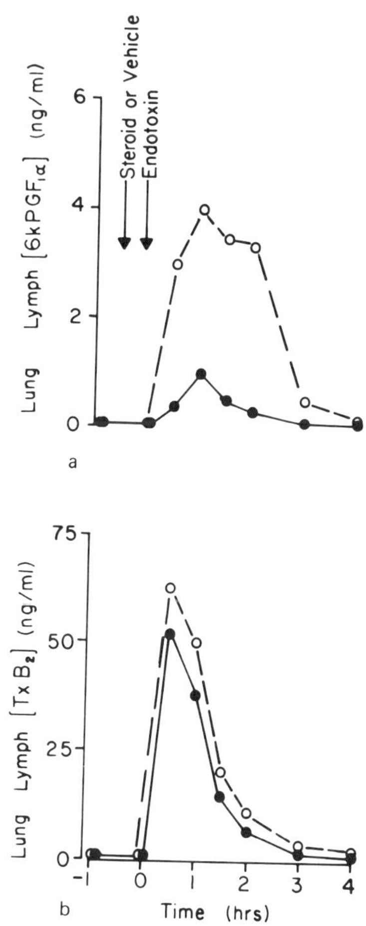

Figure 9 Lung lymph concentrations of prostacyclin and thromboxane metabolites over the course of the endotoxin response in sheep (a) with and (b) without steroid treatment. Steroid treatment largely prevented the increase in prostacyclin metabolite but reduced the thromboxane response only slightly: (○-○) vehicle; (●-●) steroid. (Redrawn and printed with permission from Ogletree et al., 1986.)

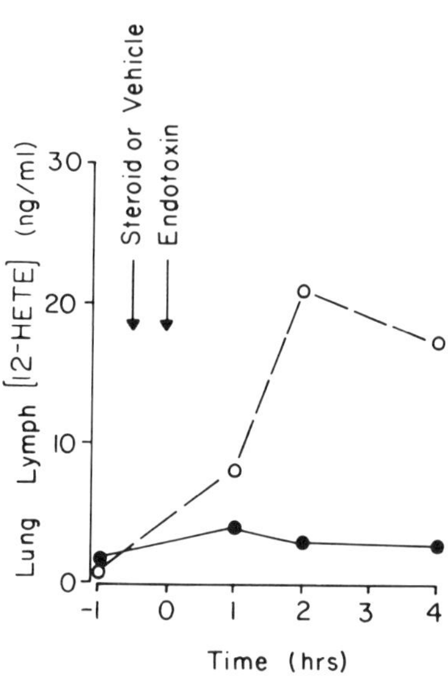

Figure 10 Lung lymph concentrations of the lipoxygenase product, 12-HETE, in sheep lung lymph over the course of the response to endotoxemia in animals with and without steroid treatment. Steroid treatment largely inhibited the increase in this lipoxygenase product in lung lymph: (○-○) vehicle; (●-●) steroid. (Redrawn and printed with permission from Ogletree et al., 1986.)

oxygenase inhibitors completely inhibit the increase in thromboxane as well as prostacyclin metabolite. The in vitro and in vivo effects of corticosteroids on eicosanoid generation may be different.

V. Clinical Trial of High-Dose Methylprednisolone in ARDS

Surprising as it may seem, in view of the widespread use of corticosteroids as treatment of ARDS over the past several years, no prospective, placebo-controlled clinical trial of efficacy was done until recently. There are at least two reasons for this. First, a firm bias that steroids were efficacious had developed in a sizable group of clinicians based on anecdotal experience. Second, because patients with ARDS are critically ill, usually in intensive care units, and have complex medical problems, some believed that it was not possible to conduct a meaningful clinical trial.

Despite these problems, a multicenter trial was conducted and reported recently (Bernard et al., 1987). The goal of the trial was to determine whether

Table 4 Criteria for Selection of Patients with ARDS

Illness associated with ARDS
Pa_{O_2} less than 70 torr on FI_{O_2} of at least 0.40 or Pa_{O_2}/Pa_{O_2} less than or equal to 0.3
Pulmonary edema on chest x-ray
Pulmonary artery wedge pressure 18 torr or less

high doses of methylprednisolone as commonly used clinically in the treatment of established ARDS altered either the eventual mortality or the course of the disease. Table 4 lists the selection criteria for entry of patients into the study. These criteria are those usually accepted for the clinical diagnosis of ARDS. Following entry into the study, patients were randomized into either steroid or placebo groups. Methylprednisolone (30 mg/kg) or placebo was administered intravenously every 6 hr for four doses, and patients were followed until recovery or death. Although no attempt was made to select specific clinical settings ("etiologies"), as has been true in most series, the largest etiologic subset of patients had sepsis either alone or in the presence of another risk factor.

Figure 11 shows cumulative survival in the steroid- and placebo-treated groups. Eventual overall mortality was similar to that reported in patient groups selected simiarly by others (Pepe et al., 1984). Corticosteroid treatment had no effect on either eventual mortality or mortality at any time point in the course of the disease.

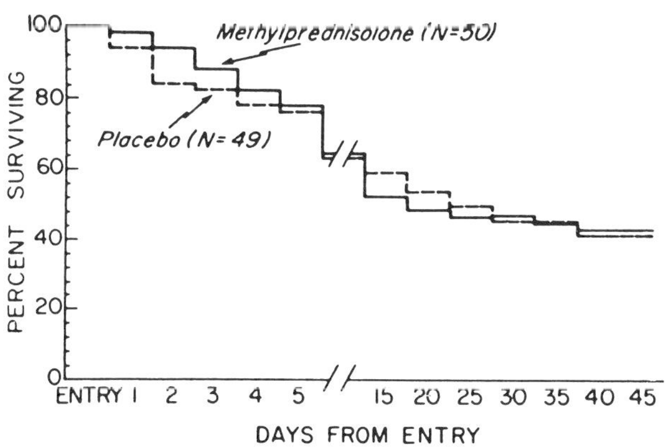

Figure 11 Percentage of patients with ARDS surviving as a function from time of entry into the study (first 45 days) for steroid-treated and untreated patients. The survival curves were virtually identical for the drug and placebo groups ($P = 0.77$). (Reprinted with permission from Bernard et al., 1987.)

Since patients with ARDS often have failure of organs other than the lungs, it is possible that mortality may not be altered even by an intervention that significantly reversed the lung injury. Figure 12 shows the fraction of patients reversing their respiratory failure over their clinical course. The steroid-treated patients were not different from the patients who received placebo.

In fact, no differences in steroid- and placebo-treated groups could be demonstrated in a long list of physiologic and biochemical measurements. Data for severity of pulmonary edema as assessed by chest radiograph, lung compliance, and oxygenation in the treated and untreated patients is shown in Figure 13. The length of stay in the medical intensive care unit was not different, either. There was absolutely no evidence for a favorable effect of high-dose corticosteroids in patients with this syndrome.

Could there be a subset of patients with ARDS who benefit from corticosteroid therapy? This is possible, although the data from a large multicenter study do not provide evidence to support this contention. The animal data described earlier provide good reason to expect that steroids should be beneficial in lung injury induced by sepsis. The largest etiologic subgroup of patients with ARDS in the multicenter study was sepsis. In this subgroup, there was no evidence for a beneficial steroid effect. Several etiologic subgroups were too small to allow any meaningful statement about steroid effects, and it remains possible that steroids would be beneficial in those patients. To determine whether this is the case would require additional similar clinical studies in which patients were selected for entry according to etiology.

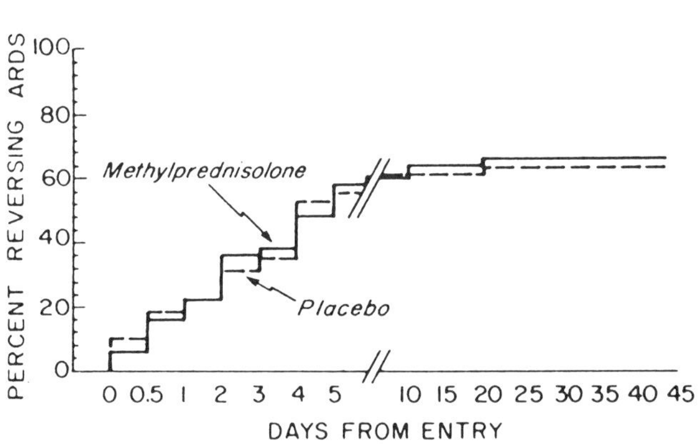

Figure 12 Percentage of patients with ARDS who reversed their respiratory failure as a function of time after entry into the study. Steroid- ($N = 50$) and placebo-treated ($N = 49$) are indistinguishable ($P = 0.74$). (Reprinted with permission from Bernard et al., 1987.)

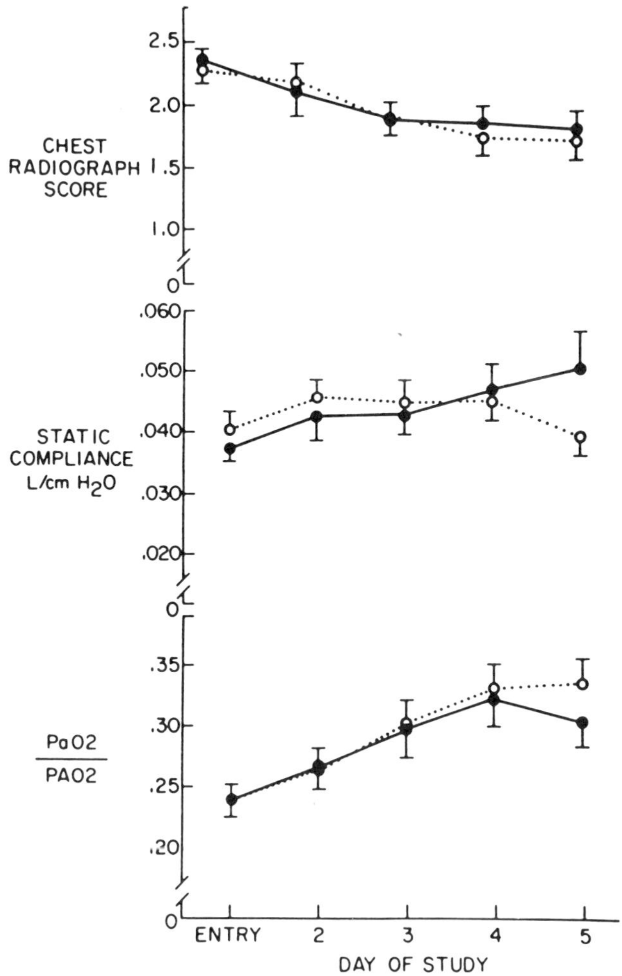

Figure 13 Chest radiograph score (0 = normal; 3 = severe pulmonary edema), lung compliance, and oxygenation in patients with ARDS over the first 5 days of their illness. There were no significant differences between steroid- (solid line, N = 50) and placebo-treated (dotted line, N = 49) groups. (Reprinted with permission from Bernard et al., 1987.)

Even the animal studies indicate that corticosteroids administered after lung injury has developed may not be beneficial. For example, the increase in vascular permeability after endotoxemia in sheep is not affected by steroid administration (Brigham et al., 1981).

Others have addressed this problem in patients by selecting a group of patients at risk for development of ARDS in which the subsequent incidence of the syndrome was predictably high (Weigfelt et al., 1985). These patients were studies in a double-blinded, placebo-controlled prospective fashion. They found no difference in incidence of ARDS between the placebo- and steroid-treated groups.

It should be noted that, in humans, it is rarely possible to treat patients before the initial insult. Even at-risk patients have already been exposed to the insult, and the question, unlike the animal studies in which true pretreatment can be done, is whether the course of the response to the insult can be altered if patients are treated early. The answer to this question, based on the cited studies, appears to be *no*. A drug that must be given to essentially healthy humans prior to exposure to insults that would place them at risk for ARDS would have limited usefulness and would have to entail little risk of undesirable effects.

VI. Summary and Conclusions

High doses of corticosteroids have been and, in some quarters still are, used liberally in treating patients with diffuse lung injury resulting in the adult respiratory distress syndrome. These drugs came into use in this setting because they are anti-inflammatory and diffuse lung injury is accompanied by inflammation in the lung periphery. The use of steroids in ARDS became rather widespread because of anecdotal impressions that they were beneficial.

There is a substantial experimental rational for using steroids in ARDS. Activated neutrophils appear to be important in the pathogenesis of ARDS, and high concentrations of corticosteroids inhibit some of the activation responses of these cells. Biologically active products of arachidonic acid (eicosanoids) also appear to mediate at least some of the pathophysiologic effects of ARDS, and in vitro, corticosteroids inhibit the generation of eicosanoids by inhibiting the liberation of free arachidonic acid through inhibition of phospholipase A_2. Lymphocytes and macrophages and their products may also participate in the pathogenesis of diffuse lung injury, and steroids can inhibit some of these responses in vitro.

In some animal models of diffuse lung injury, which are, though, analogous to the clinical syndrome of ARDS (especially gram-negative endotoxemia in sheep), high doses of corticosteroids given prior to the insult inhibit neutrophil sequestration in the lungs and inhibit the increase in lung microvascular permeability that is the basis of the pulmonary edema. However, corticosteroids do not appear to prevent pulmonary oxygen toxicity, even though this injury is also accompanied by a marked inflammatory response.

Some of the differences between the expected and the actual benefit of steroids in intact animals may derive from the fact that the in vivo effects of the drugs may differ from the in vitro effects. For example, steroids do not prevent endotoxin-induced neutropenia although the drugs may alter the sites of neutrophil sequestration. Usual clinical high doses of methylprednisolone given to sheep do not alter activation responses in neutrophils isolated from treated sheep, and the plasma from these animals does not affect the activation of neutrophils from either untreated or steroid-treated sheep. Even massive doses of corticosteroids do not prevent endotoxin-induced increases in the release of thromboxane although generation of other eicosanoids is inhibited.

A large prospective placebo-controlled double-blinded study of the efficacy of high doses of methylprednisolone in the treatment of established ARDS showed no effect of the drug. There was no effect on mortality, the course of the disease, time in the intensive care unit, or any other variable that could be measured. This study demonstrates that the routine use of steroids in the therapy of patients with established ARDS is not warranted. Further, in the largest etiologic subset of those patients, sepsis, there was no demonstrable benefit of steroid therapy. It remains possible that other etiologic subsets of these patients would benefit, but controlled studies will be necessary before that conclusion can be made.

A prospective study of effects of corticosteroids in patients at risk for developing ARDS also showed no benefit. The incidence of ARDS in these patients was similar whether or not they received steroids during the interval between the insult and the development of respiratory distress. It remains possible that the administration of high doses of corticosteroids to normal people prior to exposure to an insult that placed them at risk for ARDS would alter their response to the insult, but a study that would answer this question would be difficult to justify and even a positive conclusion would have very limited application.

A large number of studies related to the pathogenesis of diffuse lung injury are now in progress around the world. These studies have already identified several possible pharmacologic approaches to treatment of the syndrome, and clinical trials with some of these agents are underway. It is essential that, in each case, careful prospective clinical trials be conducted of sufficient size to arrive at a general conclusion about the efficacy of the drugs. It is now clear that such studies are feasible.

Acknowledgments

This work was supported by NIH, NHLBI Grant HL19153 (SCOR in Pulmonary Vascular Diseases), and grants from the John W. Cooke, Jr. and Laura W. Cooke Fund for Lung Research, the Hugh J. Morgan Fund for Cardiology donated by the Martha Washington Strauss-Harry H. Strauss Foundation, Inc., and the Bernard Werthan, Sr. Fund for Pulmonary Research. Dr. Brigham is Joe and Morris Werthan Professor of Investigative Medicine.

References

Ashbaugh, D. G., Bigelow, D. G., and Petty, T. L. (1967). Acute respiratory distress in adults. *Lancet,* **2**:319-323.

Begley, C. J., Ogletree, M. L., Meyrick, B. O., and Brigham, K. L. (1984). Modification of pulmonary responses to endotoxemia in awake sheep by steroidal and nonsteroidal anti-inflammatory agents. *Am. Rev. Respir. Dis.,* **130**(6):1140-1164.

Bernard, G. R., Harris, T., Luce, J. E., Rinaldo, J., Sibbald, W. J., Sprung, C., Tate, R. M., Higgins, S., Kariman, K., Bradley, R., and Brigham, K. L. (1987). High dose corticosteroids in patients with the adult respiratory distress syndrome: A randomized double-blind trial. *N. Engl. J. Med.,* **317**:1565-1570.

Brigham, K. L. (1986). Role of free radicals in lung injury. *Chest,* **89**(6): 859-863.

Brigham, K. L. (1987). Mechanisms of endothelial injury. In *Pulmonary Endothelium in Health and Disease*, Vol. 9. Edited by U. S. Ryan. New York, Marcel Dekker, pp. 207-236.

Brigham, K. L., Bowers, R. E., and McKeen, C. R. (1981). Methylprednisolone prevention of increased lung vascular permeability following endotoxemia in sheep. *J. Clin. Invest.,* **67**:1103-1110.

Brigham, K. L., Begley, C. J., Bernard, G. R., Hutchison, A. A., Loyd, J. E., Lucht, W. D., Meyrick, B., Newman, J. H., Niedermeyer, M. E., Ogletree, M. L., Sheller, J. R., and Snapper, J. R. (1983). Septicemia and lung injury. *Clin. Lab. Med.,* **3**(4):719-744.

Brigham, K. L., Meyrick, B., Bernard, G. R., Snapper, J. R., Berry, L. C., Tumen, J., and Hussein, A. (1986). Role of free radicals and metabolites of arachidonic acid in endotoxin induced pulmonary endothelial injury. In *Physiology of Oxygen Radicals.* Edited by A. E. Taylor, S. Matalon, and P. A. Ward. Baltimore, Waverly Press, pp. 199-206.

Brigham, K. L., Serafin, W., Zadoff, A., Blair, I., Meyrick, B., and Oates, J. (1988). Attenuation of lung vascular responses and eicosanoid release following endotoxemia in unanesthetized sheep by prostaglandin E_2. *J. Appl. Physiol.*, **64**:2568-2574.

Duke, S. S., Bolds, J. M., Loyd, J. E., and Brigham, K. L. (1989). Neutrophilic alveolitis and alveolar macrophage production of neutrophil chemotaxins following endotoxemia in unanesthetized sheep. *Am. J. Med. Sci.*, **296**(6):381-386.

Esbenshade, A. M., Newman, J. H., Lams, P. M., Jolles, H., and Brigham, K. L. (1982). Respiratory failure after endotoxin infusion in sheep: Lung mechanics and lung fluid balance. *J. Appl. Physiol.*, **53**(4):967-976.

Fantone, J., and Ward, P. (1982). Role of oxygen-derived free radicals and metabolites in leukocyte-dependent inflammatory reactions. *Am. J. Pathol.*, **107**:395-418.

Flick, M. R., Peru, A., and Staub, N. C. (1981). Leukocytes are required for increased lung microvascular permeability after microembolization in sheep. *Circ. Res.*, **48**:344-351.

Hammerschmidt, D. E., White, J. G., and Craddock, P. R. (1979). Corticosteroids inhibit complement-induced granulocyte aggregation. *J. Clin. Invest.*, **63**:798-803.

Heflin, A. C., and Brigham, K. L. (1981). Prevention by granulocyte depletion of increased lung vascular permeability of sheep lung following endotoxemia. *J. Clin. Invest.*, **68**:1253-1260.

Johnson, J. E., Meyrick, B., Jesmok, G., Wickersham, N., and Brigham, K. L. (1988). Infusion of recombinant human tumor necrosis factor alpha (rTNF) into sheep causes changes in pulmonary hemodynamics, pulmonary vascular permeability and leukocyte trafficking similar to those induced by endotoxin. *Am. Rev. Respir. Dis.*, **137**:391.

King, L. S., Kubo, K., Duke, S., Brigham, K. L., and Newman, J. H. (1987). Human recombinant interleukin 2 (IL2) infusion causes acute changes in lung vascular function in awake sheep. *Physiologist*, **30**:212.

Lewis, G. P., and Piper, P. J. (1975). Inhibition of release of prostaglandins as an explanation of some of the actions of anti-inflammatory steroids. *Nature*, **254**:308-311.

MacGregor, R. R., Spagnaolo, P. J., and Lentnek, A. L. (1974). Inhibition of granulocyte adherence by ethanol, prednisone and aspirin measured with an assay system. *N. Engl. J. Med.*, **29**:642-646.

Meyrick, B., and Brigham, K. L. (1983). Acute effects of *Escherichia coli* endotoxin on the pulmonary microcirculation of anesthetized sheep: Structure: function relationships. *Lab. Invest.*, **48**(4):458-470.

Nelson, D. H., and Ruhmann-Wennhold, A. (1978). Inhibition of leukocyte superoxide anion production by cortisol administration to normal subjects. *J. Clin. Endocrinol. Metab.*, **46**:702-706.

Newman, J. H., Loyd, J. E., English, D. K., Ogletree, M. L., Fulkerson, W. J., and Brigham, K. L. (1983). Effects of 100% oxygen on lung vascular function in awake sheep. *J. Appl. Physiol.*, **54**(5):1379-1386.

Newman, J. H., Fulkerson, W. J., Kobayashi, T., English, D., Meyrick, B., and Brigham, K. L. (1986). Effects of methylprednisolone on lung oxygen toxicity in awake sheep. *J. Appl. Physiol.,* **60**(4):1386-1392.

Ogletree, M. L., Begley, C. J., King, G. A., and Brigham, K. L. (1986). Influence of steroidal and non-steroidal anti-inflammatory agents on accumulation of arachidonic acid metabolites in plasma and lung lymph after endotoxemia in awake sheep: Measurements of prostacyclin and thromboxane metabolites and 12-HETE. *Am. Rev. Respir. Dis.,* **133**: 55-61.

Pepe, P. E., Hudson, L. D., and Carrico, L. J. (1984). Early application of positive end-expiratory pressure in patients at risk of the adult respiratory-distress syndrome. *N. Engl. J. Med.,* **311**:281-286.

Petty, T. L., and Ashbaugh, D. G. (1977). The adult respiratory distress syndrome: Clinical features influencing prognosis and principles of management. *Chest,* **60**:233-239.

Repine, J. E., Bowman, C. M., and Tate, R. M. (1982). Neutrophils and lung edema. State of the art. *Am. Rev. Respir. Dis.,* **81**:47s-50s.

Rinehart, J. J., Bolcerzak, S. P., Sagone, A. L., and LaBuglio, A. F. (1974). Effects of corticosteroids on human monocyte function. *J. Clin. Invest.,* **54**:1337-1352.

Snapper, J. R., and Brigham, K. L. (1985). Arachidonate products as mediators of diffuse lung injury. In *The Pulmonary Circulation and Acute Lung Injury.* Edited by S. I. Said. Mount Kisco, NY, Futura Publishing, pp. 321-336.

Weigfelt, J. A., Norcross, J. F., Borman, K. R., and Snyder, W. H., III (1985). Early steroid therapy for respiratory failure. *Arch. Surg.,* **120**: 536-540.

14

Proteases and Antiproteases in the Adult Respiratory Distress Syndrome

G. DEBY-DUPONT, M. LAMY, M. E. FAYMONVILLE, P. DAMAS, C. DEBY, and P. FRANCHIMONT

University of Liège
Liège, Belgium

A. ADAM

University of Montreal
Montreal, Quebec, Canada

I. Introduction

The adult respiratory distress syndrome (ARDS) was first described by Ashbaugh et al. in 1967 as acute respiratory failure clinically characterized by dyspnea, tachypnea, severe hypoxemia, decreased lung compliance, and widespread inhomogenous bilateral pulmonary infiltrates on chest x-ray (Pontoppidan et al., 1985; Brigham, 1982; Rinaldo and Rogers, 1982). Despite the continuous improvement in management of patients, ARDS still carries a 60% mortality rate (Fowler et al., 1985; Petty, 1985; Baumann et al., 1986; Hyers and Fowler, 1986; Rinaldo, 1986), increasing to above 90% in the presence of underlying diseases (Cox et al., 1985; Baumann et al., 1986), sepsis (Montgomery et al., 1985; Lancet, 1986) or other organ failure (Bell et al., 1983; Cerra, 1988). Direct lung injuries as well as indirect injuries can lead to the development of this syndrome (Petty and Ashbaugh, 1971; Fallat et al., 1980; Pepe et al., 1982; Fowler et al., 1983; Pontopiddan et al., 1985; Petty, 1985; Rinaldo, 1986), but independent of the variability of the risk factors, the central characteristic of the syndrome remains an increased permeability of the alveolar-capillary wall with edema and fluid accumulation in the interstitium and intra-alveolar spaces (Fein et al., 1979; Anderson et al., 1979; Holter et al., 1986). At first considered a lung disease per se, it now appears ARDS is a local expression of a systemic increase in permeability (Calandrino et al., 1988; Kreuzfelder et al., 1988). From this perspective, ARDS is the first manifestation of a general inflammatory reaction leading to multiple organ failure (Goris et al., 1985; Effros and Mason, 1986).

Numerous blood-borne mediators are believed to be essential factors for the development of ARDS (Bone, 1984; Hechtman et al., 1984; Simon and Ward, 1988), such as endotoxin (Brigham et al., 1979; Rinaldo et al., 1984), prostanoids, leukotrienes (Reines et al., 1982; Matthay et al., 1984; Brigham and Sherer, 1985; Slotman et al., 1985; Deby-Dupont et al., 1987), and mediators released by the activation of blood coagulation cascade (Schneider et al., 1980; Carvalho, 1985; Velsaco et al., 1986; Walshe et al., 1987) or complement cascade, which is a common phenomenon in numerous injuries (Hammerschmidt et al., 1980; Duchateau et al., 1984; Weinberg et al., 1984; Solomkin et al., 1985; Langlois and Gawryl, 1988). Excessive activation of alveolar macrophages may be responsible for the development of ARDS (Hocking and Golde, 1979; Brain, 1988; Johnston, 1988) after direct lung injury, although polymorphonuclear leukocytes (PMNs), particularly neutrophils, triggered by the activation of complement and sequestered in the lung, appear to play a major role in ARDS occurring after indirect lung injury. A clear demonstration of the essential role of the PMN has been furnished by both animal studies and observations in humans (Flick et al., 1979; Heflin and Brigham, 1981; Powe et al., 1982; Tahamont and Malik, 1983; Thommasen et al., 1984; Borg et al., 1985; Weiland et al., 1986; Worthen et al., 1987a; Simon and Ward, 1988).

In contrast, a key role of proteases in ARDS is rarely described, with the exception of granulocytic elastase. However, numerous proteases are produced in the complement and coagulation cascades and are released by stimulated macrophages and neutrophils as well as by other tissues and organs, particularly the liver and the pancreas. These enzymes possess major destructive potency for exceptionally long periods. They are normally regulated by specific antiproteases, but in critically ill patients proteases can be released in excess and antiproteases consumed in excess, leading to an imbalance between the proteases and their inhibitors.

II. Proteases Involved in ARDS

A. Classes and Mechanisms of Action

Proteases include all the enzymes that cleave the peptide bonds of protein chains: the term "protease" is thus used synonymously with endopeptidase (Barrett and McDonald, 1986). They act specifically on peptide bounds involving particular amino acids, and many proteases are synthesized in an inactive form, the proenzyme or zymogen that, when activated, releases the active enzyme capable of initiating new physiologic functions (Neurath and Walsh, 1976; Walsh and Wilcox, 1970).

Proteases can originate from different sources: plasma, blood cells, endothelial cells, and such organs as liver or pancreas. They are classified into four different families, the serine, the cysteine (or thiol), the aspartic (or acid), and the metalloproteases, according to the presence at the active site of the enzyme of either a specific amino acid (serine, cysteine, or aspartate) or a metal (such as zinc in collagenases).

Proteolytic activity is normally closely regulated to prevent inappropriate and uncontrolled degradation of proteins (Bond and Butler, 1987). Regulation is achieved by controlling the rate of synthesis and degradation of proteases, by the concentration of small ions or metabolites (such as Ca^{2+}) indispensable for enzymatic activity, by the availability of appropriate substrates, by compartmentalization in specialized environments, and by controlling the presence of activators or inhibitors.

B. Extracellular Proteases

These are present in plasma, intervene in the complement and coagulation-fibrinolysis cascades, and primarily belong to the group of serine proteases (Table 1).

Activation of the complement cascade is a well-known phenomenon in ARDS (Solomkin et al., 1985; Hammerschmidt et al., 1980; Duchateau et al., 1984; Weigelt et al., 1988; Langlois and Gawryl, 1988) and in many situations appears to predispose to ARDS (Chenoweth et al., 1981; Horn et al., 1982; Perez et al., 1983; Weinberg et al., 1984; Faymonville et al., 1987b).

The alternative pathway is usually involved; but at a later phase, the classic pathway can also be implicated by the binding of C1 to antibody-antigen complexes (Reid and Porter, 1981; Muller-Eberhard, 1988). C1 occurs in serum as a proenzyme that undergoes autoactivation (Ziccardi, 1982a) and is normally controlled by the serine C1 esterase inhibitor (C1-In) (Ziccardi, 1982b). Activated C1 is the first serine protease intervening in the classic pathway of complement activation. It catalyzes the formation of C3 convertase, another serine protease, from C2 and C4. C3 convertase generates the serine protease C5 convertase. The activity of the C3 and C5 convertases produces the potent anaphylatoxins C3a and C5a, which act upon granulocytes to promote their aggregation and sequestration in the pulmonary vasculature (Jacob and Hammerschmidt, 1982; Goldstein, 1988). The alternative pathway is a more spontaneously initiated mechanism and antibody independent and possesses a feedback amplification mechanism. Two particular serine proteases, factor D and activated B (Bb), intervene in this pathway.

Table 1 Extracellular Proteases[a]

Name	Class	Natural substrate	Role
Complement cascade			
Activated C1	Serine	C2 and C4	Classic pathway
C3 convertase	Serine	Arg-Ser bond of C3	Classic and alternative pathways
C5 convertase	Serine	Arg-Ser bond of C5	Classic and alternative pathways
Activated B	Serine	C3 and C5	Alternative pathway
Factor D	Serine	Arg-Lys bond of B	Alternative pathway
Coagulation-fibronolysis cascade			
Hageman factor (HFa)	Serine	Arg-Ile bond of XI	Coagulation cascade
		Prekallikrein	Coagulation cascade
		Plasminogen (?)	Fibrinolysis
		Complement factor C1 (?)	Complement cascade
Kallikrein	Serine	HF	Coagulation cascade
		HMWK	Bradykinin release
		Prorenin	Renin-angiotensin system
		Plasminogen (?)	Fibrinolysis
		Complement factor C5 (?)	Complement cascade
XIa	Serine	IX	Coagulation cascade
IXa	Serine	X	Coagulation cascade
Xa	Serine	Prothrombin	Coagulation cascade
Thrombin	Serine	Fibrinogen	Coagulation cascade
Plasmin	Serine	Fibrin	Fibrinolysis

[a]Data obtained in vitro only: ?.

D is the initial enzyme. It is always present in plasma in an active form and is not inhibited by serum protease inhibitors (Johnson et al., 1984). D cleaves protein B (producing Bb), but only when this latter protein is bound to C3b or hydrolyzed C3. When complexed with C3b, Bb forms the C3 convertase of the alternative pathway and is able to attack native C3 generating the C5 convertase of the alternative pathway.

In each of the two complement pathways there are two complex proteases, C3 convertase and C5 convertase, with equivalent specificity but a different composition. C3 occupies a central position: it is cleaved by two C3 convertases with the formation of C5 convertase and amplification of C3 convertase production, increasing the plasma level of serine proteases and leading to the formation of the membrane-attack complex (Langlois and Gawryl, 1988) and the production of potent mediators of inflammation (C3a, C5a, and others) (Goldstein, 1988). All the proteases involved in the cascade of complement activation have specific activity on appropriate substrates, such as protease D on the Arg-Lys bond of C3b-complexed protein B. When proteases are produced in excess, overloading their natural inhibitors, we cannot exclude unspecific or less specific activity at the level of Arg-Ser or Arg-Lys bonds in various plasma proteins.

The coagulation cascade starts with contact activation involving four proteins, Hageman factor (HF), prekallikrein, factor XI, and high-molecular-weight kininogen (HMWK) (Cochrane et al., 1973; Kozin and Cochrane, 1988). HF is autoactivated into activated HF (HFa) by contact with negatively charged surfaces, such as denuded vascular membranes, glycoproteins, glycosaminoglycans, or lipopolysaccharides (Wiggins et al., 1982).

HFa is a serine protease that is able to transform prekallikrein into kallikrein (Bouma et al., 1980) and activate coagulation factor XI. These two new serine proteases exert their proteolytic activity on several substrates; kallikrein cleaves HF (Cochrane et al., 1973) and HMWK, releasing bradykinin, a vasodilator peptide active in producing margination of leukocytes and increasing vascular permeability (Regali and Barabe, 1980). When disseminated in plasma, kallikrein activates prorenin in renin, triggering the renin-angiotensin system (Sealy et al., 1978), and seems able to act on plasminogen (Colman, 1969).

Factor XIa activates factor IX (Davie et al., 1979) into another serine protease, which acts on another coagulation factor. Thus the coagulation cascade produces a number of serine proteases, ending with the activation of prothrombin into thrombin acting on fibrinogen. HFa and kallikrein can also cleave plasminogen, releasing plasmin and activating fibrinolysis (Cochrane and Griffin, 1982, Kaplan et al., 1982) and exerting proteolytic activity in vitro on the complement factors C1 (Ghebrehiwet et al., 1981) and C5 (Wiggins et al., 1981). However, their activity on the complement cascade remains uncertain in vivo.

The presence of an excess of proteolytic enzymes in ARDS originating from the coagulation-fibrinolysis cascade is no longer hypothetical (Saldeen, 1983; Carvalho, 1985). Accumulation of platelets in lung vasculature, disseminated intravascular coagulation (Bone et al., 1976), and increased plasma concentration of fibrin or fibrinogen degradation products have been dem-

Table 2 Blood cell Proteases

Protease	Class	Natural substrate	Present in
Elastase	Serine	Elastin	PMN, macrophages
Neutral cathepsin G (chymotrypsinlike protease)	Serine	Glycoproteins, basic amino acid residues, collagen	PMN, macrophages
Collagenases	Metalloprotease	Collagen, proteoglycans, glycoproteins	PMN, eosinophils, macrophages-monocytes
Elastaselike protease	Metalloprotease	Elastin	Macrophages
Cathepsin A	Cysteine	Peptide bonds, near hydrophobic amino acid residues	PMN
Cathepsin D	Aspartic protease		PMN, eosinophils
Cathepsin E	Aspartic protease		PMN
Cathepsin F	Aspartic protease		PMN
Cathepsin L	Cysteine protease		Macrophages
Acid protease			PMN
Gelatinase	Metalloprotease	Gelatin, proteoglycan, glycoprotein	PMN
Plasminogen activator	Serine	Plasminogen	Neutrophils, macrophages
Chymase	Serine	Aromatic amino acid residues	Mast cells
Tryptase	Serine	Arg and Lys amino acid residues	Mast cells

onstrated in ARDS patients (Luterman et al., 1977; Haynes et al., 1980; Schneider et al., 1980; Saldeen, 1982) together with abnormal metabolites of fibrinolysis (Manwaring and Curreri, 1982).

C. Intracellular Proteases (Table 2)

Cellular proteolysis is a highly controlled complex process taking place in many cells. However, little is known about the physiologic substrates of cellular proteases, about their specificity, or about their regulatory processes (Bond and Butler, 1987). Many of the serine proteases are found in secretory granules, most of the cysteine proteases are present in the cytosol or lysosomes, the aspartic proteases are associated with secretory granules, membranes, or lysosomes, and the metalloproteases with endoplasmic reticulum, plasma membrane, mitochrondria, or cytosol. Most of the intracellular proteases are active only after degranulation and therefore play an extracellular role.

Proteases of Leukocytes

Polymorphonuclear leukocytes, particularly neutrophils, are implicated as mediators of tissue destruction in ARDS, and a major destructive role is also attributed to the excited oxygen species released during their respiratory burst (Fantone et al., 1982; Till et al., 1982; Cochrane et al., 1983b; Tate and Repine, 1983; Ayars et al., 1984; Klebanoff, 1988). Neutrophils also possess microbicidal peptides, proteins, proteases, and other enzymes and can release many other toxic agents: 50 toxins have already been identified in the neutrophil's armamentarium (Henson and Johnston, 1987; Weiss, 1989). The role of neutrophil proteolytic enzymes should be re-evaluated during ARDS, remembering that neither oxidants nor proteolytic enzymes alone can completely explain the role of neutrophils in this disease (Janoff et al., 1979). When the neutrophil is triggered, NADPH oxidase begins to generate and release toxic oxygen species. Simultaneously, granules fuse with the plasma membrane and discharge their contents into the phagocytic vacuole and the extracellular medium. The neutrophils use both the NADPH oxidase system and granule contents in a cooperative manner, and in the pathologic state of ARDS, normal tissues, especially lung endothelium (Warren et al., 1987; Worthen et al., 1987b), bear the brunt of the attack by activated cells.

The main proteases of neutrophils are located in the granules (azurophilic or specific) (Kane and Peters, 1975; Ohlsson et al., 1977), where they are present in an inactive form as a proenzyme or zymogen. The protease armamentarium of neutrophils consists essentially of two metalloproteases, collagenase and gelatinase (Murphy et al., 1977; Dewald et al., 1982; Weiss and Peppin, 1986), and two serine proteases, elastase and cathepsin G. Collagenase, elastase, and cathepsin G together represent about 7% of the dry weight of the PMN (Travis et al., 1978).

Collagenase and gelatinase are present in a latent inactive form, but experimental data suggest that oxidant and chlorinated species released by the activated neutrophils themselves release the protease from its proenzyme. Myeloperoxidase present in the azurophilic granules of neutrophils is largely responsible for proenzyme activation as previously proven for procollagenase; using H_2O_2 released during the activity of NADPH oxidase, myeloperoxidase generates hypochlorous acid and chlorinated species that release collagenase from its proenzyme (Weiss et al., 1985; Weiss and Peppin, 1986). The same kind of activation is hypothesized for progelatinase (Peppin and Weiss, 1986).

Collagenase and gelatinase are two metalloproteases acting on the basement membrane of endothelium in the course of PMN migration from the blood to extracellular tissues (Jaffé, 1988). Gelatinase acts on gelatin and on the connective tissues that form the extracellular matrix (Campbell et al., 1987). Collagenase specifically destroys collagen types I, II, and III (Gadek et al., 1980; Mainardi et al., 1980a; Hasty et al., 1986; Bieth, 1986; Campbell et al., 1987) but is also active on proteoglycans, glycoproteins (for example, fibronectin), and laminin, all constituents of the extracellular matrix of lung (Weiss and Peppin, 1986).

The best studied protease of neutrophils is elastase, which is present in azurophilic granules, perhaps in an inactive form (proelastase), and is activated in the same way as latent collagenase and gelatinase. Elastase is the specific protease of elastin but also attacks numerous other proteins, such as immunoglobulins, clotting factors, complement proteins, and even collagen and endothelial cells (Henson et al., 1988; Gadek et al., 1980; Clark et al., 1980). Elastase, free or bound to its specific inhbitor, α_1-protease inhibitor (α_1PI), has been measured in high concentration in plasma and bronchoalveolar lavage fluid from ARDS patients, particularly when sepsis occurs (Zheutlin et al., 1986; Wewers et al., 1988).

In a group of seven multiply injured posttrauma patients (Table 3), the plasma concentrations of elastase were measured from the first hour after

Table 3 Injury Severity Score (ISS), Evolution, and Outcome of Seven Multiply Injured Posttrauma Patients Studied from Arrival (Within 1 hr) at the Intensive Care Unit

Patients: sex (age)	ISS	ARDS (on day)	Sepsis (on day)	Survival
M (38)	70	+ (3)	+ (5)	+
F (34)	34	+ (6)	−	+
M (19)	61	+ (6)	+ (6)	+
M (61)	50	+ (7)	+ (8)	+
M (21)	50	+ (5)	+ (5)	+
M (25)	42	−	+ (1)	+
M (47)	25	+ (1)	+ (5)	+
7 (35 ± 15)	47 ± 15	6	6	7

trauma (Fig. 1). All the patients were at risk of ARDS, with a high value of the injury severity score (ISS) of Baker et al. (1974). Of these patients, six developed septic complications. Elastase values were elevated in plasma from the first hour after trauma and remained elevated for several days. A complete return to normal had not occurred 10 days after trauma. High plasma levels of elastase complexed with α_1PI can be due either to a high blood leukocyte concentration or continuous degranulation of PMNs or to abnormal persistance of α_1PI-elastase complexes in the blood (the normal half-life does not exceed 10 min to 1 hr) (Padrines et al., 1989). Elastase normally acts locally in the direct environment of the neutrophil, perhaps facilitating the diapedesis of cells through the endothelium, but in ARDS excessive elastase

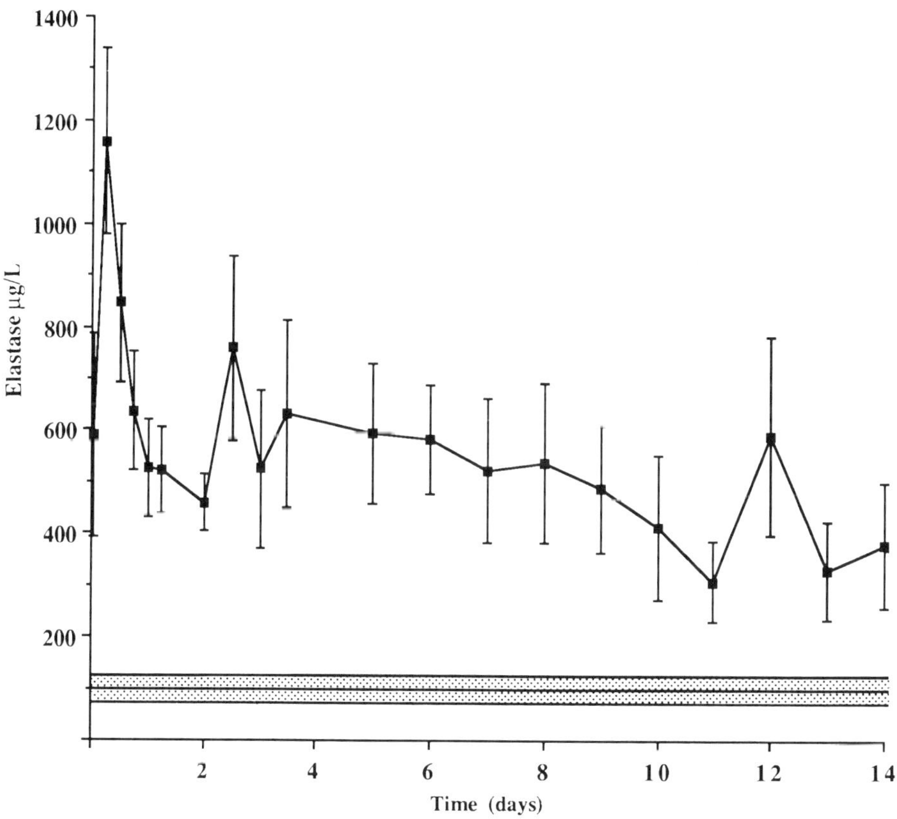

Figure 1 Sequential alterations of plasma granulocytic elastase in multiply injured posttrauma patients (n = 7; mean value ± SEM). Mean normal value ± SD shown by dotted area.

release together with oxidative inactivation of α_1PI (see later) can lead to uncontrolled proteolysis (Weiss, 1989). In recent studies, elastase is sometimes presented as a marker of complications, especially sepsis, and has prognostic value in multiple organ system failure (Duswald et al., 1985; Nuytinck et al., 1986). Among the host of additional enzymes secreted by PMNs are cathepsin G, a chymotrypsinlike serine proteinase present in azurophilic granules that is active at neutral pH on basic amino acid residues (Olsson and Venge, 1974; Feinstein and Janoff, 1975; Kane and Peters, 1975; Ohlsson et al., 1977) and depolymerizes collagen (Postlethwaite and Kang, 1988), an acid protease (Kane and Peters, 1975), a plasminogen activator (Granelli-Peperno et al., 1977), several lysosomal cysteine proteases, and the cathepsins active at acidic pH, cathepsins D (Ishikawa and Cimason, 1977), A, E, and F (which have been detected in rabbit neutrophils but not in human cells) (Henson et al., 1988). These cysteine proteases are true intracellular proteases causing proteolysis of proteins already fragmented by more specific proteases. Excessive activation of neutrophils may release the latter enzymes from the cell, producing local destructive activity, for example of endothelial cells.

Other Blood Cell Proteases

Monocytes and macrophages also produce and release proteases during phagocytosis (Adams and Hamilton, 1984; Henson et al., 1988), but the protease profile of macrophages differs from that of circulating monocytes. Macrophages secrete collagenases specific for types I, II, III, and IV collagen (Wahl et al., 1974; Mainardi et al., 1980b; Werb et al., 1980; Werb and Gordon 1984a; Welgus et al., 1985; Campbell et al., 1987; Senior et al., 1989) and gelatinase (Hibbs et al., 1987), all of which are inhibited by the tissue inhibitor of metalloproteases (see later). Cultured human macrophages also secrete an elastase metalloprotease that acts on elastin and is inhibited by α_1PI (Werb and Gordon, 1984b; Senior et al., 1989). Metalloprotease activity has been found in bronchoalveolar lavage fluid (Niederman et al., 1984). macrophages contain another elastase of the serpin family similar to the neutrophil elastase, but this protease can either be a product of macrophage synthesis or a neutrophil elastase internalized by receptor-mediated endocytosis (White et al., 1982; Campbell et al., 1987). Cathepsin L, a cysteine protease working at acidic pH, is also present in macrophages, together with a plasminogen activator involved in thrombolysis and especially present in alveolar macrophages (Unkeless et al., 1974; Chapman et al., 1984).

The protease production of other blood cells is less well studied. Eosinophils are equipped with a collagenase (Hibbs et al., 1982) and cathepsins (Archer and Hirsch, 1963; Henson et al., 1988). Human basophils produce a kallikreinlike endopeptidase acting on kininogen to generate bradykinin (Newball et al., 1979; Siraganian, 1988).

Nonblood Cell Proteases

Recent studies demonstrate that nonblood cells, such as fibroblasts (Postlethwaite and Kang, 1988) and endothelial cells (Crutchley, 1987; Jaffé, 1988; Ryan, 1987), also contain proteases. Stimulated endothelial cells can release a collagenase able to digest collagens of types I, II, III, and V and the type IV collagen of basement membrane (Moscatelli et al., 1980). Endothelial cells are attached to basement membranes containing glycosaminoglycans, elastin, laminin, and collagen. They can thus exert both normal and excessive destructive activity on these proteins (Kalebic et al., 1983). They can also secrete a protease called protein C, which inactivates factor Va and factor VIIIa by proteolysis (and should thus be considered to act as a serine protease inhibitor) (Esmon, 1983), and possess fibrinolytic activity by producing a tissue plasminogen activator (Gross et al., 1982). Fibroblasts, which synthesize connective tissue matrix, produce collagenases active at neutral pH in the presence of Ca^{2+} and Zn^{2+} ions (Postlethwaite and Kang, 1988). Mast cells (Siraganian, 1988) and lung tissues secrete tryptase (a trypsinlike protease) (Tanaka et al., 1983; Smith et al., 1984), a neutral protease present in secretory granules, and two chymotrypsinlike enzymes, chymases I and II. These two serine proteases have been found in rat mast cells from connective or mucosal tissues, but their presence in human mast cells remains uncertain.

During ARDS, when endothelial cells or fibroblasts are injured, their normal role in the controlled destruction of connective tissue may be accentuated, with the inappropriate excessive release of proteases, particularly collagenase, enhancing lung tissue destruction and edema.

Proteases from Other Organs

ARDS appears to be a particular expression of a systemic increase in permeability, and pulmonary edema is the initial manifestation of general capillary injury occurring throughout the body, especially after multiple injuries with hypovolemic shock (Fleck et al., 1985; Calandrino et al., 1988; Kreuzfelder et al., 1988). Hypoperfusion and reperfusion contribute to this systemic increase in permeability (McCord, 1987). Acute pulmonary failure is thus the first manifestation of a generalized body reaction in which other organs, such as the brain, heart, kidneys, liver, gut, and pancreas, are involved, leading to multiple organ system failure (MOSF). Ischemia and hypoxia alter the gut mucosa (Border et al., 1986; Deitch, 1988; Machiedo, 1989) owing to the toxicity of excited forms of oxygen (Roy and McCord, 1982; McCord, 1987), and leading to mucosal disruption that allows access to the systemic blood circulation by active digestive enzymes, such as the serine proteases trypsin and chymotrypsin (Diamond, 1978; Liebow and Rothman, 1975).

Liver failure, largely in relation to gut mucosal alterations (Matuschak and Rinaldo, 1988), consists of a reduction in normal Kupffer's cell function and reduced hepatic protein synthesis, possibly leading to a decreased clearance of protease-antiprotease complexes and decreased production of important antiproteases, such as α_2-macroglobulin (α_2M). Dying liver cells can release their protease contents, particularly cathepsins B, H, and L. An additional organ rich in mitochondria and susceptible to hypoxemia or ischemia (Göber, 1975; Warshaw and O'Hara, 1978; Jones et al., 1975, 1979; Jones and Dawson, 1979; Gmaz-Nikulin et al., 1981; Jones and Linhardt, 1982; Hegewald et al., 1985) is the pancreas, which is rich in potent proteases. In papers dealing with ARDS and MOSF, the pancreas is rarely mentioned, despite the early observation of hyperamylasemia both after surgery (Horton et al., 1968; Johnson and Nasbeth, 1970; Panebianco et al., 1970; Penn et al., 1970; Tilney et al., 1973; Traverso et al., 1977; Becker and Stollhoff, 1975; Morrissey et al., 1980) and in critically ill patients (Weaver et al., 1985).

In 1984 we measured the presence of large amounts of immunoreactive trypsin (IRT) circulating in plasma during ARDS and sepsis (Deby-Dupont et al., 1984). These results were confirmed by Nicod et al. in 1985 and by our subsequent reports (Lamy et al., 1985, 1987, 1988a, b; Faymonville et al., 1987a; Deby-Dupont et al., 1988a). Figures 2 and 3 present the individual plasma values of IRT measured in 52 patients divided into two groups (Table 4): a group of 31 severe polytrauma patients (22 men and 9 women; mean age $\pm$ SD, 39 $\pm$ 18 years) and a group of 21 patients (16 men and 5 women; mean age $\pm$ SD, 58 $\pm$ 15 years) with peritonitis or abdominal complications following gastrointestinal tract or abdominal aortic surgery. The incidence of ARDS was estimated using the scoring system of Morel et al. (1985), which is also quite similar to the scoring system of Murray et al. (1988). The criteria for septic complications were a need for mechanical ventilation, a body temperature above 38 °C, a blood leukocyte count above 12 $\times$ 10^9 cells per liter or below 5 $\times$ 10^9 cells per liter, a platelet level below 100 $\times$ 10^9 per liter, and a positive blood culture or an evident focus of infection (Montgomery et al., 1985). The maximal individual values of IRT were measured when ARDS was present (Fig. 2) or when septic complications occurred (Fig. 3). Large abnormal values of IRT (mean normal value $\pm$ SD 32 $\pm$ 12 μg/liter) were measured in most of the multiply injured posttrauma patients and in all the patients with peritonitis or abdominal complications after surgery. Extraordinarily high values (2300 and 4000 μg/liter) were recorded in these patients. A statistically significant difference appeared between ARDS and non-ARDS patients in the peritonitis and abdominal complications group

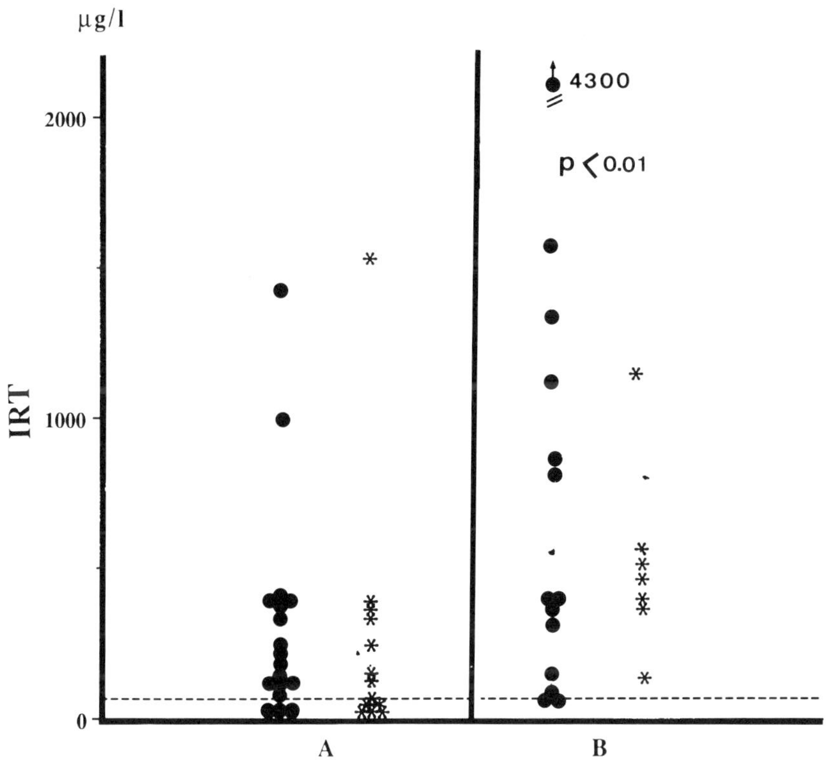

Figure 2 Maximal individual values of plasma-immunoreactive trypsin (IRT) in critically ill patients in association with ARDS. Blood sample was drawn at onset of ARDS (●) or 2-6 days after initial injury in non ARDS patients (*): (A) multiply injured posttrauma patients ($n = 31$); (B) patients with peritonitis or complications after abdominal surgery ($n = 21$). Mean normal value shown by dashed line.

(Fig. 2) and between septic and nonseptic patients in the multiply injured group (Fig. 3).

In 24 of our patients, each with a septic complication (12 multiply injured posttrauma patients and 12 peritonitis or abdominal complications patients), we also measured the level of enzymatically active trypsin (EAT) using a specific substrate for free trypsin or trypsin bound to α_2M (Fig. 4). Abnormal values (mean normal value ± SD, 284 ± 100 μg/liter) were measured in all these patients, and values of EAT above 5000 μg/liter were observed in 2 mulitply injured posttrauma patients and 7 peritonitis and abdominal complications patients with ARDS. These 2 patients died 48-72 hr later. Increased values of α-amylase and lipase were also commonly measured

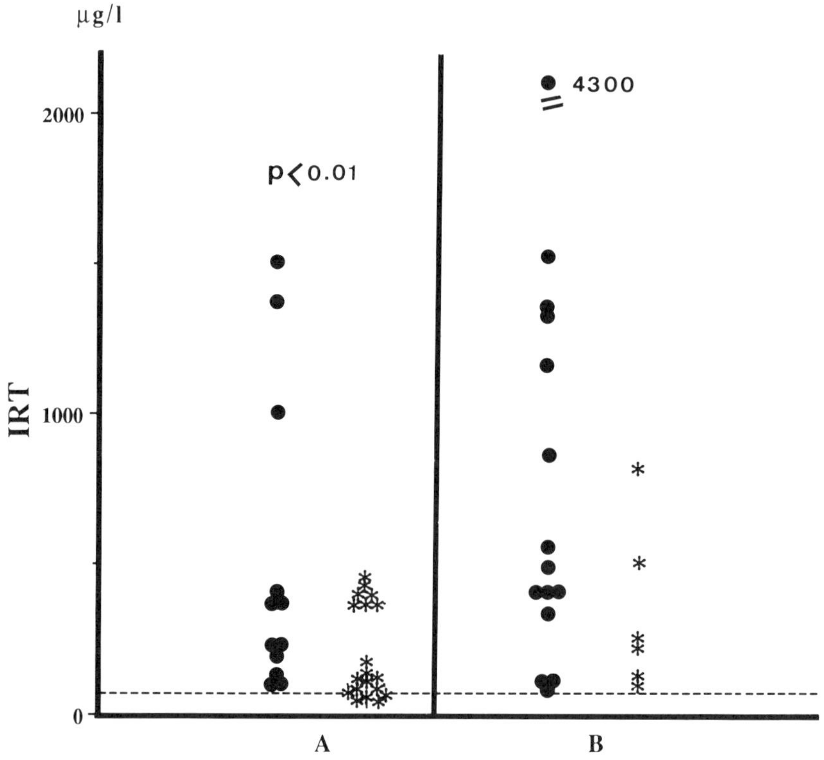

Figure 3 Maximal individual values of plasma-immunoreactive trypsin (IRT) in critically ill patients in association with sepsis. Blood sample was drawn when sepsis was present (●) or 2-6 days after initial injury in patients without sepsis (∗): (A) multiply injured posttrauma patients (n = 31); (B) patients with peritonitis or complications after abdominal surgery (n = 21). Mean normal value shown by dashed line.

Table 4 Distribution and Evolution of 52 Critically Ill Patients at Risk of ARDS

Pathology	n	ARDS	Septic complications	Death
Multiple injuries	31	18	18	8
Peritonitis or abdominal complications	21	13	15	14
	52	31	33	22
		59.6%	63.5%	42.3%

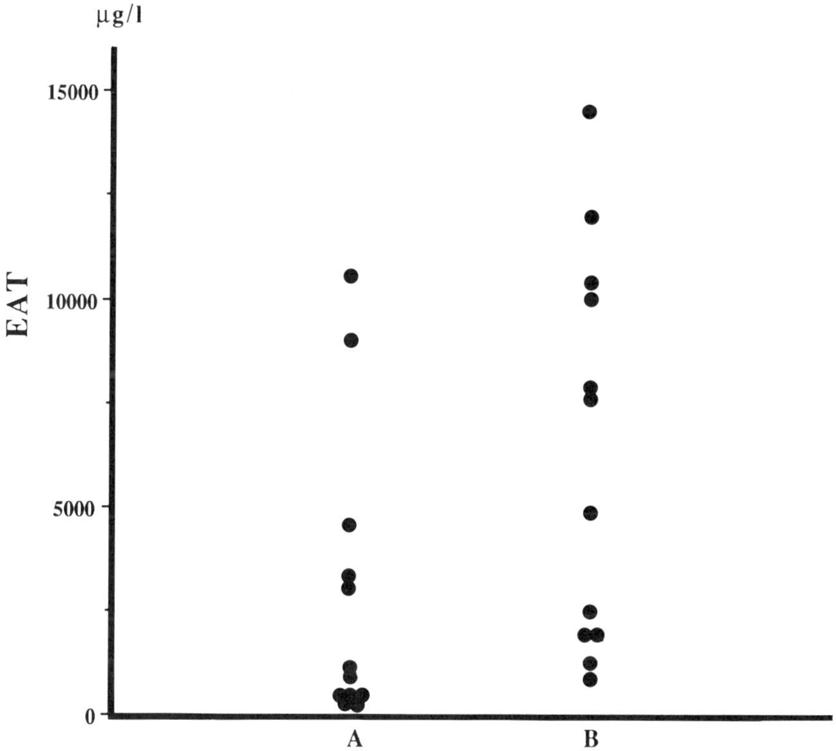

Figure 4 Maximal individual value of enzymatically active trypsin (EAT) in the plasma of septic patients ($n = 24$): (A) multiply injured posttrauma patients ($n = 12$); (B) patients with peritonitis or complications after abdominal surgery ($n = 12$). Mean normal value ± SD: 284 ± 100 μg/liter.

in blood when trypsin levels were increased (Lamy et al., 1987, 1988a; Deby-Dupont et al., 1988).

This major circulatory increase in pancreatic enzymes in association with ARDS and sepsis occurred 5-7 days after injury, but initial release (with values significantly above the mean normal value of 32 ± 12 μg/liter) was observed in the first 24 hr after injury, as shown in Figure 5 for seven multiply injured posttrauma patients (Table 3). The biphasic release of IRT is evident, the second release of trypsin beginning on day 5 and reaching a persistently high value. This increase in pancreatic enzymes in circulating blood suggests a diagnosis of acute pancreatitis; however, in our patients, this diagnosis was never established (by clinical signs, echography, or computed tomographic, CT, scan). It therefore seems reasonable to consider increased pan-

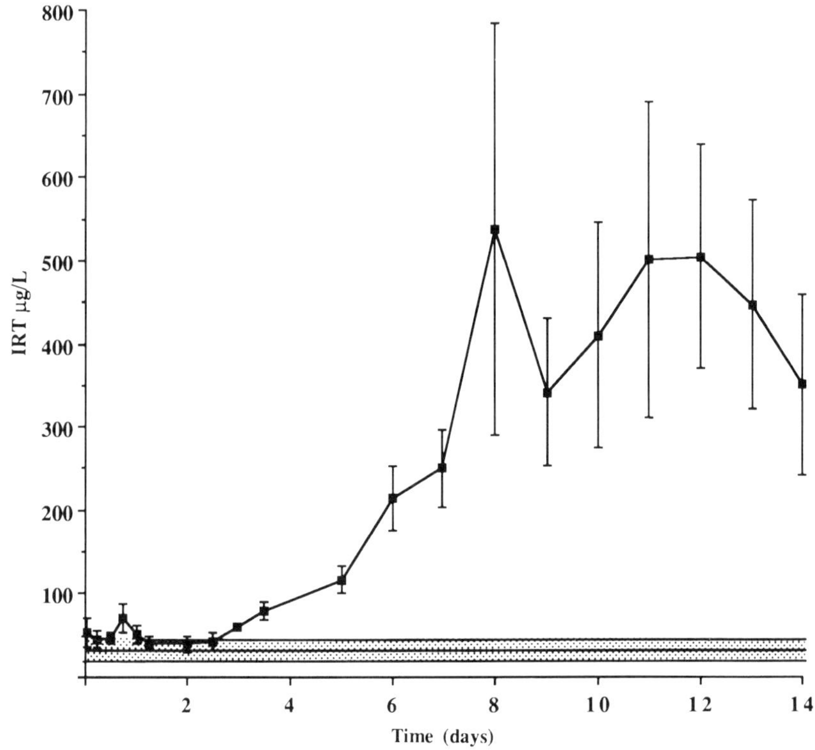

Figure 5 Sequence of plasma immunoreactive trypsin (IRT) levels in multiply injured posttrauma patients ($n = 7$; mean value ± SEM). Mean normal value ± SD shown by dotted area.

creatic enzyme permeability (a pancreatic failure) in patients with ARDS and sepsis after trauma, peritonitis, or abdominal surgery. Like the lungs, kidneys, liver, heart, and brain, the pancreas is also involved in MOSF, and the modest early pancreatic failure observed in some patients may contribute to developing ARDS and/or sepsis. The main consequence of pancreatic failure is the release into blood of numerous toxic factors and enzymes, especially the serine proteases, trypsin, chymotrypsin, elastase, kallikrein, and the metalloprotease collagenase, together with other potent enzymes, such as phospholipase (Nevalainen, 1980). A most potent enzyme is trypsin, which can activate all the other proenzymes (Ohlsson et al., 1982), inducing protein destruction (Tahamont et al., 1982) and triggering the kinin system, the coagulation cascade (Kwaan et al., 1971; Satake et al., 1973; Lasson and Ohlsson, 1986), and the complement cascade (Minta et al., 1977; Lasson and Ohlsson,

1982), with subsequent activation of polymorphonuclear leukocytes and further release of proteases causing consumption of plasma antiproteases.

III. Regulation of Protease Activity: Role of Antiproteases

Proteolytic activity needs to be highly regulated to prevent inappropriate and uncontrolled degradation of proteins. When elastase remains free, it exposes the fibrinogen receptors of platelets, causing spontaneous platelet aggregation in the presence of fibrinogen (Kornecki et al., 1986). Excessive protease activity leads to the destruction of extracellular matrix with the production of peptides that are chemotactic for inflammatory cells (Senior et al., 1980; Laskin et al., 1986). Regulation can be affected in many ways (Bond and Butler, 1987). In cells, compartmentalization largely contributes to regulation, particularly for cathepsins localized in lysosomes with an inhibitory acidic environment. When cathepsins are released into cytosol, they are quickly degraded at the high pH. Synthesis and degradation of proteases also regulate their activity in cells and in plasma, but little is known about this. The concentration of some ions (Ca^{2+}, for example) may affect protease activity as well as the availability of appropriate substrates and the presence of "abnormal" or oxidized proteins, which are degraded more rapidly than normal proteins.

An important mode of regulation of protease activity is protease inhibitors. They are numerous, localized in plasma as well as cells, and released by injured tissues and activated cells (PMNL and MN) that are recruited to the locus of inflammation. They protect tissues and cells by inactivating proteases in plasma or extravascular spaces, limiting the intravascular passage of these enzymes. Antiproteases regulate major metabolic functions—coagulation, fibrinolysis, and the complement pathway—that have been linked to the systemic inflammatory reaction observed in ARDS patients.

The antiproteases are divided into four major groups: inhibitors of serine proteases, inhibitors of thiol proteases, inhibitors of metalloproteases, and a specialized group of α-macroglobulins represented in humans by α_2-macroglobulin (Table 5).

A. Inhibitors of Serine Proteases

These form the so-called serpin family (from serine protease inhibitors) and contain α_1PI, α_1-antichymotrypsin, antithrombin III (ATIII), α_2-antiplasmin, and C1 esterase inhibitor (C1In).

The major member of the serpin group is α_1PI, a 53,000 dalton glycoprotein with genetic polymorphism (Musiani et al., 1976; Pannell et al., 1984;

Table 5 Protease Inhibitors

Name	Acts on	Specific for	Present in
α_1PI	Serine protease	Elastase	Plasma (> liver) macrophages
α_1-Antichymotrypsin	Serine protease	Chymotrypsin, cathepsin G, chymase	Plasma (> liver) macrophages
ATIII	Serine protease	Thrombin, factor XIa, HFa, kallikrein (?)	Plasma (> liver)
C1In	Serine protease	C1 esterase, HF, kallikrein	Plasma
C3INA	Serine protease	C3 convertase (classic or alternative pathway)	Plasma
α_2-Antiplasmin	Serine protease	Plasmin	Platelets
IαI	Serine protease	Trypsin	Plasma, cells
PSTI	Serine protease	Trypsin	Pancreas, plasma
Bronchial leukocyte proteinase inhibitor	Serine protease	Elastase, cathepsin G	Bronchial mucus
α_2-Cysteine inhibitor	Cysteine protease	Cathepsins B, H, L	Plasma
α_1-Cysteine protease inhibitor	Cysteine protease	Cathepsins	Plasma
α_1-TPI	Cysteine protease		
Cystatins	Cysteine protease		
HMWK, LMWK	Cysteine protease	Cathepsins	Plasma
TIMP	Metalloprotease	Collagenase	Plasma, macrophages, fibroblasts
Collagenase inhibitor (=TIMP?)	Metalloprotease	Collagenase	Endothelial cells
Plasminogen activator inhibitor	Serine protease	Plasminogen activator	Macrophages, endothelial cells
Protein C	Serine protease	Factors Va, VIIIa	Endothelial cells
Protease nexin	Serine protease	Thrombin	Endothelial cells
α_2M	Serine protease	Trypsin, elastase, chymotrypsin,	Plasma (> liver), fibroblasts
	Cysteine protease	Kallikrein, collagenase	Macrophages
	Metalloprotease	Thrombin, HF	

Carrell et al., 1982). α_1PI was first recognized as an inhibitor of trypsin and named α_1-antitrypsin (Travis and Johnson, 1981; Travis and Salvesen, 1983). It now appears to be a fast-acting inhibitor of neutrophil elastase. The normal plasma value of α_1PI ranges from 1.9 to 3.5 g/liter, with a mean value of 2.6 g/liter. It is an acute-phase protein synthesized in the liver, beginning to increase 48 hr after injury or infection and continuing its increase for 5-6 days (Colley et al., 1983; Risberg et al., 1986; Stahl, 1987; Lamy et al., 1988a, b), sometimes rising to over 7 g/liter in ARDS patients. α_1PI synthesis by cultured macrophages has also been reported (Adams and Hamilton, 1984).

The binding of elastase to α_1PI cleaves this inhibitor at the level of a methionyl residue in the active center, releasing a peptide (Travis et al., 1978; Johnson and Travis, 1978). It should be noted that α_1PI is a temporary protease inhibitor: the enzyme slowly escapes from the complex, forming inactive α_1PI with a molecular weight of 49,000 (Padrines et al., 1989); the half-life of the complex is about 4 days. The active released enzyme is quickly trapped by α_2M, and the complex is eliminated by the reticuloendothelial system. Besides its inhibitory activity against elastase, native α_1PI possesses the ability to inhibit a wide range of proteolytic enzymes, collagenase, trypsin, plasmin, thrombin, and coagulation factor XI (Scott et al., 1982b), but the reaction rate of α_1PI with these proteases is much slower than with elastase.

As a fast-acting inhibitor of neutrophil elastase, α_1PI normally affords an efficient barrier against this enzyme, particularly in the lower respiratory tract (Bieth, 1986). The active site of α_1PI contains two methionyl residues that are easily oxidizable to methionine sulfoxide derivatives. Oxidized α_1PI is generally inactive against human neutrophil elastase (Zaslow et al., 1983). Recently, Padrines et al. (1989) demonstrated that oxidized α_1PI remains active with human neutrophil elastase but reacts much more slowly than native α_1PI and forms unstable complexes. During inflammation, this slower neutralization reaction with neutrophil elastase may enable local destruction of connective tissues, enhancing the migration of PMNs out of the vascular beds. α_1PI, by delaying the inhibition of elastase, could then play a useful role.

The main enzyme oxidizing α_1PI is myeloperoxidase, which is released from azurophil granules of polymorphonuclear leukocytes (Carp and Janoff, 1979, 1980). This enzyme, in the presence of H_2O_2 and a halide, produces oxidant species, such as hypochlorous acid and *N*-chloramines (Test et al., 1984), causing the oxidation of α_1PI (Johnson and Travis, 1979; Matheson et al., 1979, 1981; Clark et al., 1981; Weiss and Regiani, 1984). α_1PI can also be inactivated by the peroxidase of eosinophils and by oxygen species produced by macrophages (Carp and Janoff, 1978; Hubbard et al., 1987; Klebanoff, 1988). Native or oxidized α_1PI is also cleaved by a metalloprotease released by activated neutrophils (Desrochers and Weiss, 1988). In the plasma and the bronchoalveolar lavage fluid of ARDS patients, an oxidized form of α_1PI has been found, witnessing important release and destruction of this antiprotease (Cochrane et al., 1982, 1983a).

The synthesis (by genetic engineering) and isolation of a nonoxidizable α_1PI affords great hope, particularly in the treatment of chronic emphysema in genetically normal α_1PI-deficient patients (Goerge et al., 1984; Rosenberg et al., 1984; Carrell and Travis, 1985; Courtney et al., 1985). However, at present only a few patients have been successfully treated (Wewers et al., 1987), and no similar treatment has been tried in ARDS patients.

α_1-Antichymotrypsin inhibits chymotrypsinlike proteases from phagocytic cells, including cathepsin G and chymase (Travis et al., 1978). It is an acute-phase inhibitory protein, and its plasma concentration may double within 8 hr after tissue damage and reaches a maximal value 4-5 days after injury (Travis and Morii, 1981). Macrophages can also produce α_1-antichymotrypsin (Adams and Hamilton, 1984).

ATIII, another acute-phase protein, is the specific inhibitor of thrombin, also inhibiting the Hageman factor (Stead et al., 1976; Chan et al., 1977), and the coagulation factors XI (Travis and Salvesen, 1983), X, and IX, as well as plasmin and kallikrein, with reduced effectiveness (Kozin and Cochrane, 1988).

α_2-Antiplasmin is the specific inhibitor of plasmin, also providing minor in vitro inhibitory activity against activated HF (Chan et al., 1977; Schapira et al., 1982; Kozin and Cochrane, 1988) and activated factor XI (Scott et al., 1982a).

C1 esterase inhibitor is the plasma inhibitor of the classic pathway of complement activation. It blocks the spontaneous activation of the proenzyme C1 but not its activation by immune complexes (Ziccardi, 1982b). C1In is an important inhibitor of activated HF (Gigli et al., 1970; De Agostini et al., 1984) and kallikrein (Gigli et al., 1970). C1In concentration increases moderately during inflammation (Lamy et al., 1988a). In ARDS patients we found an early decrease in C1In plasma level (in the first 18 hr) (Lamy et al., 1988b), indicating early consumption, perhaps due to activation of the coagulation cascade. When triggering the alternative pathway of complement activation, spontaneous activation of C3 into C3b with formation of C3 convertase plays a key role. The unique and major inhibitor of C3 convertase is C3 inactivator (C3INA), itself a serine protease specifically destroying C3b and inhibiting the formation of C3 convertase (Fearon, 1977; Reid and Porter, 1981). C3INA (with C4b binding protein as a cofactor) is also an inhibitor of C3 convertase in the classic pathway (Reid and Porter, 1981). Little is known about plasma concentrations of C3INA or their changes during inflammation.

Several other serine protease inhibitors deserve our attention: inter-α-trypsin inhibitor (IαI), pancreatic secretory trypsin inhibitor (PSTI), bronchial leukocyte protease inhibitor (BLPI), the inhibitor of plasminogen activator, and the protease nexin. IαI is a glycoprotein that is largely unstable (Steinbuch, 1976; Pratt and Pizzo, 1987), a specific inhibitor of trypsin but also active against chymotrypsin, elastase, and plasmin at a lower activity. Since IαI complexes with proteases are very unstable, any physiologic role of this antiprotease remains doubtful. IαI is present in plasma (300-500 mg/liter) (Travis and Salvesen, 1983) and appears in the upper respiratory tract in a degraded form (Hochstrassen et al., 1974; Hochstrassen and Wachter, 1983). PSTI is a specific low-molecular-weight inhibitor of trypsin but is a temporary inhibitor, releasing the intact enzyme, which is then trapped by α_2M. PSTI is produced in the pancreas (Pubols et al., 1974; Eddeland and Ohlsson, 1978), but it has been measured in plasma (17-35 μg/liter), with increased plasma concentrations in acute pancreatitis, trauma, and shock (Ogawa, 1988). BLPI is localized to secretory granules of serous cells in human bronchial mucus glands and interstitial fluids. BLPI inhibits elastase and cathepsin G (Bruch and Bieth, 1986; Dewater et al., 1986; Thompson and Ohlsson, 1986) but is readily destroyed by oxidants. The macrophages (Chapman and Stone, 1984) and endothelial cells (Ny et al., 1986) produce an inhibitor of plasminogen activator, thereby inhibiting fibrinolysis. Endothelial cells also produce the protease nexin, which inactivates thrombin as well as trypsin and urokinase (Knauer and Cunningham, 1984).

B. Inhibitors of Cysteine Proteases

The plasma cysteine protease inhibitors form another family of protease inhibitors, but we know far less about them than about the serpin family. α_2-Cysteine inhibitor acts on cathepsins B, H, and L. The α_1-thiol protease inhibitor (α_1TPI) is also a member of this group (Pagano et al., 1984). Recently, homology of structure has been evidenced between α_1TPI and HMWK (Ohkubo et al., 1988), between cystatins and HMWK (Muller-Esterl et al., 1986), and between the α_2-cysteine inhibitor and LMWK (Okhubo et al., 1984; Fung and Schreiber, 1987). Besides their role in the contact activation system as precursors of kinins, HMWK and LMWK participate in the antiprotease activity of plasma by inhibiting the cathepsins. In cells, two other types of polypeptide inhibitors have been discovered: the cystatins and the stefins (Barrett et al., 1986).

C. Metalloprotease Inhibitors

Very little is known about this family of inhibitors. One inhibitor is beginning to be studied, the tissue inhibitor of metalloprotease (TIMP), which is present in macrophages (Welgus et al., 1985; Postlethwaite and Kang, 1988), fibroblasts (Stricklin and Welgus, 1983; Murphy et al., 1985), and endothelial cells (Herron et al., 1986). It appears to be a specific inhibitor of collagenase but can be inactivated by neutrophil elastase (Weiss and Peppin, 1986; Okada et al., 1988). Another inhibitor of collagenase has been isolated from plasma, the β_1-anticollagenase (Macartney and Tschesche, 1983).

D. α_2-Macroglobulin

A well-studied inhibitor of protease is α_2-macroglobulin, a large protein (MW 725,000) with a broad spectrum of inhibitory activity on proteases of all four classes (Harpel, 1970, 1976; Barrett and Starkey, 1973; Barrett, 1980; Salvesen and Barrett, 1980; Roberts and Hall, 1983). α_2M binds to trypsin, elastase, plasma kallikrein, chymotrypsin, and collagenase and is the end point of proteases after their release from complexes with their specific antiproteases; α_2M carries the proteases to cells of the reticuloendothelial system (RES), where entire α_2M-protease complexes are trapped and catabolized (Barrett et al., 1974; Ohlsson, 1981). A main characteristic of α_2M is its ability to conserve its enzymatic activity while bound to the protease, not only against low-molecular-weight substrates, so that the complexed α_2M-protease remains active as a peptidase (Largman et al., 1977; Bieth et al., 1983), but also against fibrinogen and hemoglobin (at a slower rate) and against trypsinogen and chymotrypsin (Harpel and Mosesson, 1973; Rinderknecht and Geokas, 1973). Moreover, binding of a protease to α_2M can release peptides with immunodepressive activity (Alomran et al., 1983; Hubbard et al., 1983), suggesting an immunoregulatory role of α_2M (Koo, 1983). Exposure of activated macrophages to α_2M-protease complexes suppresses the secretion of neutral and cytolytic protease, the respiratory burst, and macrophage-mediated tumor cytolysis (Adams and Hamilton, 1984, 1988). The anergy often observed in acute and chronic disease (Cooperland et al., 1976; Constantian et al., 1977; Constantian, 1978) is attributed in part to immunosuppression due to persistence in the circulation of α_2M-protease complexes or suppressive peptides liberated from α_2M after protease binding (Alomran et al., 1983; Donnelly et al., 1983).

α_2M is mainly synthesized in the liver, but synthesis by macrophages (Hovi et al., 1977; White et al., 1980; Adams and Hamilton, 1988) and other cells, such as cultured fibroblasts, has been reported (Mosher et al., 1977; Mosher, 1983). Its mean normal concentration in plasma is 2.3 g/liter, and it was believed stable during inflammation (Daniels et al., 1974; Steinbuch and Audran, 1974; Powanda and Meyer, 1981; Nicod et al., 1985); however, recent studies report a decreased α_2M concentration in plasma (White et al., 1982; Wendt et al., 1984; Jochum et al., 1986). In ARDS patients, we measured a decreased level of α_2M levels in plasma (Faymonville et al., 1987a; Deby-Dupont et al., 1988a; Lamy et al., 1988a, b); this decrease was present in the first hour after injury and persisted for several days. A marked reduction in the plasma α_2M level is illustrated in Figure 6 in polytrauma patients. It indicates major consumption of this antiprotease. Note that major protease release into plasma can lead to protease-antiprotease imbalance. Imbalance could be aggravated by α_2M inactivation. Total or partial inactivation of α_2M by ammonium or methylamine is well studied (Steinbuch et al., 1968;

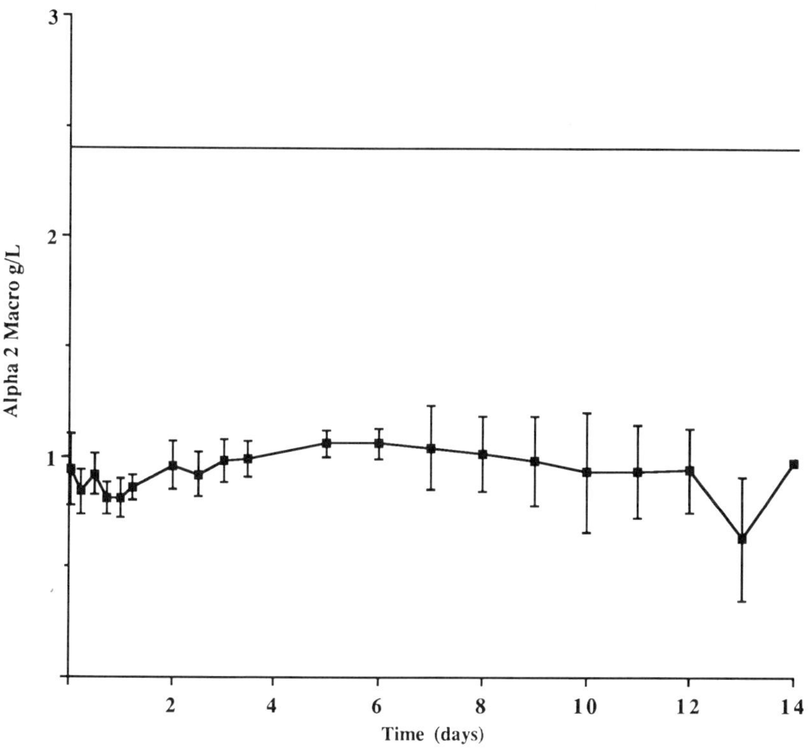

Figure 6 Sequence of plasma α_2-macroglobulin in seven multiply injured post-trauma patients (mean value ± SEM). Mean normal value: 2.3 g/liter (normal range: 1.5-3.5 g/liter).

Barrett et al., 1979), and Weiss (1989) suggested for α_2M an oxidative inactivation similar to α_1PI. We have found that α_2M, like α_1PI, is inactivated by oxidant species produced during neutrophil activation, especially by the activity of myeloperoxidase to release hypochlorous acid (unpublished results).

IV. Is a Protease-Antiprotease Imbalance Present During ARDS?

In many situations predisposing to ARDS and during ARDS, numerous proteases from various origins are carried by systemic blood flow or are locally released, particularly by neutrophils aggregating in the lungs. The capacity of various inflammatory cells to degrade components of the basement membrane and the extracellular matrix is probably essential to permit their escape from the circulation to reach distant sites and produce an inflammatory response. Such a beneficial role could become excessive and inappropriate, however, leading to connective tissue damage. Given the effectiveness, the multiplicity, and the high plasma levels of inhibitors, proteases should not be able to long remain free and mediate extracellular damage. However, during ARDS, isolates of purulent fluid, bronchoalveolar lavage fluids, ascitic fluid, lymph drained from the thoracic duct, and even plasma have been found to contain free enzymes, such as neutrophil elastase, collagenase, and trypsin (Cochrane et al., 1983b; Lee et al., 1981; Christer et al., 1985; Deby-Dupont et al., 1988b). This suggests that the antiprotease shield has been subverted and that antiprotease capacity has been overloaded or destroyed. How could this occur? It seems that plasma levels of most antiproteases are not decreased: α_1PI and α_1-antichymotrypsin increase in inflammation. We found α_1PI levels increasing 10 days after injury in multiple injured patients. ATIII, after a 2 day period of modest reduction, was stable in our ARDS patients. C1In was stable or slightly increased. However, little is known about alterations in the plasma level of other antiproteases. Locally, in tissues and interstitial fluids, the concentrations of antiproteases are unknown. Local destruction of inhibitors by proteases is possible. The close contact between neutrophils or macrophages and matrix proteins or endothelial cells can produce a microenvironment favorable to protease activity and unfavorable to inhibitor activity.

Moreover, some inhibitors are sensitive to oxidative inactivation. This sensitivity to oxidation with loss of or decrease in inhibitory power against elastase has been proven for α_1PI, and we actually know that plasminogen inactivator and BLPI are also inactivated by oxidants.

If proteases remain unregulated, they can attack other inhibitors: collagenase and gelatinase have the ability to cleave α_1PI (Weiss, 1989), and elastase can inactivate TIMP (Weiss and Peppin, 1986; Okada et al., 1988) and attack α_1-antichymotrypsin (Travis and Salvesen, 1983). It should also be kept in mind that most of the antiproteases are temporary inhibitors, which release the intact protease after a more or less long period as a complex. The released enzyme is then captured by α_2-macroglobulin, which undergoes a conformational change (Barrett et al., 1979; Dangott et al., 1983) to expose a new binding site recognized by a specific receptor expressed on a number of cells, including macrophages (Debanne et al., 1975; Van Leuven et al., 1978; Hanover et al., 1983; Mosher and Vaheri, 1980). The α_2M-protease complex is rapidly eliminated from circulating blood by the RES, but during its lifetime in tissues, plasma or other fluids, the bound protease remains active, at least against low-molecular-weight substrates. In critically ill patients, overloading the RES would prolong the lifetime of protease-α_2M complexes. α_2M is thus the end point of many proteases. In view of the large normal concentration of α_2M in plasma, one would expect sufficient antiprotease protection. However, although α_2M levels can increase during inflammation, we and others have found a dramatic decrease in the plasma level of this key antiprotease in ARDS patients (or in patients at risk for ARDS) and septic patients. This reduction in α_2M levels suggests major consumption. We also demonstrated that α_2M is sensitive to oxidative inactivation, which aggravates the protease-antiprotease imbalance of critically ill patients.

In view of a possible protease-antiprotease imbalance in ARDS patients (or patients at risk for ARDS), an early diagnosis of excessive plasma proteolytic activity would be useful and has been recently proposed (Aasen et al., 1982; Smith-Erichsen et al., 1982; Aasen, 1985). A reinforced shield of antiproteases could be useful but requires a supply of protease inhibitors. What kinds of antiproteases should be given and at what doses? Any antiprotease should be resistant to the oxidative activity of phagocytic cells or be accompanied by drugs that limit the production or the effects of toxic oxygen species.

Although a number of natural and synthetic inhibitors of proteases are available, most are toxic or have only been tried in animal studies. Low-molecular-weight chemical inhibitors of serine proteases are numerous, including azide, benzamidine, diisopropylfluorophosphate, and tosyllysylchloromethyl ketone, but all are very toxic. A few nontoxic inhibitors, such as gabexate mesilate (Hesse et al., 1984), a trypsin inhibitor, has been studied in animals and is being studied in humans (the results of these ongoing studies are still inconclusive). The effectiveness of aprotinin therapy remains uncertain (Clasen et al., 1987). A new form of this inhibitor, resistant to oxidation, has been produced that is active against elastase, but no human studies are yet available (Fritz and Wunderer, 1983). Eglin C, which is resistant to oxidants, has been proposed as an effective inhibitor of elastase, but there are no published studies of humans. The therapeutic use of α_1PI, either native or "oxidation proof," appears promising, but studies in humans remain limited to a few cases of chronic emphysema (Wewers et al., 1987). An original therapeutic approach would be to infuse purified α_2M or α_2M-enriched plasma fractions, since this antiprotease is essential for protease inhibition. However, this kind of treatment has never been tried in humans and experimental studies in animal models would first be necessary, assessing inactivation of this antiprotease by oxidants and the immunosuppressive role of peptides released by protease-antiprotease complexes (Constantian et al., 1977; Constantian, 1978).

Excessive protease release occurs during ARDS, and an important route for therapy would be to block the excessive release of proteases by excited neutrophils and excessive production by pancreas; one way would be to furnish an excess of antiproteases. In this way, normal production of proteases could be maintained, allowing their normal functions of removing clots from vessels, removing hyaline membranes from alveoli, and degrading wound tissues and protein fragments. Proteases are not solely destructive proteins; they have a beneficial role in normal and pathologic situations and play a major role in repair after injury.

Acknowledgments

The authors would like to thank Mrs. V. Salemme-Casertano, N. Bodson, M. Adam, and Mr. D. Jeuniaux for preparing the manuscript. This work was supported by the Belgian Fonds National de la Recherche Scientifique et Médicale grant 34574-89.

References

Aasen, A. O. (1985). The proenzyme functional inhibition index. A view parameter for evaluation of the severely injured and septic patients. *Acta Chir. Scand.,* **522**:211-233.

Aasen, A. O., Kierulf, P., and Ruud, T. E. (1982). Studies on pathological plasma proteolysis in patients with acute pancreatitis, a preliminary report. *Acta Clin. Scand.,* **509**:83-89.

Adams, D. O., and Hamilton, T. A. (1984). The cell biology of macrophage activation. *Annu. Rev. Immunol.,* **2**:283-318.

Adams, D. O., and Hamilton, T. A. (1988). Phagocytic cells: Cytotoxic activities of macrophages. In *Inflammation: Basic Principles and Clinical Correlates.* Edited by J. I. Gallin, I. M. Goldstein, and R. Snyderman. New York, Raven Press, pp. 471-492.

Alomram, A., Shenton, B. K., Donnelly, P. K., Francis, D. M., Proud, G., and Taylor, M. R. (1983). A possible mechanism of immunoregulation proceeded by α_2-macroglobulin. *Ann. N.Y. Acad. Sci.,* **421**:394-397.

Anderson, R. R., Holliday, R. L., Driedger, A. A., Lefcoe, M., Reid, B., and Sibbald, W. J. (1979). Documentation of pulmonary capillary permeability in the adult respiratory distress syndrome accompanying human sepsis. *Am. Rev. Respir. Dis.,* **119**:869-877.

Archer, G. T., and Hirsh, J. G. (1963). Isolation of granules from eosinophils leukocytes and study of their enzyme content. *J. Exp. Med.,* **118**: 277-285.

Ashbaugh, D. G., Bigelow, D. B., Petty, T. L., and Levine, B. E. (1967). Acute respiratory distress in adults. *Lancet,* **2**:319-323.

Ayars, G. H., Altman, L. C., Rosen, H., and Doyle, T. (1984). The injurious effect of neutrophils on pneumocytes in vitro. *Am. Rev. Respir. Dis.,* **130**:964-973.

Baker, S. P., O'Neill, B., Haddon, W., and Logon, W. B. (1974). The injury severity score: A method for describing patients with multiple injuries and evaluating emergency care. *J. Trauma,* **14**:187-196.

Barrett, A. J. (1980). α_2-Macroglobulin. *Methods Enzymol.,* **80**:737-754.

Barrett, A. J., and McDonald, J. K. (1986). Nomenclature: Protease, proteinase and peptidase. *Biochem. J.,* **237**:935.

Barrett, A., and Starkey, P. (1973). The interaction of α_2-macroglobulin with proteinases. *Biochem. J.,* **133**:709-724.

Barrett, A. J., Starkey, P. M., and Munn, E. A. (1974). The unique nature of the interaction of α_2-macroglobulin with proteinases. In *Proteinase Inhibitors.* Edited by H. Fritz, H. Tschesche, L. J. Green, and E. Truscheit. Berlin, Springer-Verlag, pp. 72-77.

Barrett, A. J., Brown, M. A., and Sayers, C. A. (1979). The electrophoretically "slow" and "fast" forms of the α_2-macroglobulin molecule. *Biochem. J.,* **181**:401-418.

Barrett, A. J., Fritz, H., Grubb, A., Isemura, S., and Jarvinen, M. (1986). Nomenclature and classification of the proteins homologous with cysteine-proteinase inhibitor chicken cystatin. *Biochem. J.,* **236**:312.

Baumann, W., Jung, R. C., Koss, M., Boylen, C. T., Navarro, L., and Sharma, O. M. (1986). Incidence and mortality of adult respiratory distress syndrome: A prospective analysis from a large metropolitan hospital. *Crit. Care Med.,* **14**:1-4.

Becker, V., and Stollhoff, K. (1985). Shock and terminal pancreatitis. *Pathol. Res. Pract.,* **179**:512-516.

Bell, R. C., Coalson, J. J., Smith, J. D., and Johanson, W. G. (1983). Multiple organ system failure and infection in adult respiratory distress syndrome. *Ann. Intern. Med.,* **99**:293-298.

Bieth, J. G. (1986). Elastases: Catalytic and biological properties. In *Biology of Extracellular Matrix. Regulation of Matrix Accumulation.* Edited by R. P. Mecham. New York, Academic Press, pp. 217-230.

Bieth, J. G., Kandel, M. J., and Zreika, M. (1983). Interaction of protein substrate and inhibitors with α_2-macroglobulin-bound proteinase. *Ann. N.Y. Acad. Sci.,* **421**:209-217.

Bond, J. S., and Butler, P. E. (1987). Intracellular proteases. *Annu. Rev. Biochem.,* **56**:333-364.

Bone, R. C. (1984). Adult respiratory distress syndrome, treatment in the next decade. In *Update in Intensive Care and Emergency Medicine.* Edited by J. L. Vincent. Berlin, Springer-Verlag, pp. 20-35.

Bone, R. C., Francis, P. B., and Pierce, A. K. (1976). Intravascular coagulation associated with adult respiratory distress syndrome. *Am. J. Med.,* **61**:585-589.

Border, J. R., Hassett, J., LaDuca, J., Seibel, R., Steinberg, S., Mills, B., Losi, P., and Border, D. (1986). The gut origin septic states in blunt multiple trauma (ISS:40) in the ICU. *Ann. Surg.*, **206**:427-448.

Borg, T., Gerdin, B., Hallgren, R., and Modig, J. (1985). The role of polymorphonuclear leucocytes in the pulmonary dysfunction induced by complement activation. *Acta Anaesthesiol. Scand.*, **29**:231-240.

Bouma, B. N., Miles, L. A., Baretta, G., and Griffin, J. H. (1980). Human plasma prekallikrein. Studies of its activation by activated factor XII and of its inactivation by diisopropyl phosphofluoridate. *Biochemistry*, **19**:1151-1160.

Brain, J. D. (1988). Lung macrophages: How many kinds are there? What do they do? *Am. Rev. Respir. Dis.*, **137**:507-509.

Brigham, K. L. (1982). Mechanisms of lung injury. *Clin. Chest Med.*, **3**: 9-24.

Brigham, K. L., and Sherer, S. D. (1985). Prostaglandins in lung disease: Adult respiratory distress syndrome. *Semin. Respir. Med.*, **7**:11-16.

Brigham, K. L., Bowers, R. E., and Haynes, J. (1979). Increased sheep lung vascular permeability caused by *Escherichia coli* endotoxin. *Circ. Res.*, **45**:292-297.

Bruch, M., and Bieth, J. G. (1986). Influence of elastin on the inhibition of leucocyte elastase by α_1-proteinase inhibitor and bronchial inhibitor: Potent inhibition of elastin-bound elastase by bronchial inhibitor. *Biochem. J.*, **238**:269-273.

Calandrino, F. S., Anderson, D. J., Mintun, M. A., and Schuster, D. P. (1988). Pulmonary vascular permeability during the adult respiratory distress syndrome. A positron emission tomographic study. *Am. Rev. Respir. Dis.*, **138**:421-428.

Campbell, E. J., Senor, R. M., and Welgus, H. G. (1987). Extracellular matrix injury during lung inflammation. *Chest*, **92**:161-167.

Carp, H., and Janoff, A. (1978). Possible mechanisms of emphysema in smokers. In vitro suppression of serum elastase-inhibitory capacity by fresh cigarette smoke and its prevention by antioxidants. *Am. Rev. Respir. Dis.*, **118**:617-621.

Carp, H., and Janoff, A. (1979). In vitro suppression of serum elastase-inhibitory capacity by reactive oxygen species generated by phagocytosing polymorphonuclear leukocytes. *J. Clin. Invest.*, **63**:793-805.

Carp, H., and Janoff, A. (1980). Potential mediators of inflammation. Phagocyte derived oxidants suppress the elastase-inhibitory capacity of α_1-proteinase inhibitor in vitro. *J. Clin. Invest.*, **66**:987-995.

Carrell, R., and Travis, J. (1985). α_1-Antitrypsin and the serpins: Variation and countervariation. *TIBS*, **10**(1):20-24.

Carrell, R. W., Jeppsson, J. O., Laurell, C. B., Brennan, S. O., Owen, M. C., Vaugham, L., and Boswell, D. R. (1982). Structure and variation of human α_1-antitrypsin. *Nature,* **298**:329-334.

Carvalho, A. A. (1985). Blood alterations in ARDS. In: *Acute Respiratory Failure.* Edited by W. Zapol and K. Falke. New York, Marcel Dekker, pp. 303-346.

Cerra, F. B. (1988). Multiple organ failure. In *Perspectives in Critical Care,* Vol. 1. Edited by F. B. Cerra. St. Louis, Quality Medical Publishing, pp. 1-22.

Chan, J. Y. C.,Burrowes, C. E., Habel, F. H., and Movat, H. Z. (1977). The inhibition of activated factor XII (Hageman factor) by antithrombin III. The effect of other plasma proteinase inhibitors. *Biochem. Biophys. Res. Commun.,* **74**:150-158.

Chapman, H. A., and Stone, O. L. (1984). A fibrinolytic inhibitor of human alveolar macrophages. Induction with endotoxin. *Am. Rev. Respir. Dis.,* **132**:569-575.

Chapman, H. A., Stone, O. L., and Vavrin, Z. (1984). Degradation of fibrin and elastin by intact human alveolar macrophages in vitro: Characterization of a plasminogen activator and its role in matrix degradation. *J. Clin. Invest.,* **73**:806-815.

Chenoweth, D. E., Cooper, S. W., Hugli, T. E., Stewart, R. W., Blackstone, E. H., and Kirklin, J. W. (1981). Complement activation during cardiopulmonary bypass. *N. Engl. J. Med.,* **304**:497-503.

Christer, P., Fein, A., Golberg, S., Lippman, M., Abrarus, W., and Weinbaum, G. (1985). Collagenase in the lower respiratory tract of patients with adult respiratory distress syndrome. *Am. Rev. Respir. Dis.,* **131**: 690-695.

Clark, J. M., Vaughan, D. W., Aiken, B. M., and Kagan, H. M. (1980). Elastase-like enzymes in human neutrophils localized by ultrastructural cytochemistry. *J. Cell Biol.,* **84**:102-119.

Clark, R. A., Stone, P. J., El Hag, A., Calore, J. D., and Franzblau, C. (1981). Myeloperoxidase-catalyzed inactivation of α_1-protease inhibitor by human neutrophils. *J. Biol. Chem.,* **256**:3348-3353.

Clasen, C., Jochum, M., and Mueller-Esterl, W. (1987). Feasibility study of very high aprotinin dosage in polytrauma patients. In *First Vienna Shock Forum. Part a. Pathophysiological Role of Mediators and Mediator Inhibitors in Shock.* Edited by R. Alan. pp. 175-183.

Cochrane, C. G., and Griffin, J. H. (1982). The biochemistry and pathophysiology of the contact system of plasma. *Adv. Immunol.,* **33**:241-304.

Cochrane, C. G., Revak, S. D., and Wuepper, K. D. (1973). Activation of Hageman factor in solid and fluid phases. A critical role of kallikrein. *J. Exp. Med.,* **138**:1564-1572.

Cochrane, C. G., Spragg, R. G., and Revak, S. D. (1982). Oxidative inactivation of α_1-proteinase inhibitor in bronchoalveolar lavage fluid of patient with the adult respiratory distress syndrome. *J. Clin. Invest.,* **71**:754-761.

Cochrane, C. G., Spragg, R. G., Revak, S. D., Cohen, A. B., and McGuire, W. W. (1983a). The presence of neutrophil elastase and evidence of oxidation activity in bronchoalveolar lavage fluid of patients with adult respiratory distress syndrome. *Am. Rev. Respir. Dis.,* **127**:S25-S27.

Cochrane, C. G., Spragg, R. G., and Revak, S. D. (1983b). Pathogenesis of the adult respiratory distress syndrome. *J. Clin. Invest.,* **71**:754-761.

Colley, C. M., Fleck, A., Goode, A. W., Muller, B. R., and Myers, M. A. (1983). Early time course of acute phase protein response in man. J. Clin. Pathol., **36**:203-207.

Colman, R. W. (1969). Activation of plasminogen by human plasma kallikrein. *Biochem. Biophys. Res. Commun.,* **35**:273-279.

Constantian, M. B. (1978). Association of sepsis with immunosuppressive polypeptide in the serum of burn patients. *Ann. Surg.,* **188**:209-215.

Constantian, M. B., Menzoian, J. O., Nimberg, R. B., Schmid, K., and Mannick, J. A. (1977). Association of a circulating immunosuppressive polypeptide with operative and accidental trauma. *Ann. Surg.,* **185**: 73-79.

Cooperland, S. R., Nimberg, K., and Mannick, A. (1976). Humoral immunosuppressive factors. *Transplant. Proc.,* **82**:225-242.

Courtney, M., Jallat, S., Tessier, L. H., Benavente, A., Crystal, R. G., and Lecocq, J. P. (1985). Synthesis in *E. coli* of $\alpha_1$antitrypsin variants of therapeutic potential for emphysema and thrombosis. *Nature,* **313**:149-151.

Cox, S. C., Norwood, S., and Duncan, C. A. (1985). Acute respiratory failure: Mortality associated with underlying disease. *Crit. Care Med.,* **13**: 1005-1008.

Crutchley, D. J. (1987). Hemostatic potential of the pulmonary endothelium. In *Pulmonary Endothelium in Health and Disease.* Edited by U. S. Ryan. New York, Marcel Dekker, pp. 237-273.

Dangott, L. J., Puette, D., and Cunningham, L. W. (1983). Change in α_2-macroglobulin conformation by reaction with trypsin and methylamine. *Ann. N.Y. Acad. Sci.,* **421**:158-159.

Daniels, J. C., Larson, D. L., Abston, S., and Ritzman, S. E. (1974). Serum protein profiles in thermal burns. *J. Trauma,* **14**:153-162.

Davie, E. W., Fujikawa, K., Kurachi, K., and Kesiel, W. (1979). The role of serine proteases in the blood coagulation cascade. *Adv. Enzymol.,* **48**:227-318.

De Agostini, A., Lijnen, H. R., Pixley, R. A., Colman, R. W., and Schapira, M. (1984). Inactivation of factor XII active fragment in normal plasma. Predominant role for C1-inhibitor. *J. Clin. Invest.,* **73**:1542-1549.

Debanne, M. T., Beel, R. J., and Dolovich, J. (1975). Uptake of proteinase-α_2-macroglobulin complexes by macrophages. *Biochim. Biophys. Acta,* **411**:295-304.

Deby-Dupont, G., Haas, M., Pincemail, J., Braun, M., Lamy, M., Deby, C., and Franchimont, P. (1984). Immunoreactive trypsin in adult respiratory distress syndrome. *Intensive Care Med.,* **10**:7-12.

Deby-Dupont, G., Braun, M., Lamy, M., Deby, C., Pincemail, J., Faymonville, M. E., Damas, P., Bodson, L., Lecart, M. P., and Goutier, R. (1987). Thromboxane and prostacyclin release in adult respiratory distress syndrome. *Intensive Care Med.,* **13**:167-174.

Deby-Dupont, G., Faymonville, M. E., Damas, F., Damas, P., and Lamy, M. (1988a). Shock pancreas. *Intensive Care News,* **1**:1-6.

Deby-Dupont, G., Reynaert, M., Damas, P., Lamy, M., and Franchimont, P. (1988b). Justification biochimique du drainage du canal thoracique au cours de la pancréatite aiguë necrotico-hémorragique. *Acta Gastroenterol. Belg.,* **51**:31-40.

Deitch, E. A. (1988). Does the gut protect or injure patients in the ICU? *Perspect. Crit. Care,* **1**(2):1-31.

Desrochers, P. E., and Weiss, S. J. (1988). Proteolytic inactivation of α_1-proteinase inhibitor by a neutrophil metalloproteinase. *J. Clin. Invest.,* **81**:1646-1650.

Dewald, B., Bretz, U., and Baggiolini, M. (1982). Release of gelatinase from a novel secretory compartment of human neutrophils. *J. Clin. Invest.,* **70**:518-525.

Dewater, R., Willems, L. N., Van Muijen, G. N., Franken, C., Fransen, J., Dijkman, J. H., and Kramps, J. A. (1986). Ultrastructural localization of bronchial antileukoprotease in central and peripheral human airways by a gold-labeling technique using monoclonal antibodies. *Am. Rev. Respir. Dis.,* **133**:882-890.

Diamond, J. M. (1978). Reabsorption of digestive enzymes: Playing with poison. *Nature,* **271**:111-112.

Donnelly, P. K., Shenton, B. K., Alomran, A., Francis, D. M., Proud, G., and Taylor, R. M. (1983). The clinical relevance of α_2-macroglobulin. *Ann. N.Y. Acad. Sci.,* **421**:382-387.

Duchateau, J., Haas, M., Schreyen, H., Radoux, L., Sprangers, L., Noël, F. X., Braun, M., and Lamy, M. (1984). Complement activation in patients at risk of developing the adult respiratory distress syndrome. *Am. Rev. Respir. Dis.,* **130**:1058-1064.

Duswald, K. H., Jochum, M., Schramm, W., and Fritz, H. (1985). Released granulocytic elastase: An indicator of pathobiochemical alterations in septicemia after abdominal surgery. *Surgery,* **98**:892-899.

Eddeland, A., and Ohlsson, K. (1978). Purification and immunochemical quantitation of human pancreatic secretory trypsin inhibitor. *Scand. J. Clin. Lab. Invest.,* **38**:261-267.

Effros, R. M., and Mason, G. R. (1986). An end to "ARDS." *Chest,* **89**: 162-163.

Esmon, C. T. (1983). Protein-C: Biochemistry, physiology and clinical implications. *Blood,* **62**:1155-1158.

Fallat, R. J., Mielke, C. H., Jr., and Rodvien, R. (1980). Editorial: Adult respiratory distress syndrome and gram-negative sepsis. *Arch. Intern. Med.,* **140**:612-613.

Fantone, C., Kunkel, J. L., and Warp, P. (1982). Chemotactic mediators in neutrophil-dependent lung injury. *Annu. Rev. Physiol.,* **44**:283-293.

Faymonville, M. E., Lamy, M., Duchateau, J., Adam, A., Deby-Dupont, G., Micheels, J., and Jacquemin, D. (1987a). Biochemical mediators in acute respiratory distress syndrome (ARDS) after burning injury. In *Lipids: Mediators in the Immunology of Shock.* Edited by M. Paubert-Braquet, P. Braquet, D. Demling, B. B. Fletcher, and M. Foegh. New York, Plenum Press, pp. 43-56.

Faymonville, M. E., Micheels, J., Bodson, L., Jacquemain, D., Lamy, M., Adam, A., and Duchateau, J. (1987b). Biochemical investigations after burning injury: Complement system, protease-antiprotease balance and acute-phase proteins. *Burns,* **13**:26-33.

Fearon, D. T. (1977). Purification of C3b inactivator and demonstration of its two polypeptide chain structure. *J. Immunol.,* **119**:1248-1252.

Fein, A., Grossman, R. F., Jones, J. G., Overland, E., Pitts, L., Murray, J. F., and Staub, N. C. (1979). The value of edema fluid protein measurements in patients with pulmonary edema. *Am. J. Med.,* **67**:32-38.

Feinstein, G., and Janoff, A. (1975). A rapid method for purification of human granulocyte cationic neutral proteases: Purification and characterization of human granulocyte chymotrypsin-like enzyme. *Biochim. Biophys. Acta,* **403**:477-485.

Fleck, A., Colley, C. M., and Myers, M. A. (1985). Liver export proteins and trauma. *Br. Med. Bull.,* **41**:265-273.

Flick, M. R., Perel, A., and Staub, N. C. (1979). Increased lung vascular permeability after microemboli in unanesthetized sheep requires circulating leukocytes. *Physiologist,* **22**:39-48.

Fowler, A. A., Hamman, R. F., Good, J. T., Benson, K. N., Baird, M., Eberle, D. J., Petty, T. L., and Hyers, T. M. (1983). Adult respiratory distress syndrome: Risk with common predispositions. *Ann. Intern. Med.,* **98**:593-597.

Fowler, A. A., Hamman, R. F., Zerbe, G. O., Benson, K., and Hyers, T. (1985). Adult respiratory distress syndrome. Prognosis after onset. *Am. Rev. Respir. Dis.,* **132**:472-478.

Fritz, H., and Wunderer, G. (1983). Biochemistry and application of aprotinin, the kallikrein inhibitor from bovine organs. *Arzneimittelforsch.,* **33**(1):479-494.

Fung, W. P., and Schreiber, G. (1987). Structure and expression of the genes for major acute phase α_1-protein (thiostatin) and kininogen in the rat. *J. Biol. Chem.,* **262**:298-305.

Gadek, J. E., Fells, G. A., Wright, D. G., and Crystal, R. G. (1980). Human neutrophil elastase functions as a type III collagen "collagenase." *Biochem. Biophys. Res. Commun.,* **95**:1815-1822.

Ghebrehiwet, B., Silverberg, M., and Kaplan, A. P. (1981). Activation of the classical pathway of complement by Hageman factor fragment. *J. Exp. Med.,* **153**:665-676.

Gigli, I., Mason, J. W., Colman, R. W., and Austen, K. F. (1970). Interaction of plasma kallikrein with C_1 inhibitor. *J. Immunol.,* **104**:574-581.

Gmaz-Nikulin, E., Nikulin, A., and Plamena, P. (1981). Pancreatic lesions in shock and their significance. *J. Pathol.,* **135**:223-236.

Göber, I. (1975). Die Auswirkung des hypovolämischen Shocks auf das Pankreas. *Wien Klin. Wochenschr.,* **87**:2-11.

Goerge, P. M., Travis, J., Visser, M. C. M., Winterbourn, C. C., and Carrell, R. N. (1984). A genetically engineered mutant of α_1-antitrypsin protects connective tissue from neutrophil damage and may be useful in lung disease. *Lancet,* **2**:22-29.

Goldstein, I. M. (1988). Complement: Biologically active products. In *Inflammation: Basic Principles and Clinical Correlates.* Edited by J. I. Gallin, I. M. Goldstein, and R. Snyderman. New York, Raven Press, pp. 55-74.

Goris, R. J. A., ten Boekhorst, T. P. A., Nuytinck, J. K. S., and Gimbrère, J. S. F. (1985). Multiple organ failure. Generalized autodestructive inflammation? *Arch. Surg.,* **120**:1109-1115.

Granelli-Peperno, A., Vassalli, J. D., and Reich, E. (1977). Secretion of plasminogen activator by human polymorphonuclear leukocytes. *J. Exp. Med.,* **146**:1693-1706.

Gross, J. L., Moscatelli, D., Jaffe, E. A., and Rifkin, D. B. (1982). Plasminogen activator and collagenase production by cultured capillary endothelial cells. *J. Cell Biol.,* **95**:974-981.

Hammerschmidt, D. A., Weaver, L. J., Hudson, L. D., Craddock, P. R., and Jacob, H. S. (1980). Association of complement activation and elevated plasma C5a with adult respiratory distress syndrome: Pathophysiologic relevance and possible prognostic value. *Lancet,* **1**:947-949.

Hanover, J. A., Willingham, M. C., and Pastan, I. (1983). Receptor-mediated endocytosis of α_2-macroglobulin: Solubilization and partial purification of the fibroblast α_2-macroglobulin receptor. *Ann. N.Y. Acad. Sci.,* **421**:410-423.

Harpel, P. C. (1970). Human plasma alpha$_2$-macroglobulin. An inhibitor of plasma kallikrein. *J. Exp. Med.,* **132**:329-352.

Harpel, P. C. (1976). Human α_2-macroglobulin. *Methods Enzymol.,* **45**: 639-653.

Harpel, P. C., and Mosesson, N. W. (1973). Degradation of fibrinogen by plasma α_2-macroglobulin enzyme complexes. *J. Clin. Invest.,* **53**:2175-2184.

Hasty, K. A., Hibbs, M. S., Kang, A. H., and Mainardi, C. L. (1986). Secreted forms of human neutrophil collagenase. *J. Biol. Chem.,* **261**: 5645-5650.

Haynes, J. B., Hyers, T. M., Giclas, P. C., Franks, J. J., and Petty, T. L. (1980). Elevated fibrin(ogen) degradation products in adult respiratory distress syndrome. *Am. Rev. Respir. Dis.,* **122**:841-847.

Hechtman, H. B., Valeri, C. R., and Shepro, D. (1984). Role of humoral mediators in adult respiratory distress syndrome. *Chest,* **86**:623-627.

Heflin, A. C., and Brigham, K. L. (1981). Prevention by granulocyte depletion of increased vascular permeability of sheep lung following endotoxemia. *J. Clin. Invest.,* **68**:1253-1260.

Hegewald, G., Nikulin, A., and Gmaz-Nikulin, E. (1985). Ultrastructural changes of the human pancreas in acute shock. *Pathol. Res. Pract.,* **179**:610-615.

Henson, P. M., and Johnston, R. B., Jr. (1987). Tissue injury in inflammation: Oxidants, proteinases and cationic proteins. *J. Clin. Invest.,* **79**: 669-674.

Henson, P. M., Henson, J. E., Fittschen, C., Kamani, G., Bratton, D. L., and Riches, D. W. H. (1988). Phagocytic cells: Degranulation and secretion. In *Inflammation: Basic Principles and Clinical Correlates.* Edited by J. I. Gallin, I. M. Goldstein, and R. Snyderman. New York, Raven Press, pp. 363-389.

Herron, G. S., Banda, M. J., Clark, E. J., Gavrilovic, J., and Werb, Z. (1986). Secretion of metalloproteinases by stimulated capillary endothelial cells. II. Expression of collagenase and stromelysin activities is regulated by endogenous inhibitors. *J. Biol. Chem.,* **261**:2814-2818.

Hesse, B., Lankisch, P. G., and Kunze, H. (1984). Effects of serine protease inhibitor gabexate mesilate on purified pancreatic phospholipase A_2. *Pharmacol. Res. Commun.,* **16**:637-645.

Hibbs, M., Mainardi, C. L., and Kang, A. M. (1982). Type-specific collagen degradation by eosinophils. *Biochem. J.,* **207**:;621-624.

Hibbs, M. S., Hoidal, J. R., and Kang, A. H. (1987). Expression of a metalloproteinase that degrades native type V collagen and denatured collagens by cultured human alveolar macrophages. *J. Clin. Invest.,* **80**: 1644-1650.

Hochstrasser, K., and Wachter, E. (1983). Kunitz-type proteinase inhibitors derived by limited proteolysis of the inter-α-trypsin inhibitor. VII. Determination of the amino-acid sequence of the trypsin-released inhibitor from bovine inter-α-trypsin inhibitor. *Hoppe Seylers Physiol. Chem.,* **364**:1679-1687.

Hochstrasser, K., Feuth, H., and Hochgesand, K. (1974). Proteinase inhibitors of the respiratory tract. Studies on the structural relationship between acid-stable inhibitors present in the respiratory tract, plasma and urine. In *Proteinase Inhibitors.* Edited by H. Fritz, H. Tschesche, L. J. Greene, and E. Truscheit. Berlin, Springer-Verlag, pp. 111-116.

Hocking, W. G., and Golde, D. W. (1979). The pulmonary-alveolar macrophage. *N. Engl. J. Med.,* **301**:639-643.

Holter, J. F., Weiland, J. E., Pacht, E. R., Gadek, J. E., and Davis, W. B. (1986). Protein permeability in the adult respiratory distress syndrome. Loss of size selectivity of the alveolar epithelium. *J. Clin. Invest.,* **78**: 1513-1522.

Horn, J. K., Ranson, J. H. C., Ong, R., Poulis, D., Perez, H. D., and Goldstein, I. M. (1982). Complement catabolism and chemotaxis in acute pancreatitis. *J. Surg. Res.,* **32**:569-575.

Horton, E. H., Murthy, S. K., and Seal, R. M. E. (1968). Haemorrhagic necrosis of small intestine and acute pancreatitis following open-heart surgery. *Thorax,* **23**:438-445.

Hovi, T., Mosher, D. F., and Vaheri, A. (1977). Cultured human monocytes synthesize and secrete α_2-macroglobulin. *J. Exp. Med.,* **145**:1580-1589.

Hubbard, W. J., Anderson, B. D., Balder, A. E., Proud, G. M., Alomran, A. M., and Shenton, B. K. (1983). Immunosuppression by human α_2-macroglobulin, a 3800 Mr peptide and other derivatives. *Ann. N.Y. Acad. Sci.,* **421**:332-339.

Hubbard, R. C., Ogushi, F., Fells, G. A., Cantin, A. M., Jallat, S., Courtney, M., and Crystal, R. (1987). Oxidants spontaneously released by alveolar macrophages of cigarette smokers can inactivate the active site of α_1-antitrypsin, rendering it ineffective as an inhibitor of neutrophil elastase. *J. Clin. Invest.,* **80**:1289-1295.

Hyers, T. M., and Fowler, A. A. (1986). Adult respiratory distress syndrome: Causes, morbidity and mortality. *Fed. Proc.,* **45**:25-29.

Ishikawa, J., and Cimason, G. (1977). Isolation of cathepsin D from human leukocytes. *Biochim. Biophys. Acta,* **480**:228-240.

Jacob, H. S., and Hammerschmidt, D. H. (1982). Tissue damage caused by activated complement and granulocytes in shock lung, post perfusion lung, and after amniotic fluid embolism: Ramifications for therapy. *Ann. Chir. Gynecol.,* **71**(suppl. 196):3-9.

Jaffé, E. A. (1988). Endothelial cells. In *Inflammation: Basic Principles and Clinical Correlates.* Edited by J. I. Gallin, I. M. Goldstein, and R. Snyderman. New York, Raven Press, pp. 559-578.

Janoff, A., White, R. Carp, H., Harel, S., Dearing, R., and Lee, D. (1979). Lung injury induced by leukocytic proteases. *Am. J. Pathol.,* **97**:111-129.

Jochum, M., Witte, J., Duswald, K. H., Inthorn, D., Welther, H., and Fritz, H. (1986). Pathobiochemistry of sepsis: Role of proteinases, proteinase inhibitors and oxidizing agents. *Behring. Inst. Mitt.,* **79**:121-130.

Johnson, D. M. A., and Travis, D. (1978). Structural evidence for methionine at the reactive site of human α_1-proteinase inhibitor. *J. Biol. Chem.,* **253**:;7142-7144.

Johnson, D. M. A., and Travis, D. (1979). The oxidative inactivation of human α_1-proteinase inhibitor: Further evidence for methionine at the reactive center. *J. Biol. Chem.,* **254**(10):4022-4026.

Johnson, D. M. A., Gagnon, J., and Reid, K. B. M. (1984). Amino acid sequence of human factor D of the complement system. Similarity in sequence between factor D and proteases of non plasma origin. *FEBS Lett.,* **166**:347-351.

Johnson, W. C., and Nasbeth, D. C. (1970). Pancreatitis in renal transplantation. *Ann. Surg.,* **171**:309-314.

Johnston, R. B. (1988). Monocytes and macrophages. *N. Engl. J. Med.,* **318**:747-752.

Jones, M. S., and Dawson, H. (1979). Studies of the ischemic pancreas in shock. *Adv. Shock Res.,* **1**:197-207.

Jones, R. T., and Linhardt, G. (1982). Pathology and pathophysiology of the exocrine pancreas in shock. In *Pathophysiology of Shock, Anoxia and Ischemia.* Edited by R. A. Cowley and B. F. Trump. Baltimore, Williams & Wilkins, pp. 309-324.

Jones, R. T., Garcia, J., Mergner, W., Pendergrass, R. E., Valigorsky, J. M., and Trump, B. F. (1975). Effects of shock on the pancreatic acinar cell. Cellular and subcellular effects in humans. *Arch. Pathol. Lab. Med.,* **99**:634-644.

Jones, R. T., Kreisberg, J. I., Linhardt, G. E., and Trump, B. F. (1979). Studies of the ischemic pancreas in shock. *Adv. Shock Res.,* **1**:197-207.

Kalebic, T., Garbisa, S., Glaser, B., and Liotta, L. A. (1983). Basement membrane collagen: Degradation by migrating endothelial cells. *Science,* **221**:281-283.

Kane, S. P., and Peters, T. J. (1975). Analytical subcellular fractionation of human granulocytes with reference to the localization of vit B_{12}-binding proteins. *Clin. Sci. Mol. Med.,* **49**:171-182.

Kaplan, A. P., Silberberg, M., Dunn, J. T., and Ghebrehiwet, B. (1982). Interaction of the clotting, kinin-forming, complement and fibrinolytic pathways in inflammation. *Ann. N.Y. Acad. Sci.,* **389**:25-32.

Klebanoff, S. J. (1988). Phagocytic cells: Products of oxygen metabolism. In *Inflammation: Basic Principles and Clinical Correlates.* Edited by J. I. Gallin, I. M. Goldstein, and R. Snyderman, New York, Raven Press, pp. 391-444.

Knauer, D. J., and Cunningham, D. D. (1984). Protease nexins: Cell-secreted proteins which regulate extracellular serine proteases. *Trends Biochem. Sci.,* **9**:231-233.

Koo, P. H. (1983). Tumor inhibition by human α_2-macroglobulin. *Ann. N.Y. Acad. Sci.,* **421**:388-390.

Kornecki, E., Ehrlich, Y. D., DeMars, D., and Lenox, R. H. (1986). Exposure of fibrinogen receptors in human platelets by proteolysis with elatase. *J. Clin. Invest.,* **77**:750-756.

Kozin, F., and Cochrane, C. G. (1988). The contact activation system of plasma: Biochemistry and pathophysiology. In *Inflammation: Basic Principles and Clinical Correlates.* Edited by J. I. Gallin, I. M. Goldstein, and R. Snyderman. New York, Raven Press, pp. 101-120.

Kreuzfelder, E., Joka, T., Keinecke, H. O., Obertacke, U., Schmidt-Neuerberg, K. P., Nakhosteen, J., Paar, D., and Scheiermann, N. (1988). Adult respiratory distress syndrome as a specific manifestation of a general permeability defect in trauma patients. *Am. Rev. Respir. Dis.,* **137**:95-99.

Kwaan, H. C., Anderson, P. S., and Grammatica, L. (1971). A study of pancreatic enzymes as a factor in the pathogenesis of disseminated intravascular coagulation during acute pancreatitis. *Surgery,* **79**:663-672.

Lamy, M., Deby-Dupont, G., Pincemail, J., Braun, M., Duchateau, J., Deby, C., Van Erck, J., Bodson, L., Damas, P., and Franchimont, P. (1985). Biochemical pathways of acute lung injury. *Clin. Respir. Physiol.,* **21**:221-229.

Lamy, M., Faymonville, M. E., and Deby-Dupont, G. (1987). Shock pancreas: A new entity? In *Update in Intensive Care and Emergency Medicine.* Edited by J. L. Vincent. Berlin, Springer-Verlag, pp. 148-154.

Lamy, M., Faymonville, M. E., Adam, A., Deby-Dupont, G., Bodson, L., Damas, P., and Franchimont, P. (1988b). Biochemical changes in patients at risk from the adult respiratory distress syndrome. Does the pancreas play a role? In *Shock and the Adult Respiratory Distress Syndrome*. Edited by W. Kox and D. Bihari. Berlin, Springer-Verlag, pp. 67-77.

Lancet (1986). Adult respiratory distress syndrome. **1**:301-303.

Langlois, P. F., and Gawryl, M. S. (1988). Accentuated formation of the terminal C5b-9 complement complex in patient plasma precedes development of the adult respiratory distress syndrome. *Am. Rev. Respir. Dis.*, **138**:368-375.

Largman, C., Johnson, J. H., Brodrick, J. N., and Geokas, H. C. (1977). Proinsulin conversion to desalanyl insuylin by α_2-macroglobulin-bound trypsin? *Nature,* **269**:168-170.

Laskin, D. L., Kimura, T., Sakakibara, S., Riley, D. J., and Berg, R. A. (1986). Chemotactic activity of collagen-like polypeptides for human peripheral blood neutrophils. *J. Leukocyte Biol.,* **39**:255-266.

Lasson, A., and Ohlsson, K. (1982). An in vivo study of the influence of plasma protease inhibitors and aprotinin on trypsin-induced C3 cleavage in human serum. *Biochim. Biophys. Acta,* **709**:227-233.

Lasson, A., and Ohlsson, K. (1986). Consumptive coagulopathy, fibrinolysis and protease-antiprotease interactions during acute human pancreatitis. *Thromb. Res.,* **41**:167-183.

Lee, C. T., Fein, A. M., Lippman, M., Holzman, H., Kimbel, P., and Weinbaum, G. (1981). Elastolytic activity in pulmonary lavage fluid from patients with adult respiratory distress syndrome. *N. Engl. J. Med.,* **304**: 192-196.

Liebow, C., and Rothman, S. S. (1975). Enteropancreatic circulation of digestive enzymes. *Science,* **189**:472-474.

Luterman, A., Manwaring, D., and Curreri, P. W. (1977). Role of fibrinogen degradation products in the pathogenesis of the respiratory distress syndrome. *Surgery,* **82**:703-709.

Macartney, H. W., and Tschesche, H. (1983). Characterisation of β_1-anticollagenase from human plasma and its reaction with polymorphonuclear leukocyte collagenase by disulfide/thiol interchange. *Eur. J. Biochem.,* **130**:95-102.

Machiedo, G. W. (1989). Sepsis and multiple organ failure: Pathogenesis and treatment. In *Update in Intensive Care and Emergency Medicine.* Edited by J. L. Vincent. Berlin, Springer-Verlag, pp. 3-10.

Mainardi, C. L., Hasty, D. L., Seyer, J. M., and Kang, A. H. (1980a). Specific cleavage of human type III collagen by human polymorphonuclear leukocyte elastase. *J. Biol. Chem.,* **255**:12006-12010.

Mainardi, C. L., Seyer, J. M., and Kang, A. H. (1980b). Type-specific collagenolysis: A type V collagen-degrading enzyme from macrophages. *Biochem. Biophys. Res. Commun.,* **97**:1108-1115.

Manwaring, D., and Curreri, P. W. (1982). Platelet and neutrophil sequestration after fragment D-induced respiratory distress. *Circ. Shock,* **9**:75-81.

Matheson, N. R., Wong, P. D., and Travis, J. (1979). Enzymatic inactivation of human α_1-proteinase inhibitor. *Biochem. Biophys. Res. Commun.,* **88**:402-409.

Matheson, N. R., Wong, P. S., Schuyler, M., and Travis, J. (1981). Interaction of human α_1-proteinase inhibitor with neutrophil myeloperoxidase. *Biochemistry,* **20**:331-336.

Matthay, M. A., Eschenbacher, W. L., and Goetzl, E. J. (1984). Elevated concentrations of leukotrienes D_4 in pulmonary edema fluid of patients with the adult respiratory distress syndrome. *J. Clin. Immunol.,* **4**:479-483.

Matuschak, G. M., and Rinaldo, J. E. (1988). Organ interaction in the adult respiratory distress syndrome during sepsis. Role of the liver in host defense. *Chest,* **94**:400-406.

McCord, J. M. (1987). Oxygen-derived radicals: A link between reperfusion injury and inflammation. *Fed. Proc.,* **46**:2402-2406.

Minta, J. O., Man, D., and Movat, H. Z. (1977). Kinetic studies on the fragmentations of the third component of complement (C_3) by trypsin. *J. Immunol.,* **118**:2192-2198.

Montgomery, A. B., Stager, M. A., Carrico, C. J., and Sludson, L. D. (1985). Causes of mortality in patients with the adult respiratory distress syndrome. *Am. Rev. Respir. Dis.,* **132**:485-489.

Morel, D. R., Dargent, F., Bachmann, M., Suter, P. M., and Junod, A. (1985). Pulmonary extraction of serotonin and propranolol in patients with adult respiratory distress syndrome. *Am. Rev. Respir. Dis.,* **132**: 479-485.

Morrissey, R., Beri, J. E., Fridhandler, L., and Pelot, D. (1980). The nature and significance of hyperamylasemia following operation. *Ann. Surg.,* **180**:67-71.

Moscatelli, D., Jaffe, E., and Rifkin, D. B. (1980). Tetradecanoyl phorbol acetate stimulates latent collagenase production by cultured human endothelial cells. *Cell,* **20**:343-351.

Mosher, D. F. (1983). Synthesis of α_2-macroglobulin by cultured adherent cells. *Ann. N.Y. Acad. Sci.,* **421**:327-331.

Mosher, D. F., and Vaheri, A. (1980). Binding and degradation of α_2 macroglobulin by cultured fibroblasts. *Biochim. Biophys. Acta,* **27**:113-122.

Mosher, D. F., Saskela, O., and Vaheri, A. (1977). Synthesis and secretion of α_2-macroglobulin by culture adherent lung cells. *J. Clin. Invest.,* **60**: 1036-1045.

Muller-Eberhard, H. J. (1988). Complement: Chemistry and pathways. In *Inflammation: Basic Principles and Clinical Correlates.* Edited by J. I. Gallin, I. M., Goldstein, and R. Snyderman. New York, Raven Press, pp. 21-53.

Muller-Esterl, W., Iwanaga, S., and Nakaninski, S. (1986). The revised kininogens. *Trends Biochem. Sci.,* **11**:336.

Murphy, G., Reynolds, J. J., Bretz, U., and Baggiolini, M. (1977). Collagenase is a component of the specific granules of human neutrophil leukocytes. *Biochem. J.,* **162**:195-197.

Murphy, G., Reynolds, J. J., and Werb, Z. (1985). Biosynthesis of tissue inhibitor of metalloproteinases by human fibroblasts in culture. *J. Biol. Chem.,* **260**:3079-3083.

Murray, J. F., Matthay, M. A., Luce, J. M., and Flick, M. R. (1988). Pulmonary perspectives. An expanded definition of the adult respiratory distress syndrome. *Am. Rev. Respir. Dis.,* **138**:720-723.

Musiani, P., Massi, G., and Piantelli, M. (1976). Separation of different molecular forms of serum α_1-antitrypsin. *Clin. Chim. Acta,* **73**:S61-S65.

Neurath, H., and Walsh, K. A. (1976). Role of proteolytic enzymes in biological regulation (a review). *Proc. Natl. Acad. Sci. USA,* **73**:3825-3832.

Nevalainen, T. J. (1980). The role of phospholipase A. *Scand. J. Gastroenterol.,* **15**:641-650.

Newball, H. H., Berninger, R. W., Talamo, R. C., and Lichtenstein, L. M. (1979). Anaphylactic release of a basophil kallikrein-like activity. I. Purification and characterization. *J. Clin. Invest.,* **64**:457-465.

Nicod, L., Leuenberger, C., Seydoux, C., Rey, F., Van Melle, G., and Perret, C. (1985). Evidence for pancreas injury in adult respiratory distress syndrome. *Am. Rev. Respir. Dis.,* **131**:696-699.

Niederman, M. S., Fritts, L. L., Merrill, W. W., Fick, R. B., Matthay, R. A., Reynolds, H. Y., and Gee, I. B. (1984). Demonstration of a free elastolytic metalloenzyme in human lung lavage fluid and its relationship to alpha$_1$-antiprotease. *Am. Rev. Respir. Dis.,* **129**:943-947.

Nuytinck, J. K., Goris, J. A., Redl, H. R., Schlagg, G., and Van Munster, P. J. (1986). Post-traumatic complications and inflammatory mediators. *Arch. Surg.,* **121**:886-890.

Ny, T., Sawdey, M., Lawrence, D., Millan, J. L., and Loskutoff, D. J. (1986). Cloning and sequence of a cDNA coding for the human beta-migrating endothelial-cell-type plasminogen activator inhibitor. *Proc. Natl. Acad. Sci. USA,* **83**:6776-6780.

Ogawa, M. (1988). Pancreatic secretory trypsin inhibitor as an acute phase reactant. *Clin. Biochem.,* **21**:19-25.

Ohkubo, I., Kurachi, K., Takasowa, T., Shiokawa, H., and Sasaki, M. (1984). Isolation of a human c-DNA for α_2-thiol proteinase inhibitor and its identity with low molecular weight kininogen. *Biochemistry,* **23**:5691-5697.

Ohkubo, I., Namikawa, C., and Kigashiyama, S. (1988). Purification and characterization of a α_1-thiol proteinase inhibitor and its identity with kinin and fragment 1-2-free high molecular weight kininogen. *Int. J. Biochem.,* **20**:243-249.

Ohlsson, K. (1981). Elimination of ^{125}I-trypsin-alpha-macroglobulin complexes from blood by reticuloendothelial cells in dog. *Acta Physiol. Scand.,* **81**:269-272.

Ohlsson, K. K., Olsson, I., and Spitznagel, J. K. (1977). Localization of chymotrypsinlike cationic protein, collagenase, and elastase in azurophilic granules of human neutrophilic polymorphonuclear leukocytes. *Hoppe Seylers Z. Physiol. Chem.,* **358**:361-366.

Ohlsson, K., Balldin, G., Borgström, A., and Genell, S. (1982). On the role of trypsin and trypsin inhibitors in acute pancreatitis. In *Role of Chemical Mediators in the Pathophysiology of Acute Illness and Injury.* Edited by R. J. McCoon. New York, Raven Press, pp. 132-150.

Okada, Y., Watanabe, S., and Nakanishi, I. (1988). Inactivation of tissue inhibitor of metalloproteinases by neutrophil elastase and other serine proteinases. *FEBS Lett.,* **229**:157-160.

Olsson, I., and Venge, P. (1974). Cationic proteins of human granulocytes. II. Separation of the cationic proteins of the granules of leukemic myeloid cells. *Blood,* **44**:235-245.

Padrines, M., Schneider-Pozzer, M., and Bieth, J. G. (1989). Inhibition of neutrophil elastase by alpha-1-proteinase inhibitor oxidized by activated neutrophils. *Am. Rev. Respir. Dis.,* **139**:783-790.

Pagano, M., Esnard, F., Engler, R., and Gauthier, F. (1984). Inhibition of human liver cathepsin L by α_2-cysteine-proteinase inhibitor and the low-Mr cysteine proteinase inhibitor from human serum. *Biochem. J.,* **220**: 147-155.

Panebianco, A. C., Scott, S. M., and Dart, C. H. (1970). Acute pancreatitis following extracorporeal circulation. *Ann. Thorac. Surg.,* **9**:562-567.

Pannell, R., Johnson, D., and Travis, J. (1974). Isolation and properties of human plasma-α_1-proteinase inhibitor. *Biochemistry,* **13**:5439-5445.

Penn, I., Durst, A. L., and Machado, M. (1970). Acute pancreatitis following extracorporeal circulation. *Ann. Thorac. Surg.,* **9**:562-569.

Pepe, P. E., Potkin, R. T., Holtman-Reus, D., Hudson, L. D., and Carrico, C. J. (1982). Clinical predictors of the adult respiratory distress syndrome. *Am. J. Surg.,* **144**:124-130.

Peppin, G. J., and Weiss, S. J. (1986). Activation of the endogenous metalloproteinase gelatinase by triggered human neutrophils. *Proc. Natl. Acad. Sci. USA,* **83**:4322-4326.

Perez, H. D., Horn, J. K., Ong, R., and Goldstein, I. M. (1983). Complement (C5)-derived chemotactic activity in serum from patients with pancreatitis. *J. Lab. Clin. Med.,* **101**:123-129.

Petty, T. L. (1985). Indicators of risk, course and prognosis in adult respiratory distress syndrome (ARDS). *Am. Rev. Respir. Dis.,* **132**:471.

Petty, T. L., and Ashbaugh, D. G. (1971). The adult respiratory distress syndrome: Clinical features, factors influencing prognosis and principles of management. *Chest,* **70**:233-239.

Pontoppidan, H., Hüttemeier, P. C., and Quinn, D. A. (1985). Etiology, demography and outcome. In *Adult Respiratory Failure.* Edited by W. Zapol and R. Falke. New York, Marcel Dekker, pp. 1-21.

Postlethwaite, A. E., and Kang, A. H. (1988). Fibroblasts. In *Inflammation: Basic Principles and Clinical Correlates.* Edited by J. I. Gallin, I. M. Goldstein, and R. Snyderman. New York, Raven Press, pp. 577-597.

Powanda, M. L., and Meyer, E. D. (1981). Plasma protein alterations during infection: Potential significance of these changes to host defense and repair systems. In *Infection: The Physiologic and Metabolic Responses of the Host.* Edited by M. C. Powanda and P. G. Canonico. Amsterdam, Elsevier, pp. 271-295.

Powe, J. E., Short, A., Sibbald, W. J., and Driedger, A. A. (1982). Pulmonary accumulation of polymorphonuclear leukocytes in the adult respiratory distress syndrome. *Crit. Care Med.,* **10**:712-718.

Pratt, C. W., and Pizzo, S. V. (1987). Mechanism of action of inter-α-trypsin inhibitor. *Biochemistry,* **26**:2855-2863.

Pubols, J. E., Bartelt, D. C., and Greene, L. (1974). Trypsin inhibitor from human pancreas and pancreatic juice. *J. Biol. Chem.,* **249**:2242-2249.

Regoli, D., and Barabe, J. (1980). Pharmacology of bradykinin and related kinins. *J. Pharmacol. Rev.,* **32**:1-45.

Reid, K. B., and Porter, R. R. (1981). The proteolytic activation systems of complement. *Annu. Rev. Biochem.,* **50**:433-464.

Reines, H. D., Halushka, P. V., Cook, J. A., Wise, W. C., and Rambo, W. (1982). Plasma thromboxane concentrations are raised in patients dying with septic shock. *Lancet,* **2**:174-175.

Rinaldo, J. E. (1986). Indicators of risk, course and prognosis in adult respiratory distress syndrome. *Am. Rev. Respir. Dis.,* **133**:343-344.

Rinaldo, J. E., and Rogers, R. M. (1982). Adult respiratory distress syndrome. *N. Engl. J. Med.,* **306**:900-912.

Rinaldo, J. E., Dauber, J. H., Christman, J., and Rogers, R. M. (1984). Neutrophil alveolitis following endotoxemia. *Am. Rev. Respir. Dis.*, **130**:1065-1071.

Rinderknecht, H., and Geokas, M. C. (1973). On the physiological role of α_2-macroglobulin. *Biochim. Biophys. Acta,* **295**:233-244.

Risberg, B. O., Medegard, A., Heideman, M., Gyzander, E., Bundsen, P., Odén, M., and Teger-Nilsson, A. C. (1986). Early activation of humoral proteolytic systems in patients with multiple trauma. *Crit. Care Med.,* **14**:917-925.

Roberts, R. C., and Hall, P. K. (1983). Specificity of proteinase for the "bait" region of α_2-macroglobulin. *Ann. N.Y. Acad. Sci.,* **421**:61-68.

Rosenberg, S., Barr, P. J., Najarian, R. C., and Hallewell, R. A. (1984). Synthesis in yeast of a functional oxidation-resistant mutant of human alpha-antitrypsin. *Nature,* **312**:77-80.

Roy, R. S., and McCord, J. M. (1982). Ischemia induced conversion of xanthine deshydrogenase to xanthine-oxidase. *Fed. Proc.,* **41**:767-772.

Ryan, U. S. (1987). Endothelial cell activation responses. In *Pulmonary Endothelium in Health and Disease.* Edited by U. S. Ryan. New York, Marcel Dekker, pp. 3-33.

Saldeen, T. (1982). Fibrin-derived peptides and pulmonary injury. *Ann. N.Y. Acad. Sci.,* **483**:310-331.

Saldeen, T. (1983). Clotting microembolism and inhibition of fibrinolysis in adult respiratory distress. *Surg. Clin. North Am.,* **63**:285-304.

Salvesen, G. S., and Barrett, A. J. (1980). Covalent binding of proteinases in their reaction with α_2-macroglobulin. *Biochem. J.,* **187**:695-701.

Satake, K., Rozmanith, J. S., Appert, H., and Howard, J. M. (1973). Hemodynamic change and bradykinin levels in plasma and lymph during experimental acute pancreatitis in dogs. *Ann. Surg.,* **178**:659-662.

Schapira, M., Scott, C. F., and Colman, R. W. (1982). Contribution of plasma protease inhibitors to the inactivation of kallikrein in plasma. *J. Clin. Invest.,* **69**:462-468.

Schneider, R. C., Zapol, W. M., and Carvalho, A. C. (1980). Platelet consumption and sequestration in severe acute respiratory failure. *Am. Rev. Respir. Dis.,* **122**:445-451.

Schwartz, L. B., Lewis, R. A., and Austen, K. F. (1981). Trypase from human pulmonary mast cells. *J. Biol. Chem.,* **256**:11939-11943.

Scott, C. F., Schapira, M., James, H. L., Cohen, A. B., and Colman, R. W. (1982a). Inactivation of factor XIa by plasma protease inhibitors. *J. Clin. Invest.,* **69**:844-852.

Scott, C. F., Schapira, M., James, H. L., Cohen, A. B., and Colman, R. W. (1982b). Inactivation of factor XIa by plasma protease inhibitors. Predominant role of alpha-1-protease inhibitor and the protective effect of high molecular weight kininogen. *J. Clin. Invest.,* **69**:844-852.

Sealy, J., Atlas, S. A., Laragh, J. H., Oza, N. B., and Ryan, J. W. (1978). Human urinary kallikrein converts inactive to active renin and is a possible physiologic activation of renin. *Nature,* **275**:144-145.

Senior, R. M., Griffin, G. L., and Mecham, R. P. (1980). Chemotactic activity of elastin-derived peptides. *J. Clin. Invest.,* **66**:859-862.

Senior, R. M., Connolly, N. L., Cury, J. D., Welgus, H. G., and Campbell, E. J. (1989). Elastin degradation by human alveolar macrophages. *Am. Rev. Respir. Dis.,* **139**:1251-1256.

Simon, R. H., and Ward, P. A. (1988). Adult respiratory distress syndrome. In *Inflammation: Basic Principles and Clinical Correlates.* Edited by J. I. Gallin, I. M. Goldstein, and R. Snyderman. New York, Raven Press, pp. 815-827.

Siraganian, R. P. (1988). Mast cells and basophils. In *Inflammation: Basic Principles and Clinical Correlates.* Edited by J. I. Gallin, I. M. Goldstein, and R. Snyderman. New York, Raven Press, pp. 513-542.

Slotman, G. J., Burchard, K. W., and Gann, D. S. (1985). Thromboxane and prostacyclin in clinical acute respiratory failure. *J. Surg. Res.,* **39**: 1-7.

Smith, J. J., Hougland, M. W., and Johnson, D. A. (1984). Human lung tryptase. Purification and characterization. *J. Biol. Chem.,* **259**:11046-11051.

Smith-Erichsen, N., Aasen, A. D., and Amundsen, E. (1982). Treatment of sepsis in the surgical patient evaluated by means of chromogenic peptide substrate assays. *Acta Clin. Scand.,* **509**:33-38.

Solomkin, J. S., Cotta, L. A., Satoh, P. S., Hurst, J. M., and Nelson, R. D. (1985). Complement activation and clearance in acute illness and injury: Evidence for C5a as a cell directed mediator of the adult respiratory distress syndrome in man. *Surgery,* **97**:668-678.

Stahl, W. M. (1987). Acute phase protein response to tissue injury. *Crit. Care Med.,* **15**:545-555.

Stead, N., Kaplan, A. P., and Rosenberg, R. D. (1976). Inhibition of activated factor XII by antithrombin-heparin cofactor. *J. Biol. Chem.,* **251**: 6481-6488.

Steinbuch, M. (1976). The inter-α-trypsin inhibitor. *Methods Enzymol.,* **45**: 760-771.

Steinbuch, M., and Audran, R. (1974). Biology and pathology of plasma proteinase inhibitors. In *Proteinase Inhibitors.* Edited by H. Fritz, H. Tschesche, L. J. Green, and E. Truscheit. Berlin, Springer-Verlag, pp. 78-95.

Steinbuch, M., Pejaudier, L., Quentin, M., and Martin, V. (1968). Molecular alteration of α_2-macroglobulin by aliphatic amines. *Biochim. Biophys. Acta,* **154**:228-231.

Stricklin, G. P., and Welgus, H. G. (1983). Human skin fibroblast collagenase inhibitor: Purification and biochemical characterization. *J. Biol. Chem.,* **258**:12252-12258.

Tahamont, M. V., and Malik, A. B. (1983). Granulocytes mediate the increase in pulmonary vascular permeability after thrombin embolism. *J. Appl. Physiol.,* **54**:1489-1495.

Tahamont, M. V., Barie, P. S., and Blumenstock, (1982). Increased lung vascular permeability after pancreatitis and trypsin infusion. *Am. J. Pathol.,* **109**:15-26.

Tanaka, T., McRae, B. J., Cho, K., Cook, R., Fraki, J. I., Johnson, D. A., and Powers, J. C. (1983). Mammalian tissue trypsin-like enzymes. Comparative reactivities of human skin tryptase, human lung tryptase and bovine trypsin with peptide 4-nitroanilide and thioester substrates. *J. Biol. Chem.,* **258**:13552-13557.

Tate, R. M., and Repine, J. E. (1983). Neutrophils and the adult respiratory distress syndrome. *Am. Rev. Respir. Dis.,* **128**:552.

Test, S. T., Lampert, M. B., and Ossanna, P. J. (1984). Generation of nitrogen-chloride oxidants by human phagocytes. *J. Clin. Invest.,* **74**: 1341-1345.

Thommasen, H. V., Boyko, W. J., Russell, J. A., and Hogg, J. C. (1984). Transient leucopenia associated with adult respiratory distress syndrome. *Lancet,* **1**:809-812.

Thompson, R. C., and Ohlsson, K. (1986). Isolation properties and complete amino acid sequence of human secretory leukocyte protease inhibitor, a potent inhibitor of leukocyte elastase. *Proc. Natl. Acad. Sci. USA,* **83**:6692-6696.

Till, G. O., Johnson, K. J., Kunkel, R., and Ward, P. A. (1982). Intravascular activation of complement and acute lung injury. Dependency on neutrophils and toxic oxygen metabolites. *J. Clin. Invest.,* **69**:1126-1135.

Tilney, N. L., Bailey, G. L., and Morgan, A. P. (1973). Sequential system failure after rupture of abdominal aortic anevrysms. *Ann. Surg.,* **178**: 117-122.

Traverso, L. W., Ferrari, B. T., Buckberg, G. D., and Tompkins, R. K. (1977). Elevated post-operative renal clearance of amylase without pancreatitis after cardiopulmonary bypass. *Am. J. Surg.,* **133**:298-303.

Travis, J., and Johnson, D. (1981). Human α_1-proteinase inhibitor. *Methods Enzymol.,* **80**:754-765.

Travis, J., and Morii, M. (1981). Human α_1-antichymotrypsin. *Methods Enzymol.,* **80**:765-771.

Travis, J., and Salvesen, G. S. (1983). Human plasma proteinase inhibitors. *Annu. Rev. Biochem.,* **52**:655-709.

Travis, J., Baugh, R., Giles, P. J., Johnson, D., Bowen, J., and Reilly, C. F. (1978). Human leukocyte elastase and cathepsin G: Isolation, characterization and interaction with plasma proteinase inhibitors. In *Neutral Proteases of Human Polymorphonuclear Leukocytes.* Edited by K. Havemann and A. Janoff. Baltimore, Urban & Schwarzenberg, pp. 118-127.

Unkeless, J. C., Gordon, S., Reich, E. (1974). Secretion of plasminogen activator by stimulated macrophages. *J. Exp. Med.,* **139**:834-850.

Van Leuven, F., Cassiman, J. J., and Van Den Berghe, H. (1978). Uptake and degradation of α_2-macroglobulin protease complexes in human cells in culture. *Exp. Cell Res.,* **117**:273-282.

Velsaco, F., Torres, A., and Guerrero, A. (1986). Behaviour of the contact phase of blood coagulation in the adult respiratory distress syndrome. *Thromb. Haemost.,* **55**:357-360.

Wahl, L. M., Wahl, S. M., Mergenhagen, S. E., and Martin, G. R. (1974). Collagenase production by endotoxin activated macrophages. *Proc. Natl. Acad. Sci. USA,* **71**:3598-3601.

Walsh, K. A., and Wilcox, P. E. (1970). Serine proteases. *Methods Enzymol.,* **19**:31-40.

Walshe, K., Mackie, I., Gallimore, M., and Machin, S. J. (1987). Perturbation of the kallikrein-kinin system in adult respiratory distress syndrome. *Thromb. Haemost.,* **58**:418.

Warren, J. S., Warp, P. A., and Johnson, K. J. (1987). Mechanisms of damage to pulmonary endothelium: In *Pulmonary Endothelium in Health and Disease.* Edited by U. S. Ryan. New York, Marcel Dekker, pp. 107-120.

Warshaw, A. L., and O'Hara, P. J. (1978). Susceptibility of the pancreas to ischemic injury in shock. *Ann. Surg.,* **188**:197-201.

Weaver, D. W., Busuito, M. J., Bouwman, D. L., and Wilson, R. F. (1985). Interpretation of serum-amylase levels in critically ill patient. *Crit. Care Med.,* **13**:532-533.

Weigelt, J. A., Chenoweth, D. E., Borman, K. R., and Norcross, J. F. (1988). Complement and the severity of pulmonary failure. *J. Trauma,* **28**: 1013-1019.

Weiland, J. E., Davis, B., Holter, J. F., Mohammed, J. R., Dorinsky, P., and Gadek, J. E. (1986). Lung neutrophils in the adult respiratory distress syndrome. Clinical and pathophysiologic significances. *Am. Rev. Respir. Dis.,* **133**:218-225.

Weinberg, P. F., Matthay, M. A., Webster, R. O., Roskos, K. V., Goldstein, I. M., and Murray, J. F. (1984). Biologically active products of complement and acute lung injury in patients with the sepsis syndrome. *Am. Rev. Respir. Dis.,* **130**:791-796.

Weiss, S. J. (1989). Tissue destruction by neutrophils. *N. Engl. J. Med.,* **320**:365-376.

Weiss, S. J., and Peppin, G. J. (1986). Collagenolytic metaloenzymes of the human neutrophil: Characteristics, regulation and pontential function in vivo. *Biochem. Pharmacol.,* **35**:3189-3197.

Weiss, S. J., and Regiani, S. (1984). Neutrophils degrade subendothelial matrices in the presence of α_1 proteinase inhibitor. Cooperative use of lysosomal proteinases and oxygen metabolites. *J. Clin. Invest.,* **73**:1297.

Weiss, S. J., Peppin, G. J., Ortiz, X., Ragsdale, C., and Test, S. T. (1985). Oxidative autoactivation of latent collagenase by human neutrophils. *Science,* **227**:747-749.

Welgus, H. G., Campbell, E. J., Bar-Shavit, Z., Senior, R. M., and Teitelbaum, S. L. (1985). Human alveolar macrophages produce a fibroblast-like collagenase and collagenase inhibitor. *J. Clin. Invest.,* **76**:219-224.

Wendt, P., Fritsch, A., and Schulz, F. (1984). Proteinases and inhibitors in plasma and peritoneal exudate in acute pancreatitis. *Hepatogastroenterology,* **31**:277-281.

Werb, Z., and Gordon, S. (1984a). Secretion of a specific collagenase by stimulated macrophages. *J. Exp. Med.,* **142**:346-360.

Werb, Z., and Gordon, S. (1984b). Elastase secretion by stimulated macrophages. *J. Exp. Med.,* **142**:361-377.

Werb, Z., Banda, M. J., and Jones, P. A. (1980). Degradation of connective tissue matrices by macrophages. I. Proteolysis of elastin, glycoproteins and collagen by proteinases isolated from macrophages. *J. Exp. Med.,* **152**:1340-1357.

Wewers, M. D., Casolari, M. A., and Crystal, R. G. (1987). Comparison of alpha-1-antitrypsin levels and antineutrophil elastase capacity of blood lung in a patient with the alpha-1-antitrypsin phenotype null-null before and during alpha-1-antitrypsin augmentation therapy. *Am. Rev. Respir. Dis.,* **135**:539-543.

Wewers, M. D., Herzyk, D. J., and Gadek, J. E. (1988). Alveolar fluid neutrophil elastase activity in the adult respiratory distress syndrome is complexed to alpha-2-macroglobulin. *J. Clin. Invest.,* **82**:1260-1267.

White, R., Janoff, A., and Godfrey, H. P. (1980). Secretion of α_2-macroglobulin by human alveolar macrophages. *Lung,* **158**:9-14.

White, R., Janoff, A., Gordon, R., and Campbell, E. J. (1982). Evidence for in vivo internalization of human leukocyte elastase by alveolar macrophages. *Am. Rev. Respir. Dis.,* **125**:779-780.

Wiggins, R. C., Gielas, P. C., and Henson, P. M. (1981). Chemotatic activity generated from the fifth component of complement by plasma kallikrein of the rabbit. *J. Exp. Med.,* **153**:1391.

Wiggins, R. C., Cochrane, C. G., and McGuire, W. W. (1982). Hageman factor: Mechanisms and consequences of activation. In *Role of Chemical Mediators in the Pathophysiology of Acute Injury.* Edited by R. McCoon. New York, Raven Press, pp. 1-12.

Witte, J., Jochum, M., and Schever, R. (1982). Disturbances of selected plasma proteins in hyperdynamic septic shock. *Intensive Care Med.,* **8**:215-222.

Worthen, G. S., Haslett, C., Ress, A. J., Gumnay, R. S., Henson, J. E., and Jenson, P. M. (1987a). Neutrophil-mediated pulmonary vascular injury. Synergistic effect of trace amounts of lipopolysaccharide and neutrophil stimuli on vascular permeability and neutrophil sequestration in the lung. *Am. Rev. Respir. Dis.,* **136**:19-28.

Worthen, G. S., Lien, D. C., Tonnesen, M. G., and Hensen, P. M. (1987b). Interaction of leukocytes with the pulmonary endothelium. In *Pulmonary Endothelium in Health and Disease.* Edited by U. S. Ryan. New York, Marcel Dekker, pp. 123-160.

Zaslow, M. C., Clark, A., Stone, P. S., Calore, J., Snider, G. L., and Franzblau, C. (1983). Human neutrophil elastase does not bind to α_1-proteinase inhibitor that has been exposed to activated human neutrophils. *Am. Rev. Respir. Dis.,* **128**:434-439.

Zheutlin, L. M., Thonar, E. J., Jacobs, E. R., Hauley, M. E., Balk, R. A., and Bone, R. C. (1986). Plasma elastase levels in adult respiratory distress syndrome. *J. Crit. Care,* **1**:39-44.

Ziccardi, R. J. (1982a). Spontaneous activation of the first component of human complement (C1) by an intramolecular autocatalytic mechanism. *J. Immunol.,* **128**:2500-2504.

Ziccardi, R. J. (1982b). A new role for C1-inhibitor in homeostasis: Control of activation of the first component of human complement. *J. Immunol.,* **128**:2505-2508.

15

Capillary Pressure Measurement in Human Lungs

AUBREY E. TAYLOR, DORIS K. COPE, RONALD C. ALLISON, and SCOTT A. BARMAN

University of South Alabama College of Medicine
Mobile, Alabama

I. Introduction

The most important determinant of lung fluid balance is the pulmonary microvascular pressure, which is usually referred to as capillary pressure. Over the past 20 years we have emhasized that any critical assessment of lung fluid balance must include a reasonable estimate of cardiac output, left atrial pressure, pre- and postcapillary resistances, and a measure of the pulmonary capillary permeability to plasma proteins. The latter represents the only major parameter related to lung fluid balance that is difficult to measure quantitatively in either the experimental animal or clinical setting; however, the recent development of new scanning techniques may help to overcome this problem in the near future (Taylor and Parker, 1985).

Recently we developed a method for the assessment of the prevailing pulmonary capillary pressure in dog lungs (Taylor et al., 1982), which Cope et al. later modified to measure pulmonary capillary pressure for the first time in human lungs (1986). Since knowledge of the effective capillary pressure is essential in determining the fluid balance status of the lung, this measurement, which is based on physiologic and physical concepts, is first described using animal models, followed by a presentation of the recent capillary pressures collected in 37 cardiac patients before and after cardiac surgery. Measurement of the effective pulmonary capillary pressure is rapid and reproducible and is a reliable estimate of the existing pulmonary capillary pressure in several animal models. In addition, it can easily be measured in patients who have indwelling pulmonary arterial Swan-Ganz catheters without placing the patient in any additional danger.

II. Capillary Pressure and Its Relation to Transcapillary Fluid Exchange

The following equation is the Starling equation, which shows the relationship of capillary pressure (Ppc), tissue pressure (PT), colloid osmotic pressure of plasma (π_P), and tissue (π_T) to the volume flow (J_V) occurring across the capillary wall:

$$J_V = K_{fc}[(Ppc - PT) - (\pi_P - \pi_T)] \tag{1}$$

The tendency for the capillary to filter is represented by the Ppc − PT term; the absorptive pressure is related to the colloid osmotic pressure term $\pi_P - \pi_T$. Usually π_P is reasonably constant and Ppc is the major force that determines capillary filtration and edema formation. Classically, pulmonary capillary pressure has been determined by assuming that the pulmonary vascular resistance can be divided into a precapillary or arterial resistance (Ra) and a postcapillary or venous resistance (Rv) as shown in Figure 1. Gaar et al. (1967), who were the first to measure capillary pressure in dog lungs,

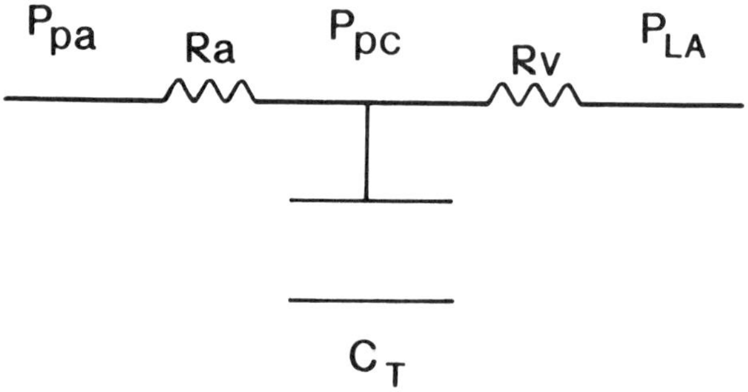

Figure 1 Electrical analog of the pulmonary circulation. Ppa is the pulmonary arterial pressure, Ra is precapillary resistance, Ppc is the pulmonary capillary pressure, Rv is the postcapillary resistance, Pla is left atrial pressure, and CT is the capacitance of the pulmonary circulation.

derived the following equation, which describes the relationship between pulmonary arterial pressure (Ppa), left atrial pressure (Pla), and the pre- and postcapillary resistances to the pulmonary capillary pressure:

$$\text{Ppc} = \text{Pla} + \frac{\text{Rv}}{\text{Ra} + \text{Rv}} (\text{Ppa} - \text{Pla}) \tag{2}$$

Equation (2) indicates that Ppc does not equal Pla. In fact, it only equals Pla when Rv = 0, which can only be approximated at high left atrial pressures. Table 1 shows how Ppc changes when total pulmonary vascular resistance (Rt) increases (shown as the second row) or decreases (shown as the third row). The examples in Table 1 were calculated for the conditions Ra = Rv, Ra > Rv, and Ra < Rv, respectively.

Several properties of the pulmonary circulation are evident from the examples shown in Table 1. When Ra = Rv, Ra > Rv, and Ra < Rv, capillary pressure always increases (rows 2 and 3) above control values when resistance is either increased or decreased! This occurs because flow is held constant, which best describes the flow conditions existing in the pulmonary circulation. Also, if Ra > Rv and total resistance is the same as in control conditions, then Ppc is decreased, but when venous resistance is higher than arterial resistance (Ra < Rv), elevation in capillary pressures results, and as can be seen, the highest capillary pressure occurs when total vascular resistance

Table 1 Calculation of Capillary Pressure (Ppc) and Arterial (Ra) and Venous (Rv) Resistance for Normal, Increased, and Decreased Rt at a Constant Cardiac Output of 5 liters/min

		Ppa	Pla	ΔP	Ra	Rv	Rt	Ppc	Change
Ra = Rv	1	20	5	15	1.5	1.5	3.0	12.5	Control
	2	35	5	30	3.0	3.0	6.0	20.0	↑
	3	20	12.5	7.5	0.75	0.75	1.5	16.25	↑
Ra > Rv	1	20	5	15	↑2.0	1.0	3.0	10.0	↓
	2	35	5	30	↑4.0	2.0	6.0	15.0	↑
	3	20	12.5	7.5	↑1.0	0.5	1.5	15.0	↑
Ra < Rv	1	20	5	15	1.0	↑2.0	3.0	15.0	↑
	2	35	5	30	2.0	↑4.0	6.0	25.0	↑
	3	20	12.5	7.5	0.5	↑1.0	1.5	17.5	↑

Source: Reproduced from Taylor, Rehder, Hyatt, and Parker, *Clinical Respiratory Physiology*, Saunders.

is elevated and left atrial pressure is unchanged. Another interesting prediction from Table 1 is that a decrease in pulmonary vascular resistance (line 3 in all examples) does not decrease Ppc because left atrial pressure increases as the pressure drop across the lung circulation is less. The heart could pump more blood, which would decrease the elevated left atrial pressure, but this is model prediction that requires further study.

The major reason for presenting the information in Table 1 is to show that capillary pressure cannot be determined only by measuring left atrial pressure (usually called the pulmonary capillary wedge pressure) or by evaluating the pressure gradient acting across the pulmonary circulation (ΔP). The pulmonary capillary pressure is a function of cardiac output, Ra, Rv, Ppa, Pla, and Ppa − Pla and the total vascular resistance Ra + Rv. Therefore, capillary pressure must be measured using the techniques described to predict this important determinant of pulmonary fluid balance.

III. Measurement of Pulmonary Capillary Pressure in Isolated Lungs

Figure 2 shows how the pulmonary arterial and venous outflow pressures respond in isolated dog lungs perfused at constant flow when either the inflow or outflow lines are clamped. This response was first observed by Hakim et al. (1979) and was critically analyzed by Dawson and Linehan's research group (Dawson et al., 1982; Linehan et al., 1982). The upper left panel in Figure 2a shows a pressure transient obtained following rapid clamping of the pulmonary artery (Ppa), which can be described by the electrical analog shown in Figure 1b: two distinct components of the arterial pressure curve tracing are observed following arterial occlusion. The first component in the pressure tracing is related to the resistance and capacitance characteristics of the larger pulmonary arteries in the lung and is of short duration. This initial pressure drop accounts for approximately 20% of the total drop occurring across the pulmonary circulation, which is 10 cmH_2O in this example. When the venous outflow (Pla) is suddenly occluded (right upper panel of Fig. 2a), a very rapid phase of the pressure transient occurs that equals 50% of the total pressure drop occurring across the pulmonary circulation, which is 25 cmH_2O in this case. This pressure drop is associated with the resistance and compliance characteristics of the larger veins.

When both arterial inflow and venous outflows are simultaneously clamped (as shown in the lower panel of Fig. 2a), both pressures equilibrate at the prevailing (or effective) capillary pressure (Ppc), which in this case is 35 cmH_2O (Dawson et al., 1982; Townsley et al., 1986). The pressure drop existing between the small arteries and the capillary pressure (Ppsa − Ppc) is only 10% of the total pressure drop (Ppa − Ppwedge) and can be calculated

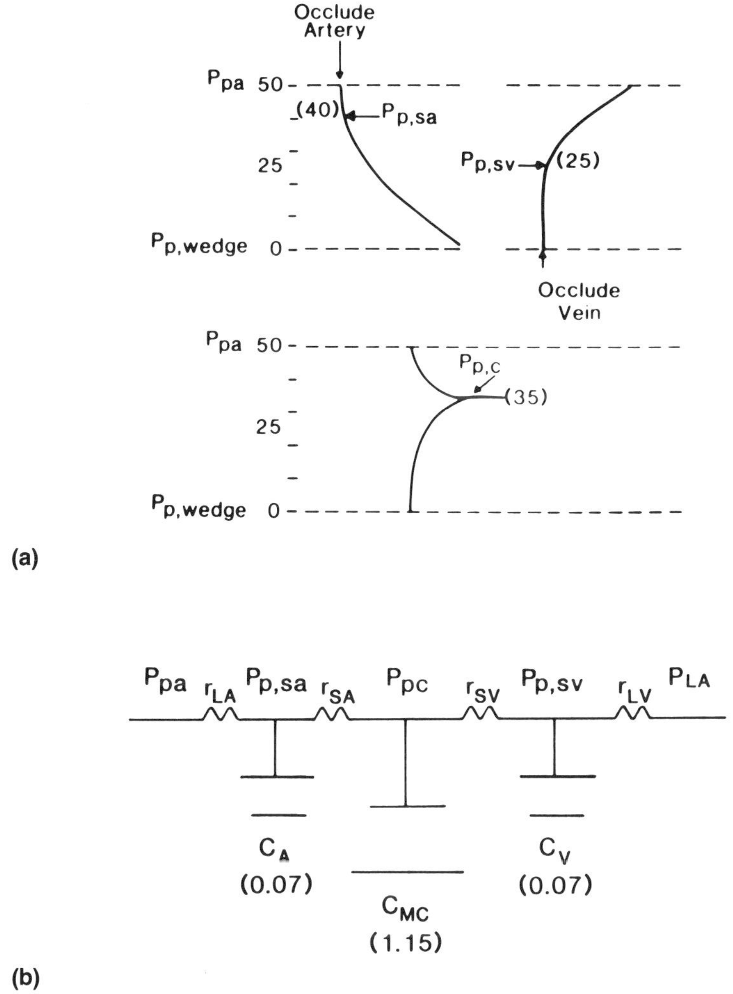

Figure 2 (a) Plot of pulmonary arterial pressure Ppa and pulmonary wedge pressure (Ppwedge) showing the rapid drop of Ppa to Ppsa when the arterial pressure line is suddenly clamped (left upper panel). The right upper panel shows the rapid rise of Ppwedge to Pssv in the Ppa tracing when the venous outflow is occluded. The lower curve shows the measurement of pulmonary capillary pressure (Ppc) when both inflow and outflow are clamped. (b) Electrical analog showing a three-compartment, four-resistance model when r_{LA} refers to large artery, r_{SA} to small artery, r_{SV} to small vein, and r_{LV} to large vein. C_A, C_V, and C_{MC} refer to compliance of the arteries, veins, and microcirculatory compartment, respectively.

by subtracting the double-occlusion capillary pressure (Ppc) from the Ppsa obtained from the rapid component of the arterial occlusion measurement. The pressure drop between the effective capillary pressure and small vein pressure is also 20% of the total pressure drop, or 10 cmH_2O. This example clearly shows that measurements of pre- and postcapillary resistances can be described by more than one pressure drop, which requires a measure of Ppc to properly analyze the system. Table 2 shows pressure drops calculated for the various vascular compartments as shown in Figure 2b when histamine (H), serotonin (5-HT), or norepinephrine (NE) is present in the pulmonary circulation (Rippe et al., 1984, 1987). The prevailing capillary pressure changes from a control value of 10-31 cmH_2O for histamine, to 20.6 cmH_2O for serotonin, and to 18.8 cmH_2O for norepinephrine, respectively. The pressure drops within the various segments of the pulmonary circulation are also different for each drug treatment. For example, the largest pressure drop that occurs with histamine is across the larger vein segment, and the smallest pressure drop for serotonin and norepinephrine is across the smaller veins. The segmental vascular compliances are also shown in Table 2. Note that the total compliance of the large arteries and veins is only 10% of the total compliance, with the largest compliance present in the microcirculation. Since the majority of the capillary filtration occurs in the most compliant region of the pulmonary

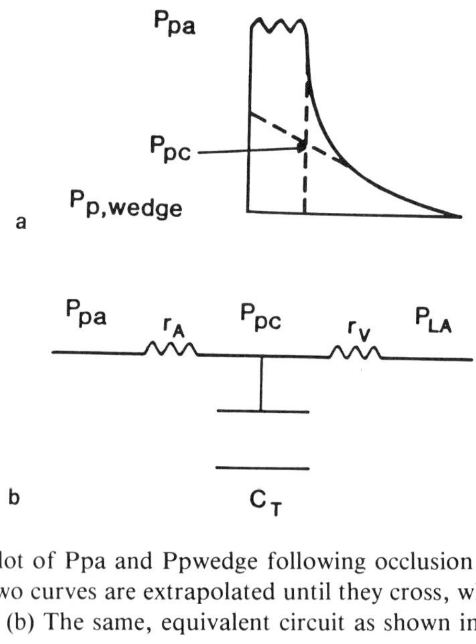

Figure 3 (a) Plot of Ppa and Ppwedge following occlusion of the pulmonary arterial line. The two curves are extrapolated until they cross, which gives a very good measure of Ppc. (b) The same, equivalent circuit as shown in Figure 1.

Table 2 Segmental Pressure Drops and Compliances in Dog Lungs

	Segmental pressure drops (cmH_2O)							Segmental compliances (ml/cmH_2O per 100 g)		
	Ppa	ΔPp,la	ΔPpsa	Ppc	ΔPpsv	ΔPp,lv	PP,wedge	Ca	Cms	Cv
Control	16.0	3.4	2.6	10.0	2.2	4.6	3.2	0.07	1.15	0.07
Histamine	41.0	4.8	5.2	31.0	2.7	25.0	3.3	0.02	0.35	0.02
Serotonin	46.5	14.2	11.7	20.6	5.5	11.9	3.2	0.015	0.37	0.015
Norepinephrine	34.3	8.9	6.6	18.8	1.7	13.8	3.3	0.05	0.75	0.05

circulation, this allows Ppc estimated by the double-occlusion technique to be identical to the classic isogravimetric capillary pressures measured by Gaar's method in an isolated perfused lung (correlation coefficients of 0.99 and slopes ≃ 1) (Holloway et al., 1983). From our earlier studies, it was shown that Ppc could be easily measured in isolated lungs, but how can Ppc be measured in lungs when their inflows and outflows cannot be simultaneously clamped, which is the situation when using a Swan-Ganz catheter in the patient?

IV. Measurement of Pulmonary Capillary Pressure Using Only Arterial Occlusion

Figure 3a shows how Ppc can be estimated following occlusion of a pulmonary arterial Swan-Ganz cathether in a closed-chest dog (Holloway et al., 1983). Remember that the early component of the arterial pressure transient is over very rapidly because of the low compliance of that segment of the circulation. This initial rapid component of the pressure tracing cannot be seen at relatively slow chart speeds because the compliance of the large arerial segment is only 5% of the total pulmonary vascular compliance. The usual recorder pressure profile is shown in the upper panel of Figure 2. Since the major compliance (capacitance) is located in the microcirculation (90% of the total compliance), when the initial transient is ignored in the arterial pressure transient following balloon expansion, the pulmonary circulation can be represented more simply as two resistances separated by a large microvascular capacitance. This electrical analog is shown in Figure 3b and is the same circuit used by Gaar for his classic study in isolated dog lungs (Gaar et

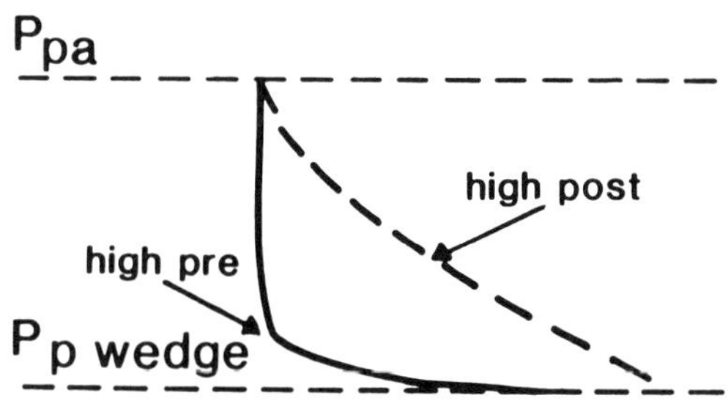

Figure 4 Plot of Ppa and Ppwedge tracing following occlusion of the arterial inflow line. When the precapillary resistance is high, which occurs with alveolar hypoxia, Ppa falls very rapidly toward Ppwedge. When postcapillary resistance is high, the approach of Ppa to wedge is much slower.

al., 1967). Capillary pressure can be more quantitatively measured by subtracting the Ppwedge from each point on the arterial pressure tracing after occluding the pulmonary artery and plotting Ppa − Ppwedge on semilogarithmic paper. The intercept of Ppa − Ppwedge can be used to calculate the capillary pressure (Holloway et al., 1983). However, in actual practice one can easily determine when the initial component of the curve is comleted by tracing lines on the two curves as shown by the dashed lines in Figure 3. When we compared this type of "eyeball" estimation of Ppc to that calculated using the proper mathematical calculation, the results were similar (Cope et al., 1986; Holloway et al., 1983). Although the most mathematically correct way of obtaining Ppc is to plot the log of Ppa − Ppwedge as a function of time and to extrapolate the line to zero time to obtain Ppc − Ppwedge, Ppc estimated as shown in Figure 3a is easily done and is accurate.

A rapid scan of the pressure transient can also indicate whether the resistance is primarily pre- or postcapillary, as shown in Figure 4. When precapillary resistance is high, Ppa drops very rapidly toward Ppwedge; consequently, when postcapillary resistance is high, the Ppa transient approaches Pwedge in a delayed fashion.

Following a determination of capillary pressure, the pre- and postcapillary resistances can be calculated as

$$\text{Precapillary resistance} = \frac{\text{Ppa} - \text{Ppc}}{\text{Q}}$$

and

$$\text{Postcapillary resistance} = \frac{\text{Ppc} - \text{Pla}}{\text{Q}}$$

V. Measurement of Pulmonary Capillary Pressure in Humans

Table 3 shows capillary pressures measured in patients undergoing coronary bypass, aortic valve replacement, and mitral valve replacement (Cope et al., 1986, 1988). Note that capillary pressure was about 10% above the wedge pressure in all the coronary artery bypass patients and cardiac patients prior to the operative procedures. Following both types of valve replacement surgery, the postoperative value of Ppc was considerably higher than the wedge measurements. The mitral valve patients show the greatest increase in capillary pressure. This increase in Ppc is related to an overall increase in total pulmonary vascular resistances located primarily in the postcapillary segment of the circulation. This set of data shows clearly that one cannot easily calculate prevailing capillary pressures using only the pulmonary arterial wedge measurement. In the critically ill patient, an increase of only a few

Table 3 Pulmonary Hemodynamic Measurements

Surgery	Ppa (mmHg)	Ppwedge (mmHg)	Ppc (mmHg)	Ppc/Ppwedge (mmHg)	CO (liters/min)	Ra/Rv (dyn/sec per cm^5)
Coronary artery bypass (n = 16)						
Preoperative	22.6 ± 1.3	16.6 ± 1.3	18.3 ± 1.3	1.11 ± 0.01	4.52 ± 0.25	2.81 ± 0.24
Postoperative	24.4 ± 2.0	17.2 ± 1.9	19.2 ± 1.9	1.14 ± 0.02	6.50 ± 0.54[a]	2.73 ± 0.22
Aortic valve replacement (n = 13)						
Preoperative	27.4 ± 2.6	20.7 ± 2.4	22.7 ± 2.5	1.11 ± 0.04	6.44 ± 0.60[b]	3.00 ± 0.41
Postoperative	23.2 ± 1.8[a]	15.3 ± 1.3[a]	17.7 ± 1.5[a]	1.16 ± 0.02[a]	6.70 ± 0.46	3.15 ± 0.51
Mitral valve replacement (n = 8)						
Preoperative	35.2 ± 4.3[b]	24.3 ± 2.1[b]	26.8 ± 3.2	1.10 ± 0.02	4.72 ± 0.82	3.36 ± 0.39
Postoperative	39.6 ± 5.1[b]	22.1 ± 1.9	28.2 ± 1.9[b]	1.28 ± 0.04[a,b]	4.82 ± 0.71	1.87 ± 0.27[a,b]

[a]$p < 0.05$, intragroup analysis.
[b]$p < 0.05$, intergroup analysis.
Source: Modified from Cope et al., *J. Cardiothorac. Anesthesiol.*, **2**:182-187, 1988.

millimeters mercury in pulmonary pressure can sometimes result in the formation of fulminating pulmonary edema.

Figure 5 illustrates how important the measurement of capillary pressure is in the assessment of lung fluid balance in the critically ill patient. In normal lungs, the pulmonary capillary pressure can increase by 20 mmHg before intra-alveolar edema results; at higher pressures, edema formation actually accelerates (B. Drake, personal communication). Often in a critically ill patient, the capillary endothelium is damaged and capillary pressure *must* be maintained at a very low level or edema results even at low capillary pressures (dashed curve). In fact, edema develops when capillary pressures are near normal. If fluid buildup occurs at low capillary pressures, as shown in

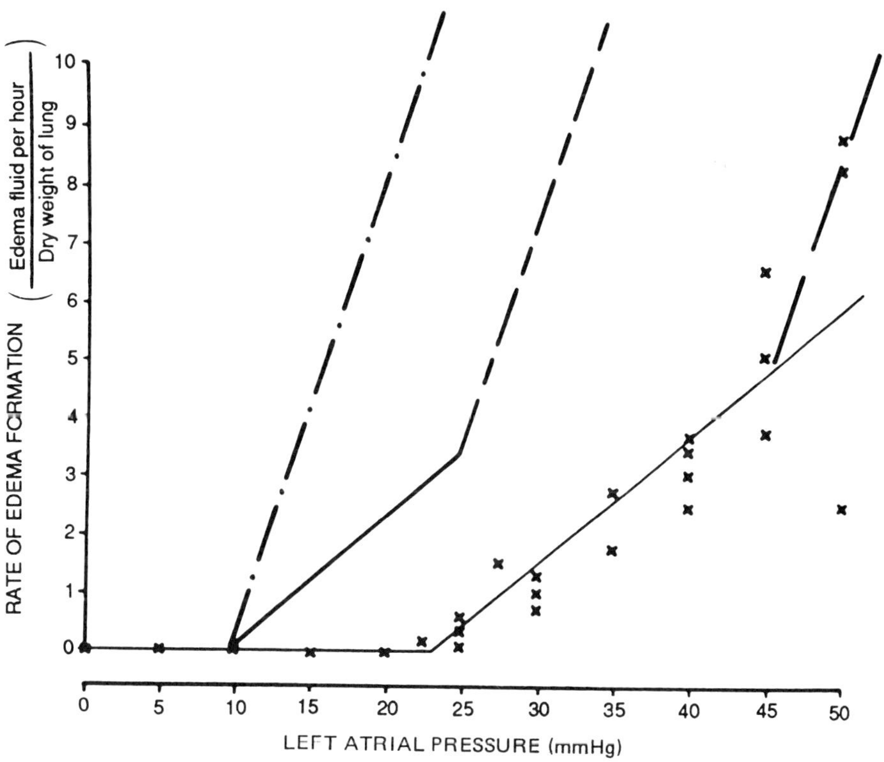

Figure 5 Plot of lung edema formation as a function of pulmonary capillary pressure for normal capillary pressures (right curve), damaged capillaries (middle curve), and damaged capillaries plus accelerated weight gain (left-hand curve). (Modified from Guyton and Lindsey, 1959.)

Figure 5 by the dashed and dotted line, then the rate of excessive edema formation accelerates (Guyton and Lindsey, 1959; Taylor, 1982).

As can be seen in Tables 1 and 2, the pulmonary arterial wedge pressure measurement is not always a good estimate of the pulmonary capillary pressure; in fact, it can greatly underestimate Ppc, as seen in the data shown in Figure 6. These data show the ratio of the capillary pressure to the wedge pressure measurement. Note that for both the coronary bypass (CABG) and aortic valve replacement (AVR) the difference between the capillary pressure and wedge pressure is that predicted by the Gaar equation. However, following mitral valve replacement, the pulmonary capillary pressure is greatly elevated above left atrial pressures. We do not recommend catheterizing a patient only to measure Ppc, but if a pulmonary arterial line is already in place, it becomes a simple matter to estimate Ppc, which provides the physician with a clearer understanding of the fluid volume status of the lung, especially when it is monitored simultaneously with therapy employed to decrease the rate of pulmonary edema formation. This method for the determination of Ppc is currently under study in other critical care units, and the usefulness of this measurement will certainly lead to the collection and dissemination of new information that will, it is hoped, relate the status of the pulmonary circulation to the critically ill patient in the near future (Collee et al., 1987).

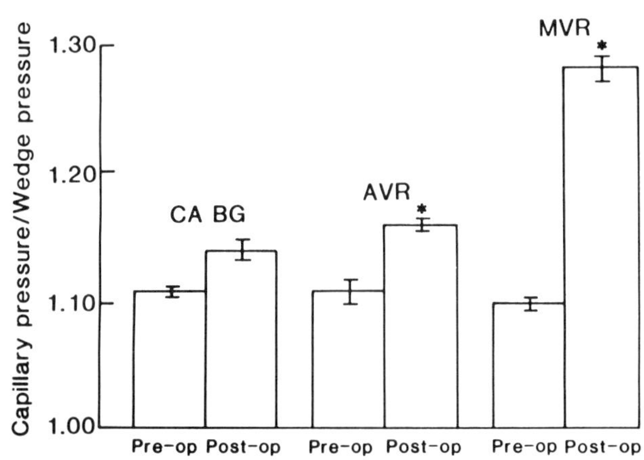

Figure 6 Plot of the ratio of capillary pressure to arterial wedge pressure measurement. Note that the wedge pressure and capillary pressures are not greatly different in a coronary artery bypass patient (CABG) from that predicted by the Gaar equation. Capillary pressure is slightly underestimated in aortic valve replacement (AVR), however, and is greatly underestimated in mitral valve replacement (MVR) compared to the pulmonary capillary wedge measurement. (Modified from Cope et al., 1986.)

Because pulmonary capillary pressure can be quickly and reproducibly measured in critically ill patients, we advocate its use to better understand the condition of the patient's pulmonary circulation. It is believed that the application of these techniques for measuring pulmonary capillary pressure and pre- and postcapillary resistances will lead to better patient care through the development of new treatment regimens coupled with the basic pulmonary and circulatory measurements.

References

Collee, G. C., Lynch, K. E., Hill, R. D., et al. (1987). Bedside measurement of pulmonary capillary pressure in patients with acute respiratory failure. *Anesthesiology,* **66**:614-620.

Cope, D. K., Allison, R. C., Parmentier, J. L., et al. (1986). Measurement of effective pulmonary capillary pressure using pulmonary artery pressure profiles after occlusion. *Crit. Care Med.,* **14**:16-23.

Cope, D. K., Allison, R. C., Dumond, M. E., and Taylor, A. E. (1988). Changes in the pulmonary capillary pressure after cardiac surgery. *J. Cardiothorac. Anesthesiol.,* **2**:182-187.

Dawson, C. A., Linehan, J. H., and Rickway, D. A. (1982). Pulmonary microcirculatory dynamics. *Ann. N.Y. Acad. Sci.,* **384**:90-106.

Gaar, K. A., Taylor, A. E., Owens, L. J., and Guyton, A. C. (1967). Pulmonary capillary pressure and filtration coefficient in the isolated perfused lung. *Am. J. Physiol.,* **213**:910-914.

Guyton, A. C., and Lindsey, A. W. (1959). Effect of elevated left atrial pressure and decreased plasma proteins concentration on the development of pulmonary edema. *Circ. Res.,* **7**:689-653.

Hakim, T. S., Dawson, C. A., and Linehan, J. H. (1979). Hemodynamic responses of dog lung lobe to lobar venous occlusion. *J. Appl. Physiol.,* **47**:145-152.

Holloway, H., Perry, M., Downey, J., and Taylor, A. E. (1983). Measurement of effective pulmonary capillary pressure in intact lungs. *J. Appl. Physiol.,* **54**:846-851.

Linehan, J. H., Dawson, C. A., and Rickway, D. A. (1982). Distribution of vascular resistance and compliance in dog lung lobe. *J. Appl. Physiol.,* **53**:158-168.

Rippe, B., Allison, R. C., Parker, J. C., and Taylor, A. E. (1984). Effects of histamine, serotonin, and norepinephrine on circulation of dog lungs. *J. Appl. Physiol.,* **57**:223-232.

Rippe, B., Parker, J. C., Townsley, M. I., Mortillaro, N., and Taylor, A. E. (1987). Segmental vascular resistance and compliance in dog lung. *J. Appl. Physiol.,* **62**:1206-1215.

Taylor, A. E. (1982). Capillary fluid filtration: Starling forces and lymph flow. *Circ. Res.,* **49**:557-575.

Taylor, A. E., and Parker, J. C. (1985). Pulmonary interstitial spaces and lymphatics. In *Handbook of Physiology, The Respiratory System, Circulatory and Non-Respiratory Function*, Sec. 3, Vol. 1, Chap. 4. Edited by Bethesda, American Physiological Society, pp. 167-230.

Taylor A. E., Parker, J. C., and Allison, R. C. (1982). Capillary exchange of fluid and protein. In *Critical Care Medicine*: *State of the Art*, Vol. 3. Fullerton, California, Soc. Crit. Care Med., pp. 1311-1326.

Townsley, M. I., Korthuis, R. J., Rippe, B., Parker, J. C., and Taylor, A. E. (1986). Validation of double vascular occlusion method for $P_{c,i}$ in lung and skeletal muscle. *J. Appl. Physiol.,* **61**:127-132.

16

The Adult Respiratory Distress Syndrome at Massachusetts General Hospital

Etiology, Progression, and Survival Rates 1978-1988

WARREN M. ZAPOL, MARK J. FRIKKER,* HENNING PONTOPPIDAN, and ROGER S. WILSON

Harvard Medical School
Massachusetts General Hospital
Boston, Massachusetts

KAREN E. LYNCH

Massachusetts General Hospital
Boston, Massachusetts

I. Introduction

Adult respiratory distress syndrome (ARDS) is a syndrome of acute respiratory failure. The diagnosis of ARDS rests on the presence of an increased right-to-left shunt, decreased pulmonary compliance, and recent bilateral and diffuse radiographic infiltrates in the absence of left atrial hypertension (usually confirmed by a pulmonary capillary wedge pressure less than 18 mmHg) (Pontoppidan et al., 1985). Mild pulmonary arterial hypertension is a usual concomitant of the syndrome; the degree of hypertension parallels the severity of the syndrome. The demographic incidence of the syndrome has been well described (Collins, 1969; Petty and Ashbaugh, 1971; Blaisdell and Schlobohm, 1973; Fulton and Jones, 1975; Petty and Newman, 1978). The precise incidence of ARDS is uncertain, with recent estimates varying from 4.5 cases/100,000 population/year in the United Kingdom (Webster et al., 1988), to 25 cases/100,000/year in San Francisco (Evans et al., 1988), to an older, 1970 estimate of 65 cases/100,000/year (Lung Program, 1972).

**Present affiliation*: William Beaumont Hospital, Royal Oak, Michigan.

While prospective identification of patients without lung disease who are likely to develop ARDS is difficult, such forecasting can be of value to the clinician. Several reports (Kaplan et al., 1979; Bell et al., 1983; Schmidt et al., 1976; Weigelt et al., 1979; Pepe et al., 1982, 1984; Fowler et al., 1983) describe an association of ARDS with one or more predisposing clinical conditions, the most common being septicemia and pneumonia (see Chapter 1, by Maunder and Hudson). Many reports provide evidence that the mortality rate of ARDS is high and increases with age and with the convergence in a single patient of more than one predisposing condition (Pepe et al., 1982; NHLBI, 1979; Bartlett et al., 1986).

A comprehensive, prospective 10-year analysis of adult acute respiratory failure has been performed at the Massachusetts General Hospital (MGH). Parts of that analysis are presented in this chapter.

From 1978 to 1988 the National Heart, Lung, and Blood Institute designated the MGH as a Specialized Center of Research (SCOR) in adult respiratory failure. This multidisciplinary SCOR group screened each patient upon admission to the Respiratory and Surgical Intensive Care Units (ICU), and, whether or not the patient developed ARDS, recorded information from that patient throughout the ICU stay.

Within 24 hr after a patient's arrival at the ICU, the severity of acute respiratory failure (ARF) was categorized as at risk, mild ARF, moderate ARDS, or severe ARDS according to the standardized radiographic, ventilatory, and arterial gas tension criteria outlined in Table 1. These criteria correspond in major part to those required for entry into the NHLBI multicenter study of ARF and extracorporeal membrane oxygenation (ECMO) (NHLBI, 1979; Zapol et al., 1979). Data recording then commenced and continued throughout the patient's ICU stay. A population of patients at high risk to develop ARF was identified and the subsequent clinical course recorded (see Table 1). These patients may later enter the ARF or ARDS groups if they meet necessary radiographic and gas exchange criteria. Survival rates of these four patient groups are presented in this report, particularly with respect to the initial etiology of lung injury, progression, and survival rates.

The reader should bear in mind three important points when considering these data. First, our categorization scheme for ARF is a simple one that was designed for easy classification at the bedside. Although ARDS can be defined with certainty, e.g., by histopathology at open lung biopsy, the clinical diagnosis of ARDS is very difficult to make in its mildest forms, and even when severe, there can be major variations in the presentation of ARDS. At times a patient can present with severe ARDS diagnosed by the criteria of Table 1, without exhibiting certain common features such as a markedly decreased pulmonary compliance, major pulmonary artery hypertension, or

Table 1 Classification of ARF (According to Severity) Used at the Massachusetts General Hospital Specialized Center of Research in Adult Respiratory Failure

Category of ARF	Chest radiograph	Tracheal intubation and positive airway pressure	Oxygenation
At risk of developing ARF (abdominal sepsis, long bone or pelvic fractures, other nonthoracic trauma)	Normal or minimal changes, e.g., segmental atelectasis	None, except for short-term routine support, e.g., postoperative therapy	O_2 administration only for short-term routine support, e.g., postoperative therapy
Mild	Minimal diffuse or lobar infiltrates or edema	May or may not be intubated and require positive airway pressure (CMV, IPS, CPAP)	$FI_{O_2} < 0.5$
Moderate (meets criteria for entry to NHLBI multicenter Additional Data Collection (25) but not criteria for severe ARF)	Panlobar alveolar infiltrates of one or both lungs	Intubated > 24 hr and need positive airway pressure (CMV, IMV, PEEP, CPAP)	$FI_{O_2} > 0.5$
Severe (meets rapid or slow criteria for entry into NHLBI multicenter study for ECMO) (18)	Bilateral panlobar alveolar infiltrates	Intubated and need CMV with PEEP	$Pa_{O_2} < 50$ mmHg with $FI_{O_2} = 1.0$ for 8 hr or longer or $FI_{O_2} \geq 0.6$ for 48 hr or longer

Abbreviations used:
CPAP: Continuous positive airway pressure
CMV: Continuous mandatory ventilation, also referred to as controlled mechanical ventilation
IMV: Intermittent mandatory ventilation
PEEP: Positive end-expiratory airway pressure
FI_{O_2}: Fraction of oxygen inspired
IPS: Intermittent pressure support

thrombocytopenia (Zapol and Snider, 1977). Eventually, patients with severe ARDS will exhibit most of these features. We chose not to use a scoring system to attempt to calibrate the degree of respiratory failure although such systems have been used for many years (Bartlett et al., 1976; Murray et al., 1988). Despite controversy over nomenclature, unilateral mild lung injury is defined here as mild ARF rather than ARDS. We made the diagnosis of ARDS only when diffuse lung injury progressed to moderate and severe ARDS.

Second, the data presented here are biased survival data. Survival in this report means the patient recovered sufficiently to be discharged from the ICU. The NHLBI ECMO study dramatically demonstrated that the likelihood of death of the ARDS patient increased markedly with concomitant failure of other major organ systems (heart, kidney, etc.) (Pepe et al., 1982; NHLBI, 1979; Bartlett et al., 1986). Although a distinction between a "respiratory" and a "nonrespiratory" death is pyrrhic for the patient, we believe the difference is important for physicians caring for acute respiratory failure patients. Respiratory deaths were defined for this report as a Pa_{O_2} equal to or less than 50 mmHg despite maximal respiratory support (i.e., mechanical ventilation with PEEP greater than 10 cm H_2O). Thus, by definition, all patients who died of respiratory failure were classified in the severe ARDS group (Table 1).

Third, because of patterns of referral to our hospital and the logistics of patient care within our hospital, patients tend to be admitted to the ICU after they require endotracheal intubation and mechanical ventilation with well-established moderate or severe ARDS. Thus much of the data reported here reflect our ICU admission pattern of patients with moderate or severe respiratory illness.

Finally, regarding definitions, in this report a septic syndrome is defined as patients with either a proven focus of infection (abcess, cellulitis, wound infection) or culture-positive septicemia. Bacterial pneumonia is diagnosed when a chest radiograph shows new infiltrates associated with bacteria and polymorphonuclear cells observed in the gram stain of the tracheal aspirate. Viral pneumonia is diagnosed by exclusion of other causes of respiratory failure and histologic evidence on lung biopsy (or autopsy), antibody titer increases, or viral cultures.

II. Results

Between December 1, 1978, and December 1, 1988, 535 patients with ARF/ARDS were admitted to the Respiratory-Surgical and Gray ICU at the Massachusetts General Hospital.

A. Etiologies of ARF

The distribution of patients based on their major predisposing illness is shown in Tables 4 and 5. Since the MGH is a major trauma center for the city of Boston, 31.9% of the ARF patients admitted had suffered major trauma (see Fig. 1). This traumatic respiratory failure group is nearly equaled by a large group of patients (33.5%) who developed ARF due to pneumonia (bacterial, viral, aspiration). Abdominal and extraabdominal sepsis (excluding pneumonias) contributed to the development of lung disease in 22% of ARF patients. A large group of patients with inhalation injuries and other noninfectious causes of lung inflammation (e.g., after radiation therapy) comprise the miscellaneous group (12.5%).

B. ICU Mortality of ARF Classified at Time of ICU Admission

Of the entire group of 762 patients we studied at admission, including 227 patients at risk of ARF, 535 patients were classified as mild ARF, moderate or severe ARDS at the time of ICU admission (Table 2 and Fig. 1). The mortality rate paralleled the degree of severity of lung inflammation at admission. The overall mortality rate was 39.3%. Upon admission of these 535 patients, 352 had mild ARF, with a mortality rate of 28.1%.

Chest trauma, abdominal sepsis, and extraabdominal sepsis were the etiologies of ARF for about half of our patients (Table 4). The highest mortality rates were due to acute lung injury caused by diffuse infectious processes and pneumonias, including certain direct pulmonary insults in the miscellaneous category. ARF either following chest trauma or associated with local abdominal sepsis was associated with a lower risk of death (21.4% and 31.8%,

Table 2 ARF Patients: Distribution and Mortality According to Severity at Time of Admission to ICU

ARF severity group	No. of patients	%	No. of dying patients	Mortality in ICU (%)
Mild	352	65.8	99	28.1
Moderate	131	24.5	72	55.0
Severe	52	9.7	39	75.0
Total	535	100.0	210	39.3

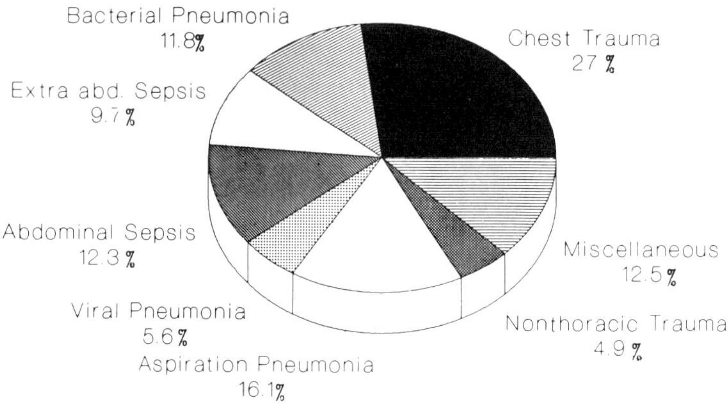

Figure 1 Percentage of 535 total patients developing ARF from various etiologies.

respectively). ARF occurring after nonthoracic trauma was infrequent (14 patients, or 4.9% of the initial ARF group) and resulted in only five deaths (19.2%).

C. Mortality Rates of Highest Severity of Acute Respiratory Failure

Table 5 provides the mortality rates of patients based on the highest degree of respiratory failure attained during the ICU course. The 535 patients admitted

Table 3 ARF Patients: Distribution and Mortality According to Highest Degree of Respiratory Failure Attained by All Patients Who Were Admitted with ARF or Developed ARF During Their Hospital Course

ARF severity group	No. of patients	%	No. of dying patients	Mortality in ICU (%)
Mild	333	52.4	63	18.9
Moderate	153	24.1	75	49.0
Severe	149	23.5	126	84.6
Total	635	100.0	264	41.6

Table 4 ARF Patients: Distribution and Mortality According to Admitting Etiology of Respiratory Failure

	Initial etiology		Mortality in ICU	
Admission diagnosis	No.	%	No.	%
Chest trauma	145	27	31	21.4
Nonthoracic trauma	26	4.9	5	19.2
Extraabdominal sepsis	52	9.7	27	51.9
Abdominal sepsis	66	12.3	21	31.8
Viral pneumonia	30	5.6	15	50
Bacterial pneumonia	63	11.8	41	65.1
Aspiration pneumonia	86	16.1	38	44.2
Miscellaneous: Smoke inhalation, lung cancer, radiation pneumonitis, etc.	67	12.5	32	47.8
Total	535	100.0	210	40.9

Table 5 ARF Patients: Distribution and Mortality for All Patients Who Developed ARF During Their Hospital Course

	Patients		Mortality in ICU	
Admission diagnosis	No.	%	No.	%
Chest trauma	157	24.7	35	22.3
Nonthoracic trauma	36	5.7	7	19.4
Extraabdominal sepsis	70	11.0	37	52.9
Abdominal sepsis	85	13.4	38	44.7
Viral pneumonia	31	4.9	16	51.6
Bacterial pneumonia	71	11.2	46	64.8
Aspiration pneumonia	89	14.0	40	44.9
Miscellaneous: Smoke inhalation, lung cancer, radiation pneumonitis, etc.	96	15.1	45	46.9
Total	635	100.0	264	41.6

with acute lung injury improved or suffered progression of respiratory disease and were joined in their respiratory disease categories by several of the 227 patients who, at the time of ICU admission, were judged to be "at risk" to develop ARF (see below). With these additional patients, the severe ARF group almost tripled in number, from 52 to 149 patients, while the moderate severity group grew only slightly (131 to 153) and the mild group was reduced in frequency (352 to 333). These data underscore the clinical observation that established ARDS frequently progresses in severity with time, while milder ARF often heals and lung function improves. However, at some early point, albeit brief, both moderate and severe ARDS patients usually can transiently be classified as mild ARF patients.

Mortality rates associated with the greatest degree of severity of these acute lung diseases (Tables 3 and 5) are generally as shown in Tables 2 and 4. However, the 18.9% mortality rate of mild ARF patients (Table 3) also reflects the loss from this group of those patients admitted with mild ARF whose lung disease progressed to a more severe category.

The overall mortality rate for all the studied patients with ARF at MGH during this 10-year period was 41.6%.

D. Patients at High Risk to Develop ARF

At the time of admission to the ICU, 227 patients were judged to be at high risk to develop ARF (Table 6). Each of these patients had suffered either abdominal or extraabdominal sepsis, chest trauma (without chest X-ray changes), or long bone or pelvic fractures, but at the time of ICU admission was not hypoxemic and had only minor pulmonary radiographic abnormalities (e.g., atelectasis). Patients with primary infectious pneumonitis in our

Table 6 Patients at Risk for ARF at Time of Admission: Distribution and Mortality According to Highest Degree of ARF During Hospital Course

ARF severity group	No. of patients	%	No. of dying patients	Mortality in ICU (%)
At risk	140	61.7	11	7.9
Mild	58	25.6	18	31.0
Moderate	11	4.9	11	100
Severe	18	7.9	16	88.9
Total	227	100.0	56	24.7

hospital generally bypassed this at-high-risk stage and were only transferred to the ICU after developing pneumonia or sepsis. Eighty-seven (38.4%) of the 227 high-risk patients developed acute lung injury and 45 of these ARF patients died, with an associated mortality of 51.7%. Twenty-nine patients (12.8% of the total at-high-risk group) developed moderate or severe ARF, and all but two died. The 140 at-high-risk patients who remained at high risk of acute lung injury but did not develop ARF had a 7.9% mortality (due to the failure of other organ systems), whereas at-high-risk patients who developed mild ARF had a fourfold increased (31.0%) mortality rate.

The mortality rates are similar for patients initially grouped as at high risk to develop acute lung injury and without radiographic signs of mild lung injury (mortality rate 24.7%) and those initially categorized as having mild ARF (mortality 28.1%). The two groups may differ only slightly and any distinction does not appear to alter their prognosis at the time of ICU admission. Our poor ability to distinguish those patients who have mild ARF from those without lung injury results from the inability of bedside radiography to detect minor increases of extravascular lung water as well as from the fact that both arterial gas tension analysis and the requirement for mechanical ventilation may not reflect minor degrees of pulmonary impairment.

Table 7 Patients at Risk for ARF at Time of Admission: Distribution and Mortality According to Admitting Diagnosis

Admission diagnosis	Total no. of patients	%	No. of dying patients	Mortality in ICU (%)
Chest trauma	26	11.5	5	19.2
Nonthoracic trauma	63	27.8	4	6.4
Extraabdominal sepsis	32	14.1	14	43.8
Abdominal sepsis	61	26.9	20	32.8
Miscellaneous: smoke inhalation, lung cancer, radiation pneumonitis, etc.	45	19.8	13	28.9
Total	227	100.0	56	24.7

At-high-risk patients admitted with extraabdominal sepsis had a 43.8% mortality (Table 7), whereas those with a miscellaneous pulmonary insult, chest trauma, or abdominal sepsis, respectively, had a 28.9, 19.2, and 32.8% risk of dying in the ICU.

III. Discussion

Acute respiratory failure is a common complication in critically ill patients. Estimates of its incidence are crude but permit an indirect assessment of its frequency. In 1982, 48,159 deaths were reportedly due to pneumonia in the United States (National Center for Health Statistics, 1982). In the 1092-bed Massachusetts General Hospital, we admitted 535 patients with acute lung injury to the Respiratory-Surgical and Gray ICU in 10 years, or about 54 patients per year. Thus we can estimate one acute lung injury patient per 17 university or referral hospital beds per year.

Hypoxic respiratory failure ($Pa_{O_2} \leq 50$ mmHg) was present before death in only 26 of 66 acute lung injury patients dying with severe ARF. For these critically ill patients ARF is only one of many causes of death. We are uncertain to what extent primary lung injury and its therapy (mechanical ventilation and barotrauma, oxygen therapy, invasive monitoring, tracheostomy, etc.) causes other organs to fail (e.g., circulatory failure, hepatic congestion) and to what extent injury to other major tissues and organs (e.g., heart, kidney) can augment injury to the lungs. It is likely that both mechanisms play important roles in increasing the mortality rate of acute lung injury. The more organ systems that fail in any critically ill patient, the greater the mortality rate (Pepe et al., 1982; NHLBI, 1979; Bartlett et al., 1986). The most common second organ to fail during acute respiratory failure is the kidney (33%) (NHLBI, 1979; Bartlett et al., 1986), perhaps because of the frequent coincidence of septic syndromes with acute respiratory failure (Bell et al., 1983). Survival from combined respiratory and anuric renal failure is uncommon and only a few patients manage this extraordinary feat.

The most common causes of acute respiratory failure vary from one hospital to another. Chest trauma, septic syndromes, and abdominal sepsis comprised the most common respiratory failure etiologies in our units admitting primarily surgical patients. In a medical intensive care unit, bacterial, viral, and aspiration pneumonia patients would predominate, whereas such patients accounted for only 33.5% of the admitting acute lung injuries in our ICUs. It is important to remember that the admitting diagnoses are the best estimates of trained nurses and physician observers. Almost all of our intubated and mechanically ventilated patients become colonized with nosocomial bacteria within a few days after admission and often have fever, leukocytosis, and radiographic abnormalities. It then becomes virtually impossible to distinguish airways colonization from invasive pneumonia. Clinical criteria are not helpful, and often only an autopsy with histopathologic analysis of the lungs allows the retrospective diagnosis of pneumonia (Bell et al., 1983; Andrews et al., 1981).

Acute lung injury due to several etiologies has decreased to extremely low frequencies in the past 10 years. Acute lung injury after nonthoracic trauma was uncommon (26/535 patients); only five nonthoracic trauma patients died. Modern methods of lung expansion, mechanical ventilation with PEEP, chest physiotherapy, suctioning, and antibiotics probably account for this high survival rate. Fat embolism was included in this etiology and respiratory failure always improved; there were no deaths from fat embolism.

Respiratory failure following cardiopulmonary bypass has a vanishingly small incidence. In this group we include acute respiratory failure after bypass without evidence of heart failure (pulmonary capillary wedge pressure less than 18 mmHg). Over several years we prospectively studied ARF at Massachusetts General Hospital; we observed only two cases immediately after cardiopulmonary bypass, both showing an elevated wedge pressure. In this period several thousand open heart bypass procedures were performed. This low incidence is significant because transient pulmonary leukosequestration and complement activation occur during cardiopulmonary bypass (as well as hemodialysis) and both have been considered possible etiologic agents of ARDS (Kirklin et al., 1983).

Our mortality rates (Table 3) for 153 patients with moderate ARDS (49.0%) and 126 patients with severe ARDS (84.6%) are similar to those reported (60 and 89%, respectively) in the NHLBI-sponsored, nine-hospital multicenter study of ARDS conducted between September 1975 and March 1977 (NHLBI, 1979; Bartlett et al., 1986). Thus there is little evidence for a major improvement of the survival rates of moderate and severe ARDS patients in the past 10 years. Indeed, there has been no major change in the respiratory therapy of severe ARF since widespread ventilation with PEEP was instituted in 1970. All of the moderate and severe ARF patients were treated with mechanical ventilation and the majority with PEEP. Our patients were treated with mechanical ventilation and PEEP with the $F_{I_{O_2}}$ no greater than necessary to maintain a safe Pa_{O_2} (50-100 mmHg). Prolonged bypass with a membrane lung was employed in only three ARF patients. Gattinoni and co-workers (1986) have suggested using prolonged membrane lung venovenous perfusion to remove CO_2 and reduce ventilator pressures, $F_{I_{O_2}}$, and lung damage. Iatrogenic causes of lung injury (barotrauma, oxygen toxicity) can increase the difficulties of treating acute lung injury. However, the major manpower requirements and minimally improved survival rates of adult ECMO, as well as fiscal restraints, have limited it to use as a research tool in a few European centers. Morris and co-workers in Utah are now carrying out a prospective randomized trial of membrane lung CO_2 removal by the venovenous route. At present most physicians caring for critically ill patients with acute respiratory failure have focused their studies on better defining the pathogenesis of ARDS, identifying early indicators, and testing novel drug therapies (anti J5 monoclonal antibodies, ibuprofen, *N*-acetylcysteine, etc.) to attempt to reduce the high mortality rate of acute inflammatory lung injury.

Acknowledgment

The authors thank the physicians and nurses of the Massachusetts General Hospital Respiratory-Surgical Intensive Care Unit and the Gray Intensive Care Unit for helping with data collection. This work was supported by NHLBI Grant HL23591.

References

Andrews, C. P., Coalson, J. J., Smith, J. D., and Johanson, W. G., Jr. (1981). Diagnosis of nosocomial bacterial pneumonia in acute, diffuse lung injury. *Chest,* **80**:254-258.

Bartlett, R. H., Brinker, P. A., Hill, J. D., Hill, R. N., and Wetmore, V. (1976). Indications for ECMO support: Quantitating pulmonary insufficiency. In *Artificial Lungs for Acute Respiratory Failure.* Edited by W. M. Zapol and J. Qvist. New York, Academic Press, pp. 373-382.

Bartlett, R. H., Morris, A. H., Fairley, H. B., Hirsch, R., O'Connor, N., and Pontoppidan, H. (1986). A prospective study of acute hypoxic respiratory failure. *Chest,* **89**:684-689.

Bell, R. C., Coalson, J. J., Smith, J. D., and Johanson, W. G. (1983). Multiple organ system failure and infection in ARDS. *Ann. Intern. Med.,* **99**:293-298.

Blaisdell, F. W., and Schlobohm, R. M. (1973). The respiratory distress syndrome: A review. *Surgery,* **74**:251-262.

Collins, J. A. (1969). The causes of progressive pulmonary insufficiency in surgical patients. *J. Surg. Res.,* **9**:685-704.

Evans, B. H., Wachter, R. M., Wiener-Kronish, J. P., and Luce, J. M. (1988). Incidence of ARDS in an urban population (Abstract). *Am. Rev. Respir. Dis.,* **137**:469.

Fowler, A. A., Hamman, R. F., Good, J. T., Benson, K. N., Baird, M., Eberle, D. J., Petty, T. L., and Hyers, T. M. (1983). Adult respiratory distress syndrome: Risk with common predispositions. *Ann. Intern. Med.,* **98**:593-597.

Fulton, R. L., and Jones, C. E. (1975). The cause of post-traumatic pulmonary insufficiency in man. *Surg. Gynecol. Obstet.*, **140**:179-186.

Gattinoni, L., Pesenti, A., Mascheroni, D., et al. (1986). Low frequency positive pressure ventilation with extracorporal CO_2 removal in severe acute respiratory failure. *JAMA*, **256**:881-886.

Kaplan, R. L., Sahn, S. A., and Petty, T. L. (1979). Incidence and outcome of the respiratory distress syndrome in gram negative sepsis. *Arch. Intern. Med.*, **139**:867-869.

Kirklin, J. K., Westaby, S., Blackstone, E. H., Kirklin, J. W., Chenoweth, D. E., and Pacifico, A. D. (1983). Complement and the damaging effects of cardiopulmonary bypass. *J. Thorac. Cardiovasc. Surg.*, **86**:845-857.

Lung Program, National Heart and Lung Institute (1972). *Respiratory Diseases: Task Force on Problems, Research Approaches, Needs.* Washington, D.C., Government Printing Office, pp. 171. [DHEW publication number (NIH) 73-432.]

Murray, J. F., Matthay, M. A., Luce, J. M., and Flick, M. R. (1988). An expanded definition of the adult respiratory distress syndrome. *Am. Rev. Respir. Dis.*, **138**:720-723.

National Heart, Lung, and Blood Institute (1979). *Extracorporeal Support for Respiratory Insufficiency: A Collaborative Study in Response to RFP NHLI 73-20.* NHLBI DLD.

Pepe, P. E., Potkin, R. T., Holtman Reus, D., Hudson, L. D., and Carrico, C. J. (1982). Clinical predictors of the adult respiratory distress syndrome. *Am. J. Surg.*, **144**:124-130.

Pepe, P. E., Hudson, L. D., and Carrico, C. J. (1984). Early application of positive end-expiratory pressure in patients at risk for the adult respiratory distress syndrome. *N. Engl. J. Med.*, **311**:281-286.

Petty, T. L., and Ashbaugh, D. G. (1971). The adult respiratory distress syndrome. *Chest*, **60**:233-239.

Petty, T. L., and Newman, J. H. (1978). Adult respiratory distress syndrome. *West. J. Med.*, **128**:339-407.

Pontoppidan, H., Huttemeier, P. C., and Quinn, D. A. (1985). Etiology, demography, and outcome. In *Acute Respiratory Failure.* Edited by W. M. Zapol and K. Falke. Lung Biology in Health and Disease series. New York, Marcel Dekker, pp. 1-21.

Schmidt, G. B., O'Neill, W. W., Kotb, K., Hwang, K. K., Bennett, E. J., and Bombeck, C. T. (1976). Continuous positive airway pressure in the prophylaxis of the adult respiratory distress syndrome. *Surg. Gynecol. Obstet.*, **143**:613-618.

Webster, N. R., Cohen, A. T., and Nunn, J. F. (1988). Adult respiratory distress syndrome—How many cases in the UK? *Anaesthesia*, **43**:923-926.

Weigelt, J. A., Mitchell, R. A., and Snyder, W. H. (1979). Early positive end-expiratory pressure in the adult respiratory distress syndrome. *Arch. Surg.,* **114**:497-501.

Zapol, W. M., and Snider, M. T. (1977). Pulmonary hypertension in severe acute respiratory failure. *N. Engl. J. Med.,* **296**:476-480.

Zapol, W. M., Snider, M. T., Hill, J. D., Fallat, R. J., Bartlett, R. H., Edmunds, L. H., Morris, A. H., Peirce, E. C., Thomas, A. N., Proctor, H. J., Drinker, P. A., Pratt, P. C., Bagniewski, A., and Miller, R. G. (1979). Extracorporeal membrane oxygenation in severe acute respiratory failure: A randomized prospective study. *JAMA,* **242**:2193-2196.

17

Abnormalities of Lung Surfactant Function in Patients with Acute Lung Injury

Implications for Therapy

ROGER G. SPRAGG

University of California
San Diego, California

I. Introduction

Physicians who provided some of the early descriptions of the adult respiratory distress syndrome (ARDS) suspected that abnormalities of the lung surfactant system might contribute to the pathophysiology of this condition (Ashbaugh et al., 1967). Despite those early suggestions, little attention has been paid to abnormalities of the lung surfactant system in patients with ARDS—or, in fact, in adult patient with almost any kind of pulmonary abnormality. In recent years, significant advances have been made in understanding the composition of lung surfactant. These advances have been stimulated by the proven efficacy of surfactant replacement therapy in the treatment of the infant respiratory distress syndrome (IRDS). As parallels between IRDS and ARDS have become clearer and as investigators have demonstrated that surfactant replacement may have a role in the therapy of acute experimental lung injury, interest in understanding abnormalities of the lung surfactant system in patients with ARDS has been rekindled.

Lung surfactant, particularly considerations relevant to replacement therapy for infants with IRDS, have been the subject of several recent excellent reviews (Jobe and Ikegami, 1987; Notter and Shapiro, 1987).

II. Surfactant System of the Healthy Lung: Composition and Structure

The term "surfactant" as used in pulmonary medicine refers to the complex mixture of phospholipids, neutral lipids, and protein that can be recovered by lung lavage or by gentle washing of lung fragments. This material may be purified by centrifugation techniques or by extraction into chloroform-methanol, in some cases followed by column chromatography. During such extraction, certain associated apoproteins are lost from the surfactant complex.

The lipid composition of adult human lung surfactant is relatively constant (Table 1). Dipalmitoylphosphatidylcholine (DPPC) is the most prominent lipid present and is thought to be largely responsible for the surface tension-lowering ability of lung surfactant. In addition, anionic phospholipids, principally phosphatidylglycerol (PG), phosphatidylinositol (PI), and phosphatidylserine (PS), may play an important role in providing necessary biophysical properties to the surfactant complex.

Surfactant-associated apoproteins, the focus of a great deal of current research, appear to exist in two classes. The first contains a single highly glycosylated protein of 32-36 kD that is synthesized and secreted by type II cells. The second class contains several hydrophobic proteins that are not glycosylated, that coextract with surfactant lipids into chloroform-methanol, and that range in molecular weight from 5 to 18 kD on sodium dodecyl sulfate-polyacrylamide gel electrophoresis (SDS-PAGE). Only these proteins are present in surfactant produced using chloroform-methanol extraction.

Table 1 Phospholipid Composition of Human Pulmonary Surfactants Recovered by Bronchoalveolar Lavage

Phospholipid	% Total phospholipid
Phosphatidylcholine	73.0
Disaturated	46.3
Phosphatidylserine	3.3
Phosphatidylinositol	2.7
Phosphatidylglycerol	12.4
Phosphatidylethanolamine	2.6
Sphingomyelin	3.7
Other	2.3

Source: From Hallman et al. (1983).

The precise function of the surfactant-associated proteins is not completely clear. The 32-36 kD protein appears to enhance absorption of phospholipid mixtures to the air/water interface (King and MacBeth, 1979) and to partially reduce minimum surface tension during dynamic in vitro testing (Revak et al., 1986). In addition, this protein may modulate the uptake of extracellular surfactant by type II cells and the secretion of surfactant by these cells (Dobbs et al., 1987; Wright et al., 1987).

The proteins of lower molecular weight appear to have a marked ability to lower absorption and minimum surface tension of phospholipid mixtures during in vitro testing (Revak et al., 1988), which is greater than that of the heavier protein. In addition, they may also modulate surfactant uptake by type II cells (Claypool et al., 1984).

Both surfactant apoproteins and phospholipids appear to be synthesized in type II cells, although the details of the intracellular organization of this process are not completely understood. Thus, events that cause type II cell injury may be expected to result in disturbance of surfactant production and/or composition.

Within the type II cell, the assembled phospholipid-apoprotein complex is stored in lamellar bodies prior to secretion. The organelles discharge their contents via an exocytotic process that may be initiated by agents that activate protein kinase A (e.g., cyclic AMP, β-adrenergic agonists, and cholera toxin), agents that activate protein kinase C (tetradecanoylphorbol acetate and 1-oleoyl-2-acetylglycerol), agents that raise intracellular calcium levels, or hyperventilation (Mason et al., 1984). The surfactant in lamellar bodies appears under electron microscopic examination to be a tightly coiled sheet with multiple lamellae or layers. Following exocytosis and in the presence of calcium, the surfactant takes the form of tubular myelin, a hydrated lattice of tubules associated with surfactant apoproteins (Benson et al., 1984; Stratton, 1984). Indeed, apoprotein appears critical for the formation of tubular myelin. It is likely that tubular myelin may spread to form a surfactant monolayer in the thin layer of fluid that lines the alveolar surface and that this monolayer is responsible for the clinically relevant biophysical properties of surfactant.

Once produced by type II cells and discharged into the alveolar lining fluid, surfactant is not simply cleared by macrophage ingestion or mucociliary means. Rather, it is able to be taken up type II cells and recycled for secretion in a process that may have some specificity for different forms of surfactant (Wright et al., 1986). The details and importance of this aspect of type II cell biology in both health and disease are not yet well understood.

III. Function

The classic experiments of Neergaard separated lung elastic forces from forces due to surface tension. He demonstrated that the retractive forces of saline-filled lungs, in which the air/liquid surface and hence surface tension is abolished, are much less than the retractive forces in gas-filled lungs. Clements extended these observations by demonstrating that gas-filled lungs from which surfactant function had been removed collapsed much more readily than did normal gas-filled lungs. Thus, it has been taught that the creation of an air/liquid interface with *high* surface tension during ventilation (as seen in surfactant-depleted lungs) is responsible for diminished compliance, and that the surfactant lining layer functions to minimize surface tension and increase lung compliance (Clements and Tieney, 1965). As a consequence, the work of breathing is reduced.

Using a very simplistic model, one may view the alveolus as an isolated bubble and apply the law of Laplace. This model predicts that if alveolar surface tension does not decrease during expiration as alveolar size decreases, then the pressure from surface tension (which tends to reduce alveolar volume) exceeds the transpulmonary distending pressure and alveolar collapse ensues. It has been concluded that a critical function of surfactant is to stabilize alveoli of different sizes during expiration and prevent the colapse of small alveoli. In addition, equalization of alveolar surface tension during inspiration may prevent undue difficulty in expanding small alveoli and promote homogeneous alveolar recruitment (Notter and Schapiro, 1987).

A theoretical consequence of lowering alveolar surface tension that may be distinct from alveolar stabilization is the ability to retard fluid flux into alveoli. Lowered alveolar surface tension results in a lesser pressure differential between the alveolar lining fluid and the alveolar gas; hypophase pressure is less subatmospheric than it would be in the absence of surfactant. This difference may be reflected directly to interstitial pressure, with the consequence that the hydrostatic pressure differential favoring fluid movement out of alveolar capillaries is decreased. There is some experimental evidence that supports these considerations (Guyton and Moffatt, 1981; Nieman and Bredengerg, 1985).

The importance of the dynamic aspects of the surface-lowering ability of lung surfactant have been well accepted and are a critical component of most in vitro tests of surfactant function. In the bubble surfactometer developed by Enhorning (1973), a bubble of known size is formed within the surfactant-containing liquid and then cyclically subjected to known changes in volume. Pressure within the bubble is continuously measured. The time from bubble formation to maintenance of stable pressure is taken as a measure of the ability of the surfactant material to absorb to the air/liquid interface, and the minimum surface tension during dynamic cycling is taken as a reflection of surface tension-lowering ability.

In addition to its biophysical properties, lung surfactant may be capable of modulating both lymphocyte and macrophage function. Natural killer cell function, as well as lymphocyte proliferation in response to mitogens or antigens, is decreased by lung surfactant (Ansfield et al., 1979; Richman et al., 1986), but opsonization and microbial killing by rat alveolar macrophages have been reported to be enhanced (LaForce et al., 1977). On the other hand, human lung surfactant appears neither to be toxic to *Hemophilus influenzae* or *Diplococcus pneumoniae* nor to alter alveolar macrophage uptake or killing of bacteria in vitro (Jonsson et al., 1986). The extent to which changes in lung surfactant during disease modulate macrophage and lymphocyte function is unknown.

IV. Abnormalities of Lung Surfactant in ARDS

Observations by Petty et al. (1979) on lavage fluid obtained post mortem from patients with ARDS suggested abnormal biophysical function of the lung surfactant. Studies by Hallman et al. (1982) of both the function and chemical composition of surfactant recovered from bronchoalveolar lavage of patients with ARDS showed both biochemical and functional abnormalities. The fractional composition of phosphatidylcholine and phosphatidylglycerol and the phosphatidylcholine-sphingomyclin ratio were decreased, and there was a marked loss of surface activity. Biochemical abnormalities of lung surfactant were present early in respiratory failure and tended to normalize during recovery.

As phospholipid synthesis is a function of type II cells, the observation that surfactant composition is altered in ARDS strongly suggests abnormality of type II cell function during ARDS. Surfactant recovered from ARDS patients was compared to surfactant from infants with IRDS who had an equivalent depression of the phosphatidylcholine-sphingomyelin ratio. This comparison showed a relatively constant and depressed fractional content of phosphatidylinositol in the ARDS surfactant relative to the IRDS surfactant, suggesting that the type II cell abnormalities of ARDS may be distinct from the abnormal function seen in the immature lung.

Abnormal function of surfactant in the lungs of patients with ARDS is likely to be partially (or perhaps primarily) due to the presence of inhibitors in the alveolar lining fluid. These are apt to include albumin (Holm et al., 1985), hemoglobin (Holm and Notter, 1987), fibrin monomer (Seeger et al., 1985), fibrinogen (Taylor and Abrams, 1966), glycolipids (Raurala and Hallman, 1984), and an inhibitor protein found in airway samples of patients with IRDS or ARDS (Berry, 1985). Many of these inhibitors are known to be present in bronchoalveolar lavage (BAL) from patients with ARDS.

V. Possible Causes of Surfactant Abnormalities in Patients with ARDS

Although the causes of ARDS remain obscure, mechanisms of acute lung injury likely to be of clinical importance have been defined. ARDS is an acute

Table 2 Causes of Dysfunctional Surfactant in Patients with ARDS

Inhibitors originating in plasma
Locally produced inhibitors
Injury of type II cells
Oxidation of apoprotein or phospholipid
Cleavage of apoprotein

inflammatory event characterized by polymorphonuclear leukocyte (PMN) infiltration of the lung with recovery of PMN in BAL (McGuire et al., 1982; Schlag et al., 1976); recovery in BAL of PMN proteases, including elastase and collagenase, which have the potential to cause lung injury (Christner et al., 1985; McGuire et al., 1982); and evidence of oxidant generation resulting in increased levels of H_2O_2 in exhaled breath condensate (Baldwin et al., 1986) and in oxidation of BAL proteins, including α_1-proteinase inhibitor, the major inhibitor in the lower airway of neutrophil elastase (Cochrane et al., 1983). Oxidant-induced lung injury may result from cellular (Schraufstatter et al., 1986; Spragg et al., 1985) or extracellular matrix injury.

There are several possible mechanisms by which surfactant abnormalities may arise in the lungs of patients with ARDS (Table 2). First, as permeability of the alveolar-capillary barrier is increased, functional inhibitors found in BAL may gain access to the airspace from plasma. Other inhibitors, such as fibrin monomer, may be generated locally as part of the inflammatory reaction. Second, type II cells may be injured by oxidants generated within the inflamed lung, and this injury may result in aberrant cell function with production of dysfunctional phospholipid or apoprotein.

Finally, oxidant and/or proteolytic attack directed against surfactant components may result in loss of surfactant function. Preliminary data indicate that the 35 kD apoprotein undergoes proteolytic cleavage with elastase or collagenase with consequent loss of function (Merritt et al., 1987; Pison et al., 1988). Whether protein oxidation enhances this cleavage or alters protein function is yet unknown. However, one would predict that the highly hydrophobic apoproteins would be protected from the enzymes present in the aqueous environment.

VI. Surfactant Replacement in Patients with IRDS

Preterm neonates are considered at risk for IRDS because of the inability of their lungs to produce a functionally adequate surfactant. Several investigators have successfully shown that exogenous surfactant from either human or bovine sources is successful in decreasing the incidence and severity of IRDS (Enhorning et al., 1985; Kwong et al., 1985; Merritt et al., 1986a; Shapiro et al., 1985). In addition to prophylactic efficacy, exogenous surfactant is also of therapeutic value in the setting of established IRDS (Collaborative European Multicenter Study Group, 1988; Gitlin et al., 1987; Hallman et al., 1985; Raju et al., 1987). These latter studies are of particular interest because of the similarities between established IRDS and ARDS. Both are characterized by evidence of neutrophil elastase release and recovery in BAL of evidence of oxidant activity (Merritt et al., 1986b). In both, dysfunction of type II cell metabolism may occur. Finally, in both syndromes, evidence of inhibitor(s) of surfactant function may be found in BAL. Thus, the therapeutic success of surfactant replacement in patients with established IRDS represents not only the ability to supply surfactant function to the immature lung but also the ability to overcome inhibitors in the inflamed lung. From this latter aspect, the therapeutic efficacy of exogenous surfactant in the setting of IRDS suggests the possibility of successful intervention in the patient with ARDS.

The therapeutic efficacy of surfactant replacement in established IRDS was well demonstrated in a large multicenter prospective randomized trial. Treatment of 146 patients with either porcine lung surfactant (purified by chloroform-methanol extract and column chromatography) or nothing showed that a single dose of surfactant (200 mg/kg) had dramatic effects. Oxygenation was improved within 5 min, with an increase in Pa_{O_2} from 57 to 148 torr (FI_{O_2} averaged 0.80). This improvement was sustained. Therapy with surfactant lowered mortality at 28 days by 40% and decreased the incidence of bronchopulmonary dysplasia by more than 50% (Collaborative European Multicenter Study Group, 1988).

VII. Animal Models for Evaluation of Surfactant Therapy of Acute Adult Lung Injury

Although the use of premature laboratory animals, for example rabbits (Obladen et al., 1985) or lambs (Jobe and Ikegami, 1984), provides a sound model for the study of the immature human lung, investigators concerned with studies of ARDS are at a disadvantage, for there are no clear animal models of acute human lung injury. Therefore, models must be chosen that aid the investigator in addressing specific hypotheses. These models may be divided into two groups: (1) those that produce a lung depleted of functional surfactant, and (2) those that produce a lung injury in which surfactant inhibitors predominate.

Models in the first group have been generated using repeated lavage (Berggren et al., 1986; Ikegami et al., 1977; Suzuki, 1982). In these studies, surfactant replacement by either instillation or aerosol is effective in restoring lung function. To separate the effects of lavage from those of surfactant depletion, lavage with a surfactant-rich fluid may be performed so that there is no net loss of surfactant from the lung (Richman et al., 1986). A second model in this group is that used by Nieman and Bredengerg (1985) in which surfactant function is removed by aerosol administration of detergent. Such treatment results in pulmonary edema, presumably the result of more negative perimicrovascular pressures.

All acute lung injury models that produce a high-permeability edema fall into the second group. The efficacy of surfactant replacement has been studied in only a few of these. Matalon et al. (1987) produced hyperoxic lung injury in adult (2 kg) rabbits by exposing them to 100% O_2 for 64 hr. Animals treated with two doses of 125 mg calf lung surfactant extract had greater lung expansion, less protein in BAL, less lung edema, and greater blood oxygenation 24 hr after hyperoxic exposure than did controls.

Berry et al. (1986) described a model of high-permeability lung injury produced in adult rabbits by bilateral cervical vagotomy. Although lung wash showed no difference in PC content between experimental and sham-generated animals, the minimum surface tension of this material was greatly elevated in experimental animals. This elevation was due to the presence of surfactant inhibitors, as surfactant isolated from lung wash by centrifugation retained full surface tension-lowering ability. Surfactant treatment with 50 mg/kg of sheep lung surfactant resulted in improvement in lung compliance and gas exchange.

As seen in the successful therapy of neonates with IRDS, these studies demonstrate that surfactant replacement may be capable of overcoming the effect of inhibitors present in alveolar lining fluid. Holm et al. (1985) demonstrated this phenomenon nicely in vitro by showing that the increase in minimum dynamic surface tension or adsorption facility of lung surfactant caused by the addition of albumin could be abolished at increased surfactant concentrations even when large amounts of albumin were added.

VIII. Surfactants Available for Therapeutic Administration

Surfactants available for therapeutic administration are divided between those derived from naturally occurring lung surfactants and those synthesized from component materials (Table 3).

The only naturally derived surfactant that has not been subjected to organic extraction and, therefore, retains the 35 kD apoprotein is that purified from human amniotic fluid (Hallman et al., 1983). Amniotic fluid from three term pregnancies is required to treat a single 1000 g infant, suggesting that

Table 3 Surfactants for Possible Therapeutic Use

Naturally occurring
Human surfactant from amniotic fluid (Merritt et al., 1986a)
Processed or synthesized
Mixtures of DPPC + hexadacanol + nonionic detergent (Durand et al., 1985)
Bovine or porcine lung lavage or wash extract (Collaborative European Multicenter Study Group, 1888; Enhorning et al., 1985; Shapiro et al., 1985)
Bovine lung surfactant extract supplemented with DPPC, tripalmitin, and palmitate (Fujiwara, 1984)
Combination of phospholipids and apoprotein (Dobbs et al., 1987; Notter et al., 1988; Revak et al., 1986, 1988; Wright et al., 1987; Yu and Possmayer, 1986)

fluid from several hundred pregnancies might be required for treatment of an adult patient. Thus, although effective clinically, this material is likely to be impractical for the clinical therapy of ARDS.

Surfactants recovered from bovine or porcine lungs and subjected to organic extraction appear equally effective as human surfactant in the therapy or prevention of IRDS, although no rigorous comparative trials have been performed. Although more available than human surfactant, lungs from approximately 50 pigs are required to prepare one dose of 100 mg/kg for a 70 kg adult. The results of biophysical and clinical testing of these surfactants are reported by Jobe and Ikegami (1987).

Synthetic surfactants are attractive because of the possibilities for enhanced availability, freedom from immunogenic proteins, and ease of sterility. Although mixtures of DPPC and PG are effective in vitro, they appear to be less effective in vivo than natural surfactants and have been ineffective in the therapy of established IRDS (Wilkinson et al., 1985). These observations illustrate the disparity that may exist between apparently excellent in vitro physical properties and poor in vivo effect.

DPPC supplemented with hexadecanol and tyloxapol (a nonionic detergent) also shows good in vitro surface tension-lowering ability and has apparent activity in vivo as well (Durand et al., 1985). Trials in infants with IRDS are in progress.

Of great current interest is the possibility of producing a clinically useful surfactant from component lipids and apoprotein. The latter might be synthesized or produced using recombinant DNA methodologies. As demonstrated by the clinical efficacy of surfactants produced from chloroform-methanol extracts of natural surfactant, the presence of low-molecular-weight apoproteins is sufficient for excellent in vitro and in vivo function. Several investigators have now demonstrated that inactive or minimally active surfactant components (phospholipid or apoprotein) may be recombined into a mixture with high in vitro surface activity and in vivo ability to improve lung compliance of preterm rabbit fetuses (Notter et al., 1988; Yu and Possmayer, 1986).

IX. Use of Exogenous Surfactants in the Therapy of ARDS

Exogenous surfactant may be delivered by direct instillation into the trachea or lobar bronchi or by jet nebulization. The latter technique, however, may take almost 20 hr to deliver a dose of 50 mg/kg to a 70 kg adult, but direct instillation has the advantage of being rapid and efficient.

The number of adults with ARDS who have been treated with exogenous surfactant is very small. Lachmann used direct instillation to treat several terminally ill patients with ARDS (B. Lachmann, personal communication), and three adults with ARDS have been treated with Curosurf. In that experience, it was found that intrabronchial administration of surfactant (50 mg/kg), given in divided doses given via a bronchoscope to each lobar bronchus, was well tolerated and caused a modest improvement in gas exchange (Richman et al., 1987). After receiving surfactant, patients had a modest (30-80 torr) increase in Pa_{O_2} that was transient ($\leqslant 1$ hr) in two and sustained in the third. No significant changes in lung compliance or chest radiograph were seen. Bronchoalveolar lavage was obtained several times during the course of the intervention and showed no change in albumin, α_1-proteinase inhibitor-specific activity, or cell count. BAL phospholipid concentrations were elevated at 3 hr and fell by 24 hr (in two patients) following therapy. In addition there was reduced activity of inhibitor of surfactant in BAL after surfactant replacement.

These studies were performed using porcine lung surfactant. Preliminary studies focused on the possibility that allergic reactions to porcine surfactant might occur. It was established that the cutaneous wheal and flare seen in normal adults to >0.1 mg surfactant were nonspecific and were not accomplished by blood lymphocyte sensitivity to porcine surfactant. Specifically, blood lymphocytes from persons reacting to intradermal surfactant showed no augmentation of proliferation or interleukin-2 production when stimulated in vitro.

X. Conclusion

Understanding of the adult lung surfactant system is in its infancy. As more is learned about factors modulating type II cell function, about the structure of the phospholipid-apoprotein complex and its components, and about the interactions between surfactant and surfactant inhibitors, more will be understood about the nature of surfactant dysfunction in the patient with ARDS. Fortunately, as more is learned about the structure of lung surfactant and about how to produce synthetic surfactant, clinical experience is being gained in the therapeutic use of exogenous surfactant. It is hoped that these separate efforts may combine to provide a useful therapeutic intervention for the patient with ARDS.

References

Ansfield, M. J., Benson, B. J., and Kaltreider, H. B. (1979). Immunosuppression by surface active material: Lack of species specificity. *Am. Rev. Respir. Dis.,* **120**:949-952.

Ashbaugh, D. G., Bigelow, D. B., Petty, T. L., et al. (1967). Acute respiratory distress in adults. *Lancet,* **2**:319-323.

Baldwin, S. R., Simon, R. H., Grum, C. M., Ketai, L. H., Boxer, L. A., and Devall, L. J. (1986). Oxidant activity in expired breath of patients with adult respiratory distress syndrome. *Lancet,* **1**:11-14.

Benson, B. J., Hawgood, S., and Williams, M. C. (1984). Role of apoprotein and calcium ions in surfactant function. *Exp. Lung Res.,* **6**:223-236.

Berggren, P., Lachmann, B., Curstedt, T., Grossmann, G., and Robertson, B. (1986). Gas exchange and lung morphology after surfactant replacement in experimental adult respiratory distress syndrome induced by repeated lung lavage. *Acta Anaesthesiol. Scand.,* **30**:321-328.

Berry, D. (1985). Adult respiratory distress syndrome: Surfactant inhibition. *J. Jpn. Med. Soc. Biol. Interface,* **16**:43-50.

Berry, D., Ikegami, M., and Jobe, A. (1986). Respiratory distress and surfactant inhibition following vagotomy in rabbits. *J. Appl. Physiol.,* **61**:1741-1748.

Christner, P., Fein, A., Goldberg, S., Lippman, M., Abrans, W., and Weinbaum, G. (1985). Collagenase in the lower respiratory tract of patients with adult respiratory distress syndrome. *Am. Rev. Respir. Dis.,* **131**: 690-695.

Claypool, W. D., Wang, D. L., Chander, A., and Fisher, A. B. (1984). "Hydrophobic" surfactant apoproteins and augmentation of phospholipid recycling. *Exp. Lung. Res.,* **6**:215-222.

Clements, J. A., and Tierney, D. F. (1965). Alveolar instability associated with altered surface tension. In *Handbook of Physiology, Respiration,* Vol. 2. Edited by W. O. Fennand and H. Rahn. Bethesda, American Physiological Society.

Cochrane, C. G., Spragg, R. G., and Revak, S. (1983). Pathogenesis of the adult respiratory distress syndrome: Evidence of oxidant activity in bronchoalveolar lavage fluid. *J. Clin. Invest.,* **71**:754-761.

Collaborative European Multicenter Study Group (1988). Surfactant replacement therapy for severe neonatal respiratory distress syndrome: an international randomized clinical trial. *Pediatrics,* **82**:683-691.

Dobbs, L. G., Wright, J. R., Hawgood, S., Gonzalez, R., Venstrom, K., and Nellenbogen, J. (1987). Pulmonary surfactant and its components inhibits secretions of phosphatidylcholine from cultured rat alveolar type II cells. *Proc. Natl. Acad. Sci. USA,* **84**:1010-1014.

Durand, D. J., Clyman, R. I., and Heymann, M. A., et al. (1985). Effects of a protein-free, synthetic surfactant on survival and pulmonary function in preterm lambs. *J. Pediatr.,* **107**:775-780.

Enhorning, G. (1973). Pulsating bubble technique for evaluating pulmonary surfactant. *J. Appl. Physiol.,* **43**:198-203.

Enhorning, G., Shennan, A., and Possmayer, F., et al. (1985). Prevention of neonatal respiratory distress syndrome by tracheal instillation of surfactant: A randomized clinical trial. *Pediatrics,* **76**:145-153.

Fujiwara, T. (1984). Surfactant replacement in neonatal RDS. In *Pulmonary Surfactant.* Edited by B. Robertson, L. M. G. Van Golde, and J. J. Battenburg. Amsterdam, Elsevier Science Publishers, pp. 479-503.

Gitlin, J. D., Soll, R. F., and Parad, R. B., et al. (1987). Randomized controlled trial of exogenous surfactant for the treatment of hyaline membrane disease. *Pediatrics,* **79**:31-37.

Guyton, A. C., and Moffatt, D. F. (1981). Role of surface tension and surfactant in the transepithelial movement of fluid and in the development of pulmonary edema. *Prog. Respir. Dis.,* **15**:62-75.

Hallman, M., Spragg, R. G., Harrell, J. H., Moser, K. M., and Gluck, L. (1982). Evidence of lung surfactant abnormality in respiratory failure. *J. Clin. Invest.,* **70**:673-683.

Hallman, M., Merritt, T. A., Schnieder, H., et al. (1983). Isolation of human surfactant from amniotic fluid and a pilot study of its efficacy in respiratory distress syndrome. *Pediatrics,* **71**:473-482.

Hallman, M., Merritt, T. A., Jarvenpaa, A. L., et al. (1985). Exogenous surfactant for treatment of severe respiratory distress syndrome: A randomized prospective clinical trial. *J. Pediatr.,* **106**:963-969.

Holm, B. A., and Notter, R. H. (1987). Effects of hemoglobin and cell membrane lipids on pulmonary surfactant activity. *J. Appl. Physiol.,* **63**: 1434-1442.

Holm, B. A., Notter, R. H., and Finkelstein, J. N. (1985). Surface property changes from interactions of albumin with natural lung surfactant and extracted lung lipids. *Chem. Phys. Lipids,* **38**:287-298.

Ikegami, M., Hesterberg, T., and Nozaki, M., et al. (1977). Restoration of lung pressure-volume characteristics with surfactant: Comparison of nebulization versus instillation and natural versus synthetic surfactant. *Pediatr. Res.,* **11**:178-182.

Jobe, A., and Ikegami, K. (1984). The prematurely delivered lamb as a model for studies of neonatal adaptation. In *Animal Models in Fetal Medicine.* Edited by P. W. Nathanielsz. Ithaca, New York, Perinatology Press. pp. 1-30.

Jobe, A., and Ikegami, M. (1987). Surfactant for the treatment of respiratory distress syndrome. *Am. Rev. Respir. Dis.,* **136**:1255-1275.

Jonsson, S., Musher, D. M., Goree, A., and Lawrence, E. C. (1986). Human alveolar lining material and antibacterial defenses. *Am. Rev. Respir. Dis.,* **133**:136-140.

King, R. G., and MacBeth, M. C. (1979). Physiochemical properties of dipalmitoyl phosphatidylcholine after interaction with an apolipoprotein of pulmonary surfactant. *Biochim. Biophys. Acta,* **557**:86-101.

Kwong, M. S., Egan, E. A., and Notter, R. H., et al. (1985). Double-blind clinical trial of calf lung surfactant extract for the prevention of hyaline membrane disease in extremely premature infants. *Pediatrics,* **76**:585-592.

LaForce, F. M., Kelly, W.J., and Huber, G. L. (1977). Inactivation of staphlococci by alveolar macrophages with preliminary observations on the importance of alveolar lining material. *Am. Rev. Respir. Dis.,* **108**: 784-790.

Mason, R. J., Cott, G. R., Robinson, P. C., Sugahara, K., Leslie, C. C., and Dobbs, L. G. (1984). Pharmacology of alveolar type II cells. *Prog. Respir. Res.,* **18**:279-287.

Matalon, S., Holm, B. A., and Notter, R. H. (1987). Mitigation of pulmonary hyperoxic injury by administration of exogenous surfactant. *Am. Physiol. Soc.,* **62**:756-761.

McGuire, W. W., Spragg, R. G., Cohen, A. B., and Cochrane, C. G. (1982). Studies on the pathogenesis of the adult respiratory distress syndrome. *J. Clin. Invest.,* **69**:543-553.

Merritt, T. A., Hallman, M., and Bloom, B. T., et al. (1986a). Prophylactic treatment of very premature infants with human surfactant. *New Engl. J. Med.,* **315**:785-790.

Merritt, T. A., Hallman, M., Holcomb, K., Strayer, D., Bloom, B., and Revak, S. (1986b). Human surfactant treatment of severe respiratory distress syndrome: Pulmonary effluent indicators of lung inflammation. *J. Pediatr.,* **108**:741-748.

Merritt, T. A., Revak, S., Hallman, M., and Cochrane, C. G. (1987). Elastolytic degradation of surfactant 35kD apoprotein. *Pediatr. Res.,* **21**:460.

Nieman, G. F., and Bredengerg, C. E. (1985). High surface tension pulmonary edema induced by detergent aerosol. *J. Appl. Physiol.,* **58**: 129-136.

Notter, R. H., and Shapiro, D. L. (1987). Lung surfactants for replacement therapy: Biochemical, biophysical, and clinical aspects. *Clin. Perinatol.,* **14**:433-479.

Notter, R. H., Shapiro, D. L., and Ohning, B., et al. (1988). Biophysical activity of synthetic phospholipids combined with purified lung surfactant 6,000 dalton apoprotein. *Chem. Phys. Lipids,* **44**:1-17.

Obladen, M., Kampanann, W., Zimmermann, I., and Lachmann, B. (1985). Artificial surfactant in preterm rabbits with and without respiratory distress syndrome: Difference of in vitro and in vivo activities. *Eur. J. Pediatr.,* **144**:195-199.

Petty, T. L., Silvers, G. W., Paul, G. W., and Stanford, R. E. (1979). Abnormalities in lung elastic properties and surfactant function in adult respiratory distress syndrome. *Chest,* **75**:571-574.

Pison, U., Hawgood, S., Tam, L., and Caughey, G. (1988). Proteolytic cleavage of lung surfactant 28-36 kDA protein (SPA) and effect on surfactant absorbtion. *FASEB J.,* **2**:A1183.

Raju, T. K., Vidyasagar, D., and Bhat, R., et al. (1987). Double-blind controlled trial of single-dose treatment with bovine surfactant in severe hyaline membrane disease. *Lancet,* **1**:651-656.

Rauvala, H., and Hallman, M. (1984). Glycolipid accumulation inbroncho-alveolar space in adult respiratory distress syndrome. *J. Lipid Res.,* **25**: 1357-1262.

Revak, S., Merritt, T. A., Hallman, M., and Cochrane, C. G. (1986). Reconstitution of surfactant activity using purified human apoprotein and phospholipids measured in vitro and in vivo. *Am. Rev. Respir. Dis.,* **134**:1258-1365.

Revak, S. D., Merritt, T.A., Degryse, E., Stefani, L., Courtney, M., Hallman, M., and Cochrane, C. G. (1988). Use of human surfactant low molecular weight apoproteins in the reconstitution of surfactant biologic activity. *J. Clin. Invest.,* **81**:826-833.;

Richman, P., Batcher, S., and Catanazaro, A. (1986). Immunoregulation by pulmonary surfactant in vitro. *Am. Rev. Respir. Dis.,* **133**:A312.

Richman, P. S., Spragg, R. G., Merritt, T. A., Robertson, B., and Curstedt, T. (1987). Administration of porcine-lung surfactant to humans with ARDS: Initial experience (abstract). *Am. Rev. Respir. Dis.,* **135**:A5.

Schlag, G., Voigt, W. H., Schnells, G., and Glatzl, A. (1976). Ultrastructure of the human lung in shock. *Anesthetist,* **25**:512-521.

Schraufstatter, I. U., Hyslop, P. A., Hinshaw, D. B., Spragg, R. G., Sklar, L. A., and Cochrane, C. G. (1986). Oxidant-induced injury of cells and its prevention by inhibitors of poly-ADP-ribose polymerase. *Proc. Natl. Acad. Sci. USA,* **83**:3908-3912.

Seeger, W. G., Stohr, G., Wolf, H. R. D., and Neuhof, H. (1985). Alteration of surfactant function due to protein leakage: Special interaction with fibrin monomer. *J. Appl. Physiol.,* **58**:326-338.

Shapiro, D. L., Notter, R.H., and Morin, F. C., III, et al. (1985). Double-blind, randomized trial of a calf lung surfactant extract administered at birth to very premature infants for prevention of respiratory distress syndrome. *Pediatrics,* **76**:593-599.

Spragg, R. G., Hinshaw, D. B., Hyslop, P. A., Schaufstatter, I. U., and Cochrane, C. G. (1985). Alterations in adenosine triphosphate levels and energy charge in P388D1 macrophages and endothelial cells following oxidant injury. *J. Clin. Invest.,* **76**:1471-1476.

Stratton, C. J. (1984). Morphology of surfactant producing cells and of the alveolar lining layer. In *Pulmonary Surfactant.* Edited by B. Robertson, L. M. G. van Golde, and J. J. Batenburg. Amsterdam: Elsevier, pp. 67-118.

Suzuki, Y. (1982). Effect of protein, cholesterol, and phosphatidylglycerol on the surface activity of the lipid-protein complex reconstituted from pig pulmonary surfactant. *J. Lipid Res.,* **23**:62-69.

Taylor, F. B., and Abrams, M. E. (1966). Effect of surface active lipoprotein on clotting and fibrinolysis, and of fibrinogen on surface tension of surface active lipoprotein. *Am. J. Med.,* **40**:346-350.

Wilkinson, A., Jenkins, P. A., and Jeffrey, J. A. (1985). Two controlled trials of day artificial surfactant: Early effects and later outcome in babies with surtactant deficiency. *Lancet,* **2**:287-291.

Wright, J. R., Wager, R. G., Hamilton, R. L., et al. (1986). Uptake of lung surfactant subfractions into lamellar bodies of adult rabbit lungs. *J. Appl. Physiol.,* **60**:817-825.

Wright, J. R., Wager, R. E., Hawgood, S., Dobbs, L., and Clements, J. A. (1987). Surfactant apoprotein M_r = 26,000-36,000 enhances uptake of liposomes by type II cells. *J. Biol. Chem.,* **262**:2888-2894.

Yu, S.H., and Possmayer, F. (1986). Reconstitution of surfactant activity by using the 6kD a apoprotein associated with pulmonary surfactant. *Biochem. J.,* **236**:85-89.

18

Humoral Aspects of Endotoxin Neutralization

H. SHAW WARREN

Shriners Burns Institute
Massachusetts General Hospital
Harvard Medical School
Boston, Massachusetts

I. Introduction

The morbidity and mortality caused by gram-negative infections have not substantially diminished over the last two decades. Much of the pathophysiology of these infections has been attributed to endotoxin (lipopolysaccharide, LPS) released from the outer bacterial cell wall. During infection LPS is believed to be partially or wholly responsible for fever, leukocytosis, activation of complement, disseminated intravascular coagulation, adult respiratory distress syndrome (ARDS), acute renal failure, acute hepatic failure, hypotension, and shock. These clinical findings and certain characteristic hemodynamic responses are collectively grouped together to form what has been called the septic syndrome. It should be emphasized, however, that the precise role of LPS in producing these conditions during infection has not been rigorously proven but rather is an assumption based on the ability of an infusion of killed gram-negative bacteria or chemically purified LPS to induce similar pathophysiology in animals (and in selected human studies). Nonetheless, the potency and diversity of the biologic effects following endotoxin administration and their similarity to the clinical findings seen in severe gram-negative infection has prompted numerous investigators to study the host factors that affect the toxicity induced by LPS. Interest in the response to LPS continues because the development of new antibiotics that are highly efficacious in killing gram-negative bacteria has not substantially altered the sequellae of gram-negative infection. In fact there are recent data suggesting that the administration of bactericidal antibiotics may release LPS from the walls of dying bacteria into the circulation, thereby worsening the syndrome (Schenep and Morgan, 1984).

It has been known for almost a century that animals receiving small doses of gram-negative bacterial cell walls or endotoxin become relatively resistant to subsequent challenge. Indeed this phenomenon, called endotoxin tolerance, was a hindrance in the so-called fever therapy for neurosyphilis early in this century, in which an attempt was made to maintain a febrile state in patients by frequent or constant intravenous infusions of killed gram-negative bacteria. Ever-increasing doses of bacteria were needed to induce a given degree of fever (Heyman, 1945). That this response presumably represents a protective adaptation against the toxic effects of gram-negative bacteria did not go unnoticed; clinicians and researchers over the last 40-50 years have been trying to understand the mechanisms responsible for tolerance to LPS with the hope that they might be manipulated for therapeutic benefit. The literature pertaining to this endeavor is extensive.

Studies on the biologic effects of LPS are difficult to interpret for several reasons. First, until the recent availability of synthetic compounds it was necessary to work with material that was partially purified by the chemical extraction of gram-negative bacteria. Such preparations differ widely in purity. The situation is made worse by the fact that the chemical structure of LPS, being part lipid and part polysaccharide, is amphipathic and therefore forms micelles in aqueous buffers that have varying degrees of solubility. It is not surprising that no two preparations are identical. Since each preparation is different, comparison of experiments between laboratories is difficult or impossible. A second problem is that different species of experimental animals vary markedly in their response to LPS as dosed by body mass. For example, rabbits, sheep, and humans are extremely sensitive to LPS, whereas dogs, rodents, and chickens are quite resistant. Consequently, studies using different animal species for experimental models cannot easily be compared. A third difficulty is that the lipid moiety of the LPS molecule results in a high degree of adsorption of LPS to glassware, plasticware, and intravenous tubing. Because of the marked potency of LPS, the amount lost to adsorption is often in the range of the sensitivity of the assay being utilized, thereby generating erroneous results.

There has been much debate on the respective contributions of the humoral and cellular branches of the immune system in mediating tolerance to endotoxin. Although there are considerable data suggesting that the reticuloendothelial system (RES) plays a major role, our laboratory has concentrated on humoral mechanisms of tolerance. A strong incentive for studying humoral factors capable of decreasing the activity or toxicity of LPS is that identification of such factors may lead to substances that could be infused prophylactically or therapeutically for gram-negative sepsis. In this chapter I review the evidence that there is LPS detoxification by plasma elements. This is, however, not to imply by omission that cellular mechanisms are not important or do not dominate host tolerance to LPS. An excellent review of cellular mechanisms contributing to endotoxin tolerance has recently been published (Johnston and Greisman, 1985).

II. Neutralization of Endotoxin by Normal Serum

It was reported 30 years ago that incubation of LPS in fresh normal serum resulted in alterations of its antigenicity (Cluff, 1956) and a loss of biologic activity (Landy et al., 1957). In a series of studies it has been shown that when chemically extracted endotoxin is exposed to serum it is first disaggregated and then binds to lipoproteins, in particular high-density lipoprotein (HDL) (Skarnes and Chedid, 1964; Ulevitch et al., 1979). The binding is both time and temperature dependent. The disaggregation is inhibited by divalent cations (Skarnes, 1966; Munford et al., 1981) and antibody to the O-polysaccharide of LPS (Munford and Dietschy, 1985). The serum element responsible for the disaggregation has not been definitively identified. It can be replaced by deoxycholate, however (Munford et al., 1981b). Two serum protein candidates that have been proposed are a beta globulin (Johnson et al., 1977) and an anion-dependent α lipoprotein with esterase activity (Skarnes, 1966).

Radiolabeled LPS that is bound to lipoproteins can be separated by ultracentrifugation or chromatography and studied for biologic activity. Although the lipoprotein-bound LPS appears to be chemically unchanged, it is markedly less active than unbound LPS in most tests of endotoxin activity, including pyrogenicity, induction of neutropenia and thrombocytopenia, lethality of actinomycin D-stimulated mice, and induction of interleukin-1 and colony stimulating factor (Ulevitch and Johnston, 1978; unpublished studies in our laboratory). Once LPS is bound to HDL, it circulates in the bloodstream in a less toxic form with a relatively long half-life (hours) compared to unbound LPS (minutes) and follows cholesterol metabolic pathways in that it is taken up by cellular HDL receptors rather than by the RES (Mathison and Ulevitch, 1979; Munford et al., 1981a).

We have developed an assay to measure the neutralizing ability of a given serum sample (Novitsky et al., 1985). The assay is based on the ability of serum to prevent the coagulation of *Limulus* amebocyte lysate in response to LPS. Whereas earlier studies reported that this phenomenon reflected inhibition of the lysate by serum proteins, we have shown that the loss of lysate reactivity represents neutralization of LPS by serum (Novitsky et al., 1985; Warren et al., 1985), presumably by disaggregation of the LPS followed by binding to HDL. Using the assay we screened 209 aliquots of plasma obtained from normal human blood donors. We measured a 100-fold variation in neutralizing ability. Exogenous LPS incubated in a pool of plasma formed from donors who were "low" neutralizers induced more fever in the rabbit pyrogen test than LPS incubated in a pool formed from donors who were "high" neutralizers, demonstrating that the assay is able to predict the degree of LPS neutralization in another biologic assay of LPS activity (Warren et al., 1985).

These studies were performed with LPS that was chemically extracted, usually with hot phenol, from gram-negative bacteria that were previously cultured in vitro. An important question is whether extracted LPS (which has an altered physicochemical form) behaves in a similar manner to LPS released from the surface of growing or dying organisms during gram-negative infection. Although there have been no studies to date concentrating on the neutralization of LPS in its native form by normal serum, it is reassuring that the lipoprotein binding behavior of bacterial membrane fragments shed from the surface of gram-negative organisms appears to be similar to that of chemically extracted LPS (Munford et al., 1982).

Collectively, these data support the notion that there are elements in normal serum and/or plasma that act to diminish the biologic activity of LPS in the host.

III. Neutralization of Endotoxin by Immunoglobulins

The lipopolysaccharide molecule consists of three parts: a toxic hydrophobic lipid moiety (lipid A) that is inserted into the bacterial membrane, a linking core oligosaccharide moiety (common core), and a long hydrophilic polysaccharide chain that is unique to each bacterial stain and is the dominant immunogen (O antigen). Polyclonal and, more recently, monoclonal antibodies have been made to epitopes on each of the three parts and tested in animal models of LPS toxicity. Surprisingly, despite that lipid A is the toxic moiety of the molecule, antibodies directed to lipid A are not protective (Mullan et al., 1974; McCabe et al., 1977).

In contrast, small amounts of type-specific polyclonal (Tate et al., 1966; Braude et al., 1973; Greisman et al., 1973) or monoclonal (Kirkland and Zeigler, 1984) antibodies directed to the O-polysaccharide chain are protective in animal models of challenge with LPS from the homologous strain. Antibodies to the O-polysaccharide moiety are not protective for challenge with LPS from heterologous strains. The large number of bacterial strains (e.g., greater than 100 for *Escherichia coli* alone) make the prophylactic or therapeutic use of these antibodies problematic unless protection is sought for a single specific gram-negative pathogen.

Polyclonal antibodies can also be induced against the "common core" regions of LPS by immunizing animals with vaccines made from killed mutant gram-negative organisms that cannot incorporate the polysaccharide chains onto the LPS. Such mutant organisms, which are called rough mutants because of the irregular appearance of the colonies on agar, have the deeper core structures of LPS exposed on the surface of the bacteria. The core structure has been conserved in the LPS from gram-negative organisms. Only six different LPS cores have been described, each of which is almost identical to the others (Jann and Jann, 1984). Because the core region is a common structure on LPS that is not lipid, attention has focused on it as a part of the molecule that could provide a cross-protective epitope for immunotherapy.

A series of investigations over the last two decades has demonstrated that passively transferred antisera raised to rough mutant gram-negative organisms, such as *E. coli* J5 and *Salmonella minnesota* Re 595 consistently protect against challenge with heterologous LPS in animal models (McCabe et al., 1977; Johns et al., 1983; Ziegler et al., 1973; Young et al., 1975). The importance of these studies is that although protection requires the passive transfer of a greater volume of antiserum than type-specific antiserum raised to the O-polysaccharide, this antiserum protects against LPS from most bacterial strains. These promising studies in animals led to a double-blind clinical trial in 1982 in which passively transferred sera drawn from human volunteers vaccinated with killed rough mutant *E. coli* J5 significantly decreased mortality from 77 to 44% in patients with gram-negative shock (Ziegler et al., 1982). As in the animal studies, the antiserum protected against shock and death from *all* strains of gram-negative bacteria, proving it was possible to successfully, and dramatically, treat gram-negative sepsis in humans with passive immunotherapy. Similar findings were obtained in a subsequent double-blinded clinical trial performed with surgical patients treated with plasma obtained from plasmaphoresed volunteers who had been vaccinated with *E. coli* J5 (Baumgartner et al., 1985).

Two lines of evidence suggest that the protective element in this antiserum is antibody directed against a common epitope in the LPS core. First, purified IgG and IgM immunoglobulin fractions prepared from the polyclonal antisera protect in animal models (Ziegler et al., 1975; Davis et al., 1978). Second, the protective activity in the antiserum can be absorbed with immobilized rough mutant LPS or bacteria but not with control heterologous LPS or bacteria (Johns et al., 1983; McCabe, 1972; Marks et al., 1982; Sakulramrung and Domingue, 1985). On the other hand, many of the animal experiments did not use highly purified antibody preparations, and a recent clinical trial failed to show protection using purified IgG prepared from volunteers who were vaccinated with *E. coli* J5 (Calandra et al., 1988). Also, the absorption experiments are unclear because of possible nonspecific removal of substances from serum and because during absorption LPS may escape into the antisera, thereby contaminating it (Marks et al., 1982). At this time the exact nature of the protective factor remains uncertain.

At present no in vitro test correlates closely with protection in animal models. Development of a test specific for cross-reactive anticore antibody has been difficult because there are a large number of very immunogenic epitopes on the surface of rough mutant bacterial vaccines. The protective epitopes have not yet been identified and are likely to be weak immunogens. Since polyclonal antisera to rough mutant bacteria presumably have high titers of antibody directed to numerous irrelevant antigens and lower titers of extremely protective antibody directed to the desired common epitope, assays using the vaccine itself as an antigen measure many irrelevant antibodies. Another difficulty that has complicated the development of assays measuring anticore antibody is that the amphipathic nature of LPS results in large physicochemical changes in molecular conformation depending upon the milieu. In aqueous buffers, LPS is micellar. In serum and in vivo the LPS micelles disaggregate, and then approximately half the LPS binds to lipoproteins through hydrophobic interactions (Ulevitch and Johnston, 1978; Munford et al., 1982). Since the core region bridges the lipid A and O antigen moieties of the LPS molecule, such conformational changes almost certainly result in altered exposure of the protective epitope. Furthermore, antibody assays in which the antigen is bound to a fixed surface, such as enzyme-linked immunosorbant assays (ELISA) or Western blotting techniques, probably utilize molecular conformations of LPS not found in nature. In particular, with ELISA assays using LPS as antigen (with which most prior work has been done) the lipid A portion of the molecule probably has a high affinity for plastic surfaces, thereby hiding the core epitopes and extending the polysaccharide chains into the aqueous buffer. Because of this, ELISA assays using smooth LPS as the antigen are especially sensitive to anti-O-polysaccharide antibody (Siber et al., 1985). In contrast, polyclonal antibodies raised to rough mutants do not recognize complete heterologous LPS in either ELISA (Siber et al., 1985; Baumgartner et al., 1987) or Western blotting systems (De Jongh-Leuvenink et al., 1985). The lack of an in vitro test for cross-reactive antibody recognizing heterologous LPS has been an obstacle to developing monoclonal antibodies that should be protective. Until very recently, it was assumed that all antibodies directed to LPS extracted from rough mutant bacteria, such as *E. coli* J5, would be cross-reactive and, consequently, cross-protective. Therefore, numerous groups have produced monoclonal antibodies to LPS from *E. coli* J5 utilizing direct ELISA assays in which the LPS was coated onto the microtiter plate as antigen (Teng et al., 1984; Nelles and Niswander, 1984; Gigliotti and Shenep, 1985; Miner et al., 1986; Mutharia et al., 1984; Bogard et al., 1987; Pollack et al., 1987). For the most part these monoclonal antibodies bind well to LPS from *E. coli* J5 but variably or not at all to heterologous LPS. One such monoclone is believed to protect in animal models of LPS toxicity (Teng et al., 1984).

Despite the considerable controversy that surrounds many of the studies involving the use of anticore antibodies to LPS, an obvious hope is that monoclonal antibodies will be produced that can be developed for use as a prophylactic or therapeutic agent for endotoxemia. At this time there are two ongoing double-blinded clinical trials studying the ability of such monoclonal antibodies to decrease morbidity and mortality in septic shock.

IV. Neutralization of Endotoxin by Inflammatory Factors in Serum

Since the studies of Greisman several decades ago on the pyrogenic effects of LPS (Greisman et al., 1969, 1973), tolerance to endotoxin has been divided into two temporal phases. The "early" phase is present for 5-6 days following administration of endotoxin (even in minute doses) and is a phase during which experimental animals are tolerant to challenge with LPS from either homologous or heterologous bacterial strains. The "late" phase begins approximately 1 week after LPS administration, during which experimental animals are tolerant to challenge with LPS from homologous but not heterologous gram-negative strains. Late, strain-specific tolerance is believed to be mediated by immunoglobulin directed to the O-polysaccharide chain and has already been discussed. The mechanisms responsible for the "early" phase are not yet understood and are probably numerous. There is uncertainty about whether circulating serum factors that are not antibody can contribute to early tolerance. Classically, early pyrogenic tolerance is not mediated by factors in serum. However, several studies have described that tolerance can be passively transferred with large amounts of serum from animals made tolerant to LPS in the absence of antibody (Freedman, 1959; Wolff et al., 1965; Greisman et al., 1973). These studies suggest that there may be inducible humoral factors that are capable of augmenting the detoxification of LPS.

The mechanisms of the increased neutralization of LPS in tolerant or inflammatory sera have been studied by several investigators. In 1973, Moreau and Skarnes reported that LPS was rapidly detoxified by tolerant rabbit sera. They developed an assay system that measured the ability of serum to transfer LPS from a toxic and slowly diffusing precipitation band on immunodiffusion plates to a nontoxic and rapidly diffusing band. Sera from tolerant rabbits transformed the LPS completely and more rapidly than sera from normal rabbits. Since the bands containing the rapidly diffusing nontoxic LPS stained with Sudan black, they concluded that detoxification was due to the formation of LPS-lipoprotein complexes. They also reported that injection of LPS into tolerant rabbits resulted in an in vivo decrease in ionized calcium that was not present in control rabbits. Such a change would favor the formation of LPS-lipoprotein complexes. The detoxification was hypothesized to be related to a heat-stabile esterase associated with low-density lipoprotein. It is notable that an inducible esterase associated with HDL that also binds LPS was subsequently described by another laboratory (Bog-Hansen et al., 1978), although its relationship to LPS neutralization remains unclear.

We have employed the *Limulus* neutralization assay described in the last section to study inflammatory sera and noted that sera obtained from tolerant rabbits neutralized 5- to 10-fold more LPS than normal sera (Warren et al., 1986). The tolerant sera neutralized LPS from several gram-negative strains. Neutralization did not correlate with either anti-O-polysaccharide or anticore antibody as measured by ELISA. Increased LPS neutralization by rabbit sera was also measured 24 hr after administration of recombinant human interleukin-1 (Riveau et al., 1987). In another project we examined human sera obtained in different clinical settings. Sera obtained from patients following gram-positive or gram-negative bacteremia or from patients with gram-negative shock neutralized significantly more LPS than sera from normal control patients or from patients with cardiogenic shock (Warren et al., 1987).

We also examined the binding of biosynthetically radiolabeled LPS to serum lipoproteins in normal and tolerant rabbit sera by analyzing isopycnic density gradients generated by ultracentrifugation in the presence of cesium chloride (Warren et al., 1986). The LPS bound much more rapidly and to a greater extent to lipoproteins in tolerant sera compared to normal sera. In other studies we found that augmented lipoprotein binding was present within 8 hr after intravenous injection of heterologous LPS or LPS-free activated macrophage supernatants (Warren et al., 1988). Fractionation and reconstitution experiments suggest that the responsible factor for the phenomenon has the same density as serum lipoproteins (Warren et al., 1988).

There may be several factors that modulate LPS-protein binding. Tobias et al. recently decribed a glycoprotein in inflammatory serum of MW 60,000 that binds to LPS extracted from rough mutant *S. minnesota* Re 595, thereby slowing its binding to lipoproteins (Tobias and Ulevitch, 1983; Tobias et al.,

1986). Interestingly, this glycoprotein appears to be homologous to certain cationic antibacterial proteins found in neutrophils (Tobias et al., 1988).

Another factor that may be important is serum amyloid A. It has been shown that immunoaffinity-purified complexes of HDL-LPS formed in inflammatory serum contain serum amyloid A, whereas control complexes formed in normal serum do not (Tobias et al., 1982). Serum amyloid A is an apoprotein of HDL induced during the inflammatory response. It is unclear if serum amyloid A plays an active role in the binding of LPS or is simply present on HDL particles binding to LPS.

Although many details remain to be clarified, these data collectively suggest that inflammatory sera contain factors capable of neutralizing LPS, at least in part by modulating the binding of LPS to lipoproteins.

V. Conclusions

A major reason to examine the humoral mechanisms of LPS detoxification is that they could perhaps be manipulated for the therapeutic advantage of patients with endotoxemia or the septic syndrome. That this might be possible is most evident from the results of many animal experiments and clinical trials demonstrating protection against the toxic effects of gram-negative bacteria by administering polyclonal antisera raised to rough mutant bacterial vaccines. Despite 20 years of intensive investigation, the protective element(s) in these antisera remain uncertain, controversial, and elusive. Nonetheless, there remain optimism and enthusiasm among investigators that the protective factors can be identified, characterized, and produced in a form suitable for clinical use. To this end an increasingly large array of monoclonal antibodies are being generated to different epitopes on the common core of LPS. In addition it seems probable that there will be progress in understanding the interaction of LPS with inflammatory proteins generated during the acute-phase response. It is hoped that one or more of these differing approaches will result in an effective therapeutic substance to neutralize endotoxin.

Acknowledgments

The skillful secretarial assistance of Mrs. Marlene O'Donnell is gratefully acknowledged. This work was supported in part by grant 15861 from the Shriners Hospital for Crippled Children.

References

Baumgartner, J. D., McCutchan, J. A., van Melle, G., Vogt, M., Luethy, R., Glauser, M. P., Aiegler, E. J., Klauber, M. R., Muehlen, E., Chiolero, R., and Geroulanos, S. (1985). Prevention of gram-negative shock and death in surgical patients by antibody to endotoxin core glycolipid. *Lancet,* **2**:59-63.

Baumgartner, J. D., O'Brien, T. X., Kirkland, T. N., Glauser, M. P., and Ziegler, E. J. (1987). Demonstration of cross-reactive antibodies to smooth gram-negative bacteria in antiserum to *Escherichia coli* J5. *J. Infect. Dis.,* **156**:136-143.

Bogard, W. C., Jr., Dunn, D. L., Abernethy, K., Kilgarriff, C., and Kung, P. C. (1987). Isolation and characterization of murine monoclonal antibodies specific for gram-negative bacterial lipopolysaccharide: Association of cross-genus reactivity with lipid A specificity. *Infect. Immun.,* **55**:899-908.

Bog-Hansen, T. C., Krog, H. H., and Back, U. (1978). Plasma lipoprotein-associated arylesterase is induced by bacterial lipopolysaccharide. *FEMS Lett.,* **93**:86-90.

Braude, A. I., Douglas, H., and Davis, C. E. (1973). Treatment and prevention of intravascular coagulation with antiserum to endotoxin. *J. Infect. Dis.,* **128**:S157-S164.

Calandra, T., Glauser, M. P., Schellekens, J., Verhoef, J., and the Swiss-Dutch J5 Immun. Study Group (1988). Treatment of gram-negative septic shock with human IgG antibody to *Escherichia coli* J5: A prospective, double-blind, randomized trial. *J. Infect. Dis.,* **158**:312-316.

Cluff, L. E. (1956). A study of the effect of serum on the immunological reaction of a bacterial endotoxin. *J. Exp. Med.,* **103**:439-452.

Davis, C. E., Zeigler, E. J., and Arnold, K. F. (1978). Neutralization of meningococcal endotoxin by antibody to core glycolipid. *J. Exp. Med.,* **147**:1007-1017.

De Jongh-Leuvenink, J., Vreede, R. W., Marcelis, J. H., De Bos, M., and Verhoef, J. (1985). Detection of antibodies against lipopolysaccharides of *Escherichia coli* and Salmonella R and S strains by immunoblotting. *Infect. Immun.,* **50**:716-720.

Freedman, H. H. (1959). Passive transfer of protection against lethality of homologous and heterologous endotoxins. *Proc. Soc. Exp. Biol. Med.,* **102**:504-506.

Gigliotti, F., and Shenep, J. L. (1985). Failure of monoclonal antibodies to core glycolipid to bind intact smooth strains of *Escherichia coli. J. Infect. Dis.,* **151**:1005-1011.

Greisman, S. E., Young, E. J., and Carozza, F. A., Jr. (1969). Mechanisms of endotoxin tolerance. V. Specificity of the early and late phases of pyrogenic tolerance. *J. Immunol.,* **103**:1223-1236.

Greisman, S. E., Young, E. J., and DuBuy, J. B. (1973). Mechanisms of endotoxin tolerance. VIII. Specificity of serum transfer. *J. Immunol.,* **111**: 1349-1360.

Heyman, A. (1945). The treatment of neurosyphilis by continuous infusion of typhoid vaccine. *Vener. Dis. Inform.*, **26**:51-57.

Jann, K., and Jann, B. (1984). Structure and biosynthesis of O-antigens. In *Handbook of Endotoxin,* Vol. I, *Chemistry of Endotoxin.* Edited by E. T. Rietchel. New York, Elsevier,

Johns, M., Skehill, A., and McCabe, W. R. (1983). Immunization with rough mutants of*Salmonella minnesota.* IV. Protection by antisera to O and rough antigens against endotoxin. *J. Infect. Dis.*, **147**:57-67.

Johnson, K. J., Ward, P. A., Goralnick, B. S., and Osborn, M. J. (1977). Isolation from human serum of an inactivator of bacterial lipopolysaccharide. *Am. J. Pathol.*, **88**:559-574.

Johnston, C. A., and Greisman, S. E. (1985). Mechanisms of endotoxin tolerance. In *Handbook of Endotoxin,* Vol. 2. Edited by L. B. Hinshaw. Amsterdam, Elsevier Science Publishers,

Kirkland, T. N., and Ziegler, E. J. (1984). An immunoprotective monoclonal antibody to lipopolysaccharide. *J. Immunol.*, **132**:2590-2592.

Landy, M., Skarnes, R. C., Rosen, F. S., Trapani, R.-J., and Shear, M. J. (1957). Inactivation of biologically active ("endotoxic") polysaccharides by fresh human serum. *Proc. Soc. Exp. Biol. Med.*, **96**:744-747.

Marks, M. I., Ziegler, E. J., Douglas, H., Corbeil, L. B., and Braude, A. I. (1982). Induction of immunity against lethal *Haemophilis influenza* type b infection by *Escherichia coli* core lipopolysaccharide. *J. Clin. Invest.*, **69**:742-749.

Mathison, J. C., and Ulevitch, R. J. (1979). The clearance, tissue distribution, and cellular localization of intravenously injected lipopolysaccharide in rabbits. *J. Immunol.*, **123**:2133-2143.

McCabe, W. R. (1972). Immunization with R mutants of *S. minnesota*. I. Protection against challenge with heterologous gram-negative bacilli. *J. Immunol.*, **108**:601-610.

McCabe, W. R., Bruins, S. C., Craven, D. E., and Johns, M. (1977). Cross-reactive antigens: Their potential for immunization-induced immunity to gram-negative bacteria. *J. Infect. Dis.*, **136**(S):161-166.

Miner, K. M., Manyak, C. L., Williams, E., Jackson, J., Jewell, M., Gammon, M. T., Ehrenfreund, C., Hayes, E., Callahan, L., Zweerink, H., and Sigal, N. H. (1986). Characterization of murine monoclonal antibodies to *Escherichia coli* J5. *Infect. Immun.*, **52**:56-62.

Moreau, S. C., and Skarnes, R. C. (1973). Host resistance to bacterial endotoxemia: Mechanisms in endotoxin-tolerant animals. *J. Infect. Dis.*, **128**(S):122-133.

Mullan, N. A., Newsome, P. M., Cunnington, P. G., Palmer, G. H., and Wilson, M. E. (1974). Protection against gram-negative infections with antiserum to lipid A from *Salmonella minnesota* R595. *Infect. Immun.*, **10**:1195-1201.

Munford, R. S., and Dietschy, J. M. (1985). Effects of specific antibodies, hormones, and lipoproteins on bacterial lipopolysaccharides injected into the rat. *J. Infect. Dis.,* **152**:177-184.

Munford, R. S., Andersen, J. M., and Dietschy, J. M. (1981a). Sites of tissue binding and uptake in vivo of bacterial lipopolysaccharide-high-density lipoprotein complexes: Studies in the rat and squirrel monkey. *J. Clin. Invest.,* **68**:1503-1513.

Munford, R. S., Hall, C. L., and Dietschy, J. M. (1981b). Binding of *Salmonella typhimurium* lipopolysaccharides to rat high-density lipoproteins. *Infect. Immun.,* **34**:835-843.

Munford, R. S., Hall, C. L., Lipton, J. M., and Dietschy, J. M. (1982). Biological activity, lipoprotein-binding behavior, and in vivo disposition of extracted and native forms of *Salmonella typhimurium* lipopolysaccharides. *J. Clin. Invest.,* **70**:877-888.

Mutharia, L. M., Crockford, G., Bogard, W. C., and Hancock, R. E. W. (1984). Monoclonal antibodies specific for *Escherichia coli* J5 lipopolysaccharide: Cross reaction with other gram-negative bacterial species. *Infect. Immun.,* **45**:631-636.

Nelles, M. J., and Niswander, C. A. (1984). Mouse monoclonal antibodies reactive with J5 lipopolysaccharide exhibit extensive cross reaction with a variety of gram-negative bacteria. *Infect. Immun.,* **46**:677-681.

Novitsky, T. J., Roslansky, P. F., Siber, G. R., and Warren, H. S. (1985). Turbidometric method for quantifying serum inhibition of limulus amoebocyte lysate. *J. Clin. Microbiol.,* **21**:211-216.

Pollack, M., Raubitschek, A. A., and Larrick, J. W. (1987). Human monoclonal antibodies that recognize conserved epitopes in the core-lipid-A region of lipopolysaccharides. *J. Clin. Invest.,* **79**:1421-1430.

Riveau, G. R., Novitsky, T. J., Roslansky, P. F., Dinarello, C. A., and Warren, H. S. (1987). Role of interleukin-1 in augmenting serum neutralization of bacterial lipopolysaccharide. *J. Clin. Microbiol.,* **25**:889-892.

Sakulramrung, R., and Domingue, G. J. (1985). Cross-reactive immunoprotective antibodies to *Escherichia coli*:0111 rough mutant J5. *J. Infect. Dis.,* **151**:995-1004.

Schenep, J. L., and Morgan, K. A. (1984). Kinetics of endotoxin release during antibiotic therapy for experimental gram-negative bacterial sepsis. *J. Infect. Dis.,* **150**:380-388.

Siber, G. R., Kania, S., and Warren, H. S. (1985). Cross reactivity of rabbit antibodies to lipopolysaccharides of *Escherichia coli* J5 and other gram-negative bacteria. *J. Infect. Dis.,* **152**:954-964.

Skarnes, R. C. (1966). The inactivation of endotoxin after interaction with certain proteins of normal serum. *Ann. N.Y. Acad. Sci.,* **133**:644-662.

Skarnes, R. C., and Chedid, L. C. (1964). Biological degradation and inactivation of endotoxin (chromate-labeled). In *Bacterial Endotoxins.* Edited by M. Landy and W. Braun. New Brunswick, N.J., Institute of Microbiology, Rutgers.

Tate, W. J., Douglas, H., and Braude, A. I. (1966). Protection against lethality of *E. coli* endotoxins with "O" antiserum. *Ann. N.Y. Acad. Sci.,* **133**:746-762.

Teng, N. N. H., Kaplan, H. S., Hebert, J. M., Moore, C., Douglas, H., Wunderlich, A., and Braude, A. I. (1984). Protection against gram-negative bacteremia and endotoxemia with human monoclonal antibodies. *Proc. Natl. Acad. Sci. USA,* **82**:1790-1794.

Tobias, P. S., and Ulevitch, R. J. (1983). Control of lipopolysaccharide-high-density lipoprotein binding by acute-phase protein(s). *J. Immunol.,* **131**:1913-1916.

Tobias, P. S., McAdam, K. P. W. J., and Ulevitch, R. J. (1982). Interactions of bacterial lipopolysaccharide with acute-phase rabbit serum and isolation of two forms of rabbit serum amyloid A. *J. Immunol.,* **128**:1420-1427.

Tobias, P. S., Soldau, K., and Ulevitch, R. J. (1986). Isolation of a lipopolysaccharide-binding acute-phase reactant from rabbit serum. *J. Exp. Med.,* **164**:777-793.

Tobias, P. S., Mathison, J. C., and Ulevitch, R. J. (1988). A family of lipopolysaccharide binding proteins involved in responses to gram-negative sepsis. *J. Biol. Chem.,* **263**:13479-13481.

Ulevitch, R. J., and Johnston, A. R. (1978). The modification of biophysical and endotoxic properties of bacterial lipopolysaccharides by serum. *J. Clin. Invest.,* **62**:1313-1324.

Ulevitch, R. J., Johnston, A. R., and Weinstein, D. B. (1979). New function for high-density lipoproteins: Their participation in intravascular reactions of bacterial lipopolysaccharides. *J. Clin. Invest.,* **64**:1516-1524.

Warren, H. S., Novitsky, T.J., Ketchem, P. A., Roslansky, P. F., Kania, S., and Siber, G. R. (1985). Neutralization of bacterial lipopolysaccharides by human plasma. *J. Clin. Microbiol.,* **22**:590-595.

Warren, H. S., Knights, C. V., and Siber, G. R. (1986). Neutralization and lipoprotein binding of lipopolysaccharides in tolerant rabbit serum. *J. Infect. Dis.,* **154**:784-791.

Warren, H. S., Novitsky, T. J., Martin, P., Roslansky, P. F., and Siber, G. R. (1987). Endotoxin neutralizing capacity of sera from different patient populations assessed by limulus lysate test. In *Second International Conference on Endotoxins and Their Detection with Limulus Lysate.* Edited by S. W. Watson. New York, Alan R. Liss.

Warren, H. S., Riveau, G. R., de Deckker, F. A., and Chedid, L. A. (1988). Control of endotoxin activity and interleukin-1 production by regulation of lipopolysaccharide-lipoprotein binding by a macrophage factor. *Infect. Immun.,* **56**:204-212.

Wolff, S. M., Mulholland, J. H., Ward, S. B., Rubenstein, M., and Mott, P. D. (1965). Effect of 6-mercaptopurine on endotoxin tolerance. *J. Clin. Invest.,* **44**:1402-1409.

Young, L. S., Stevens, P., and Ingram, J. (1975). Functional role of antibody against "core" glycolipid of Enterobacteriaecae. *J. Clin. Invest.,* **56**:850-861.

Ziegler, E. T., Douglas, H., Sherman, J. E., Davis, C. E., and Braude, A. I. (1973). Treatment of *E. coli* and *Klebsiella* bacteremia in agranulocytopenic animals with antiserum to a UDP-Gal eperimase-deficient mutant. *J. Immunol.,* **111**:433-438.

Ziegler, E. J., McCutchan, J. A., Douglas, H., and Braude, A. I. (1975). Prevention of lethal pseudomonas bacteremia with epimerase-deficient *E. coli* antisera. *Trans. Am. Assoc. Phys.,* **88**:101-108.

Ziegler, E. J., McCutchan, J. A., Fierer, J., Glauser, M. P., Sadoff, J. C., Douglas, H., and Braude, A. I. (1982). Treatment of gram-negative bacteremia and shock with human antiserum to mutant *Escherichia coli. N. Engl. J. Med.,* **307**:1225-1230.

19

Pulmonary Nuclear Magnetic Resonance
Potential Applications in ARDS

ALAN H. MORRIS

University of Utah and LDS Hospital
Salt Lake City, Utah

ANTONIO G. CUTILLO, DAVID C. AILION, CARL H. DURNEY, and KRISHNAMURTHY GANESAN

University of Utah
Salt Lake City, Utah

I. Introduction

Nuclear magnetic resonance (NMR) imaging is in widespread use in most major medical centers. Because of the widespread distribution and consequently the availability of this expensive, noninvasive technology (to date unassociated with any harmful biologic effects), it is attractive to consider for lung study those quantitative NMR applications that would complement the routine images obtained in most commercial NMR systems. The global and regional NMR measurement of lung water has the potential to become the absolute standard for lung water measurement and its spatial distribution. If this goal is achieved, NMR would provide the first technique permitting an in vivo, noninvasive, repetitive, relatively rapid means of measuring absolute lung water and its distribution without exposing patients to harmful x-rays.

In addition, because of its foamlike structure, the inflated lung exhibits a unique NMR behavior that distinguishes it from all other body tissues. This unique behavior can be explored by applying a modified NMR pulsing technique that, when combined with the standard NMR pulsing technique, allows the generation of a difference signal D (see later). The difference signal D is produced by that fraction of lung water sensitive to the presence of an air/tissue (air/water) interface. This feature may provide a remarkably powerful tool for the evaluation of atelectasis and for the distinction between recruitment and distention of already open alveoli in the ordinary pressure-volume behavior of the lung. This unique behavior, due to water that senses the air/tissue interface, provides information about lung water at a microscopic level (alveolar structural level), interestingly without requiring optical resolution of the structures concerned.

Among less well evaluated but still attractive possible applications of NMR studies of lung water are nonspatial distributions of NMR information, both of absolute water content and of the difference signal D. These distributions may provide characteristic patterns of specific injuries or pulmonary responses to injury. Studies of D may allow identification of that water in the alveolar structure that is sensitive to the air/tissue interface effect and may enable distinction between alveolar septal water and the water located in the corner regions where alveolar septae intersect. This latter application may allow indirect estimations of pulmonary vascular pressures, perhaps most effectively with short-term well-defined perturbations carried

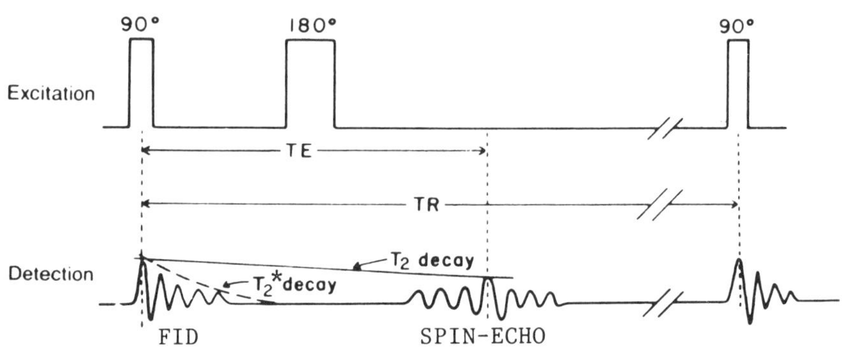

Figure 1 Spin-echo pulse sequence (simplified); 90° and 180° refer to RF pulses of magnitudes and duration sufficient to tip the net magnetic moment of the specimen 90° or 180° away from the direction of the dc magnetic field. FID = free induction decay characterized by time constant T_2^* (includes irreversible and reversible signal losses; the reversible losses are recovered in the spin-echo NMR signal). Spin echo = NMR signal produced when the dephased nuclear magnetic moments become rephased. TE = spin-echo time. TR = repetition time (time from beginning of one 90° to 180° RF pulse sequence to the beginning of the following 90° to 180° RF pulse sequence). T_2 decay = curve describing the irreversible transverse signal loss characterized by time constant T_2. (From Scherzinger and Hendee, 1985, with permission.)

out by the patient within the magnet. Geometric modeling of the lung holds promise for obtaining simple morphometric and geometric information from analysis of the NMR signal. The evaluation of the NMR relaxation times (longitudinal relaxation time T_1 describing the rate of recovery of magnetization of the specimen after a perturbation, and transverse relaxation time T_2 (Fig. 1) describing the rate at which the NMR signal irreversibly decays as a result of the dephasing of nuclear magnetic moments due to variations in local magnetic fields) may provide important diagnostic and therapeutic information when combined with measurements of water (proton) density.

All these possibilities are applicable both to the whole lung and to lung regions. The ability to address these issues regionally will, we expect, open avenues of investigation and clinical application that have previously been unapproachable. Much systematic and carefully controlled work in animals and humans remains to be done. At the present time, it is not possible to define which of the potential contributions will be realized in the application of NMR to the study of edematous lung states like the adult respiratory distress syndrome (ARDS), but the probability of successful application of some of these appears to us to be high.

II. Basic NMR Phenomena

Basic principles and applications of NMR imaging have been reviewed elsewhere (Kaufman et al., 1981; Gadian, 1982; Partain et al., 1983; Young, 1984; Mansfield and Morris, 1982; Morris, 1986; Fullerton, 1982; Pykett et al., 1982; Hendee and Morgan, 1984; Budinger and Margulis, 1986; Scherzinger and Hendee, 1985). Both quantum mechanical and classical physical explanations are available. In quantum mechanical terms, the nuclear magnetic resonance phenomenon involves induced transitions between discrete energy states of nuclei possessing magnetic moments through absorption and radiation of electromagnetic energy in a magnetic field. For the proton, only two energy states are allowed, the low-energy state being, roughly, a parallel orientation of the proton magnetic moment with respect to the direction of the externally applied magnetic field H_0 and the high-energy state an antiparallel orientation. The energy difference ΔE between these states corresponds to an electromagnetic frequency ω in the radio range $\Delta E = \hbar\omega$. Both ΔE and ω are directly proportional to the magnetic field intensity. From the classical physical perspective, the frequency ω is the frequency with which the nuclear magnetic moment precesses about the direction of the external magnetic field H_0.

The NMR behavior of a specimen is observed by perturbing the specimen after it has been magnetized in a large static magnetic field H_0. The perturbation is carried out by applying a radiofrequency (RF) magnetic field at the resonant frequency ω that corresponds to ΔE. The time constant T_1 characterizes the time required to establish the equilibrium magnetization of the specimen after placement in the magnetic field H_0. At equilibrium, the net magnetic moment of the specimen is aligned along the direction of the magnetic field H_0. The RF magnetic field (usually applied perpendicular to H_0) displaces the specimen net magnetic moment away from the direction of H_0. This RF field can be applied for a short time interval (an RF pulse), and the product of its intensity and duration determines the angular displacement of the specimen net magnetic moment away from the direction of H_0. The RF pulse is identified by the angular displacement produced (e.g., a 90° RF pulse rotates the specimen net magnetic moment 90° so that it is perpendicular to the direction of H_0 when the RF pulse is terminated). The time constant T_2^* characterizes the decay, called the free induction decay (FID), of the NMR signal following an RF magnetic field pulse (Fig. 1). This NMR signal decay is caused by inhomogeneity of the magnetic field seen by the protons in the specimen. As a result of this nonuniform magnetic field the protons resonate at slightly different frequencies, and the signal disappears as a result of the subsequent dephasing of the magnetic moments of the different protons. It is only when the vector sum of all the contributions from the nuclear magnetic moments of the precessing protons is >0 (the net magnetic moment is >0) that a signal is detected. Once complete dephasing occurs, the net magnetic moment of the specimen is zero even though the different nuclear magnetic moments are still precessing. The NMR signal loss characterized by T_2^* includes irreversible and reversible contributions. The reversible component can be recovered with a spin echo (see later).

Among the techniques used for NMR data acquisition, the spin-echo RF pulse sequence (the application of a 90° RF pulse followed by a 180° RF pulse in the presence of external magnetic field gradients) is of particular interest (Fig. 1). In the 90° to 180° RF pulse sequence technique, the 180° RF pulse inverts magnetic dipoles in the plane transverse to the direction of H_0 and thus reverses the direction of dephasing nuclear magnetic moments. Those nuclear magnetic moments experiencing the highest local magnetic fields were moving away from the direction of the net magnetization vector of the specimen with the greatest speed. They now, with direction reversed, move toward this net magnetization vector with the greatest speed. They, and therefore all other nuclear magnetic moments, reconverge (refocus) and produce an NMR signal (the spin echo) at a time TE called the echo time.

Most nuclei with odd-numbered nucleons have magnetic moments. A number of these are available for NMR studies in biologic systems (Table 1). The proton is the nucleus most commonly used for NMR studies, particularly imaging, since it not only has the highest NMR signal-to-noise ratio but is

Table 1 Nuclei of Biologic Interest Exhibiting the NMR Phenomenon[a]

Nucleus	Resonant frequency (MHz/T)
^{1}H	42.58
^{13}C	10.71
^{17}O	5.77
^{19}F	40.05
^{23}Na	11.26
^{31}P	17.24

[a]T = tesla (10^4 gauss).

present in the body at a concentration (approximately 80 M) that exceeds by more than two orders of magnitude those of all other nuclei of interest.

III. NMR Imaging: Frequency Encoding of Position

The energy content and RF used in NMR imaging are much lower than those utilized for optical imaging with either visible light or x-rays. The wavelength of the electromagnetic radiation is consequently much longer than that associated with light or x-rays (Table 2). The wavelength (about 10 m) of the RF used in a typical NMR measurement in biologic systems is so large that direct resolution of the spatial elements of the structure being studied is not possible using the techniques employed in optical imaging. The approach used in NMR imaging produces a correspondence of each position in space to a specific and distinct RF associated with the NMR phenomenon. This correspondence of position and frequency is based on the fact that both ΔE and ω are directly proportional to the magnetic field H_0 within which the sample is placed, according to

$$\Delta E = \hbar\omega = \frac{\hbar\gamma H_0}{2\pi} \tag{1}$$

where γ is the magnetogyric ratio and $\hbar$ is Planck's constant. By superimposing a small linear magnetic field gradient on the uniform magnetic field H_0, every point in space along the direction of the field gradient has a unique local field equal to the sum of H_0 and the value of the gradient at that point.

Table 2 Comparison of Electromagnetic Radiation Employed in X-ray and NMR Imaging[a]

	X-ray	NMR
E (eV)	10^4-10^6	10^{-11}-10^{-6}
f (Hz)	10^{18}-10^{20}	10^3-10^8
λ (m)	10^{-10}-10^{-12}	10^5-10^0

[a]E = energy in electron volts; f = frequency in Hz (sec^{-1}); λ = wavelength in meters.

Each of these points is therefore associated with a different and specific ω. After recording the NMR signal in the time domain, a Fourier transform of the signal to the frequency domain assigns a magnitude to each frequency capable of resolution. The magnitude of the NMR signal at a given frequency corresponds to the number of protons resonating at that frequency. The frequency itself corresponds to a particular and specific position in space. By applying gradients in the three directions (or intermediate directions) in space, it is possible to resolve spatially the resonating protons in a three-dimensional object, such as a human chest. The data so resolved are used to construct, through computer tomographic (CT) techniques, an image.

IV. NMR of Lung Water: An Absolute Standard?

The NMR technique for measuring lung water offers some attractive advantages. Lung water measurements by NMR are nondestructive and noninvasive. They are relatively rapid and easily repeatable. They are independent of ventilation and perfusion of the lung, and they involve no ionizing radiation. NMR imaging techniques are well suited to the regional quantitation of lung water. Among the limitations of the NMR technique must be included susceptibility to motion-induced error (from both heart and chest movement) and the current inability to discriminate between intravascular and extravascular water compartments.

In isolated rat lungs (Cutillo et al., 1984), NMR quantitation of lung water was as accurate and precise as was the gravimetric technique when applied to lung slices of 0.076 ml containing 4-40 mg H_2O. With careful attention to the details of data acquisition, the NMR technique appears capable of fulfilling the theoretical promise of absolute lung water measurement. The specific techniques used in rat have yet to be extended to larger animals, including humans.

Among the technical requirements for the use of NMR for absolute lung water measurements must be included the reduction of noise due to tissue motion, careful calibration of the system with appropriate water standards, attention to the temporal symmetry of the RF pulsing sequence (see later), use of an adequately long repetition time (time between the beginnings of identical RF pulse sequences) and/or correction for incomplete recovery of sample magnetization (T_1 signal loss), correction for NMR signal loss due to transverse dephasing (T_2 signal loss), and appropriate control and characterization of the physiologic preparation, particularly with reference to the stability of lung water and its distribution. With the exception of quantitative analysis of plain chest x-rays (Pistolesi et al., 1985; Milne et al., 1985), the clinical potential of measurements of lung water content and distribution by noninvasive, relatively rapid, and easily repeatable analytic methods is virtually unexplored. Equally unknown is the relative value of lung water content measurements with respect to measurements of liquid and solute exchange, particularly in terms of important patient outcome variables, such as survival.

V. Unique NMR Behavior of Inflated Lung and the Difference Signal D

The free-induction decay (FID) is much shorter in inflated lung than in airless lung or other solid body tissues (Fig. 2) (Morris et al., 1985). This rapid temporal loss of NMR signal corresponds to a distribution of emitted RF energy over a broad range of frequencies ω. This frequency-domain representation of the NMR signal is called the NMR line. Such an increase in frequency content is termed NMR line broadening. In inflated lung in a perfectly uniform external magnetic field, the NMR line broadening is due solely to the structure of the water-containing tissue. Inflated lung tissue resembles a foam, and NMR line broadening is a general property of foams (e.g., detergent-water foam or aerosol shaving cream) (Morris et al., 1985). The NMR line broadening (short FID in the time domain) results from the magnetic susceptibility difference between water and air. A shell of water, representing a single alveolus, when placed in a uniform external magnetic field H_0 produces a sample-induced internal magnetic field inhomogeneity. As a result of the diamagnetism of water, the magnetic field is reduced within the water in that part of the shell oriented parallel to the direction of H_0. In contrast, the magnetic field is unaltered within the water in that part of the shell oriented perpendicular to the direction of H_0 (Fig. 3). Water protons in the shells of foams (or inflated lung) therefore experience different local magnetic fields,

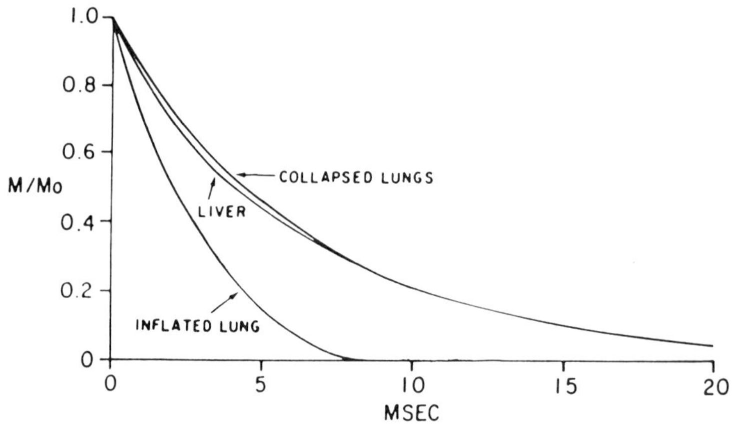

Figure 2 NMR free induction (FID) of inflated lung, collapsed lung, and liver. M/M_0 = magnetization as a fraction of initial (maximum) magnetization M_0. Collapsed lungs = airless, degassed lungs prepared in vacuo. (From Morris et al., 1985, with permission.)

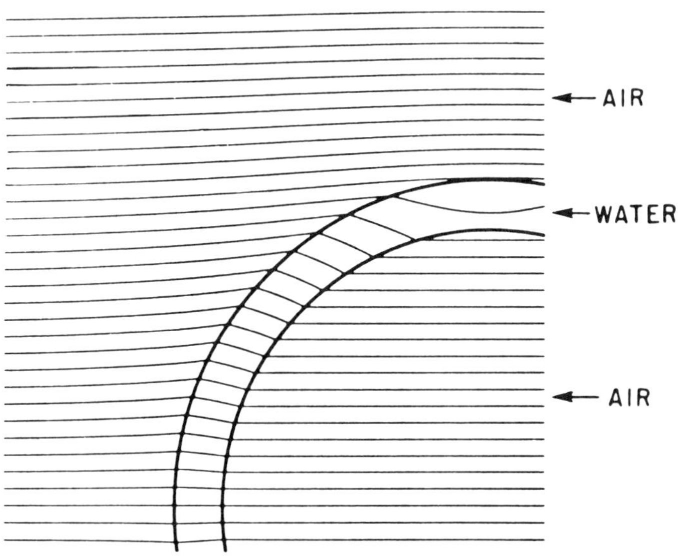

Figure 3 Magnetic field perturbations caused by a spherical shell of water in air. Water in that part of the shell oriented parallel to the field direction repels the field and reduces the field within the shell. Water in that part of the shell oriented perpendicular to the field direction does not change the field strength. (From Case et al., 1987, with permission.)

resulting in NMR line broadening and a short FID. The theoretical and experimentally observed NMR line broadening produced by a single spherical shell of water are almost identical (Fig. 4) (Case et al., 1987).

The reversible sample-induced magnetic field inhomogeneity can also be detected using NMR spin-echo sequences that are temporally symmetric or asymmetric with respect to the time intervals between the 90° and 180° RF pulses and between the 180° pulse and the spin echo (Fig. 5). A symmetric sequence is one in which the time τ is equal to the time τ'. An asymmetric sequence is one in which τ is not equal to τ'. Typically, there are two sources of transverse dephasing in inflated lung. The dephasing due to the external field gradient rephases at a time $\tau + \tau'$ when the area under the gradient curve G_x before the 180° pulse is equal to the area under the gradient curve after the 180° pulse. In contrast, the dephasing due to the sample-induced internal magnetic inhomogeneity rephases at 2τ (twice the time between the 90° and 180° pulses). The combined effect of these two sources of dephasing determines the amplitude of the spin echo. In a symmetric sequence, these two dephasings are refocused at the same time, since $\tau + \tau'$ equals 2τ, and the maximum spin-echo amplitude is obtained. In an asymmetric spin-echo RF pulse sequence, the dephasing due to the reversible sample-

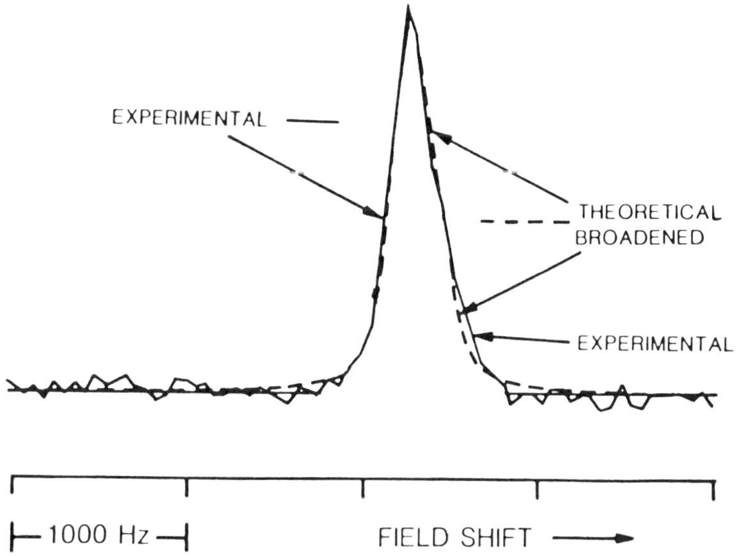

Figure 4 Comparison of the theoretical and experimental (observed) NMR line shape of a spherical water shell in air. Vertical displacement represents NMR signal magnitude. (From Case et al., 1987, with permission.)

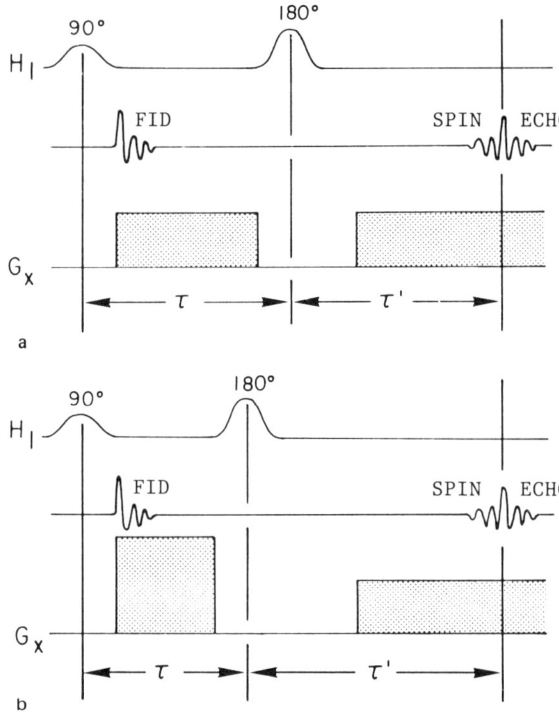

Figure 5 (a) Symmetric and (b) asymmetric spin-echo sequences. H_1 = RF magnetic field (90° and 180° pulses). FID = free induction decay. G_x = external magnetic field gradient applied in the x direction (stippled area). Horizontal axis = time. (From Blatter et al., 1985, with permission.)

induced internal magnetic field inhomogeneity would be refocused at 2τ but would no longer be coincident with the refocusing of the dephasing due to the external field gradients at $\tau + \tau'$. In a tissue like the liver, without significant reversible sample-induced internal magnetic field inhomogeneity, the echo heights in the symmetric and in the asymmetric RF pulse sequence are equal. In contrast, in inflated lung, within which significant sample-induced internal magnetic field inhomogeneity exists because of the air/water interface, the asymmetric RF pulse sequence spin-echo amplitude is reduced relative to the symmetric RF pulse sequence spin-echo amplitude. The difference between the asymmetric and symmetric spin echo heights we call the difference signal D.

These difference signals D can be utilized to construct images (subtraction or difference images) of the water experiencing the air/water interface

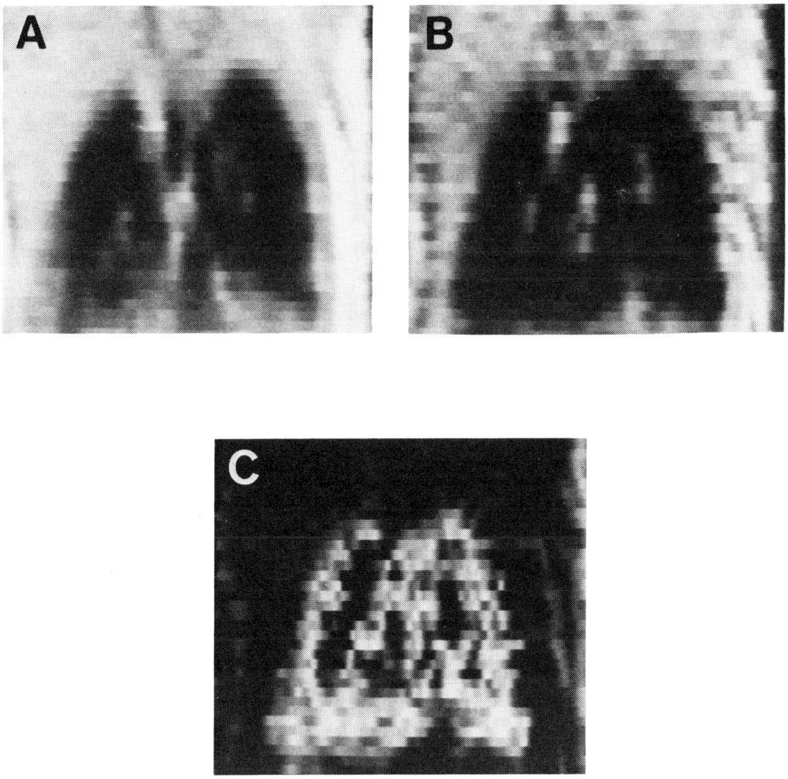

Figure 6 In vivo spontaneously breathing rat: three spin-echo images of the chest. (A) Symmetric RF pulse spin-echo sequence image; (B) asymmetric RF pulse spin-echo sequence image; (C) difference image (voxel by voxel) in which D = (A − B)/A. Note that A is the usual or standard spin-echo imaging technique. (From Morris et al., 1985, with permission.)

phenomenon in inflated lung (Fig. 6) (Morris et al., 1985; Ailion et al., 1984a, b; Blatter et al., 1985). We are currently exploring the possibility that D is provided by water in the "thin" portions of the alveolar wall, in contrast to corner water (at the junctions between alveoli), which we suspect is less sensitive to the air/water interface effect. The interesting potential benefits of distinguishing alveolar septal from corner water remain to be explored.

For appropriate asymmetry times, D dramatically increases coincidently with the increase in lung volume when isolated lungs are inflated from the airless (degassed) state (Fig. 7).

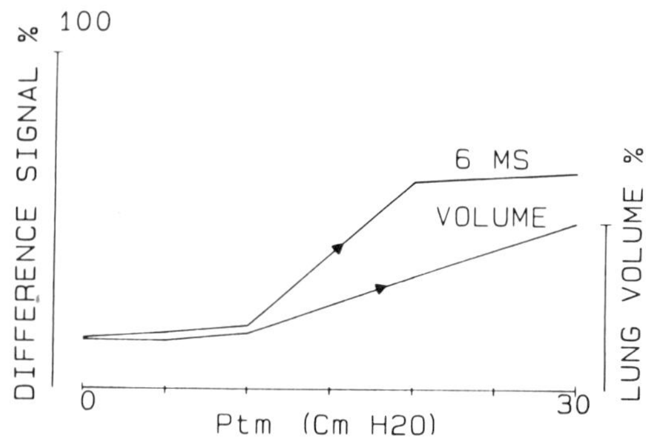

Figure 7 Isolated rat lungs, initially airless after degassing in vacuo. Measurements made during a single inflation from the degassed state (P_{TM} = 0) to full inflation (P_{TM} = 30). Difference signal D at 6 msec asymmetric RF spin-echo pulse sequence compared with lung volume (100% lung volume defined at P_{TM} = 30 cmH_2O). P_{TM} = transpulmonary pressure.

VI. Nonspatial Distributions of Lung Water

The representation of lung water distribution as a function of spatial position is a conventional approach, analogous to ventilation and perfusion maps obtained by radioisotopic techniques. In addition to this approach, a new display of the NMR data has recently been proposed (Cutillo et al., 1988) that describes the distribution of lung water as a function of water density ρH_2O. The new method displays the distribution of fractional lung volume V_f (number of voxels at a given density divided by the total number of voxels) with respect to water density ρH_2O (water content per unit lung volume). Therefore, the display is a normalized frequency distribution of ρH_2O. Theoretically, ρH_2O is expected to vary from 0 (air) to about 0.8 (blood and solid lung tissue). Studies in excised rat lungs and in living rats showed that pulmonary edema induced by oleic acid injection or rapid saline injection was associated with marked changes in the V_f versus ρH_2O distribution (Fig. 8). These changes reflect both the increased lung water content and, in the case of the oleic acid model, the marked spatial inequality of the injury. Abnormal V_f versus ρH_2O distributions have also been obtained in other types of experimental pulmonary edema, including intrabronchial instillation of saline, and the V_f versus ρH_2O distribution method has also been used successfully in rats to follow the time course of experimental lung injury (Cutillo et al., 1988). The conventional spatial display and the V_f versus ρH_2O distribution are complementary (rather than competitive) approaches, each defining a different aspect of lung water distribution.

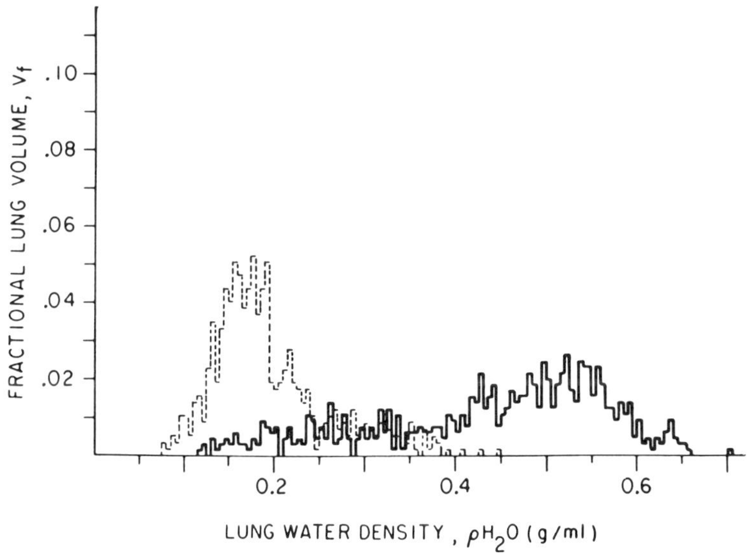

Figure 8 Spontaneously breathing rat, before (dashed line) and after (solid line) intravenous injection of oleic acid. Distribution of fractional lung volume Vf [(number of voxels at ρH_2O)/(total number of voxels)] as a function of lung water density ρH_2O. Average ρH_2O (g H_2O/ml) = 0.19 before and 0.44 after oleic acid injection. Gravimetric lung water content after oleic acid ((wet lung weight − dry lung weight)/dry lung weight) = 6.09 g H_2O/g dry lung. (From Cutillo et al., 1988, with permission.)

The V_f versus ρH_2O distribution is analogous to the distributions of ventilation and perfusion as a function of the ventilation-perfusion ratio (Wagner et al., 1974). Gattinoni et al. (1987) have utilized a similar approach in describing the distribution of x-ray CT scan voxels as a function of density in ARDS patients.

VII. Geometric Information About Lung Structure Without Requiring Optical Resolution

One of the most fascinating factors of NMR studies of lung is the possibility that, using appropriate geometric models, basic morphometric or structural information may be obtained from the NMR line shape (the frequency-domain NMR signal). Preliminary work with a simple model consisting of an array of hexagonally close-packed spherical airspaces in a water medium has provided promising results (Case et al., 1987). The intriguing possibility of distinguishing corner from thin alveolar septal water by analysis of the NMR line shape seems theoretically achievable without the addition of markers and therefore without the necessity of invading the patient through either the vascular or the airway routes. Although not intuitively obvious, this information, if obtainable, will not require optical resolution of the structures of interest (e.g., the alveolar septum, the alveolar corners, or alveoli themselves). The extraction of such information from NMR line shape analysis would be possible both globally and regionally, the limitations being primarily determined by the signal-to-noise ratio, a function of the size of the spatial lung region from which NMR data are acquired.

VIII. Relaxation Times T_1 and T_2

Advantage is frequently taken of the dependence of the NMR signal intensity upon T_1 and T_2 in NMR imaging to enhance tissue differentiation (Kaufman et al., 1981; Partain et al., 1983; Young, 1984). In animal tissues, T_1 and T_2 (or their reciprocals, the relaxation rates) vary with water content (Lauterbur, 1976; Skalina et al., 1984; Schmidt et al., 1985, 1986; Wexler et al., 1985). This is predictable from models describing the state of water in biologic systems (Mansfield and Morris, 1982; Taylor and Bore, 1981). Relaxation time and proton density measurements have generally been used as alternative measures of lung water content. Recent studies, however, suggest the interesting possibility that T_1 and T_2 measurements may complement the proton density data, thus providing a more comprehensive assessment of lung water and pulmonary edema. According to these studies, the determination of T_1 (and/or T_2) in addition to proton density might be valuable in differentiating lung edema from other causes of increased proton density (e.g., vascular congestion or atelectasis) and in defining the pathogenetic type of pulmonary edema (hydrostatic versus increased permeability) (Skalina et al., 1984; Schmidt et al., 1986; Moore et al., 1986; Podgorski et al., 1986). This hypothesis is based upon relaxation time mechanisms and the state of water in biologic systems. The relaxation times T_1 and T_2 in biologic tissues are affected not only by water content but also, among other factors, by the interactions between water and macromolecules (Mansfield and Morris, 1982; Mathur-De Vré, 1984; Bottomley et al., 1984). According to simple two-state models, biologic tissues contain two fractions of water: free water and water bonded to macromolecules (bound water). If a rapid exchange exists between the free-water compartment and the bound water compartment, the spin-lattice relaxation rate $1/T_1$ is the weighted average of the relaxation rates of the two compartments:

$$\frac{1}{T_1} = \left(\frac{1}{T_1}\right)_b F_b + \left(\frac{1}{T_1}\right)_f (1 - F_b) \tag{1}$$

where $(1/T_1)_b$ and $(1/T_1)_f$ are the relaxation rates for the bound and free water and F_b is the bound-water fraction. According to the equation, T_1 is dependent on the ratio of bound to free water. The dependence of T_1 on water-macromolecule interactions is reflected by the close correlation between $1/T_1$ and protein concentration in water solutions (Mansfield and Morris, 1982; Taylor and Bore, 1981; Bottomley et al., 1984; Daszkiewicz et al., 1963; Allen et al., 1986; Menon and Allen, 1987) and likely is an important cause of T_1 variation among different biologic tissues (Taylor and Bore, 1981). Water motion in normal lung has recently been shown to be more restricted than that of free water (Kveder et al., 1988).

A fraction of interstitial lung water is associated with the macromolecules that constitute the matrix of the lung (collagen, elastin, proteoglycans, and fibronectin) (Prockop, 1979; Taylor et al., 1982; Crystal et al., 1984; Turino, 1985; Gil, 1983), with cellular macromolecules, and with other molecules (including plasma proteins). This fraction corresponds to the bound water fraction F_b in Equation (2). In pulmonary edema, the accumulation of water in the interstitial space can be expected to cause an increase in the free-water fraction and should increase the value of T_1. Since the bound-water fraction is proportional to protein concentration (Mansfield and Morris, 1982; Taylor and Bore, 1981; Bottomley et al., 1984), the equation also predicts that, for the same lung water content, T_1 should vary according to the pathogenetic type of pulmonary edema. Podgorski and associates (1986) tested these concepts by measuring the relaxation times of lung lymph obtained from chronically instrumented unanesthetized sheep after administration of *Escherichia coli* endotoxin or insertion of a left atrial balloon. As predicted, they found that the lymph T_1 value was higher when pulmonary hydrostatic pressure was elevated than when capillary permeability was increased. However, Huber and Adams (1984) found no difference between the lung T_1 values obtained from rabbit models of hydrostatic (aortic balloon and saline infusion) and increased permeability (oleic acid) pulmonary edema.

Other investigators have also tested the hypothesis that T_1 measurements may differentiate pulmonary edema from other pathologic conditions, with inconclusive results in rabbit models of lung hemorrhage and edema (Huber and Adams, 1984) and in NMR imaging studies of patients (Moore et al., 1986). Nevertheless, in rats exposed to high concentrations (80-100%) of oxygen, T_1 increased with water content during the acute phase of the injury but decreased more markedly than did water content during the repair stage (Shioya et al., 1985). The initial increase in T_1 may reflect an increase in the free-water fraction due to edema; the subsequent disproportionate decrease in T_1 may reflect an increased bound-water fraction due to structural changes associated with the repair stage of the injury (proliferation of interstitial cells with accumulation of new collagen and elastin) (Frank, 1985). An increased bound-water fraction due to increased concentration of macromolecules may also partly account for the decreased T_1 values observed by Vinitski and associates (1986) in rat lungs with bleomycin-induced injury.

Since the spin-spin relaxation time T_2 is, like T_1, dependent on tissue type (Mathur-De Vré, 1984; Bottomley et al., 1984), it also appears to be a potentially useful complement to proton density data. Although some experimental evidence supports this prediction, there are inconsistencies in the published data. T_2 was found to differ between hydrostatic and increased permeability edema (Schmidt et al., 1986) and to be shorter in bleomycin-induced pulmonary fibrosis (Vinitski et al., 1986). Exponential components of the lung T_2 decay obtained from rats exposed to high oxygen concentrations showed changes similar to those of T_1 (Schmidt et al., 1986). However, other studies showed no significant differences in T_2 between pulmonary edema and other pathologic conditions or between hydrostatic and permeability lung edema (Huber and Adams, 1984; Moore et al., 1986; Podgorski et al., 1986).

Although, on the whole, these experimental results suggest that relaxation time measurements can complement the proton density data, at least under certain experimental conditions, they are not conclusive. Overlap between relaxation times obtained in different pathologic conditions is a possible limitation. The practical value of the combined T_1, T_2, and proton density approach remains to be proved.

IX. Potential Applications in ARDS

To date, only limited data are available concerning the application of NMR techniques to the evaluation of lung edema. Most of the work has been restricted to in vitro specimen studies or animal model work. A systematic evaluation of the many factors involved and the ultimate applicability of NMR data to the diagnosis and treatment of patients with lung edema is a matter for the future.

Although pulmonary edema is an extremely common occurrence, the clinical significance of lung water measurements is controversial. Emphasis has recently been placed on the need to develop clinical methods capable of assessing the dynamic aspects of lung liquid and solute exchange (Staub, 1986; Cutillo, 1987). Compared with static lung water content measurements, dynamic methods appear to detect abnormalities of liquid balance at an earlier stage of disease. However, since the effects of protective factors (e.g., lymph flow) are at present not clinically measurable or quantitatively predictable, determinations of lung water content to assess the extent of fluid accumulation may be equally important. With respect to the prediction of patient outcome, the value of lung water content measurements compared to that of determinations of liquid and solute exchange is undefined, and little information is available. In patients with lung edema and acute respiratory failure (Brigham et al., 1983), in critically ill patients (Laggner et al., 1984), and in animals (Mihm et al., 1982), extravascular lung water measured by an indicator dilution technique was poorly correlated with arterial oxygenation and did not predict the outcome (Brigham et al., 1983). The poor correlation has been attributed to a compensatory mechanism preserving oxygenation (decreased perfusion to poorly ventilated edematous regions of the lung) (Brigham et al., 1983), thereby suggesting that water accumulation is not the sole determinant of respiratory impairment in pulmonary edema. However, these observations may merely be a consequence of limitations of the indicator dilution technique. Although the prognostic value of lung water measurements may be limited, the dissociation reported between lung water content and arterial oxygenation justifies the application of lung water measurements in patients with pulmonary edema, provided these measurements become sufficiently practical and reliable. Additional clinical studies in larger series of subjects and at multiple stages of water accumulation are clearly needed. Determinations of regional lung water distribution as a function of time (during water accumulation and recovery) in different types of pulmonary edema (e.g., high-pressure versus increased permeability edema) are also required.

It seems probable that the NMR evaluation of lung water will eventually provide useful information in patients with edematous lungs, such as ARDS patients. Recent studies have shown that standard NMR techniques can quantify relative changes in lung water content in various types of experimental lung injury (Hayes et al., 1982; Schmidt et al., 1985, 1986; Carrol et al., 1985; Cutillo et al., 1988). Preliminary data show that these techniques can be used for studies in living human subjects (Lallemand et al., 1984; Carrol et al., 1985; Ailion et al., 1986; Moore et al., 1986; MacLennan et al., 19876). Therefore, the application of NMR to the detection and quantification of clinical lung edema and its regional distribution should be feasible both for single measurements and for multiple determinations as a function of time. The measurement of absolute lung water content, although requiring special attention to technical details, seems feasible as well (Cutillo et al., 1984).
In addition, new techniques recently developed to detect the unique NMR behavior of inflated lung can be used to isolate the lung water signal from that of other body tissues and, more importantly, to explore the air/tissue interface phenomenon. These techniques provide not only a means for distinguishing very dense lung (which is usually partially aerated) from solid tissues, thus aiding in the definition of atelectasis, but coupled with evaluation of the difference signal D, they may also provide new and informative data about lung structure and the distribution of water within the gas-exchanging region.

The application of nonspatial distributions, such as the V_f versus ρH_2O distribution, may allow distinctions between different kinds of lung injury. Such information would follow in the footsteps of contributions that have come from the analysis of ventilation and perfusion as a function of $\dot{V}/\dot{Q}$ ratios. The ultimate usefulness of this approach, particularly the possibility of defining "fingerprints" of particular diseases or pulmonary derangements, remains to be explored.

The possibility of obtaining geometric information about lung structure without requiring optical resolution remains exciting. Should it prove feasible in the clinical setting to separate the signal from corner water from that of thin alveolar septal water, it may be possible to utilize the NMR line shape as an indicator of corner vessel size and, therefore, of pulmonary venous pressure. Discrete and rapidly effected forcing functions (e.g., hand grip exercise) may provide a practical means to take advantage of this possibility.

The combination of NMR information obtained from proton density and that obtained from relaxation time studies may also prove fruitful. The enhancement of sensitivity, specificity, and predictive value that may come from a combination of proton density and T_1 and T_2 assessment (and perhaps other relaxation times or variables) carries with it the burden of greater complexity. The usefulness of such a combined approach will depend heavily upon the performance of carefully controlled and systematically conducted animal and human studies.

In summary, the potential applications of NMR studies of lung in edematous states in general and in ARDS patients in particular appear interesting and exciting but, to date, undefined. The great attraction of NMR imaging lies, in part, in that much greater contrast is possible between tissues of interest because of the multiple variables that operate upon the final product (the NMR image), in contrast with x-ray images, which depend almost exclusively upon much smaller variations in electron density. This remarkable attractiveness of NMR imaging brings with it a marked increase in complexity because of the increased number of variables of importance. Ultimate applicability will depend upon definitions obtained through carefully controlled systematic studies.

Acknowledgments

Supported by NIH grants HL-23746, HL-31216, CA-44972, and RR-02316, by the University of Utah, and by the LDS Hospital.

References

Ailion, D. C., Blatter, D. D., Case, T. A., Morris, A. H., Cutillo, A. G., and Durney, C. H. (1984a). Asymmetric imaging. In *Proceedings of the*

XXII Congress Ampere. Edited by K. A. Muller, R. Kind, and J. Roos. Zurich, Zurich Ampere Committee, University of Zurich, pp. 510-511.

Ailion, D. C., Case, T. A., Blatter, D. D., Morris, A. H., Cutillo, A. G., Durney, C. H., and Johnson, S. A. (1984b). Applications of NMR spin imaging to the study of lungs. *Bull. Magn. Res.*, **6**:130-139.

Ailion, D. C., Case, T. A., Blatter, D. D., Morris, A. H., Cutillo, A. G., and Durney, C. H. (1986). New imaging techniques for lung and fat. In *New Developments in Nuclear Magnetic Resonance and Magnetic Resonance and Quantum Electronics*. Edited by I. Ursu and K. H. Hausser. Bucharest, CIP Press, pp. 1-20.

Allen, P. S., Castro, M. E., Treiber, E. O., Lunt, J. A., and Boisvert, D. P. J. (1986). A proton NMR relaxation evaluation of a model of brain oedema fluid. *Phys. Med. Biol.*, **31**:699-711.

Blatter, D. D., Morris, A. H., Ailion, D. C., Cutillo, A. G., and Case, T. A. (1985). Asymmetric spin echo sequences. A simple new method for obtaining NMR ^{1}H spectral images. *Invest. Radiol.*, **20**:845-853.

Bottomley, P. A., Foster, T. H., Argersinger, R. E., and Pfeifer, L. M. (1984). A review of normal tissue hydrogen NMR relaxation time and relaxation mechanisms from 1-100 MHz: Dependence on tissue type, NMR frequency, temperature, species, excision, and age. *Med. Phys.*, **11**:425-448.

Brigham, K. L., Kariman, K., Harris, T. R., Snapper, J. R., Bernard, G. R., and Young, S. L. (1983). Correlation of oxygenation with vascular permeability-surface area but not with lung water in humans with acute respiratory failure and pulmonary edema. *J. Clin. Invest.*, **72**:339-349.

Budinger, T. F., and Margulis, A. R., editors (1986). *Medical Magnetic Resonance Imaging and Spectroscopy. A Primer*. Berkeley, Society of Magnetic Resonance in Medicine.

Carroll, F. E., Jr., Lloyd, J. E., Nolop, K. E., and Collins, J. C. (1985). MR imaging parameters in the study of lung water. A preliminary study. *Invest. Radiol.*, **20**:381-387.

Case, T. A., Durney, C. H., Ailion, D. C., Cutillo, A. G., and Morris, A. H. (1987). A mathematical model of diamagnetic line broadening in lung tissue and similar heterogeneous systems: Calculations and measurements. *J. Magn. Reson.*, **73**:304-314.

Crapo, J. D., Barry, B. E., Foscue, H. A., and Shelburne, J. (1980). Structural and biochemical changes in rat lungs occurring during exposures to lethal and adaptive doses of oxygen. *Am. Rev. Respir. Dis.*, **122**:123-143.

Crystal, R. G., Bitterman, P. B., Rennard, S. I., Hance, A. J., and Keogh, B. A. (1984). Interstitial lung diseases of unknown cause. Disorders characterized by chronic inflammation of the lower respiratory tract (first of two parts). *N. Engl. J. Med.*, **310**:154-166.

Cutillo, A. G. (1987). The clinical assessment of lung water. *Chest,* **92**:319-325.

Cutillo, A. G., Morris, A. H., Blatter, D. D., Case, T. A., Ailion, D. C., Durney, C. H., and Johnson, S. A. (1984). Determination of lung water content and distribution by nuclear magnetic resonance. *J. Appl. Physiol.,* **57**:583-588.

Cutillo, A. G., Morris, A. H., Ailion, D. C., Case, T. A., Durney, C. H., Ganesan, K., Watanabe, F., and Akhtari, M. (1988). Assessment of lung water distribution by nuclear magnetic resonance. A new method for quantifying and monitoring experimental lung injury. *Am. Rev. Respir. Dis.,* **137**:1371-1378.

Daszkiewsicz, O. K., Hennel, J. W., Lubas, B., and Szczepkowski, T. W. (1963). Proton magnetic relaxation and protein hydration. *Nature,* **200**:1006-1007.

Frank, L. (1985). Oxydant injury to pulmonary endothelium. In *The Pulmonary Circulation and Acute Lung Injury.* Edited by S. I. Said. Mount Kisko, New York, Futura Publishing, pp. 283-305.

Fullerton, G. D. (1982). Basic concepts for nuclear magnetic resonance imaging. *Magn. Reson. Imaging,* **1**:39-55.

Gadian, D. G. (1982). *Nuclear Magnetic Resonance and Its Applications to Living Systems.* Oxford, Clarendon Press.

Gattinoni, L., Pesenti, A., Avalli, L., Rossi, F., and Bombino, M. (1987). Pressure-volume curve of total respiratory system in acute respiratory failure. Computed tomographic scan study. *Am. Rev. Respir. Dis.,* **136**:730-736.

Gil, J. (1982). Alveolar wall relations. *Ann. N.Y. Acad. Sci.,* **384**:31-43.

Hayes, C. E., Case, T. A., Ailion, D. C., Morris, A. H., Cutillo, A., Blackburn, C. W., Durney, C. H., and Johnson, S. A. (1982). Lung water quantitation by nuclear magnetic resonance imaging. *Science,* **216**:1313-1315.

Hendee, W. R., and Morgan, C. J. (1984). Magnetic resonance imaging. Part I. Physical principles. *West. J. Med.,* **141**:491-500.

Huber, D. J., and Adams, D. F. (1984). Proton NMR of acute pulmonary edema and hemorrhage. *Invest. Radiol.,* **19**:S21.

Kaufman, L., Crooks, L., and Margulis, A. R., editors (1981). *Nuclear Magnetic Resonance Imaging in Medicine.* New York, Igaku-Shoin.

Kveder, M., Lahajnar, G., Blinc, R., and Zupancic, I. (1988). Non-Brownian water self-diffusion in lung tissue. *Magn. Reson. Med.,* **6**:194-198.

Laggner, A., Kleinberger, G., Sommer, G., Haller, J., Lenz, K., Base, W., and Druml, W. (1985). Bestimmung des extravaskularen Lungenwassergehalts bei Intensivepatienten: Gegenubenstellung mit radiologischen, hamodynamischen und funktionellen Lungenbefunden. *Schweiz. Med. Wochenschr.,* **115**:210-213.

Lallemand, D. P., Brasch, R. C., Gooding, C. A., Wesbey, G. E., and Higgins, C. B. (1984). NMR imaging of lung parenchyma. *Magn. Reson. Med.,* **1**:190-191.

Lauterbur, P. C. (1976). Feasibility of NMR zeugmatographic imaging of the heart and lungs. Presented at the Engineering Foundation Conference on Comparative Productivity of Techniques for Noninvasive Medical Diagnosis, Henniker, New Hampshire, New England College, August 15-20.

MacLennan, F. M., Foster, M. A., Smith, F. W., and Crosher, G. A. (1986). Measurement of total lung water from nuclear magnetic resonance images. *Br. J. Radiol.,* **59**:553-560.

Mansfield, P., and Morris, P. G. (1982). *NMR Imaging in Biomedicine.* Supplement 2. *Advances in Magnetic Resonance.* New York, Academic Press.

Mathur-De Vré, R. (1984). Biomedical implications of the relaxation behavior of water related to NMR imaging. *Br. J. Radiol.,* **57**:955-976.

Menon, R. S., and Allen, P. S. (1987). Proton relaxation in aqueous solutions of fibrinogen and α_2-macroglobulin. In book of abstracts, *6th Annual Meeting, Society of Magnetic Resonance in Medicine,* Berkeley, California, p. 436.

Mihm, F. G., Feeley, T. W., Rosenthal, M. H., and Lewis, F. (1982). Measurement of extravascular lung water in dogs using the thermal-green dye indicator dilution method. *Anesthesiology,* **57**:116-122.

Milne, E. N. C., Pistolesi, M., Miniati, M., and Giuntini, C. (1985). The radiologic distinction of cardiogenic and noncardiogenic edema. *AJR,* **144**:879-894.

Moore, E. H., Webb, W. R., Muller, N., and Sollitto, R. (1986). MRI of pulmonary airspace disease: Experimental model and preliminary clinical results. *AJR,* **146**:1123-1128.

Morris, A. H., Blatter, D. D., Case, T. A., Cutillo, A. G., Ailion, D. C., Durney, C. H., and Johnson, S. A. (1985). A new nuclear magnetic resonance property of lung. *J. Appl. Physiol.,* **58**:759-762.

Morris, P. G. (1986). *Nuclear Magnetic Resonance Imaging in Medicine and Biology.* Oxford, Clarendon Press.

Partain, C. L., James, A. E., Jr., Rollo, F. D., and Price, R. R. (1983). *Nuclear Magnetic Resonance (NMR) Imaging.* Philadelphia, W. B. Saunders.

Pistolesi, M., Miniati, M., Milne, E. N. C., and Giuntini, C. (1985). The chest roentgenogram in pulmonary edema. *Clin. Chest Med.,* **6**:315-344.

Podgorski, G. T., Carroll, F. E., and Parker, R. E. (1986). MR evaluation of pulmonary interstitial and intravascular fluids. *Invest. Radiol.,* **21**:478-482.

Prockop, D. J. (1979). Collagen, elastin, and proteoglycans: Matrix for fluid accumulation in the lung. In *Pulmonary Edema.* Edited by A. P. Fishman and E. M. Renkin. Bethesda, American Physiological Society, pp. 125-135.

Pykett, I. L., Newhouse, J. H., Buonanno, F. S., Brady, T. J., Goldman, M. R., Kistler, J. P., and Pohost, G. M. (1982). Principles of nuclear magnetic resonance imaging. *Radiology,* **143**:157-168.

Scherzinger, A. L., and Hendee, W. R. (1985). Basic principles of magnetic resonance imaging—an update. *West. J. Med.,* **143**:782-792.

Schmidt, H. C., McNamara, M. T., Brasch, R. C., and Higgins, C. B. (1985). Assessment of severity of experimental pulmonary edema with magnetic resonance imaging. Effect of relaxation enhancement by Gd-DTPA. *Invest. Radiol.,* **20**:687-692.

Schmidt, H. C., Tsay, D.-G., and Higgins, C. B. (1986). Pulmonary edema: An NMR study of permeability and hydrostatic types in animals. *Radiology,* **158**:297-302.

Shioya, S., Haida, M., Fukuzaki, M., Tsuji, C., Ohta, Y., and Yamabayashi, H. (1985). Detection of oxygen lung injury by NMR method. *Kokyu-To-Junkan,* **33**:603-607.

Skalina, S., Kundel, H. L., Wolf, G., and Marshall, B. (1984). The effect of pulmonary edema on proton nuclear magnetic resonance relaxation times. *Invest. Radiol.,* **19**:7-9.

Staub, N. C. (1986). Clinical use of lung water measurements. Report of a workshop. *Chest,* **90**:588-594.

Taylor, D. G., and Bore, C. F. (1981). A review of the magnetic resonance response of biological tissue and its applicability to the diagnosis of cancer by NMR radiology. *CT,* **5**:122-134.

Taylor, A. E., Parker, J. C., Kvietys, P. R., and Perry, M. A. (1982). The pulmonary interstitium in capillary exchange. *Ann. N.Y. Acad. Sci.,* **384**:146-165.

Turino, G. M. (1985). The lung parenchyma—a dynamic matrix. *Am. Rev. Respir. Dis.,* **132**:1324-1334.

Vinitski, S., Pearson, M. G., Karlik, S. J., Morgan, W. K. C., Carey, L. S., Perkins, G., Goto, T., and Befus, D. (1986). Differentiation of parenchymal lung disorders with in vitro proton nuclear magnetic resonance. *Magn. Reson. Med.,* **3**:120-125.

Wagner, P. D., Saltzman, H. A., and West, J. B. (1974). Measurement of continuous distributions of ventilation-perfusion ratios: Theory. *J. Appl. Physiol.,* **36**:588-599.

Wexler, H. R., Nicholson, R. L., Prato, F. S., Carey, L. S., Vinitski, S., and Reese, L. (1985). Quantitation of lung water by nuclear magnetic resonance imaging. A preliminary study. *Invest. Radiol.,* **20**:583-590.

Young, S. W. (1984). *Nuclear Magnetic Resonance Imaging.* New York, Raven Press.

20

Lung Overinflation

Physiologic and Anatomic Alterations Leading to Pulmonary Edema

DIDIER DREYFUSS and GEORGES SAUMON

Hôpital Louis Mourier
Colombes
and INSERM U82
Paris, France

I. Introduction

The deleterious effects on the lung of overinflation are known as "barotrauma." This term usually includes the consequences of air leakage during mechanical ventilation (i.e., pulmonary interstitial emphysema, pneumomediastinum, and pneumothorax, among others). In addition to such immediately life-threatening lesions, alterations in lung structures leading to pulmonary edema have now been demonstrated in animal models. Pulmonary edema due to barotrauma results from increased permeability of the alveolar capillary barrier and is accompanied by alveolar cellular damage.

II. Pathways for Pulmonary Edema Due to Lung Distention

A. Increased Filtration of Fluid

Alterations in Pulmonary Surfactant

The effects of cyclic lung distention on pulmonary surfactant properties have been extensively studied (Faridy et al., 1966; Forrest, 1972; Wyszogrodski et al., 1975). They invariably result in changes in lung pressure-volume curves that were attributed to an increased air/liquid surface tension. The observed reduction in pulmonary compliance was directly related to the tidal volume and the duration of ventilation, being prevented by positive end-expiratory pressure (PEEP) (Faridy et al., 1966). Some uncertainty exists as to the mechanism of increased surface activity since large tidal volume ventilation can promote surfactant secretion (Oyarzun and Clements, 1978; Nicholas and Barr, 1983). The proposed explanations include modification of surfactant properties because of rupture of the surface film following compression and re-expansion (Faridy et al., 1966) or loss of surface-active material from alveoli to airways (Faridy, 1976).

A low air/liquid interface tension is mandatory to prevent both alveolar collapse and fluid accumulation in the lung interstitium. An increased surface tension lowers the perimicrovascular pressure of extra-alveolar vessels, thus increasing the transmural pressure and fluid filtration rate (Albert et al., 1979; Bredenberg et al., 1986). This favors the occurrence of pulmonary edema but has no effect on microvascular permeability (Bredenberg et al., 1986).

Effects of Alveolar Distention on the Pulmonary Vasculature

Intrapulmonary vessels are classified as alveolar and extra-alveolar vessels depending upon their anatomic localization and the stress applied to their outer surface (Howell et al., 1961; Permutt, 1979). The transmural pressure of alveolar microvessels is determined mainly by alveolar pressure, but that of extra-alveolar vessels depends on transpulmonary (pleural) pressure. The effects of lung distention differ for alveolar and extra-alveolar vessels since the increase in lung volume increases the alveolar to pleural pressure difference. Extra-alveolar vessels thus enlarge because of increased transmural pressure with lung volume but alveolar vessels are compressed (Howell et al., 1961; Permutt, 1979; Taylor and Parker, 1985).

Pulmonary distention is therefore likely to enhance fluid filtration at the extra-alveolar level during either hydrostatic or permeability edema (Illif, 1971; Albert et al., 1980).

B. Alveolar-Capillary Barrier Alterations

Increase in Microvascular Permeability

Parker et al. (1984) demonstrated in isolated blood-perfused lobes of canine lungs that ventilation with high peak airway pressures (45-65 cmH_2O) for 20 min results in increased microvascular permeability. This is manifested by an increased capillary filtration coefficient K_{fc} and a decreased protein osmotic reflection coefficient as assessed by decreases in both the isogravimetric capillary pressure and the critical capillary pressure for exhaustion of tissue safety factors. Noteworthy are that the increase in K_{fc} was immediate and continued after cessation of distention in some of the lobes. A curvilinear relationship was observed between the level of peak airway pressure and K_{fc} (Fig. 1). These findings have been confirmed in rabbit lungs removed after 1 hr of high peak airway pressure ventilation in vivo (Hernandez et al., 1988).

Increased Epithelial Permeability

Alveolar epithelial permeability during lung distention has been extensively studied (Egan et al., 1976; Egan, 1980, 1982). The permeability of large and small solutes across the epithelial barrier was estimated during static inflation of fluid-filled in situ sheep lobes (Egan et al., 1976). The equivalent pore radius of the epithelium obtained by this method increased from about 1 nm

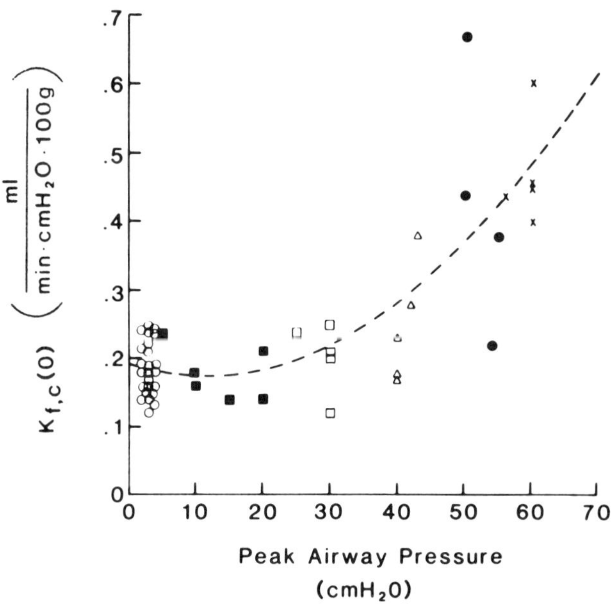

Figure 1 Effect of high peak airway pressures on the capillary filtration coefficient K_{fc} of isolated, blood-perfused lobes of dog lungs. The lobes were ventilated at 6 breaths per min for 20 min, with peak airway pressures ranging from 5 to 60 cmH_2O. K_{fc} measured immediately after the challenge remained roughly unchanged up to 40 cmH_2O peak airway pressure and then increased for larger pressures. Range of peak airway pressures in cmH_2O: (x) 55-65; (●) 45-55; (Δ) 35-45; (□) 25-35; (■) 5-25; (O) 3 (control). r = 0.72. (Reproduced from Parker et al., 1984, with permission.)

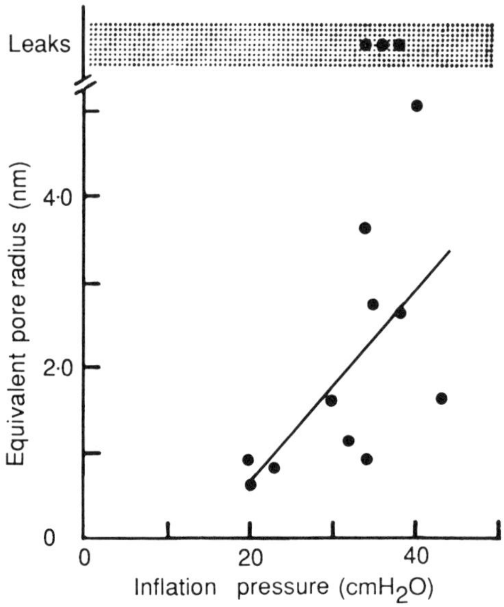

Figure 2 Static inflation of a sheep segment in vivo results in an increased epithelial permeability. The permeability was characterized in this experiment by the equivalent pore radius, calculated assuming that the epithelial membrane contains uniform cylindrical water-filled pores. There was a significant correlation ($r = 0.624$) between inflating pressure and pore radius. At the highest pressures, the sieving properties of the alveolar epithelium were in some instances lost, which was interpreted as resulting from membrane leaks. (Reproduced from Egan et al., 1976, with permission.)

at a low inflating pressure (20 cmH_2O) to 5 nm at 40 cmH_2O alveolar pressure. In some instances free diffusion of albumin was observed, indicating large leaks (Fig. 2). These observations have been confirmed in dogs (Egan, 1980). The alterations did not reverse after cessation of inflation, and even increased, suggesting irreversible lung injury. The distention of in situ lobes with large airway pressures resulted in supraphysiologic overinflation. To evaluate the effects of distention in the physiologic range, Egan (1982) performed experiments in situ of both lobes and entire rabbit lungs. Static segmental inflation resulted in a 6- to 12-fold increase in lung volume from functional residual capacity (because of compression of the surrounding parenchyma) and in a permeable epithelium to the test solutes (albumin, cytochrome c, and cyanocobalamin). In contrast, whole-lung inflation resulting in a 3- to 4-fold increase in lung volume produced less escape from the alveolar spaces of the smallest solutes and a negligible increase in albumin permeability. Hence, major increases in alveolar volume-surface area were mandatory to produce significant permeability changes in large molecules. This concept has been further strengthened by Kim and Crandall (1982), who showed in isolated bullfrog lungs that epithelial permeability was not modified by inflation within the physiologic range but was increased after overinflation.

As previously mentioned, these experiments were conducted during static inflation. An increased epithelial permeability to small solutes was also observed during intermittent positive-pressure ventilation (IPPV) at 40 cmH_2O peak airway pressure in rats (Fiorica et al., 1988). Increasing functional residual capacity by increasing PEEP levels during mechanical ventilation in sheep similarly produced an increase in aerosolized ^{99m}Tc-DTPA clearance (Cooper et al., 1987). The augmentation of DTPA clearance at high lung volume was larger than expected from the increased alveolar exchange surface area, suggesting increased permeability to small solutes would occur.

Using the same approach in humans, it has been found that ^{99m}Tc-DTPA clearance increased at high lung volume (Marks et al., 1985) whether such an increase was obtained by positive- or negative-pressure breathing (Nolop et al., 1986).

III. Pulmonary Edema Due to Mechanical Ventilation

A. Pulmonary Edema After Intermittent Positive-Pressure Ventilation

Webb and Tierney (1974) demonstrated in mechanically ventilated rats that high inflation pressures could promote pulmonary edema. They ventilated rats with IPPV at high peak airway pressures of 30-45 cmH_2O (HIPPV) Interstitial edema (e.g., peribronchovascular edema) was found by light microscopic examination in animals ventilated with 30 cmH_2O peak pressure. At 45 cmH_2O peak pressure, alveolar flooding occurred. Interestingly, when 10 cmH_2O PEEP was applied in conjunction with 45 cmH_2O HIPPV, the amount of edema was decreased and alveolar flooding was prevented.

The explanations proposed by Webb and Tierney (1974) to account for this edema were modifications of surfactant activity together with increased fluid filtration due to lung distention. As mentioned earlier, these mechanisms could only be responsible for the hydrostatic type of edema.

B. Microvascular Permeability and Cellular Alterations During HIPPV Edema

We have demonstrated that HIPPV edema is of the permeability type and is accompanied by severe ultrastructural alterations (Dreyfuss et al., 1985).

We ventilated rats with HIPPV of 45 cmH_2O for increasing durations (5, 10, and 20 min). Controls were ventilated with IPPV at 7 cmH_2O peak airway pressure. Pulmonary edema was assessed by postmortem measurement of extravascular lung water content (Qwl). Microvascular permeability alterations were evidenced by the dry lung weight measurement (DLW) and by the pulmonary distribution space of ^{125}I-labeled albumin.

Pulmonary edema was present as early as 5 min of HIPPV and was accompanied by an increased microvascular permeability to proteins (Fig. 3). During additional experiments (unpublished observations) we performed bronchoalveolar lavage after 5 min of HIPPV. We calculated the volume of alveolar subphase that diluted with lavage fluid using a modification of the method of Rennard et al. (1986). The rat lungs were lavaged with a Na- and K-free solution (choline chloride), and the calculations were performed using the sum of these cation concentrations in the retrieved fluid and in plasma

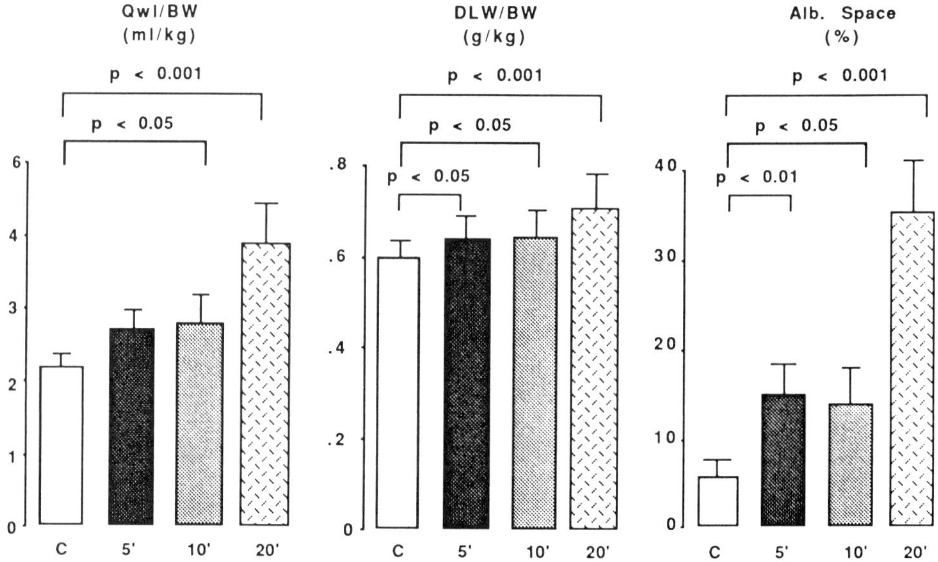

Figure 3 Effect of 45 cmH_2O peak airway pressure ventilation of increasing duration on indices of pulmonary edema in rats. Extravascular lung water Qwl/BW, dry lung weight DLW/BW, and the distribution space in lungs of ^{125}I-labeled albumin (Alb. Space) progressively increased as ventilation was continued. After 20 min of mechanical ventilation, there was a dramatic increase in all edema indices ($p < 0.01$ versus other groups). Moreover, at this stage, proteinaceous tracheal fluid was regularly found in the trachea. (Adapted from Dreyfuss et al., 1985, with permission.)

instead of the levels of urea described in the original method. The volume of alveolar subphase was significantly increased after only 5 min of HIPPV (Fig. 4).

After 20 min of HIPPV there was a major increase in all the edema indices (Fig. 3). Another criterion for the severity of pulmonary edema in these animals was the presence of tracheal fluid. This fluid had a high albumin content, further attesting to the occurrence of augmented permeability edema.

Severe pathologic damage accompanied the edema. Hence, at gross examination, the lungs of the rats ventilated for 20 min were enlarged and very congested. Light microscopy disclosed interstitial edema, but not alveolar edema, after 5 and 10 min of HIPPV; after 20 min widespread alveolar flooding was present. The most striking alterations were found at the ultrastructural level. In early stages, interstitial edema was obvious in peribronchovascular spaces and alveolar septa (Fig. 5). The thin parts of endothelial cells

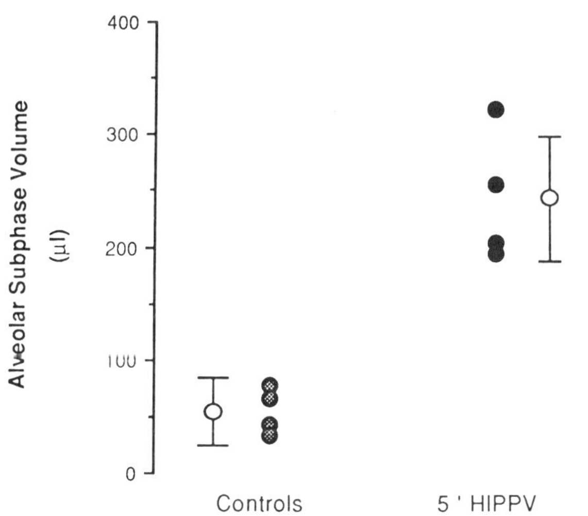

Figure 4 Effect of 45 cmH_2O IPPV for 5 min on alveolar subphase volume. The volume of bronchoalveolar subphase is estimated assuming that a particular solute (absent from the lavage fluid) was at the same concentration in alveolar subphase as in plasma (Rennard et al., 1986). Rat lungs were lavaged twice with 3 ml isotonic choline chloride. Na and K concentrations were measured in bronchoalveolar lavage fluid and plasma, and the sum of these cations was used to calculate the volume of bronchoalveolar subphase that diluted with the lavage solution. Individual (and mean $\pm$ SD) results of the second lavage are presented. After 5 min of HIPPV, there was a significant ($p < 0.001$) increase in subphase volume. Our data suggest either that edema liquid entered airways or alveoli or that a larger distribution volume (such as peribronchovascular cuffs) was accessible for lavage.

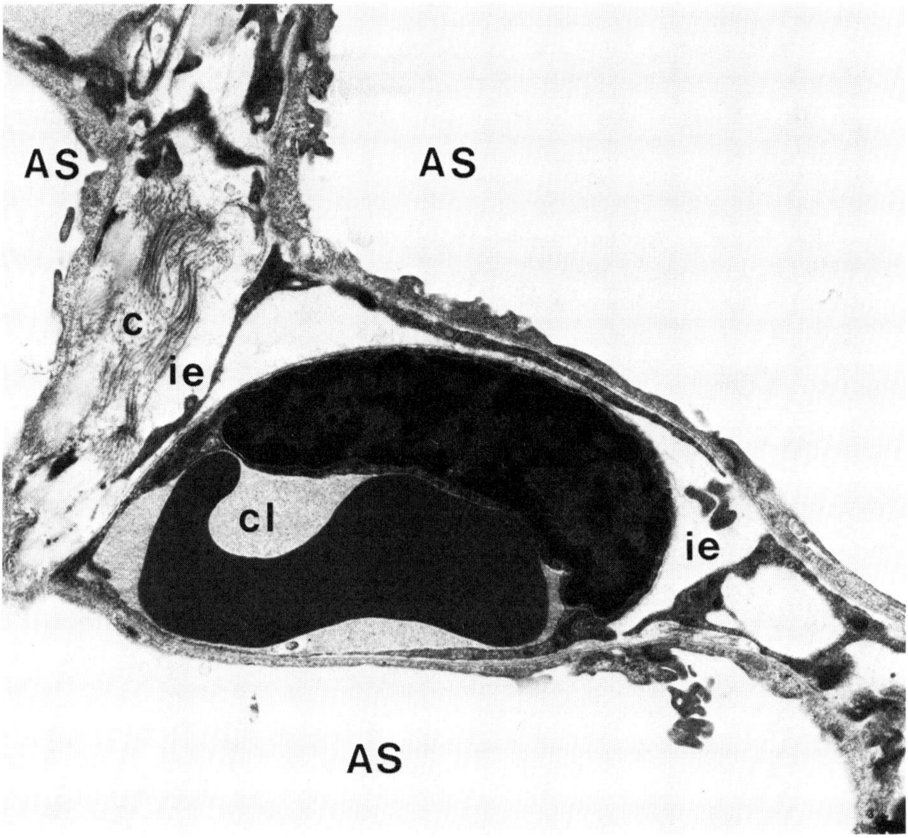

Figure 5 Ultrastructural aspects of the blood-air barrier after 5 min of 45 cmH_2O HIPPV in a rat: alveolar wall with interstitial edema (ie) and dissociating collagen fibers (c). The epithelial lining appears normal at this stage: cl, capillary lumen; AS, alveolar space. Original magnification ×7100. (By courtesy of Dr. Paul Soler.)

were frequently found detached from their basement membrane, protruding into the capillary lumen (Fig. 6). Such blebs have frequently been described in other types of experimental increased permeability edema (Teplitz, 1979; Hurley, 1982), but not during hydrostatic edema (Cottrell et al., 1967). At these early stages, no alteration was found in the alveolar epithelium. In contrast, severe diffuse alveolar damage was observed after 20 min (Fig. 7). Swelling and disruption of type I cells was present, leading to denudation of the basement membrane, and hyaline membranes were found in alveoli. Such diffuse alveolar damage was comparable to that described during experimental

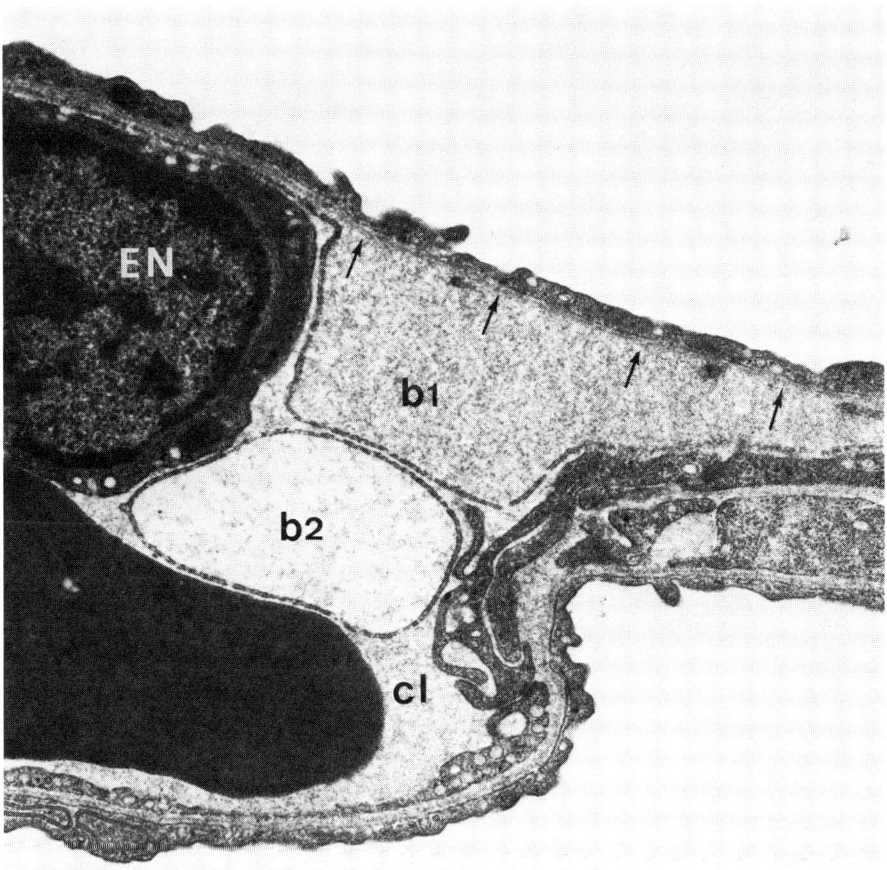

Figure 6 Abnormal alveolar capillary. The thin part of the endothelial cell is detached from the basal lamina (arrows), resulting in a bleb (b1) filled with electron-dense material (e.g., plasma). Another bleb (b2) appears isolated inside the capillary lumen (cl), probably because of the plane of this section. EN, endothelial cell. Original magnification ×13,000. (By courtesy of Dr. Paul Soler.)

high-permeability edema (Teplitz, 1979; Hurley, 1982; Cottrell et al., 1967) and the adult respiratory distress syndrome in patients (Bachofen and Weibel, 1982).

C. Separating the Effects of High Airway Pressures from Those of High Lung Volumes

We have addressed this point (Dreyfuss et al., 1988) by comparing the effects of high-pressure-high-volume ventilation (HIPPV) with those of high-

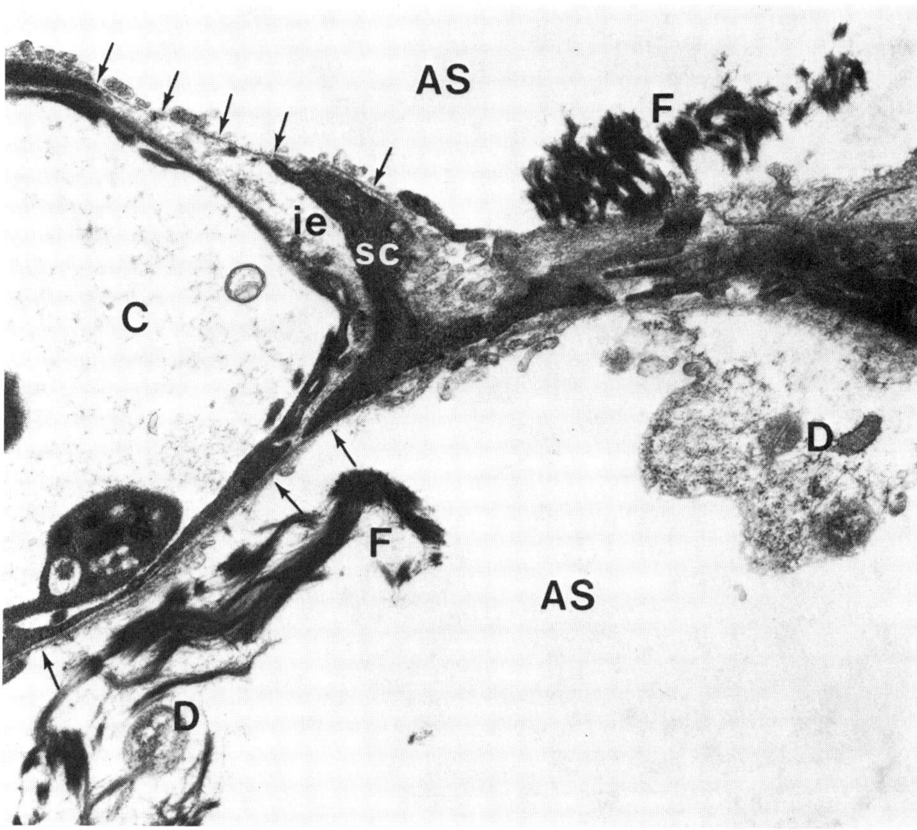

Figure 7 Severe injury of the epithelial lining. Type I cells are destroyed, leading to denudation of the basal lamina (arrows). Cell debris (D) and fibrin (F) are found in the alveolar space (AS). Interstitial edema (ie) surrounds a dilated capillary. sc, septal cell. Original magnification ×10,000. (By courtesy of Dr. Paul Soler.)

volume-low-pressure ventilation (iron lung) and of high-pressure-low-volume ventilation (45 cmH_2O peak pressure, the tidal volume being limited by thoracoabdominal strapping). Permeability edema occurred only when rats were ventilated with high tidal volumes, irrespective of airway pressure (i.e., positive or negative; Fig. 8).

As previously shown by Webb and Tierney (1977), when PEEP was applied during HIPPV, the amount of edema was reduced. Moreover, the severity of microvascular permeability alterations was diminished (Fig. 9).

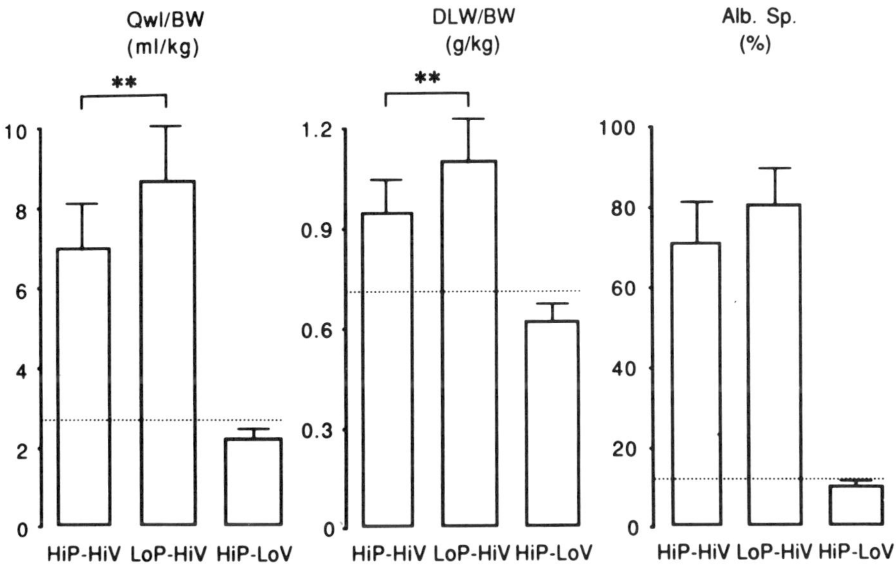

Figure 8 Respective effects of high-pressure-high-volume ventilation (HiP-HiV), low-pressure-high-volume ventilation (LoP-HiV, iron lung), and high-pressure-low-volume ventilation (HiP-LoV, thoracoabdominal strapping during 45 cmH_2O IPPV). The dotted line represents the upper 95% confidence limit for control values. There was no edema in the animals that were not distended, but those with pulmonary distention presented high-permeability edema irrespective of airway pressure ($p < 0.001$ versus controls). (Reproduced from Dreyfuss et al., 1988, with permission.)

It is noteworthy that whatever type of pulmonary distention was produced (iron lung or positive pressure with or without PEEP) there was always the same proportion of proteins and water in the extravasated fluid (Fig. 10). The slope of the relationship between DLW and Qwl was about 0.07 g/ml, which corresponded to the protein content of plasma. This indicated that the microvascular barrier had lost its protein-sieving properties, attesting to the presence of large leaks. Lung damage following iron lung ventilation was similar to that observed after HIPPV.

In keeping with the absence of edema, the lungs of rats ventilated with thoracoabdominal strapping were normal. Application of PEEP not only reduced the amount of edema but also modified the pathologic effects. Indeed, neither alveolar edema nor epithelial lesions were produced.

In summary, mechanical ventilation can produce high-permeability pulmonary edema. This is not to due to high airway pressures but is the consequence of pulmonary distention. Permeability edema occurs within a few

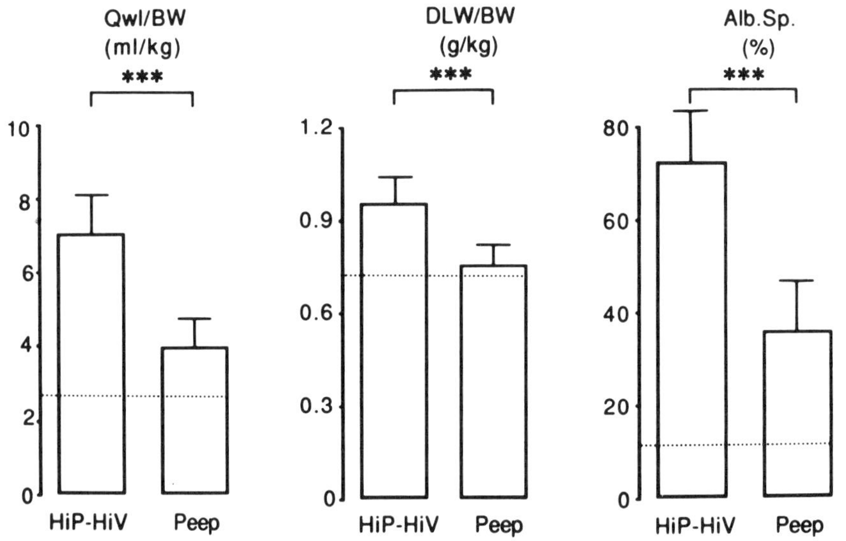

Figure 9 Effect of 10 cmH_2O positive end-expiratory pressure (PEEP) on HIPPV-induced pulmonary edema. When PEEP was applied, all indices of edema were diminished ($p < 0.001$) although remaining significantly different from controls ($p < 0.05$). These findings were corroborated by microscopic examination, which disclosed only interstitial edema, in contrast to the diffuse alveolar edema found in the high-volume groups. (Reproduced from Dreyfuss et al., 1988, with permission.)

minutes in rats. Continued overinflation results in alveolar epithelial damage similar to that observed during ARDS in patients.

It has been demonstrated in sheep that IPPV with 50 cmH_2O resulted in severe alterations in lung mechanics and gas exchange, very severe lung damage at gross examination, and the death of some animals (Kolobow et al., 1987). Unfortunately the authors did not measure indices of either lung edema or permeability and did not report microscopic examinations of the lungs. However, it seems probable that the impaired lung function observed was due to pulmonary edema.

D. Possible Explanations for Lung Distention Edema

Can the mechanisms of HIPPV edema be deduced from experiments dealing with pulmonary distention? Indeed, even if none of these experiments precisely defines the pathogenesis of high-permeability edema, some information can still be derived. Hence, the increased filtration coefficient together with the decreased reflection coefficient for proteins in isolated dog (Parker et al.,

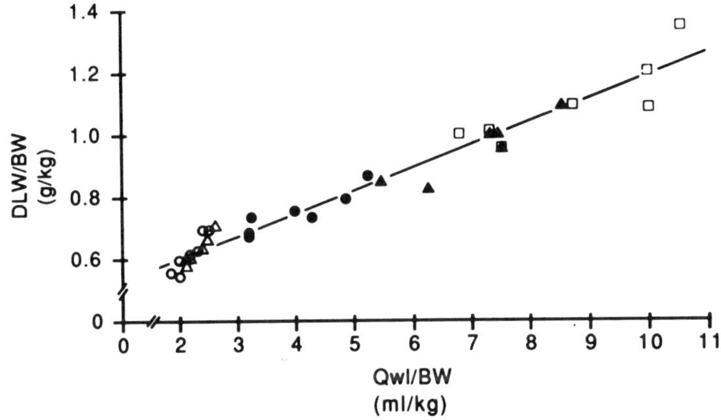

Figure 10 Correlation observed between dry lung weight and extravascular lung water ($r = 0.981$; $p < 0.001$): (△) Controls; (○) high airway pressure-low tidal volume (thoracoabdominal strapping); (▲) high airway pressure-high tidal volume; (□) low airway pressure-high tidal volume; and (●) high airway pressure + PEEP. This correlation suggests that the extravasated fluid always contained the same protein concentration (given by the slope of the regression line: 0.07 g/ml, corresponding to the protein concentration of plasma). Permeability edema was present after all conditions of ventilation with distention. (Reproduced from Dreyfuss et al., 1988, with permission.)

1984) and rabbit (Hernandez et al., 1988) lungs at distending pressures of comparable magnitude may not be sufficient to explain the free passage of proteins through microvessels occurring during HIPPV edema. Similarly, epithelial leakiness after inflation volumes and pressures that remained within the physiologic range was modest, and increases were restricted to relatively small solutes (Egan, 1982). Therefore, large increases in lung volume were mandatory to produce a protein-permeable epithelium. This may be related to the larger increase in alveolar surface area at high lung volumes (Gil et al., 1979). Egan (1982) proposed that at high pulmonary volume the tension on cell connections may become so important that the tight junctions are stretched, allowing the free passage of macromolecules. No ultrastructural study has substantiated this hypothesis. It is very unlikely that the overinflations leading to protein leakage could be attained during HIPPV. Tidal volume during 45 cmH_2O HIPPV in rats was about 40 ml/kg (Dreyfuss et al., 1988); thus the maximal volume was probably only slightly above total lung capacity. Nevertheless, the diffuse alveolar damage observed in our studies appeared greater than that produced by simple stretching of cell junctions. The discrepancy between the consequences of moderate overdistention and the cell lysis produced by HIPPV suggests that distention may not be the sole effect responsible for increased permeability and pathologic changes. As a matter of fact, the salutary effect of PEEP in addition to HIPPV (Webb and Tierney, 1974; Dreyfuss et al., 1988) argues for this hypothesis. Indeed, in these experiments, although maximal lung distention was similar during HIPPV without PEEP, there was decreased pulmonary edema and preservation of the epithelial lining. PEEP may have reduced the amount of edema by diminishing cardiac output, but its "protective" effect on alveolar epithelium remains unexplained. Moreover, in a recent study (Bshouty et al., 1988) conducted on in situ perfused canine lobes, at equivalent flows and microvascular hydrostatic pressures, the rate of hydrostatic edema formation was higher with large than with small tidal volumes. Furthermore, when the same increase in mean airway pressure was achieved either with large tidal volumes or by applying PEEP, the rate of edema formation was less in the latter condition, despite maintaining identical flows and microvascular pressures. This suggests that the amplitude of cyclic changes in lung volume favors the development of edema.

In conclusion, lung overdistention produces high-permeability pulmonary edema. Increased transmural microvascular pressure as a consequence of high lung volume and surfactant alterations might compound its effects, with increased epithelial and endothelial permeabilities to promote a profuse, protein-rich edema (Brigham et al., 1974; Prewitt et al., 1981). When lung lesions are unevenly distributed, as has recently been shown in the adult respiratory distress syndrome (Maunder et al., 1986), regional overdistention may occur during mechanical ventilation owing to the great inhomogeneity of mechanical time constants. Spared lung zones may receive overventilation with resultant damage. It would be very difficult to separate those lesions due to the primary offending process from those produced by mechanical ventilation. Moreover, during the infant respiratory distress syndrome it has been hypothesized that lung injury and permeability alterations were the result of overdistending surfactant-deficient lungs (Froese and Bryan, 1987). These speculations led to testing new ventilatory techniques, such as low-frequency ventilation with extracorporeal CO_2 (Gattinoni et al., 1980) or high-frequency oscillatory ventilation (McCulloch et al., 1988). The rationale for such techniques is to avoid large tidal volume ventilation, which may be more deleterious than low tidal volume ventilation at the same lung volume (Hamilton et al., 1983; McCulloch et al., 1988). If this approach proves valuable, it may be possible to reduce iatrogenic injury during the ventilator treatment of patients with ARDS.

References

Albert, R. K., Lakshminarayan, S., Hildebrandt, J., Kirk, W., and Butler, J. (1979). Increased surface tension favors pulmonary edema formation in anesthetized dogs' lungs. *J. Clin. Invest.*, **63**:1015-1018.

Albert, R. K., Lakshminarayan, S., Kirk, W., and Butler, J. (1980). Lung inflation can cause pulmonary edema in zone I of in situ dog lungs. *J. Appl. Physiol.,* **49**:815-819.

Bachofen, M., and Weibel, E. R. (1982). Structural alterations of lung parenchyma in the adult respiratory distress syndrome, ARDS. *Clin. Chest Med.,* **3**:35-56.

Bredenberg, C. E., Nieman, G. F., Paskanik, A. M., and Hart, A. K. E. (1986). Microvascular membrane permeability in high surface tension pulmonary edema. *J. Appl. Physiol.,* **60**:253-259.

Brigham, K. L., Woolverton, W. C., Blake, L. H., and Staub, N. C. (1974). Increased sheep lung vascular permeability caused by *Pseudomonas* bacteremia. *J. Clin. Invest.,* **54**:792-804.

Bshouty, Z., Ali, J., and Younes, M. (1988). Effect of tidal volume and PEEP on rate of edema formation in in situ perfused canine lobes. *J. Appl. Physiol.,* **64**:1900-1907.

Cooper, J. A., Van Der Zee, H., Line, B. R., and Malik, A. B. (1987). Relationship of end-expiratory pressure, lung volume, and ^{99m}Tc-DTPA clearance. *J. Appl. Physiol.,* **63**:1586-1590.

Cottrell, T. S., Levine, O. R., Senior, R. M., Weiner, J., Spiro, D., and Fishman, A. P. (1967). Electron microscopic alterations at the alveolar level in pulmonary edema. *Circ. Res.,* **21**:783-797.

Dreyfuss, D., Basset, G., Soler, P., and Saumon, G. (1985). Intermittent positive-pressure hyperventilation with high inflation pressures produces pulmonary microvascular injury in rats. *Am. Rev. Respir. Dis.,* **132**:880-884.

Dreyfuss, D., Soler, P., Basset, G., and Saumon, G. (1988). High inflation pressure pulmonary edema. Respective effects of high airway pressure, high tidal volume, and positive end-expiratory pressure. *Am. Rev. Respir. Dis.,* **137**:1159-1164.

Egan, E. A. (1980). Response of alveolar epithelial solute permeability to changes in lung inflation. *J. Appl. Physiol.,* **49**:1032-1036.

Egan, E. A. (1982). Lung inflation, lung solute permeability, and alveolar edema. *J. Appl. Physiol.,* **53**:121-125.

Egan, E. A., Nelson, R. M., and Olver, R. E. (1976). Lung inflation and alveolar permeability to non-electrolytes in the adult sheep in vivo. *J. Physiol.* (*Lond.*), **260**:409-424.

Faridy, E. E. (1976). Effect of ventilation on movement of surfactant in airways. *Respir. Physiol.,* **27**:323-334.

Faridy, E. E., Permutt, S., and Riley, R. L. (1966). Effect of ventilation on surface forces in excised dogs' lungs. *J. Appl. Physiol.,* **21**:1453-1462.

Fiorica, N. O., Oberdoerster, G., Morse, P. A., Hyde, R. W., and Utell, M. J. (1988). Evaluation of intravenous Tc-DTPA as a measure of lung epithelial permeability. *Am. Rev. Respir. Dis.,* **137**(Suppl):A143.

Forrest, J. B. (1972). The effect of hyperventilation on pulmonary surface activity. *Br. J. Anaesthesiol.,* **44**:313-319.

Froese, A. B., and Bryan, A. C. (1987). High frequency ventilation. *Am. Rev. Respir. Dis.,* **135**:1363-1374.

Gattinoni, L., Agostoni, A., Pesenti, A., Pelizzola, A., Rossi, G. P., Langer, M., Vesconi, S., Uziel, L., Fox, U., Longoni, F., Kolobow, T., and Damia, G. (1980). Treatment of acute respiratory failure with low-frequency positive-pressure ventilation and extracorporeal removal of CO_2. *Lancet,* **2**:292-294.

Gil, J., Bachofen, H., Gehr, P., and Weibel, E. R. (1979). Alveolar volume-surface area relation in air- and saline-filled lungs fixed by vascular perfusion. *J. Appl. Physiol.,* **47**:990-1001.

Hamilton, P. P., Onayemi, A., Smyth, J. A., Gillan, J. E., Cutz, E., Froese, A. B., and Bryan, A. C. (1983). Comparison of conventional and high-frequency ventilation: Oxygenation and lung pathology. *J. Appl. Physiol.,* **55**:131-138.

Hernandez, L. A., Peevy, K., and Parker, J. C. (1988). Effect of high peak airway pressure on the normal rabbit lung. *FASEB J.,* **2**:A1184.

Howell, J. B. L., Permutt, S., Proctor, D. F., and Riley, R. L. (1961). Effect of inflation of the lung on different parts of the pulmonary vascular bed. *J. Appl. Physiol.,* **16**:71-76.

Hurley, J. V. (1982). Types of pulmonary microvascular injury. *Ann. N.Y. Acad. Sci.,* **384**:269-285.

Iliff, L. D. (1971). Extra-alveolar vessels and edema development in excised dog lungs. *Circ. Res.,* **28**:524-532.

Kim, K. J., and Crandall, E. D. (1982). Effects of lung inflation on alveolar epithelial solute and water transport properties. *J. Appl. Physiol.,* **52**: 1498-1505.

Kolobow, T., Moretti, M. P., Fumagalli, R., Mascheroni, D., Prato, P., Chen, V., and Joris, M. (1987). Severe impairment in lung function induced by high peak airway pressure during mechanical ventilation. An experimental study. *Am. Rev. Respir. Dis.,* **135**:312-315.

Marks, J. D., Luce, J. M., Lazar, N. M., Wu, J. N., Lipavsky, A., and Murray, J. F. (1985). Effect of increases in lung volume on clearance of aerosolized solutes from human lungs. *J. Appl. Physiol.,* **59**:1242-1248.

Maunder, R. J., Shuman, W. P., McHugh, J. W., Marglin, S. I., and Butler, J. (1986). Preservation of normal lung regions in the adult respiratory distress syndrome. Analysis by computed tomography. *JAMA,* **255**: 2463-2465.

McCulloch, P. R., Forkert, P. G., and Froese, A. B. (1988). Lung volume maintenance prevents lung injury during high frequency oscillatory ventilation in surfactant-deficient rabbits. *Am. Rev. Respir. Dis.,* **137**: 1185-1192.

Nicholas, T. E., and Barr, H. A. (1983). The release of surfactant in rat lung by brief periods of hyperventilation. *Respir. Physiol.,* **52**:69-83.

Nolop, K. B., Maxwell, D. L., Royston, D., and Hughes, J. M. B. (1986). Effect of raised thoracic pressure and volume on ^{99m}Tc-DTPA clearance in humans. *J. Appl. Physiol.,* **60**:1493-1497.

Oyarzun, M. J., and Clements, J. A. (1978). Control of lung surfactant by ventilation, adrenergic mediators, and prostaglandins in the rabbit. *Am. Rev. Respir. Dis.,* **117**:879-891.

Parker, J. C., Townsley, M. I., Rippe, B., Taylor, A. E., and Thigpen, J. (1984). Increased microvascular permeability in dog lungs due to high peak airway pressures. *J. Appl. Physiol.,* **57**:1809-1816.

Permutt, S. (1979). Mechanical influences on water accumulation in the lungs. In *Pulmonary Edema.* Edited by A. P. Fishman and E. M. Renkin. Bethesda, Clinical Physiology Series, American Physiological Society, pp. 175-193.

Prewitt, R. M., McCarthy, J., and Wood, L. D. H. (1981). Treatment of acute low pressure pulmonary edema in dogs. Relative effects of hydrostatic and oncotic pressure, nitroprusside, and positive end-expiratory pressure. *J. Clin. Invest.,* **67**:409-418.

Rennard, S. I., Basset, G., Lecossier, D., O'Donnell, K. M., Pinkston, P., Martin, P. G., and Crystal, R. G. (1986). Estimation of volume of epithelial lining fluid recovered by lavage using urea as marker of dilution. *J. Appl. Physiol.,* **60**:532-538.

Taylor, A. E., and Parker, J. C. (1985). Pulmonary interstitial spaces and lymphatics. In *Handbook of Physiology,* Section 3, *The Respiratory System,* Vol. 1, *Circulation and Nonrespiratory Functions.* Edited by A. P. Fishman, Bethesda, American Physiological Society, pp. 167-230.

Teplitz, C. (1979). Pulmonary cellular and interstitial edema. In *Pulmonary Edema.* Edited by A. P. Fishman and E. M. Renkin. Bethesda, Clinical Physiology Series. American Physiological Society, pp. 97-111.

Webb, H. H., and Tierney, D. F. (1974). Experimental pulmonary edema due to intermittent positive pressure ventilation with high inflation pressures. Protection by positive end-expiratory pressure. *Am. Rev. Respir. Dis.,* **110**:556-565.

Wyszogrodski, I., Kyei Aboagye, K., Taeusch, H. W., Jr., and Avery, M. E. (1975). Surfactant inactivation by hyperventilation: Conservation by end-expiratory pressure. *J. Appl. Physiol.,* **38**:461-466.

21

Adverse Heparin-Protamine Neutralization Interactions and the Lung

ERNI KREIL, GILLES MONTALESCOT DWIGHT R. ROBINSON, and WARREN M. ZAPOL

Harvard Medical School and
Massachusetts General Hospital
Boston, Massachusetts

KAREN E. LYNCH

Massachusetts General Hospital
Boston, Massachusetts

EDWARD LOWENSTEIN

Harvard Medical School and
Beth Israel Hospital
Boston, Massachusetts

I. Introduction

Inclusion of a chapter devoted to adverse cardiopulmonary responses to protamine reversal of heparin anticoagulation in a book focused upon acute respiratory failure appears on initial inspection to require a defense. The authors believe it is warranted for the following reasons. A significant pathophysiologic component of the adult respiratory distress syndrome (ARDS) is acute pulmonary hypertension leading to right heart failure. The proximate cause of the right ventricular failure in ARDS is pulmonary vascular obliteration (Zapol and Snider, 1977). Although the mechanisms of vascular injury are incompletely known, a variety of events, including complement activation, leukocyte activation and pulmonary leukosequestration, release of reactive oxygen species, and increased lipid peroxidation, arachidonic acid metabolism, and eicosanoid generation, may contribute to injury and the development of pulmonary hypertension. Activation of many of these pathways has been demonstrated in experimental animals when protamine interacts with heparin. In some species, this drug interaction predictably causes intense pulmonary vasoconstriction. However, this interaction has not been shown to cause pulmonary tissue damage. We therefore believe the heparin-protamine interaction provides an important prospective human and experimental animal model that will lead to a better understanding of the biology of acute pulmonary vasoconstriction. Furthermore, if we can learn why activation by heparin and protamine of many of these same pathways does not cause acute lung injury, then we may understand why these activated mediators do not always cause ARDS and thereby point the way toward potential therapeutic strategies to prevent both syndromes.

II. Overview

We first review animal studies of the heparin-protamine (HP) interaction, focusing on the cellular and biochemical mediators that may contribute to HP-induced pulmonary vasoconstriction, since our primary effort has been to elucidate the mechanism of this pulmonary hemodynamic event. After this review, we briefly compare some of the major pulmonary and known mediator responses to HP and lipopolysaccharide challenge in sheep. We focus on the sheep because it is among the species in which both these challenges have been most thoroughly studied. A discussion of the HP syndrome in humans completes our chapter. We only briefly discuss true, IgE-mediated allergy to protamine because it is a separate entity from HP-induced pulmonary vasoconstriction and occurs far less frequently in humans (Weiss et al., 1989). We refer readers to recent reviews for other aspects of protamine-associated toxicity (Horrow, 1985, 1988a, b). We also refer readers to more thorough reviews of the biology of the heparin molecules (Jacques, 1980; O'Reilly, 1985).

III. Animal Models of Heparin-Protamine-Associated Pulmonary Vasoconstriction

Adverse responses to protamine neutralization of heparin anticoagulation have been studied in numerous animal species, including sheep (Morel et al., 1988; Montalescot et al., 1989; Kreil et al., 1989), pigs (Stefaniszyn et al., 1984; Fiser et al., 1985; Rogers et al., 1983; Hobbhahn et al., 1988; Schumacher et al., 1988; Degges et al., 1987; Conzen et al., 1989), dogs (Goldman et al., 1969; Jacques, 1949; Casthely, 1986; Radegran et al., 1971a, 1974; Radegran and McAshan, 1972; Wakefield, 1984, 1986, 1987; Lindblad et al., 1987, 1988; Taylor et al., 1986; Gourin et al., 1971; Fadali et al., 1976), isolated perfused cat lungs (Jastrzebski et al., 1975), rats (Chang et al., 1987; Fairman et al., 1987; unpublished studies from our laboratory), rabbits (Jacques, 1949; Fehr and Rohr, 1983), and *Macaca cynomulgus* monkeys (unpublished studies from our laboratory). Most investigators anticoagulated the animals with 150-1000 IU/kg of either porcine gut or bovine lung heparin and reversed the heparin during the subsequent 30 min with intravenous (IV) salmine protamine sulfate, 1-10 mg/kg, thereby utilizing a protamine-heparin ratio between 0.6 and 2:1. The rate of protamine reversal, the doses of heparin and protamine administered, the route of protamine administration (intravenous versus intra-arterial) (Horrow, 1985, 1988a, 1988b), and the source of heparin (beef lung versus pork intestinal mucosal heparin) (Fiser et al., 1985) have all been reputed to influence the subsequent pulmonary hemodynamic response to HP challenge.

The hemodynamic responses to HP challenge also appear species dependent. In awake sheep and anesthetized pigs, HP challenge consistently causes marked but transient pulmonary vasoconstriction. In the anesthetized pig systemic hypotension may occur (Stefaniszyn et al., 1984; Fiser et al., 1985; Conzen et al., 1989; Rogers et al., 1983; Hobbhahn et al., 1988), whereas systemic vasodilation appears rare at these doses of heparin and protamine (Rogers et al., 1983). Awake sheep challenged with comparable doses of heparin and protamine develop neither systemic vasodilation nor hypotension. Protamine reversal of heparin anticoagulation in the dog rapidly causes pulmonary vasoconstriction and both systemic vasodilation and hypotension (Goldman et al., 1969; Casthely et al., 1986; Radegran et al., 1971a, 1974; Radegran and McAshan, 1972; Wakefield et al., 1984, 1986, 1987; Lindblad et al., 1988; Gourin et al., 1971), although protamine alone caused these changes in some studies (Goto et al., 1985; Radegran et al., 1971a; Goldman et al., 1969) but not all (Wakefield et al., 1986). Importantly, in the dog, systemic vasodilation may be due in part to mechanisms other than those that cause pulmonary vasoconstriction (Radegran and McAshan, 1972; Lindblad et al., 1988), including histamine release (Casthely et al., 1986). In contrast, HP challenge at these doses caused neither pulmonary vasoconstriction nor systemic hypotension in two *M. cynomulgus* monkeys (unpublished studies) nor pulmonary vasoconstriction in rats (Chang et al., 1987; unpublished studies from our laboratory).

Our laboratory utilizes principally the model of Morel and co-workers (1988). Commercial bovine lung heparin, 200 U/kg, is rapidly infused via a central venous catheter and neutralized 5 min later with IV salmine protamine sulfate, 2 mg/kg. Anticoagulation and its reversal are monitored with the activated clotting time (Hatterslea, 1966), although other measurements of coagulation, such as thrombin clotting time (Wakefield et al., 1986; Lindblad et al., 1987) and activated partial thromboplastin time (Lindblad et al., 1987), have been monitored in other studies. In contrast to the sporadic occurrence of HP-induced pulmonary vasoconstriction in humans (Lowenstein et al., 1983; Lowenstein, 1989; Morel et al., 1987), HP challenge with this protocol reproducibly causes pulmonary vasoconstriction in sheep, even when repeated up to three times at 90 min intervals.*

A. Pulmonary Vascular Physiology

At the doses noted, HP challenge consistently increases pulmonary vascular resistance within 0.5-5 min after protamine infusion in awake sheep (Morel et al., 1988; Montalescot et al., 1989; Kreil et al., 1989), anesthetized pigs (Stefaniszyn et al., 1984; Fiser et al., 1985; Rogers et al., 1983; Hobbhahn et al., 1988; Degges et al., 1987; Conzen et al., 1989), dogs (Goldman et al., 1969; Casthely et al., 1986; Radegran et al., 1971a, 1974; Radegran and McAshan, 1972; Wakefield et al., 1984, 1986, 1987; Lindblad et al., 1988; Gourin et al., 1971), and isolated perfused cat lung (Jastrzebski et al., 1975) but, as noted previously, does not cause pulmonary vasoconstriction either in rats or in a primate model of pulmonary vasoconstriction utilizing two *M. cynomolgus* monkeys. In sheep, pulmonary vascular resistance typically increases 2- to 4.5-fold and mean pulmonary artery pressure 2- to 3.5-fold above baseline values (Fig. 1). The pulmonary artery pressure and vascular resistance return to preprotamine levels within the next 5-20 min. In association with pulmonary vasoconstriction, cardiac output generally decreases in awake sheep (Morel et al., 1988; Montalescot et al., 1989), anesthetized pigs (Stefaniszyn et al., 1984; Fiser et al., 1985; Rogers et al., 1983; Hobbhahn et al., 1988), and dogs (Goldman et al., 1969; Wakefield et al., 1984, 1986; Gourin et al., 1971; Radegran et al., 1971a; Radegran and McAshan, 1972), although isolated animal studies reported either no change (Conzen et al., 1989; Kreil et al., 1989) or an increase in cardiac output (Casthely et al., 1986). Some of these differences in output may be partly related to the degree of pulmonary vasoconstriction produced. Pulmonary artery balloon occlusion pressure (Pw) increases transiently in sheep (Fig. 1) (Morel et al., 1988; Montalescot et al., 1989; Kreil et al., 1989), pigs (unpublished study), and dogs (Casthely et al., 1986; Wakefield et al., 1984) concomitantly with the peak increase in pulmonary vascular resistance. The increase in Pw may be artefactual and may reflect bronchoconstriction rather than an elevated transmural left ventricular filling pressure, or it may reflect pulmonary venoconstriction (Radegran, 1974) with an increased Pw-left atrial pressure gradient. Left atrial pressure does not increase in either sheep (Morel, 1988) or dogs (Radegran and McAshan, 1972; Radegran et al., 1974). Similarly, other studies report that left ventricular end-diastolic pressure remained stable in dogs (Radegran et al., 1971a) and either decreased (Hobbhahn et al., 1988)

*Radegran also reported that HP rechallenge in dogs reproducibly causes pulmonary vasoconstriction (Radegran et al., 1971a).

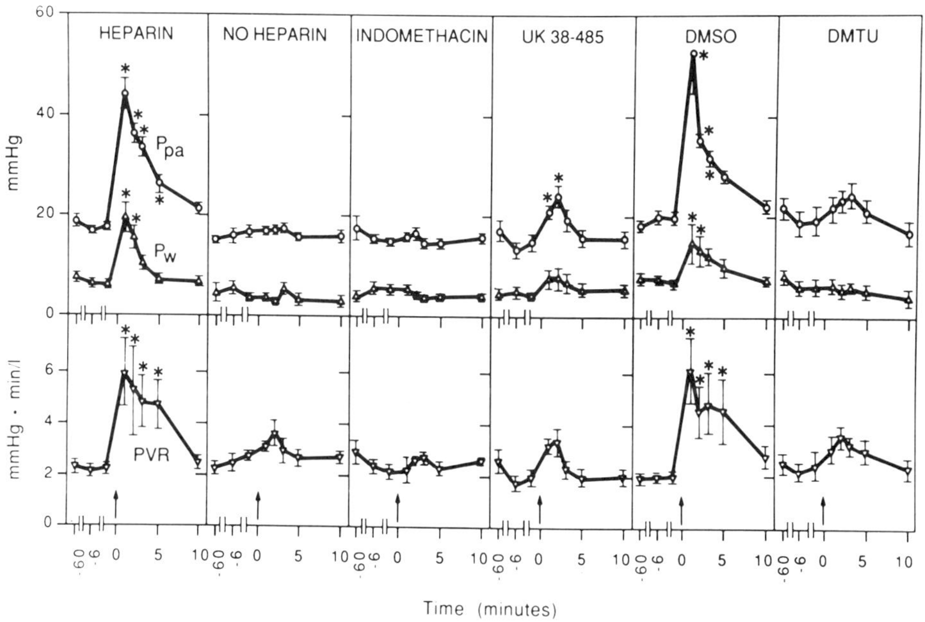

Figure 1 Effect of a bolus injection of protamine (arrow) on mean pulmonary arterial pressure (Ppa), pulmonary capillary wedge pressure (Pw), and pulmonary vascular resistance (PVR) in the six treatment groups. Heparinized controls, $n = 4$; unheparinized controls, $n = 10$ (except for times +1 and +2 min for PVR values, where $n = 6$ and 7, respectively); indomethacin-pretreated heparinized sheep, $n = 3$; UK 38-485-pretreated heparinized sheep, $n = 5$; DMSO-pretreated heparinized sheep, $n = 4$; DMTU-pretreated heparinized sheep, $n = 6$. Values are the mean ± SEM. *$p < 0.05$ value differs from before protamine injection. (Reprinted from *Circ. Res.*, **62**:908, 1988.)

or remained stable in pigs (Stefaniszyn et al., 1984; Fiser et al., 1985; Rogers et al., 1983; Conzen et al., 1989).

Results from a number of studies suggest that the sequence of infusion of heparin and protamine influences the pulmonary vascular response to the heparin-protamine interaction. In sheep, we infused heparin and protamine in a reversed sequence, that is, protamine (2 mg/kg) first and heparin (200 IU/kg) 5 min later (Kreil et al., 1989). The activated clotting time increased only slightly (from 153 ± 5 to 170 ± 6 sec, mean ± SEM), but pulmonary vascular resistance did not increase. Thus, protamine-heparin complexes formed but did not cause pulmonary vasoconstriction. Similarly, canine studies with protamine pretreatment (2.25 mg) 5-7 min before heparin infusion (150 U/kg), to prevent pulmonary vasoconstriction caused by a subsequent reversal dose of protamine (1.5 mg/kg), did not report pulmonary vasoconstriction (Wakefield et al., 1986, 1987). In all five dogs in one of these studies (Wakefield et al., 1986), additional heparin administration (75-150 U/kg) was required to increase the thrombin time above 100 sec, demonstrating that a substantial portion of the heparin complexed with the initial protamine dose. In pigs, infusing protamine (3 mg/kg) prior to heparin (3 mg/kg) also failed to increase pulmonary vascular resistance (Stefaniszyn et al., 1984).

We do not know why reversing the sequence of heparin and protamine infusion fails to increase the pulmonary vascular resistance in these animal species. This result in the dog and sheep cannot be due to total inactivation of the protamine prior to heparin infusion; otherwise, the subsequently infused heparin would effectively anticoagulate the blood. It is possible that other factors, such as the binding of polycationic protamine to polyanionic surfaces of either circulating (Al-Mondhiry et al., 1985) or other intravascular cells, may modulate the response to HP challenge in vivo. This issue is discussed further elsewhere (Kreil et al., 1989).

Infusing preformed heparin-protamine complexes to learn whether circulating HP complexes cause pulmonary vasoconstriction is difficult because of the character of the infusate. Prolonged in vitro mixing of commercially available heparin and protamine produces a gelatinous precipitate that, if infused, may either behave as an embolus or appear hemodynamically inactive (Goldman et al., 1969). However, studies with pigs (Stefaniszyn et al., 1984) and isolated cat lungs (Jastrzebski et al., 1975) reported that infusing a solution of heparin and protamine immediately after the compounds were mixed caused variable increases in pulmonary vascular resistance. We challenged sheep with a modified heparin-protamine solution. Protamine was added to a dilute mixture of heparin and dextran-40, producing slight turbidity without a precipitate (unpublished observations). Infusing this solution into sheep rapidly increased pulmonary vascular resistance, whereas infusing heparin and dextran or protamine and dextran did not (unpublished study).* Thus, these studies support the hypothesis that circulating HP complexes can induce pulmonary vasoconstriction.

---

*In contrast, protamine (5 mg/kg) caused comparable increases in pulmonary vascular resistance in isolated cat lung perfused with either acellular, nonheparinized dextran-70 or heparinized whole blood (10 mg/kg body weight) (Jastrzebski et al., 1975). It is possible that a complex of polyanionic dextran and polycationic protamine caused pulmonary vasoconstriction in this species. The authors did not report studies infusing protamine into lungs perfused without blood or dextran.

Interestingly, neutralizing heparin anticoagulation (200 U/kg) in sheep with hexadimethrine bromide (1.4 mg/kg), another polycation polymer (MW approximately 5000), produces an increase in pulmonary vascular resistance comparable to the increase caused by standard HP challenge (Montalescot, in preparation). Anticoagulating sheep with 1 mg/kg of a low-molecular-weight heparin (enoxaparine, PK 10169, MW approximately 4500) and subsequently neutralizing this heparin with 1.5 mg/kg of protamine (MW approximately 4000) similarly increases the pulmonary vascular resistance (Montalescot, in preparation). However, infusing low-molecular-weight heparin (3 mg/kg) and neutralizing this with hexadimethrine (3 mg/kg) has minimal pulmonary vascular effect. These results suggest that a variety of polyanion-polycation interactions, although not all heparin neutralization reactions, may cause pulmonary vasoconstriction. The absence of systemic hypotension in these studies suggests that the ovine hemodynamic response to these compounds is primarily nonallergic.

Protamine alone (1-3 mg/kg) does not increase pulmonary vascular resistance in either sheep (Morel et al., 1988; Montalescot et al., 1989; Kreil et al., 1989) or pigs (Stefaniszyn et al., 1984; Fiser et al., 1985; Rogers et al., 1983; Hobbhahn et al., 1988), suggesting that, in these species, both heparin and protamine are important to the pulmonary vascular response to HP challenge. In dogs, slightly higher doses of protamine alone (2-10 mg/kg) may cause pulmonary vasoconstriction (Radegran et al., 1971a; Goldman et al., 1969), although this was not found in all studies (Wakefield et al., 1986). In isolated rat lungs perfused with physiologic salt solution (Chang et al., 1987; Fairman et al., 1987) and also in vivo (Fairman et al., 1987), larger doses of protamine (estimated range 4-80 mg/kg body weight) cause both pulmonary vasoconstriction and increased lung water content. Surprisingly, administering heparin (100 U/mg protamine) before protamine (100 μg/ml salt solution) prevents protamine-induced pulmonary vasoconstriction in the isolated rat lung (Chang et al., 1987). Furthermore, infusing heparin (90 U/mg protamine) into rats after protamine severely blunts the pulmonary vascular response to protamine (Fairman et al., 1987). Heparin also blocks the pulmonary hypertensive effect of the polycationic molecules hexadimethrine and poly-L-lysine. These results suggest that the charge of the infused molecules may play an important role in the pulmonary vascular response to these agents in the rat (Chang et al., 1987).

Summary of Animal Physiology Studies

Heparin-protamine challenge consistently causes pulmonary vasoconstriction without systemic vasodilation in sheep and pigs, suggesting a common mechanism of action that does not depend upon protamine allergy. Heparin-protamine challenge in dogs causes both pulmonary vasoconstriction and systemic vasodilation, documenting the species-dependent variability in systemic hemodynamic responses to HP challenge. However, the pulmonary and systemic hemodynamic responses to HP challenge may involve different mechanisms in the dog. Animal species also differ in the pulmonary hemodynamic response to protamine alone. Whereas protamine alone does not appear to influence pulmonary vascular resistance in the sheep or pig, infusing heparin-protamine mixtures causes pulmonary vasoconstriction in both these species, as well as in isolated perfused cat lung, suggesting that formation of the HP complex may be a prerequisite to this pulmonary hemodynamic response in these animals. Ovine studies with heparin and hexadimethrine, as well as with low-molecular-weight heparin and protamine, suggest that a variety of nonallergic, polyanion-polycation interactions can increase pulmonary vascular resistance. We do not yet know why the sequence of heparin and protamine infusion influences the subsequent pulmonary hemodynamic response in the sheep, pig, and dog. With the possible exception of the rat, in which very large doses of protamine alone caused an increase in lung weight associated with pulmonary vasoconstriction, none of the aforementioned heparin-protamine studies reported evidence of acute lung injury.

B. Cellular Elements

Leukocytes

A transient decrease in circulating leukocyte concentration accompanies HP-induced pulmonary vasoconstriction in sheep (Morel et al., 1988; Montalescot et al., 1989; Kreil et al., 1989), pigs (Conzen et al., 1989; unpublished data from our laboratory), and dogs (Wakefield et al., 1986; Lindblad et al., 1987; Radegran et al., 1971a). Pulmonary leukosequestration may also occur in sheep (Morel et al., 1988). In contrast, comparable doses of heparin and protamine cause leukopenia without pulmonary vasoconstriction in rats (unpublished study) and *M. cynomolgus* monkeys (unpublished study). Infusing protamine alone produces varying but generally lesser decreases in leukocyte concentrations in dog (Radegran et al., 1971a), pig (Conzen et al., 1989), and rabbit (Fehr and Rohr, 1983). Protamine alone does not consistently cause leukopenia in sheep (Morel et al., 1988; Kreil et al., 1989). Administering heparin after protamine in sheep (i.e., in reverse sequence) does not produce either pulmonary vasoconstriction or leukopenia (Kreil et al., 1989). These results suggest that the heparin-protamine interaction, rather than heparin or protamine alone, is the principal cause of leukopenia in these animal species. For unknown reasons, the reverse sequence of heparin and protamine infusion impairs the leukocyte response.

The implication of leukocytes in the HP syndrome is of particular interest because activated leukocytes may release vasoactive agents, including thromboxane (Goldstein et al., 1978; Tahamont et al., 1984) and peroxide (Milligan et al., 1988), which are proposed mediators of HP-induced pulmonary vasoconstriction. Studies with inhibitors of several proposed mediators of this syndrome (more thoroughly discussed later) suggest that if neutrophil activation is important, it probably occurs proximal to the release of these mediators. Pretreating sheep with either an antioxidant (dimethylthiourea) (Morel et al., 1988) or a protease inhibitor (nafamstat mesilate; 6-amidino-2-napthyl-*p*-quanidinobenzoate dimethanesulfonate) (Kreil et al., 1989) markedly attenuates the HP-induced increase in pulmonary vascular resistance but not the decrease in leukocyte concentrations. In addition, administering either thromboxane receptor blockers or cyclooxygenase inhibitors prevents pulmonary vasoconstriction in sheep and pig (see Eicosanoids in Sec. III.C) but does not modify the leukopenia. Pretreating dogs with protamine prior to subsequent HP challenge also prevents the pulmonary hemodynamic response to HP challenge but has little effect on the leukocyte concentrations (Wakefield et al., 1986).

However, several studies suggest that the role of leukocytes in HP-induced pulmonary vasoconstriction is limited. Of major importance is the demonstration that HP challenge increased pulmonary vascular resistance comparably in isolated pig lungs perfused with either acellular dextran or whole blood, suggesting that the leukocyte is not an essential mediator of pulmonary vasoconstriction in pigs (Degges et al., 1987). That protamine caused comparable increases in pulmonary vascular resistance in isolated cat lungs perfused with either nonheparinized dextran or heparinized whole blood (Jastrzebski et al., 1975) reinforces our belief in the independence of pulmonary vasoconstriction from leukocytes. Confirming this hypothesis in sheep will require either similar studies with isolated perfused lungs or studies with neutrophil depletion.

It is likely that HP-induced activation of the complement anaphylatoxin C5a, which binds to polymorphonuclear leukocytes (PMN) (Chenoweth and Hugli, 1978) and enhances PMN chemotaxis and aggregation (Webster et al., 1980; Fernandez et al., 1978), causes this leukopenia (Fehr and Rohr, 1983). However, studies to confirm this hypothesis have produced mixed results. Rabbits treated with cobra venom factor to deplete complement do not develop leukopenia during protamine neutralization of heparin (Fehr and Rohr, 1983). We studied two sheep treated intravenously with 70 mg/kg of *Naja haje* cobra venom factor (in seven divided doses over 3 days), a dose that lowered plasma CH_{50} titers to undetectable levels and plasma C3a levels to 4 ± 2% of baseline and prevented leukopenia and pulmonary vasoconstriction caused by cardiopulmonary bypass in a previous ovine study (Wonders et al., 1983). HP challenge in both these sheep caused increased pulmonary vascular resistance and leukopenia, suggesting that cobra venom factor did not completely block C5a generation (unpublished study). Difficulties with total complement depletion were also noted in a study of sheep challenged with endotoxin: *N. haje* cobra venom factor treatment reduced plasma CH_{50} titers to undetectable levels but failed to eliminate C5a-derived chemotactic activity and prevent endotoxin-induced leukopenia (Flick et al., 1986).

In summary, we believe leukocytes probably are not essential mediators of HP-induced pulmonary vasoconstriction. Rather, transient decreases in circulating leukocyte concentrations more likely reflect activation or release of other mediators, including complement C5a, which may or may not increase pulmonary vascular resistance.

Platelets

We studied HP challenge in sheep both before and after marked platelet depletion (Montalescot et al., 1989). A total of six sheep received one to two intramuscular injections per day of rabbit antisheep platelet antibodies, reducing circulating platelet concentrations by about 99%. Heparin-protamine challenge in control sheep caused pulmonary vasoconstriction without thrombocytopenia. In comparison to control HP studies, severe platelet depletion did not modify the HP-induced increases in plasma thromboxane B_2 levels and pulmonary vascular resistance, the 20% decrease in cardiac output, leukopenia (to 60-70% of baseline value), or the decrease in Pa_{O_2} (by approximately 34 mmHg). In vitro, neither heparin nor protamine nor heparin and protamine together caused either ovine platelet thromboxane release or platelet aggregation, suggesting that platelets were not activated. Thus, platelets do not mediate pulmonary vasoconstriction in HP-challenged sheep.

Platelets appear to play a more important role in the canine response to infusion of heparin and protamine. Heparin-protamine challenge causes pulmonary accumulation of radiolabeled platelets (Radegran et al., 1971a; Wakefield et al., 1987) and thrombocytopenia (Radegran et al., 1971a, 1974; Radegran and McAshan, 1972; Wakefield et al., 1987) that accompany the increase in pulmonary vascular resistance. Protamine alone also may cause increased pulmonary vascular resistance and thrombocytopenia (Radegran et al., 1971a), although not consistently (Wakefield et al., 1986). In vitro studies of the canine platelet response to heparin and protamine suggest that HP complexes activate platelets and cause aggregation (Wakefield et al., 1984). Yet the central role of platelets in the dog is most convincingly demonstrated by studies in which platelet depletion prevents HP-induced pulmonary vasoconstriction (Lindblad et al., 1988). For unknown reasons, protamine pretreatment of dogs before HP challenge prevents both the pulmonary vasoconstriction and intrapulmonary accumulation of radiolabeled platelets (Wakefield et al., 1987).

Studies with isolated porcine and cat lungs perfused with either whole blood or dextran, as noted earlier, suggest that platelets are not essential for HP-induced pulmonary vasoconstriction in these species.

Pulmonary Intravascular Macrophages

An intriguing possibility is that pulmonary intravascular macrophages mediate or contribute to acute pulmonary vasoconstriction during HP challenge. They have been described in numerous cloven-hoofed animal species, including sheep (Warner et al., 1986, 1988; Wheeldon and Hansen-Flaschen, 1986) and pigs (Bertram et al., 1988; Winkler and Cheville, 1985), but appear less common in dogs (Crocker et al., 1981a) and rats (Warner et al., 1987, 1988). Notably, pulmonary intravascular macrophages may be up to five times as numerous as neutrophils in sheep lung (Albertine et al., 1987) and occupy up to 15% of the pulmonary intracapillary volume (Warner et al., 1986). These macrophages may play an important role in the pulmonary hemodynamic responses following the infusion of a variety of foreign particles, including lipopolysaccharide (Staub, 1988; Warner et al., 1988) and liposomes (Miyamoto et al., 1988). Porcine pulmonary intravascular macrophages challenged in vitro with either gram-negative bacteria (Bertram et al., 1989) or the calcium ionophore A23187 (Bertram et al., 1988) release a variety of pulmonary vasoactive eicosanoids, including the vasoconstrictor thromboxane. Furthermore, activated ovine pulmonary intravascular macrophages appear to be able to generate or release both superoxide radical and peroxide (Staub et al., 1987), which may in turn induce thromboxane release (Tate et al., 1984). These results may explain why pigs, which have greater numbers of pulmonary intravascular macrophages than dogs (Crocker et al., 1981a, b), also demonstrate markedly greater pulmonary clearance of infused *Pseudomonas* bacteria and subsequently develop greater pulmonary vasoconstriction. Similarly, in newborn pigs, development of the pulmonary intravascular macrophage and monocyte population parallels the pulmonary vascular response to the infusion of bacteria (Winkler and Cheville, 1985). Differences in the pulmonary population of these macrophages may also explain why infusing either 1 μg/kg of endotoxin or 0.1-5 μmol/kg of liposomes causes greater thromboxane release and pulmonary vasoconstriction in sheep than in dogs (Staub, 1988). It is notable that ovine pulmonary intravascular macrophages appear to be activated rapidly (within 10 min) following exposure to lipopolysaccharide (Warner et al., 1988).

Because the Morel and co-workers model of HP challenge causes pulmonary vasoconstriction consistently in sheep and pigs but rarely in rats or *M. cynomolgus* monkeys, we speculated that pulmonary intravascular macrophages may play an important role in the pulmonary response to HP challenge. To learn whether animals with a substantial population of these macrophages sequester a greater proportion of infused heparin and protamine in the lung than animals that lack these macrophages, we infused ^{111}In-radiolabeled protamine into heparinized sheep and rats. Using gamma camera scanning, we noted that radiolabeled protamine uptake in three rats occurred primarily in the liver, whereas uptake in sheep occurred primarily in the lung. These results parallel the fate of infused endotoxin in these species (Warner et al., 1988). Rats display predominantly hepatic uptake of lipopolysaccharide and do not easily develop lipopolysaccharide-induced pulmonary vasoconstriction or lung injury; in contrast, sheep sequester most of the infused lipopolysaccharide in the lung and quickly develop pulmonary vasoconstriction and acute lung injury (Warner et al., 1987). The parallel between the organ entrapment of protamine and lipopolysaccharide in these two species and the subsequent pulmonary hemodynamic response suggest that the pulmonary response to these agents depends on which organ (and macrophage) entraps the majority of the molecules or complexes. This idea is reinforced by studies that demonstrate that hepatic uptake of gram-negative bacteria provides partial protection against lung injury in sheep (Warner et al., 1989b).

If our hypothesis is correct—that is, HP challenge induces pulmonary intravascular macrophages to release mediators, which cause pulmonary vasoconstriction—then it is possible to speculate that we might identify human reactors to HP challenge by measuring the pulmonary uptake of infused, radiolabeled compounds, such as sulfur colloids, which are readily ingested by macrophages. Pulmonary intravascular macrophages appear to be less prevalent in humans than in either sheep or pig (Dehring and Wismar, 1989), which may explain why human reactors to HP challenge are infrequent. However, the pulmonary intravascular macrophage population in primates may change under certain stresses. Pulmonary intravascular macrophages in healthy baboons occupy approximately 1.8% of the capillary intravascular volume; this value increased to 6.3% after prolonged hyperoxic exposure (Francica et al., 1988). Similarly, in other species that generally lack these macrophages, endotoxemia can promote the conversion of circulating mononuclear cells into resident pulmonary intravascular cells that resemble macrophages (Warner et al., 1989a).

The pulmonary intravascular macrophage hypothesis also may explain why HP challenge in isolated porcine lung perfused with acellular dextran causes thromboxane release and pulmonary vasoconstriction. Resident intravascular macrophages may not have been cleared from the lung by instituting dextran perfusion and may have contributed to these HP-induced events. In dogs, the role of pulmonary intravascular macrophages is uncertain. Pulmonary intravascular macrophages are less common in dogs than in sheep or pigs; nevertheless, HP challenge causes pulmonary vasoconstriction. It is possible that canine pulmonary intravascular macrophages interact with platelets to produce pulmonary vasoconstriction during HP challenge.

The role of the pulmonary vascular endothelium and its interaction with other possible mediators of HP-induced pulmonary vasoconstriction, including these macrophages, remain to be defined.

C. Biochemical Mediators

Eicosanoids

Vasoactive eicosanoids play an important role in HP-induced pulmonary vasoconstriction in the sheep and pig and probably also in the dog. Rapid intravenous protamine reversal of heparin anticoagulation in sheep (Morel et al., 1988; Montalescot et al., 1989; Kreil et al., 1989) and pig (Hobbhahn et al., 1988; Schumacher et al., 1988; Conzen et al., 1989) causes marked thromboxane release into plasma accompanied by intense pulmonary vasoconstriction. Administering protamine to reverse anticoagulation with low-molecular-weight heparin in dogs (Lindblad et al., 1987) and sheep (Montalescot, in preparation) also releases thromboxane. In sheep challenged with standard heparin and protamine, the peak increase in plasma thromboxane B_2 (TxB_2) levels correlates with the concomitant peak increase in pulmonary artery pressure (r = 0.83-0.84) (Morel et al., 1988; Kreil et al., 1989). In addition, infusing sheep with protamine before heparin fails to cause either increased plasma thromboxane B_2 levels or elevated pulmonary vascular resistance, supporting the association between thromboxane release and pulmonary vasoconstriction (Kreil et al., 1989). Transpulmonary arteriovenous gradients of plasma TxB_2 (Degges et al., 1987) and prostaglandin $F_{2\alpha}$ ($PGF_{2\alpha}$) (Hobbhahn et al., 1988) levels in pigs suggest that the lung releases these vasoactive eicosanoids although these gradients were not found in other porcine studies (Conzen et al., 1989).

Stronger evidence for the causal relationship between HP challenge, thromboxane release, and pulmonary vasoconstriction is provided by studies utilizing inhibitors of eicosanoid synthesis and function. Pretreating sheep with either a cyclooxygenase blocker (indomethacin, 10 mg/kg) (Morel et al., 1988) or a thromboxane synthetase blocker (UK38485, 10 mg/kg) (Morel et al., 1988) prevents both HP-induced thromboxane release and increased pulmonary vascular resistance (Fig. 1). Similarly, cyclooxygenase inhibition in pigs with either indomethacin (Hobbhahn et al., 1988; Conzen et al., 1989) or acetylsalicylic acid (Degges et al., 1987) blocks both the HP-induced release of vasoactive eicosanoids, including thromboxane (Hobbhahn et al., 1988; Degges et al., 1987; Conzen et al., 1989), $PGF_{2\alpha}$, and $KH_2PGF_{2\alpha}$ (Hobbhahn et al., 1988; Conzen et al., 1989), and the increase in pulmonary vascular resistance. Pretreating dogs with acetylsalicyclic acid also blocks pulmonary vasoconstriction during HP challenge (Radegran and McAshan, 1972). Of particular importance is the demonstration that pretreatment with a thromboxane receptor blocker in both sheep (SQ30741), (Montalescot, in preparation) and pigs (BM 13.177 and SQ30741) (Conzen et al., 1989; Schumacher et al., 1988) prevents the HP-induced increase in pulmonary vascular resistance but not the thromboxane release.

Thus, these studies strongly support the hypothesis that thromboxane A_2 is the key pulmonary vasoconstrictor released during HP challenge in several animal species. The cellular source of the thromboxane remains unknown and may differ in various species.

Complement

Viewed together, numerous studies of widely differing nature suggest that complement activation by HP challenge contributes to pulmonary vasoconstiction. First, studies of cardiac surgical patients demonstrated increased plasma levels of complement anaphylatoxins C3a, C4a (Morel et al., 1987; Kirklin et al., 1986; Cavarocchi et al., 1985; Best et al., 1984), C3 split products (Best et al., 1983), and C5a (Morel et al., 1987) after protamine infusion to reverse heparin anticoagulation. Second, infusing zymosan-activated plasma and complement into sheep causes pulmonary leukosequestration (Klausner et al., 1988; Meyrick and Brigham, 1984), thromboxane release, and increased pulmonary vascular resistance (Gee et al., 1986; Perkowski et al., 1983; McDonald et al., 1983) similar to the response to HP challenge in sheep. Third, infusing the complement fragment $C5a_{desArg}$ into pigs causes leukopenia and pulmonary vasoconstriction (Cheung et al., 1986); also, infusing the anaphylatoxin C5a into isolated guinea pig lung induces the release of the pulmonary vasoconstrictor thromboxane (Pavek et al., 1979). Fourth, depleting plasma complement with cobra venom factor prevents the thromboxane release and pulmonary vasoconstriction caused by venovenous bypass in sheep (Wonders et al., 1983). Finally, in vitro studies document that heparin-protamine complexes activate the classic complement pathway, primarily at the level of C1 (Rent et al., 1975; Fiedel et al., 1976), via nonimmunologic mechanisms. Both complement activation in human serum (Rent et al., 1975) and HP-induced leukopenia in rabbit (Fehr and Rohr, 1983) are maximal when approximately equivalent quantities of heparin and protamine, or with a slight protamine excess, are combined. Either protamine or heparin alone activates complement to a much lesser degree (Rent et al., 1975). Interestingly, high concentrations of heparin may limit complement activation by several mechanisms, including the potentiation of C1 esterase inhibitor activity (Rent et al., 1976). For unknown reasons, the preformed HP complex causes less complement activation in vitro than does mixing heparin and protamine in the presence of serum (Claus et al., 1977).

Based upon human studies of protamine reversal of heparin anticoagulation after cardiopulmonary bypass (described later in this chapter), Morel and co-workers (1987) postulated that C5a may be a major factor in HP-induced pulmonary vasoconstriction. Although C5a-derived products may increase pulmonary vascular resistance in some animals, Morel subsequently studied inhibitors of cyclooxygenase and thromboxane synthetase in sheep (see Eicosanoids earlier in this section) and demonstrated that thromboxane, not complement anaphylatoxin C5a, is the principal circulating pulmonary vasconstrictor released during HP challenge in this species. They then proposed that HP challenge in both human (Morel et al., 1987) and sheep (Morel et al., 1988) activates complement anaphylatoxins, which subsequently triggers thromboxane release and pulmonary vasoconstriction.

We therefore examined whether we could prevent HP-induced pulmonary vasoconstriction in sheep by infusing nafamstate mesilate (FUT-175), a synthetic broad-spectrum protease inhibitor with potent activity against both the classic and alternative complement pathways (Aoyama et al., 1984), prior to protamine reversal of heparin. Because radioimmunoassay (RIA) for ovine C5a was unavailable at the time of study, we measured plasma C3a levels. HP challenge increased plasma C3a levels, whereas sheep treated with a reversed HP sequence, that is, protamine first, followed by heparin, experienced neither increased plasma C3a levels nor a change in pulmonary vascular resistance (Fig. 2) (Kreil et al., 1989). Treatment with FUT-175 markedly attenuated the HP-induced increases in plasma C3a and TxB_2 levels and almost completely prevented the increase in pulmonary vascular resistance. FUT-175 did not prevent either the rise in plasma TxB_2 levels or pulmonary vasoconstriction caused by subsequent infusion of arachidonic acid, suggesting that FUT-175 did not reduce pulmonary vascular resistance by directly inhibiting eicosanoid production.

Interestingly, plasma C3a levels in these sheep increased after the peak increase in arterial plasma TxB_2 levels and pulmonary vascular resistance, which occurred 1 min after protamine infusion. Moreover, the increase in C3a levels correlated only weakly with the increase in pulmonary artery pressure during the peak pulmonary vascular response ($r = 0.53; p < 0.02$) and did not correlate with the peak increase in plasma TxB_2 levels. The conflict between these results and the hypothesis that HP-induced complement activation triggers thromboxane release and pulmonary vasoconstriction may arise for several reasons. FUT-175 did not block leukopenia, suggesting FUT-175 incompletely inhibited C5a formation. Furthermore, because plasma levels of C3a and C5a may not correlate well (Chenoweth, 1987), the increase in plasma C3a levels may not correspond to the C5a-induced increase in plasma TxB_2 levels. It is also possible that small quantities of rapidly generated C3a may suffice to activate C5a and cause leukopenia, thromboxane release, and increased pulmonary vascular resistance within the first minute after protamine infusion to reverse heparin anticoagulation. Subsequent increases in plasma C3a and C5a levels may cause little additional thromboxane release

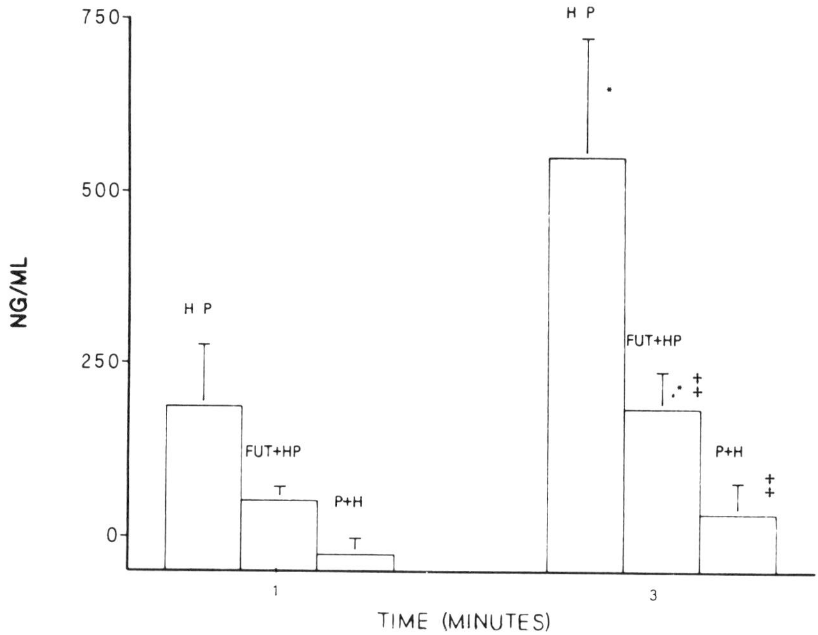

Figure 2 Increase in arterial plasma complement C3a concentrations in control heparin-protamine (HP) sheep ($n = 6$), FUT + HP sheep ($n = 10$), and in sheep treated with protamine first followed by heparin (P + H, $n = 5$). Plasma C3a levels did not change in sheep give FUT-175 alone; thus the data are not shown. $^*p < 0.05$ significant increase from t = −1 min (plasma C3a levels did not change significantly from t = −6 to t = −1 min in any study group). $^‡p < 0.05$: significant change in C3a concentrations compared to the concomitant change in HP sheep. (Reprinted from *J. Appl. Physiol.*, **67**:1467, 1989.)

and increase in pulmonary vascular resistance because C5a receptors may remain saturated. Finally, it is possible that activated complement may not be a key mediator in this model of acute pulmonary vasoconstriction. Our data are consistent with the possibility that FUT-175 may block pulmonary vasoconstriction by mechanisms other than inhibition of complement pathways. Thus, these studies do not define a clear role for complement activation in HP-induced pulmonary vasoconstriction.

In subsequent studies, we treated two sheep with *N. haje* cobra venom factor to deplete plasma complement prior to HP challenge. As described earlier (see Leukocytes in Sec. III.B.), we administered doses that, in a previous ovine study, reduced sheep plasma C3a levels to 4 ± 2% of baseline value and plasma CH_{50} liters to undetectable levels and prevented the leukopenia, thromboxane release, and pulmonary vasoconstriction caused by venovenous bypass (Wonders et al., 1983). However, in both HP-challenged sheep, cobra venom factor treatment failed to prevent thromboxane release, increase in pulmonary vascular resistance, and leukopenia (unpublished study). Although the leukopenia suggests that cobra venom factor did not completely prevent complement activation, these results also suggest that activated complement may not be a key mediator of HP-induced pulmonary vasoconstriction in sheep.

To learn whether C5a plays a key role in pulmonary vasoconstriction in pigs, we performed pilot studies of HP challenge both before and after treating two pigs with a murine monoclonal antiporcine C5a antibody. Infusing 1.5, 5, and 12 mg/kg of the antibody during three separate trials did not block the leukopenia and increase in pulmonary vascular resistance during HP challenge (unpublished study). Although we do not know why anti-C5a antibody appeared ineffective in these studies, our results are consistent with the results of prior studies of HP challenge in pigs: pulmonary vascular resistance increased comparably during HP challenge in isolated pig lungs perfused with either whole blood or acellular dextran-40. Thus, HP-induced pulmonary vasoconstriction in pigs probably does not depend upon complement activation (Degges et al., 1987).

Similar studies of HP challenge in isolated perfused cat lung (Jastrzebski et al., 1975) also suggest that complement activation is not necessary to cause pulmonary vasoconstriction in this species. In dogs, HP challenge did not decrease plasma CH_{50} levels in one study (Wakefield et al., 1986), although this measurement may be less sensitive to complement activation than measurements of specific complement factors (Rent et al., 1975). Heparin-protamine challenge of two dogs in another study failed to significantly modify plasma C3a levels (Lindblad et al., 1987).

Thus, activated complement does not appear to be an essential mediator of ovine pulmonary vasoconstriction during HP challenge, although the persistence of C5a-derived activity in these studies, despite anticomplement treatment, suggests that more definitive studies are required. Complement activation does not appear mandatory for the HP-induced release of pulmonary vasoconstrictors in either pigs or cats, whereas the precise role of complement in the dog remains unknown.

D. Reactive Oxygen Species

Sheep studies with infused zymosan-activated complement suggest that complement activation releases reactive oxygen species (Perkowski et al., 1983). Chemically generated reactive oxygen species may in turn induce thromboxane release and pulmonary vasoconstriction (Tate et al., 1984). Based on these studies, Morel and co-workers (1988), during their initial investigations of HP-induced pulmonary vasoconstriction, postulated that HP challenge in sheep activates complement and stimulates the release of reactive oxygen species, causing both thromboxane release and pulmonary vasoconstriction. They demonstrated that pretreating sheep with 0.5-1.0 g/kg of dimethylthiourea (DMTU), a scavenger of both hydroxyl radicals and peroxide, abolished HP-induced thromboxane release and the increase in pulmonary vascular resistance (Fig. 1) but not the leukopenia (Morel et al., 1988). Plasma DMTU levels decreased concomitantly with this effect on pulmonary vascular resistance, suggesting that DMTU was consumed during this reaction. DMTU did not block the thromboxane release and rise in pulmonary vascular resistance caused by infusing arachidonic acid, suggesting that DMTU did not prevent either thromboxane production or eicosanoid-induced pulmonary vasoconstriction. In contrast, pretreating sheep with dimethylsulfoxide (DMSO), a scavenger of hydroxyl radicals, did not block HP-induced thromboxane release or the increase in pulmonary vascular resistance (Fig. 1) (Morel et al., 1988), although secondary radicals may have been formed from the combination of DMSO with the hydroxyl radical (Raleigh and Kremers, 1981). These studies therefore provided indirect evidence that at least one reactive oxygen species, peroxide, contributes to pulmonary vasoconstriction during HP challenge in sheep.

To further test the hypothesis that reactive oxygen species mediate HP-induced pulmonary vasoconstriction, we intravenously pretreated sheep with other antioxidants prior to protamine infusion (Table 1). All these agents failed to block the increase in pulmonary vascular resistance. Superoxide dismutase (SOD), which catalyzes the conversion of superoxide anion to peroxide, augmented pulmonary vascular resistance during HP challenge, supporting the hypothesis that peroxide plays a key role in this syndrome (Kreil et al., 1987). However, infusing catalase, which catalyzes the conversion of peroxide to water, also failed to modify the increase in pulmonary vascular resistance (Kreil et al., 1987). Furthermore, pretreating two sheep with both SOD and catalase did not modify the pulmonary hemodynamic changes caused by HP challenge (unpublished data). Neither allopurinol, which inhibits xanthine oxidase generation of O_2^- and peroxide from O_2, nor desferroxamine, which decreases the availability of catalytic iron to participate in the generation of reactive oxygen species, including hydroxyl radical and hypoiodous acid, blocked the increase in pulmonary vascular resistance in pilot studies (unpublished data). *N*-acetylcysteine (NAC), which attenuates endotoxin-induced pulmonary hypertension in sheep, presumably either by scavenging hydroxyl radicals or by replenishing intracellular antioxidant supplies (Bernard et al., 1984), also did not modify the increase in pulmonary vascular resistance (unpublished data).

Thus, the hypothesis that reactive oxygen species mediate HP-induced pulmonary vasoconstriction in sheep remains tenuous and is supported solely

Table 1 Effect of Antioxidant Therapies on Heparin-Protamine-Induced Pulmonary Vasoconstriction (PVC) and Leukopenia[a]

Therapy	No. sheep	Dose per kg	Completion of therapy (min before protamine)	Effect of Rx on PVC
DMTU	3	1 g	15	Blocked
DMTU	3	0.5 g	15	Attenuated
DMSO	4	1 g	15	No block
SOD	5	16,000-17,000 U	11	Augmented
Catalase	5	200,000 U	11	No block
SOD + catalase	2	200,000 U	11	No block
Allopurinol	1	50 mg	15	No block
Desferroxamine	1	20 mg	30	No block
NAC	1	200 mg	5	No block

[a]None of the drugs modified the leukopenia, which probably reflects complement activation.

by the results of the DMTU studies. The conflicting results with other antioxidant studies may be due to several factors.

1. Reactive oxygen species may be generated intracellularly (Freeman, and Crapo, 1982) during HP challenge. Small antioxidant molecules, such as DMTU and DMSO, may penetrate cells more easily than larger charged molecules, such as SOD and catalase. The decrease in plasma DMTU levels during HP challenge suggests that DMTU was consumed; however, the decrease does not define whether the scavenging occurred intracellularly or whether DMTU scavenged reactive oxygen species that may have been generated or released intravascularly.
2. Higher doses of the larger peroxide scavengers, such as catalase, may be necessary to block HP-induced pulmonary vasoconstriction.
3. Reactive oxygen species other than peroxide may contribute to this HP syndrome.
4. DMTU may block thromboxane release and pulmonary vasoconstriction in sheep by a mechanism that does not involve its antioxidant function.

E. Other Mediators

Histamine

Histamine release after protamine infusion appears species dependent. In sheep, plasma histamine levels increased markedly and systemic blood pressure decreased during anaphylaxis (D.R. Morel et al., in preparation) but not during HP challenge (Morel et al., 1988). In dogs, histamine release may contribute to HP-induced systemic vasodilation and hypotension, although histamine appears to be released only if protamine is infused through a central venous catheter but not if it is infused into a peripheral vein or via the left atrium (Casthely et al., 1986). Notably, studies with antihistamines in pigs (Degges et al., 1987) and histamine depletion in dogs (Fadali et al., 1986), as well as the eicosanoid studies discussed earlier, suggest that histamine does not play an important role in the pulmonary response to HP challenge in these species.

Carboxypeptidase N

Plasma carboxypeptidase N (CPN, also called kininase I and anaphylatoxin inactivator, MW 280,000) is an enzyme produced in the liver that cleaves C-terminal basic amino acids from peptides (Matthews, 1986). This enables CPN to inactivate complement anaphylatoxins, including C3a and C5a, which have been suspected of contributing to HP-induced pulmonary vasoconstriction (see Complement in Sec. III.C). Both CPN deficiency, which may be genetically determined, and protamine, which may inhibit human CPN (Skidgel et al., 1988; Tan et al., 1989), may limit inactivation of complement anaphylatoxins.

We found normal plasma CPN levels in sheep and in three human reactors (unpublished studies). Moreover, although protamine may inhibit human CPN, pulmonary vasoconstriction occurs in only a small proportion of patients who receive protamine. Thus, we believe it is unlikely that HP-induced pulmonary vasoconstriction in either sheep or human is due to a deficiency or inhibition of CPN enzymatic activity.

Platelet Activating Factor

Platelet activating factor (PAF, also called acetylglyceryl ether phosphorylcholine) is released by a variety of cells, including leukocytes, platelets, vascular endothelial cells, and macrophages (O'Flaherty and Wykle, 1987; Henson and Lynch, 1983). Infusing PAF (2-20 μg) into sheep causes thromboxane release, pulmonary vasoconstriction, leukopenia, and thrombocytopenia (Smallbone et al., 1987). Infusing PAF (28 μg/kg) into baboons also caused these changes, as well as systemic hypotension and increased vascular permeability (McManus et al., 1981). Based on these studies, we examined PAF levels during HP challenge in sheep. We found that PAF levels (by bioassay) did not increase during the peak increase in pulmonary vascular resistance (unpublished study). Furthermore, infusing 20 mg/kg of the PAF receptor blocker BN52021 (courtesy Institut H. Beaufour, Paris, France) into four sheep 30 min before protamine infusion did not block either the increase in pulmonary vascular resistance or leukopenia. Thus, we believe PAF does not mediate HP-induced pulmonary vasoconstriction in sheep.

F. Summary of Animal Mediator Studies

Thromboxane A_2 appears to be the key pulmonary vasoconstrictor released by HP challenge in the sheep and pig and probably also in the dog. The cascade of mediators activated by HP challenge, which leads directly to thromboxane release and pulmonary vasoconstriction, remains unidentified. Complement and leukocyte activation do not appear essential to this response, although further study is required to prove this hypothesis for all animal species. Evidence for a causal role for reactive oxygen species is limited and indirect. Pulmonary intravascular macrophages may play an important role in HP-induced pulmonary vasoconstriction in several species, including sheep and pig. Platelets appear to have an important role only in the dog but not in pig, sheep, or cat.

IV. Heparin-Protamine, Lipopolysaccharide, and Lung Injury in Sheep

The ovine response to HP challenge partially resembles the initial response to LPS infusion. Both treatments cause pulmonary leukosequestration, decreases in circulating leukocyte concentrations, and marked thromboxane release with intense pulmonary vasoconstriction, which can be severe enough to substantially impede cardiac output. Both HP and LPS activate complement pathways. Furthermore, reactive oxygen species appear to play a major role in the response to LPS infusion (Brigham and Meyrick, 1986; Said and Foda, 1989); limited evidence suggests that they may also contribute to the adverse responses to HP challenge. Yet, despite these similarities, major pulmonary vascular endothelial injury has been documented only after challenge with LPS but not HP.

Ovine studies with zymosan-activated complement and plasma (ZAP) demonstrate that leukocyte activation and pulmonary leukosequestration, in association with activated complement, do not necessarily cause major pulmonary vascular endothelial injury (Meyrick and Brigham, 1984). These results suggest that HP-induced leukocyte and complement activation, per se, also may not cause major lung injury, although a minor increase in endothelial permeability cannot be excluded. In contrast, activated complement (Said and Foda, 1989) and leukocytes (Brigham and Meyrick, 1986) appear to contribute to LPS-induced endothelial injury.

This comparison of the HP, ZAP, and LPS studies suggests that factors in addition to complement and leukocyte activation, pulmonary leukosequestration, and thromboxane release determine the evolution of major vascular endothelial injury. These factors may also account for the differences in timing of the corresponding responses to HP and LPS. HP-induced leukopenia, thromboxane release, and pulmonary vasoconstriction occur quickly, within the first few minutes after protamine infusion, and resolve quickly, returning toward prechallenge levels within the next 5-10 min. In contrast, the corresponding LPS-induced responses generally begin more than 10 min after LPS infusion, peak (or reach nadir) after 30-60 min, and subsequently recover toward baseline values, although the increased pulmonary vascular resistance and a severe leukopenia may persist for hours.

Similar comparisons of other cellular and biochemical mediators activated by HP and LPS may help to identify factors that either cause or modify injury. However, the direct effect of HP and LPS on the vascular endothelium must also be considered because mediators may have differing effects on intact and previously injured cells. LPS rapidly causes endothelial cell damage in the absence of circulating mediators, and serum enhances this effect (Meyrick and Brigham, 1986). As yet, the effect of HP complexes on vascular endothelium has not been studied. Furthermore, the mechanism of mediator activation needs to be considered. For example, the release of reactive oxygen species during HP challenge may occur as a by-product of cyclooxygenase pathway activation. Because this pathway appears to be activated for only a brief period, the vascular endothelial cell may be exposed only briefly to reactive oxygen species. In this case, it is possible that native scavenging systems may suffice to limit or prevent injury. Although these considerations complicate the interpretation of mediator effects, they also suggest that HP studies may complement other studies, including those with ZAP, in learning the causes of lung injury.

V. The Clinical Syndrome of Heparin-Protamine-Associated Acute Pulmonary Vasoconstriction in Humans

Normally, protamine reversal of heparin in humans is not associated with detectable cardiocirculatory changes. Sporadically, administration of protamine to neutralize heparin in humans is followed by transient pulmonary vasoconstriction (Lowenstein et al., 1983). This has been observed most frequently after separation from cardiopulmonary bypass (CPB) during cardiac surgical operations. The vasoconstriction may be sufficiently intense to prevent virtually all blood transfer across the pulmonary circulation. Since systemic venous return continues to the right heart, right ventricular and pulmonary hypertension occur. The right ventricle becomes distended and ventricular failure occurs, as reflected by an elevated right ventricular diastolic and right atrial pressure. Moreover, since blood does not traverse the lungs and reach the left side of the heart, left atrial and left ventricular pressure and volume decline and systemic hypotension occurs. This may be so severe that CPB is reinstituted (Fig. 3).

An initial report of five patients documenting HP-associated pulmonary vasoconstriction was composed primarily of patients with mitral valve disease and pre-existing pulmonary hypertension who received small boluses of protamine (5-20 mg) into a central venous line (Lowenstein et al., 1983). It also included one patient with coronary artery disease and one whose protamine was injected into a peripheral vein. An addendum to the article described an identical event after left-sided (i.e., intra-aortic) infusion of protamine. Nevertheless, we hypothesized that bolus infusion of large quantities of protamine into patients with pre-existing pulmonary hypertension would be most likely to elicit the acute pulmonary vasoconstriction.

To define the incidence of acute pulmonary vasoconstriction in cardiac surgical patients, we prospectively surveyed 925 adult patients whose pulmonary artery pressures were monitored for clinical indications. An increase in mean pulmonary artery pressure of 7 mmHg and/or an increase in mean right atrial pressure of 4 mmHg during protamine administration was considered evidence of acute pulmonary vasoconstriction. In all cases, 120 mg protamine was given by slow, regulated infusion into the superior vena cava-right atrium at a rate of approximately 10 mg/min.

A total of 14 incidents of acute pulmonary vasoconstriction were documented in these 925 patients, an incidence of 1.5%. Table 2 presents data from this survey. Most striking is that the survey failed to identify or confirm any demographic risk factors. For instance, although 4 of 5 patients in the first reported series had valvular heart disease and underlying pulmonary vascular disease, the incidence of reactions in the prospective survey was directly proportional to their percentage in the study population. Diabetes mellitus or pretreatment with histamine blockers or steroids also did not affect the incidence of this adverse reaction. We concluded that the incidence of HP-induced pulmonary vasoconstriction was over 1%, far higher than we had suspected, and the factors predisposing to its occurrence were not understood.

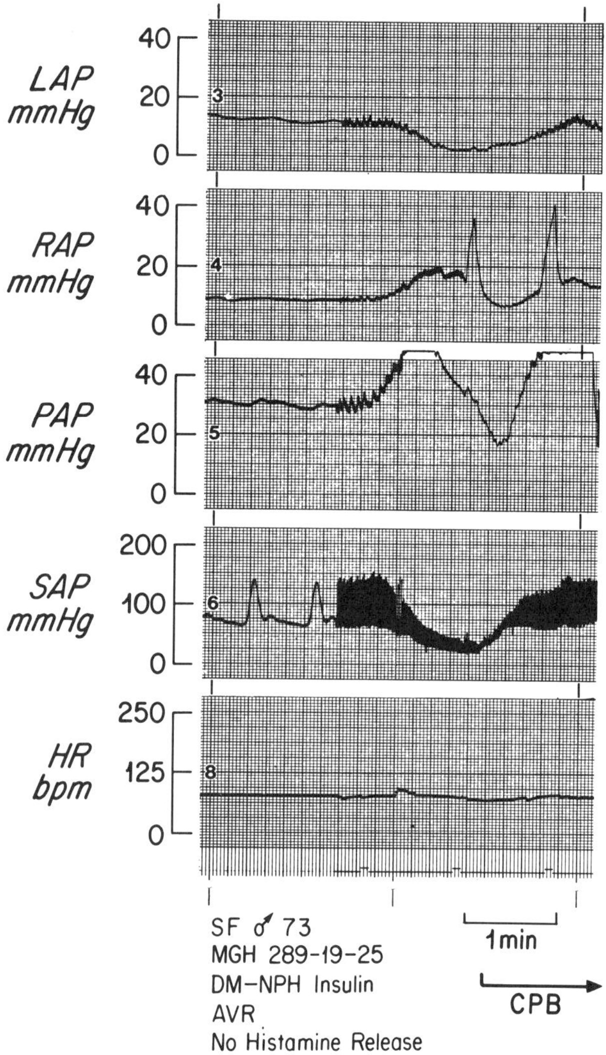

Figure 3 Anaphylactoid response to protamine reversal of heparin. Catastrophic pulmonary vasoconstriction after 10 mg protamine administered over 3 min. Note the sequential elevation of pulmonary arterial pressure (PAP) and right atrial pressure (RAP), followed by the decline of left arterial pressure (LAP). CPB was reinstituted to treat systemic hypotension. The transients in the RAP recording represent injection of heparin. The initial decline in PAP recording may represent a functional pulmonary capillary wedge recording. SAP: systemic arterial pressure. (Stripchart recording courtesy of N. Sims, M.D. Reprinted from *J. Cardiothorac. Anesth.*, **3**: 101, 1989.)

Table 2 Incidence of Reputed Risk Factors and Prophylactic Therapy with Antihistamines and Steroids upon Incidence of Heparin-Protamine-Associated Pulmonary Vasoconstriction in Cardiac Surgical Patients[a]

Patient group	Population (*n*/%)	Reactors (*n*/%)
CABG	669/75	11/79
Heart valve disease	133/15	3/21
Diabetes mellitus	159/18	1/7
DM-insulin	64/7	1/7
PAP > 20 (preoperative)	156/18	2/14
H_1 blockers (intraoperative)	248/28	4/29
H_2 blockers (intraoperative)	149/17	3/21
Steroids (intraoperative)	228/26	5/36

[a]The incidence of pulmonary vasoconstriction was not affected by the type of cardiac disease, diabetes, chronic treatment with protamine-insulin, or prophylaxis.

A. Mediators Associated with Acute Pulmonary Vasoconstriction in Humans

Morel and associates (1987) conducted a prospective study in humans to determine the mediators associated with acute pulmonary vasoconstriction occurring episodically with protamine reversal of heparin. The study was conducted in 48 adult patients scheduled to undergo cardiac surgery utilizing cardiopulmonary bypass. Patients included those undergoing elective coronary artery bypass grafting or mitral valve replacement. Patients with a documented hypersensitivity to protamine who had received either a nonsteroidal or steroidal anti-inflammatory agent during the 2 weeks prior to operation were excluded. In these studies, protamine sulfate was injected over a 10 sec period into the right atrium. All patients received 100 mg protamine, except those with mitral valve disease and pre-existing pulmonary hypertension, who were given 20 mg.

Of these 48 patients, 2 developed pulmonary hypertension, increased airway pressure, and systemic hypotension following protamine administration. Data from patient 49, who was not selected for study in advance, are included in the analysis. Blood sampling from this patient was initiated as soon as increased airway pressure and pulmonary hypertension were recognized

Table 3 Hemodynamics Associated with Protamine Reversal of Heparin[a]

Patient group[b]	Variable	Time relative to protamine injection[c]			
		−5 Min	−1 Min	+3 Min	+10 Min
CABG	Heart rate (beats per min)	84 ± 2	82 ± 3	83 ± 2	84 ± 2
	Mean arterial pressure (mmHg)	62 ± 3	68 ± 3	69 ± 5	72 ± 5
	Mean pulmonary arterial pressure (mmHg)	15 ± 1	15 ± 1	16 ± 1	13 ± 1
	Central venous pressure (mmHg)	4 ± 1	4 ± 1	4 ± 4	4 ± 1
	Left atrial pressure (mmHg)	6 ± 1	5 ± 1	6 ± 1	4 ± 1
	Cardiac index (liter × m^2/min)	2.6 ± 0.1	2.5 ± 0.1	2.4 ± 0.1	2.4 ± 0.1
	Systemic vascular resistance index (mmHg × min/liter × m^2)	27 ± 2	28 ± 3	27 ± 3	30 ± 4
	Pulmonary vascular resistance index (mmHg × min/liter × m^2)	3.6 ± 0.3	4.3 ± 0.4	4.0 ± 0.4	3.7 ± 0.4
MVR	Heart rate (beats per min)	91 ± 6	89 ± 6	88 ± 6	91 ± 6
	Mean arterial pressure (mmHg)	71 ± 3	73 ± 3	73 ± 4	75 ± 4
	Mean pulmonary arterial pressure (mmHg)	22 ± 2	22 ± 2	21 ± 2	22 ± 2
	Central venous pressure (mmHg)	6 ± 1	6 ± 1	5 ± 1	5 ± 1
	Left atrial pressure (mmHg)	10 ± 1	10 ± 1	10 ± 1	10 ± 1

Table 3 Continued

Patient group[b]	Variable	Time relative to protamine injection[c] −5 Min	−1 Min	+3 Min	+10 Min
	Cardiac index (liter × m²/min)	3.0 ± 0.2	3.0 ± 0.2	2.9 ± 0.2	2.9 ± 0.2
	Systemic vascular resistance index (mmHg × min/liter × m²)	23 ± 2	24 ± 2	24 ± 3	26 ± 3
	Pulmonary vascular resistance index (mmHg × min/liter × m²)	4.1 ± 0.4	3.8 ± 0.5	3.9 ± 0.6	4.1 ± 0.5

[a]No statistically significant changes were observed despite three episodes of systemic hypotension and two of pulmonary hypertension and pulmonary vasoconstriction.
[b]CABG, coronary artery bypass graft patients, $n = 18$; MVR, mitral valve replacement patients, $n = 9$.
[c]Data are means ± SEM. No statistically significant changes were observed over time.
Source: Reprinted from *Anesthesiology,* **66**:600 (1987).

(1 min after protamine administration). Increased peak airway pressure, indicative of bronchoconstriction, preceded the pulmonary vasoconstriction in all reactors and occurred in no other patients. These 3 patients constituted the initial database from which the mediator profiles of HP-associated pulmonary vasoconstriction were defined.

Table 3 presents the hemodynamic data from 18 coronary artery bypass graft patients and 9 mitral valve replacement patients in whom plasma thromboxane B_2 levels were measured. It is striking that the data presented in this standard fashion do not reveal any change in vascular pressures.

The most striking mediator response in this study was the increase in the plasma thromboxane B_2 levels. The mean plasma thromboxane B_2 level prior to protamine administration was 0.17 ± 0.12 ng/ml (±SD). In the three reactors, the levels rose between one and two orders of magnitude, to between 7.4 and 18.6 ng/ml, and remained elevated at 10 min (mean 5.01 ng/ml; range 2.78-9.03), whereas thromboxane B_2 levels did not change in the remaining patients (mean 0.15 ± 0.07 ng/ml). Figure 4 shows the association of plasma thromboxane B_2 levels and peak changes in mean pulmonary artery pressure and peak airway pressure. Plasma C5a anaphylatoxin levels

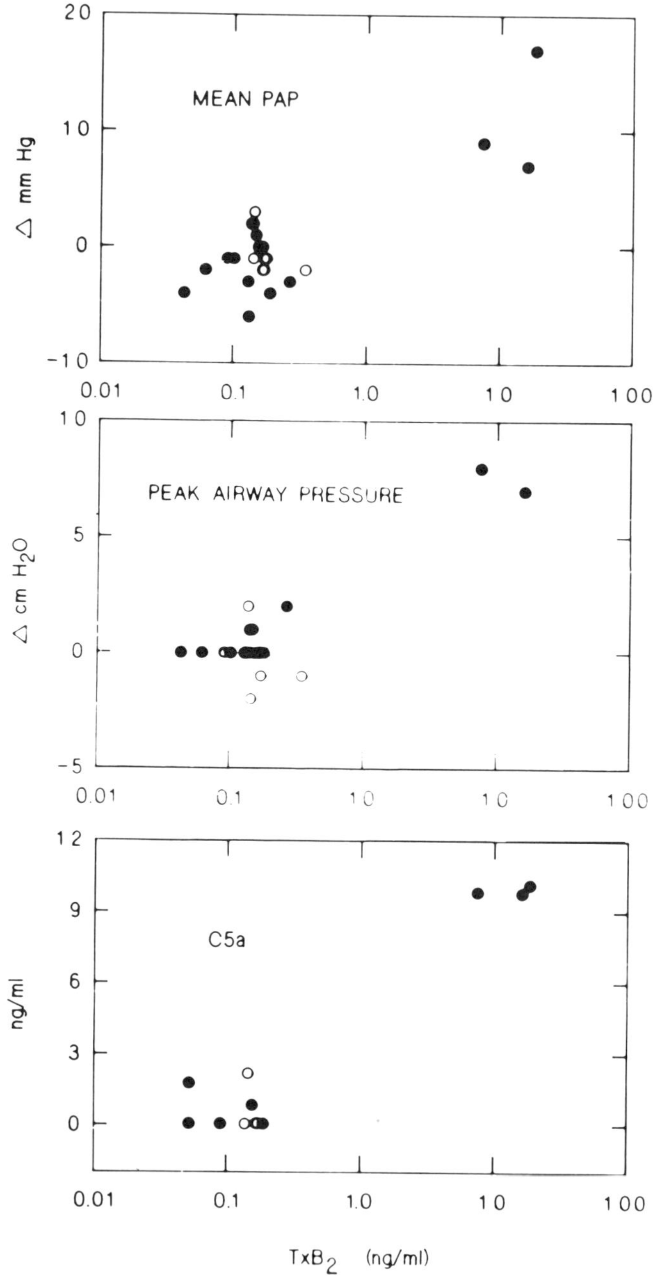
MEAN PAP
Δ mm Hg
PEAK AIRWAY PRESSURE
Δ cm H2O
C5a
ng/ml
TxB2 (ng/ml)

were measured in the 3 reactors and 9 nonreactors; these data are also included in Figure 4. Plasma C5a levels increased (approximately 10-fold) only in the reacting patients. Thus, there was no overlap between reactors and nonreactors in either measurement. In addition, no consistent transpulmonary arteriovenous gradient of either plasma thromboxane B_2 or C5a levels was demonstrated.

Plasma levels of 6-keto-$PGF_{1\alpha}$, a stable metabolite of prostacyclin, were undetectable before protamine and increased in only one of three reacting patients. Plasma PGE_2 concentrations were undetectable in all subjects.

Arterial plasma levels of C3a and C4a increased significantly from prebypass values to the control preprotamine values (Table 4). Patients who received the 100 mg dose had a significant further increase in both C3a and C4a levels after protamine infusion. In addition, the 100 mg protamine dose produced acute leukopenia that was maximal at 1 min with a mean decrease of approximately 29 ± 21% at its nadir. The degree of arterial leukopenia 1 min after protamine injection was proportional to the transpulmonary leukocyte concentration gradient and correlated with the maximum increase in C3a and C4a concentrations. The 100 mg protamine dose also significantly decreased the platelet count (−19 ± 14% of preinjection values) at the 10 min sampling period. However, no transpulmonary platelet gradient was demonstrated for platelets.

Arterial plasma histamine levels increased slightly although significantly with protamine administration (from 0.14 ± 0.12 to 0.28 ± 0.24 ng/ml). One patient demonstrated a major elevation of plasma histamine from 0.7 to 10.4 ng/ml in arterial blood and 5.9 ng/ml in mixed venous blood 1 min after a 100 mg dose of protamine. Notably, plasma TxB_2, C5a, 6-keto-$PGF_{1\alpha}$, and PGE_2 concentrations did not change. This patient immediately became hypotensive, with mean arterial pressure declining to 37 mmHg, apparently due to a decreased systemic vascular resistance. In contrast to the patients with plasma TxB_2 elevations, mean pulmonary artery pressure and pulmonary vascular resistance in this patient decreased from 25 to 15 mmHg and from 4.4 to 1.7 mmHg × liter/min per m^2, respectively. Airway pressure did not change. Hypotension was treated with epinephrine, and no sequellae were recognized.

Figure 4 Relationship between plasma TxB_2 levels 1 min after protamine, peak changes in mean pulmonary arterial pressure and peak airway pressure, and absolute plasma C5a levels. Note that TxB_2 levels are shown on a logarithmic scale. Each point represents the data from one patient. Closed circles = 100 mg protamine; open circles = 20 mg protamine. The three patients who reacted are clearly separated from the others. One reactor had no preprotamine airway pressure recorded. (Reprinted from *Anesthesiology,* **66**:601, 1987.)

Table 4 Plasma Levels (ng/ml) of C3a and C4a Anaphylatoxins

Anaphyla-toxin type	Dose of protamine[a] (mg)	Time relative to protamine injection							F_{ratio}[c]	*P*
		Pre-bypass[b]	−5 Min	−1 Min	+1 Min	+3 Min	+5 Min	+10 Min		
C3a	100									
	Mean[d]	360	1283	1082	1822	1600	1956	2137	2.81	0.02
	Limits[e]	286-453	1109-1485	950-1233	1496-2219	1395-1836	1631-2345	1813-2520		
	20									
	Mean[d]	±471	1513	1341	1586	1459	1517	1394	0.09	>0.1
	Limits[e]	353-630	1318-1738	1154-1559	1288-1953	1174-1813	1205-1909	1086-1788		
C4a	100									
	Mean[d]	574	1160	1181	3573	2650	3273	3405	4.61	<0.001
	Limits[e]	479-687	941-1429	985-1417	2629-4856	2058-3413	2492-4298	2707-4290		
	20									
	Mean[d]	730	1353	1288	1896	1724	1863	1822	1.09	>0.1
	Limits[e]	654-816	1163-1573	1097-1512	1620-2219	1431-2077	1578-2199	1555-2136		

[a]For 100 mg, $n = 19$; for 20 mg, $n = 9$.
[b]Prebypass levels were significantly different from postbypass values in all four groups (paired *t*-test).
[c]Prebypass data not included in this calculation.
[d]These calculations represent the antilogarithm of mean values subjected to logarithmic transformation.
[e]These limits represent 68% confidence intervals for the mean, equivalent to ±1 SEM.
Source: Reprinted from *Anesthesiology*, **66**:601 (1987).

Thus, this study documented that patients who respond to protamine neutralization of heparin with pulmonary hypertension and bronchoconstriction demonstrate a characteristic mediator profile that differs from the profile of nonreactors. Thromboxane generation leading to elevated arterial plasma levels of thromboxane B_2 was observed only in patients who manifested this reaction. Complement activation was present in all patients who received the large dose of protamine, but marked elevations of plasma C5a levels were observed only in the pulmonary vasoconstrictor reactors. Major histamine release did not occur in these reactors.

We measured plasma thromboxane B_2, 6-keto-$PGF_{1\alpha}$, and histamine concentrations 1-10 min after detection of the adverse cardiopulmonary response and also 1 day postoperatively in 10 additional patients who demonstrated HP-associated pulmonary vasoconstriction. In these patients, pulmonary artery pressure increased from 19 $\pm$ 7 (SD) to 35 $\pm$ 11 mmHg and right atrial pressure increased from 6 $\pm$ 2 to 12 $\pm$ 5 mmHg, but mean systemic arterial pressure decreased from 78 $\pm$ 15 to 53 $\pm$ 18 mmHg and left atrial pressure decreased from 10 $\pm$ 4 to 2 $\pm$ 2 mmHg. All these patients demonstrated abnormally high arterial plasma thromboxane B_2 levels at the time of sampling (peak levels of 11.6 $\pm$ 10.5 ng/ml compared to 0.63 $\pm$ 0.28 ng/ml 1 day postoperatively). Plasma 6-keto-$PGF_{1\alpha}$ levels increased slightly, although significantly, to 0.95 $\pm$ 0.88 ng/ml, compared to postoperative values of 0.14 $\pm$ .12 ng/ml. Plasma histamine levels were not elevated in any patient. These additional data lend strong support to the role of thromboxane A_2 as the principal mediator of the HP-induced pulmonary vasoconstrictor response in humans.

B. True Allergic Reactions to Protamine

We recently described specific antiprotamine IgE and IgG antibodies (Weiss et al., 1989). The former were found exclusively in patients with diabetes mellitus receiving protamine-insulin preparations who had experienced an adverse protamine reaction. In a case control study, this antibody was associated with a greatly increased risk for a protamine reaction (relative risk, 95; $P = 10^{-5}$). The reactions associated with IgE appeared clinically to be true type 1 anaphylaxis, although mediator profiles have not yet been defined.

Antiprotamine IgG antibodies were found both in patients who had or had not experienced an adverse protamine reaction and in patients with or without protamine-insulin-dependent diabetes mellitus. Thus, they appear far less specific for a reaction, although they were also associated with a somewhat increased relative risk.

These data reconcile some apparent contradictions in the literature. They support the hypothesis that allergic and nonallergic protamine reactions exist. In our experience, nonallergic, thromboxane-mediated reactions far outnumber true allergic reactions. In the past 3 years, in which approximately 3500 cardiac surgical patients have received protamine, we recognized and validated only one true IgE-mediated protamine reaction. This explains why diabetes mellitus did not appear to be a risk factor for protamine reactions in the survey of 925 consecutive patients reported here. At present we are defining the incidence of antiprotamine IgE and IgG antibodies in protamine-insulin-dependent diabetic cardiac surgical patients.

VI. Summary

Acute pulmonary vasoconstriction is associated with protamine neutralization of heparin anticoagulation in a variety of species. In some species, such as sheep and pigs, the pulmonary hypertensive response is consistent and predictable. In humans, the response appears sporadically, with an incidence of approximately 1.5%. The precise factors that influence the incidence of response have not been identified. In all species studied, thromboxane appears to cause the pulmonary vasoconstriction. The role of complement activation in this response is uncertain but is probably not essential. Effective prophylactic pharmacologic strategies in experimental animals include cyclooxygenase inhibition and thromboxane receptor blockade. A short-lived thromboxane synthesis inhibitor or thromboxane receptor blocker is vital to allow a clinical trial of drug prophylaxis.

References

Albertine, K. H., Decker, S. A., Schultz, E. L., and Staub, N. C. (1987). Clearance of monastral blue by intravascular macrophages in pulmonary microvessels of sheep, goat, and pig (abstract). *Anat. Rec.*, **218**:6A.

Al-Mondhiry, H., Pierce, W. S., and Basarab, R. M. (1985). Protamine-induced thrombocytopenia and leukopenia. *Thromb. Haemost.*, **53**: 60-64.

Aoyama, T., Ino, Y., Ozeki, M., Oda, M., Sato, T., Koshiyama, Y., Suzuki, S., and Fujita, M. (1984). Pharmacological studies of FUT-175, nafamstat mesilate. I. Inhibition of protease activity in vitro and in vivo experiments. *Jpn. J. Pharmacol.*, **35**:203-227.

Bernard, G. R., Lucht, W. D., Niedermeyer, M. E., Snapper, J. R., Ogletree, M. L., and Brigham, K. L. (1984). Effect of *N*-acetylcysteine on the pulmonary response to endotoxin in the awake sheep and upon in vitro granulocyte function. *J. Clin. Invest.*, **73**:1772-1784.

Bertram, T. A., Overby, L. H., Danilowicz, R., Eling, T. E., and Brody, A. R. (1988). Pulmonary intravascular macrophages metabolize arachidonic acid in vitro. *Am. Rev. Respir. Dis.*, **138**:936-944.

Bertram, T. A., Thigpen, J., Eling, T. E., and Brody, A. R. (1989). Bacterial phagocytosis and consequent arachidonic acid metabolism by pulmonary intravascular and alveolar macrophages in vitro. *Am. Rev. Respir. Dis.*, **139**:A159.

Best, N., Teisner, B., Grudzinskas, J. G., and Fisher, M. M. (1983). Classical pathway activation during an adverse response to protamine sulfate. *Br. J. Anaesthesiol.*, **55**:1149-1153.

Best, N., Sinosich, M. J., Teisner, B., Grudzinskas, J. G., and Fisher, M. M. (1984). Complement activation during cardiopulmonary bypass by heparin-protamine interaction. *Br. J. Anaesthesiol.*, **56**:339-343.

Brigham, K. L., and Meyrick, B. (1986). State of art: Endotoxin and lung injury. *Am. Rev. Respir. Dis.*, **133**:913-927.

Casthely, P. A., Goodman, K., Fyman, P. N., Abrams, L. M., and Aaron, D. (1986). Hemodynamic changes after the administration of protamine. *Anesth. Analg.*, **65**:78-80.

Cavarocchi, N. C., Schaff, H. V., Orszulak, T. A., Homburger, H. A., Schnell, W. A., Jr., and Pluth, J. R. (1985). Evidence for complement activation by protamine-heparin interaction after cardiopulmonary bypass. *Surgery*, **98**:525-530.

Chang, S.-W., Westcott, J. Y., Henson, J. E., and Voelkel, N. F. (1987). Pulmonary vascular injury by polycations in perfused rat lungs. *J. Appl. Physiol.*, **62**:1932-1943.

Chenoweth, D. E. (1987). Complement activation in extracorporeal circuits. *Ann. N.Y. Acad. Sci.*, **516**:306-313.

Chenoweth, D. E., and Hugli, T. E. (1978). Demonstration of specific C5a receptor on intact human polymorphonuclear leukocytes. *Proc. Natl. Acad. Sci. USA*, **75**:2943.

Cheung, A. K., LeWinter, M., Chenoweth, D. E., Lew, W. Y. W., and Henderson, L. W. (1986). Cardiopulmonary effects of cuprophane-activated plasma in the swine: Role of complement products. *Kidney Int.*, **29**:799-806.

Claus, D. R., Siegel, J., Petras, K., Skor, D., Osmand, A. P., and Gewurz, H. (1977). Complement activation by interaction of polyanions and polycations. III. Complement activation by interaction of multiple polyanions and polycations in the presence of C-reactive protein. *J. Immunol.*, **118**:83-87.

Conzen, P. F., Habazettl, H., Gutmann, R., Hobbhahn, J., Goetz, A. E., Peter, K., and Brendel, W. (1989). Thromboxane mediation of pulmonary hemodynamic responses after neutralization of heparin by protamine in pigs. *Anesth. Analg.*, **68**:25-31.

Crocker, S. H., Edy, D. O., and Lowery, B. D. (1981a). Bacteremia: Host-specific lung clearance and pulmonary failure. *J. Trauma*, **21**:215-220.

Crocker, S. H., Lowery, B. D., Eddy, D. O., Wismar, B. L., Bueschine, W. J., and Obenant, R. N. (1981b). Pulmonary clearance of blood borne bacteria. *Surg. Gynecol. Obstet.,* **153**:845-851.

Degges, R. D., Foster, M. E., Dang, A. Q., and Read, R. C. (1987). Pulmonary hypertensive effect of heparin and protamine interaction: Evidence for thromboxane B_2 release from the lung. *Am. J. Surg.,* **154**:696-699.

Dehring, D. J., and Wismar, B. L. (1989). Intravascular macrophages in pulmonary capillaries of humans. *Am. Rev. Respir. Dis.,* **139**:1027-1029.

Fadali, M. A., Papacostas, C. A., Duke, J. T., Ledbetter, M., and Osbakken, M. (1976). Cardiovascular depressant effect of protamine sulphate: Experimental study of clinical implications. *Thorax,* **31**:320-323.

Fairman, R. P., Sessler, C. N., Bierman, M., and Glauser, F. L. (1987). Protamine sulfate causes pulmonary hypertension and edema in isolated rat lungs. *J. Appl. Phys.,* **62**:1363-1367.

Fehr, J., and Rohr, H. (1983). In vivo complement activation by polyanion-polycation complexes: Evidence that C_{5a} is generated intravascularly during heparin-protamine interaction. *Clin. Immunol. Immunopathol.,* **29**:7-14.

Fernandez, H. N., Henson, P. M., Otani, A., and Hugli, T. E. (1978). Chemotactic response to human C3a and C5a anaphylatoxins. I. Evaluation of C3a and C5a leukotaxis in vitro and under simulated in vivo conditions. *J. Immunol.,* **120**:109-115.

Fiedel, B. A., Rent, R., Myhrman, R., and Gewurz, H. (1976). Complement activation by interaction of polyanions and polycations. II. Precipitation and role of IgG, Clq and C1-INH during heparin-protamine-induced consumption of complement. *Immunology,* **30**:161-169.

Fiser, W. P., Fewell, J. E., Hill, D. E., Barnes, R. W., and Read, R. C. (1985). Cardiovascular effects of protamine sulfate are dependent on the presence and type of circulating heparin. *J. Thorac. Cardiovasc. Surg.,* **89**:63-70.

Flick, M. R., Horn, J. K., Hoeffel, J. M., and Goldstein, I. M. (1986). Reduction of total hemolytic complement activity with *Naja haje* cobra venom factor does not prevent endotoxin-induced lung injury in sheep. *Am. Rev. Respir. Dis.,* **133**:62-67.

Francica, P., Bertram, T. A., Knapp, M., and Crapo, J.D. (1988). Pulmonary intravascular macrophages in normal and oxygen injured baboon lung (abstract). *Clin. Res.,* **36**:591A.

Freeman, B. A., and Crapo, J. D. (1982). Biology of disease: Free radicals and tissue injury. *Lab. Invest.,* **47**:412-426.

Gee, M. H., Perkowski, S. Z., Tahamont, M. V., Flynn, J. T., and Wasserman, M. A. (1986). Thromboxane as a mediator of pulmonary dysfunction during intravascular complement activation in sheep. *Am. Rev. Respir. Dis.,* **133**:269-273.

Goldman, B. S., Joison, J., and Austen, W. G. (1969). Cardiovascular effects of protamine sulfate. *Ann. Thorac. Surg.,* **7**:459-471.

Goldstein, I. M., Malmsten, C. L., Kindahl, H., Kaplan, K. B., Rodmark, O., Samuelsson, B., and Weissman, G. (1978). Thromboxane generation by human peripheral blood polymorphonuclear leukocytes. *J. Exp. Med.,* **148**:787-792.

Goto, H., Kushihashi, T., Benson, K. T., Hitashi, K., Fox, D. K., and Arakawa, K. (1985). Heparin, protamine, and ionized calcium in vitro and in vivo. *Anesth. Anal.,* **64**:1081-1084.

Gourin, A., Streisand, R.L., Greineder, J. K., and Stuckey, J. H. (1971). Protamine sulfate administration and the cardiovascular system. *J. Thorac. Cardiovasc. Surg.,* **62**:193-204.

Hatterslea, P. G. (1966). Activated coagulation time in whole blood. *JAMA,* **196**:436.

Henson, P. M., and Lynch, J. M. (1983). Cellular origins of PAF. In *Platelet-Activating Factor and Structurally Related Ether-Lipids.* From the Proceedings of the 1st International Symposium on Platelet-activating Factor (PAF-acether, AGPEPC) and Structurally Related Ether-Lipids. Edited by J. Benveniste and B. Arnoux. Amsterdam, Elsevier Science Publishers, pp. 75-82.

Hobbhahn, J., Conzen, P. F., Zenker, B., Goetz, A. E., Peter, K., and Brendel, W. (1988). Beneficial effect of cyclooxygenase inhibition on adverse hemodynamic responses after protamine. *Anesth. Analg.,* **67**: 253-260.

Horrow, J. C. (1985). Protamine: A review of its toxicity. *Anesth. Analg.,* **64**:348-361.

Horrow, J. C. (1988a). Protamine allergy. *J. Cardiothorac. Anesth.,* **2**:225-242.

Horrow, J. C. (1988b). Protamine: A necessary evil? In *Effective Hemostasis in Cardiac Surgery.* Edited by N. Ellison and D. Jobes. Philadelphia, Grune & Stratton, pp. 15-39.

Jacques, L. B. (1949). A study of the toxicity of the protamine, salmine. *Br. J. Pharmacol.,* **4**:135-144.

Jacques, L. B. (1980). Heparins—anionic polyelectrolytic drugs. *Pharmacol. Rev.,* **31**:99-166.

Jastrzebski, J., Hilgard, P., and Sykes, M. K. (1975). Pulmonary vasoconstriction produced by protamine and protamine-heparin complex in the isolated cat lung perfused with blood or dextran. *Cardiovasc. Res.,* **9**: 691-696.

Kirklin, J. K., Chenoweth, D. E., Naftel, D. C., Blackstone, E. W., Kirklin, J. W., Bitran, D. D., Curd, J. G., Reeves, T. G., and Samuelson,

P. N. (1986). Effects of protamine administration after cardiopulmonary bypass on complement, blood elements, and the hemodynamic state. *Ann. Thorac. Surg.,* **41**:193-199.

Klausner, J. M., Kobzik, L., Valeri, C. R., Shepro, D., and Hechtman, H. B. (1988). Selective lung leukosequestration after complement activation. *J. Appl. Physiol.,* **65**:80-88.

Kreil, E., Robinson, D., Lowenstein, E., and Zapol, W. (1987). Antioxidant enzymes and the heparin-protamine neutralization reaction (abstract 2044). *Fed. Proc.,* **46**:666.

Kreil, E., Montalescot, G., Greene, E. M., Fitzgibbon, C., Robinson, D., Chenoweth, D. E., and Zapol, W. M. (1989). Nafamstat mesilate attenuates pulmonary hypertension during protamine reversal of heparin anticoagulation. *J. Appl. Physiol.,* **67**:1463-1471.

Lindblad, B., Borgstrom, A., Wakefield, T. W., Whitehouse, W. M., Jr., and Stanley, J. C. (1987). Protamine reversal of anticoagulation achieved with a low molecular weight heparin. The effects on eicosanoids, clotting, and complement factors. *Thromb. Res.,* **48**:31-40.

Lindblad, B., Wakefield, T. W., Whitehouse, W. M., Jr., and Stanley, J. C. (1988). The effect of protamine sulfate on platelet function. *Scand. J. Thorac. Cardiovasc. Surg.,* **22**:55-59.

Lowenstein, E. (1989). Lessons from studying an infrequent event: Adverse hemodynamic response associated with protamine reversal of heparin anticoagulation. *J. Cardiothorac. Anesth.,* **3**:99-107.

Lowenstein, E., Johnston, W. E., Lappas, D. G., D'Ambra, M. N., Schneider, R. C., Daggett, W. M., Akins, C. W., and Philbin, D. M. (1983). Catastrophic pulmonary vasoconstriction associated with protamine reversal of heparin. *Anesthesiology,* **59**:470-473.

Matthews, K. P. (1986). Deficiencies in regulator proteins. 4. Anaphylatoxin inactivator. *Prog. Allergy,* **39**:344-351.

McDonald, J. W. D., Ali, M., Morgan, E., Townsend, E. R., and Cooper, J. D. (1983). Thromboxane synthesis by sources other than platelets in association with complement-induced pulmonary leukostasis and pulmonary hypertension in sheep. *Circ. Res.,* **52**:1-6.

McManus, L. M., Pinckard, R. N., Fitzpatrick, F. A., O'Rourke, R. A., Crawford, M. H., and Hanahan, D. J. (1981). Acetyl glyceryl ether phosphorylcholine: Intravascular alterations following intravenous infusion into the baboon. *Lab. Invest.,* **45**:303-307.

Meyrick, B., and Brigham, K. L. (1984). Effect of a single infusion of zymosan activated plasma on the pulmonary microcirculation of sheep: Structure function relationships. *Am. J. Pathol.,* **114**:32-45.

Milligan, S. A., Hoeffel, J. M., Goldstein, I. M., and Flick, M. R. (1988). Effect of catalase on endotoxin-induced acute lung injury in anesthetized sheep. *Am. Rev. Respir. Dis.,* **137**:420-428.

Miyamoto, K., Schultz, E., Heath, T., Mitchell, M. D., Albertine, K. H., and Staub, N. C. (1988). Pulmonary intravascular macrophages and hemodynamic effects of liposomes in sheep. *J. Appl. Physiol.,* **64**:1143-1152.

Montalescot, G., Kreil, E., Lynch, K., Greene, E. M., Torres, A., Carvalho, A., Fitzgibbon, C., Robinson, D. R., Lowenstein, E., and Zapol, W. M. (1989). Effect of platelet depletion on lung vasoconstriction in heparin-protamine reactions. *J. Appl. Physiol.,* **66**:2344-2350.

Morel, D. R., Zapol, W. M., Thomas, S. J., Kitain, E. M., Robinson, D. R., Moss, J., Chenoweth, D. E., and Lowenstein, E. (1987). C5a and thromboxane generation associated with pulmonary vaso- and bronchoconstriction during protamine reversal of heparin. *Anesthesiology,* **66**:597-604.

Morel, D. R., Lowenstein, E., Nguyenduy, T., Robinson, D. R., Repine, J. E., Chenoweth, D. E., and Zapol, W. M. (1988). Acute pulmonary vasoconstriction and thromboxane release during protamine reversal of heparin anticoagulation in awake sheep: Evidence for the role of reactive oxygen metabolites following nonimmunological complement activation. *Circ. Res.,* **62**:905-915.

O'Flaherty, J. T., and Wykle, R. L. (1987). Metabolic origin and fate of platelet-activating factor. *Agents Actions* (*Suppl.*), Vo. **21**:59-66.

O'Reilly, R. A. (1985). Anticoagulants, antithrombotics, and thrombolytic drugs. In *Pharmacological Basis of Therapeutics.* Edited by A. S. Gilman, L. S. Goodman, T. W. Rall, and F. Murad. New York, Macmillan, pp. 1338-1344.

Pavek, K., Piper, P. J., and Smedegard, G. (1979). Anaphylatoxin-induced shock and two patterns of anaphylactic shock: Hemodynamics and mediators. *Acta Physiol. Scand.,* **105**:393-403.

Perkowski, S. Z., Havill, A. M., Flynn, J. T., and Gee, M. H. (1983). Role of intrapulmonary release of eicosanoids and superoxide anions as mediators of pulmonary dysfunction and endothelial injury in sheep with intermittent complement activation. *Circ. Res.,* **53**:574-584.

Radegran, K., and McAshan, C. (1972). Circulating and ventilatory effects of induced platelet aggregation and their inhibition by salicylic acid. *Acta Anesthesiol. Scand.,* **16**:76-84.

Radegran, K., Taylor, G. A., and Olsson, P. (1971a). Mode of action of protamine in regard to its circulatory and respiratory side effects. *Eur. Surg. Res.,* **3**:139-148.

Radegran, K., Drugge, U., and Olsson, P. (1974). Pulmonary venoconstriction by induced platelet aggregation. *Acta Anesthesiol. Scand.,* **18**:243-247.

Raleigh, J. A., and Kremers, W. (1981). DMSO does not protect against hydroxyl radical induced peroxidation in model membranes. *Int. J. Radiat. Biol.,* **39**:441-444.

Rent, R., Ertel, N., Eisenstein, R., and Gewurz, H. (1975). Complement activation by interaction of polyanions and polycations. I. Heparin-protamine induced consumption of complement. *J. Immunol.,* **114**: 120-124.

Rent, R., Myhrman, R., Fiedel, B. A., and Gewurz, H. (1976). Potentiation of Cl-esterase inhibitor activity by heparin. *Clin. Exp. Immunol.,* **23**: 264-271.

Rogers, K., Milne, B., and Salerno, T. A. (1983). The hemodynamic effects of intra-aortic versus intravenous administration of protamine for reversal of heparin in pigs. *J. Thorac. Cardiovasc. Surg.,* **85**:851-855.

Said, S. I., and Foda, H. D. (1989). State of the art: Pharmacologic modulation of lung injury. *Am. Rev. Respir. Dis.,* **139**:1553-1564.

Schumacher, W. A., Heran, C. L., and Ogletree, M. L. (1988). Effect of thromboxane receptor antagonism on pulmonary hypertension caused by protamine-heparin interaction in pigs. *Circulation,* **78**(4):A825.

Skidgel, R. A., Tan, F., Jackman, H., Zsigmond, E. K., and Erdös, E. G. (1988). Protamine inhibits plasma carboxypeptidase N (CPN), the inactivator of anaphylatoxins and kinins (abstract). *FASEB J.,* **2**:A1382.

Smallbone, B. W., Taylor, N. E., and McDonald, J. W. D. (1987). Effects of L-652-731, a platelet-activating factor (PAF) receptor antagonist, on PAF- and complement-induced pulmonary hypertension in sheep. *J. Pharmacol. Exp. Ther.,* **242**:1035-1040.

Staub, N. (1988). Pulmonary intravascular macrophages. *Chest,* **93**(3):84S.

Staub, N. C., Schultz, E., Milligan, S., Wang, T., Enzan, K., Clarkson, S., and Goldstein, I. (1987). Isolation, primary culture, and properties of pulmonary intravascular macrophages from goats and sheep (abstract). *Fed. Proc.,* **46**:329.

Stefaniszyn, H. J., Novick, R. J., and Salerno, T. A. (1984). Toward a better understanding of the hemodynamic effects of protamine and heparin interaction. *J. Thorac. Cardiovasc. Surg.,* **87**:678-686.

Tahamont, M. V., Gee, M. H., and Flynn, J. T. (1984). Aggregation and thromboxane synthesis and release in isolated sheep neutrophils and lymphocytes in response to complement stimulation. *Prostaglandins Leukotrienes Med.,* **16**:181-190.

Tan, F., Jackman, H., Skidgel,R., Zsigmond, E. K., and Erdös, E. G. (1989). Protamine inhibits plasma caboxipeptidase N, the inactivator of anaphylatoxins and kinins. *Anesthesiology,* **70**:267-275.

Tate, R. M., Morris, H. G., Schroeder, W. R., and Repine, J. E. (1984). Oxygen metabolites stimulate thromboxane production and vasoconstriction in isolated saline-perfused rabbit lungs. *J. Clin. Invest.,* **74**: 608-613.

Taylor, R. L., Little, W. C., Freeman, G. L., Avery, D. M., Norris, S. E., Trinkle, J. K., and Grover, F. L. (1986). Comparison of the cardiovascular effects of intravenous and intraaortic protamine in the conscious and anesthetized dog. *Ann. Thorac. Surg.,* **42**:22-26.

Wakefield, T. W., Whitehouse, W. M., and Stanley, J. C. (1984). Depressed cardiovascular function and altered platelet kinetics following protamine sulfate reversal of heparin activity. *J. Vasc. Surg.,* **1**:346-355.

Wakefield, T. W., Lindblad, B., Whitehouse, W. M., Hantler, C. B., and Stanley, J. C. (1986). Attenuation of hemodynamic and hematologic effects of heparin-protamine sulfate interaction after aortic reconstruction in a canine model. *Surgery,* **100**:45-51.

Wakefield, T. W., Bouffard, J. A., Spaulding, S., Petry, N. A., Gross, M. D., Lindblad, B., and Stanley, J. C. (1987). Sequestration of platelets in the pulmonary circulation as a consequence of protamine reversal of the anticoagulant effects of heparin. *J. Vasc. Surg.,* **5**:187-193.

Warner, A. E., Barry, B. E., and Brain, J. D. (1987). Pulmonary intravascular macrophages in sheep: Morphology and function of a novel constituent of the mononuclear phagocyte system. *Lab. Invest.,* **55**:276-288.

Warner, A. E., Molina, R. M., and Brain, J. D. (1987). Uptake of blood-borne bacteria by pulmonary intravascular macrophages and consequent inflammatory responses in sheep. *Am. Rev. Respir. Dis.,* **136**:683-690.

Warner, A. E., DeCamp, M. M., Jr., Molina, R. M., and Brain, J. D. (1988). Pulmonary removal of circulating endotoxin results in acute lung injury in sheep. *Lab. Invest.,* **59**:219-230.

Warner, A. E., DeCamp, M. M., Bellows, C. F., and Brain, J. D. (1989a). Endotoxemia enhances lung uptake of circulating particles in species lacking pulmonary intravascular macrophages. *Am. Rev. Respir. Dis.,* **139**:A158.

Warner, A. E., DeCamp, M. M., Molina, R. M., and Brain, J. D. (1989b). Hepatic uptake of circulating gram negative bacteria in sheep partially protects the lungs from acute injury. *Am. Rev. Respir. Dis.,* **139**:A252.

Webster, R. O., Hong, S. R., Johnston, R. B., and Henson, P. M. (1980). Biological effects of the human complement fragments C5a and $C5a_{des\ Arg}$ on neutrophil function. *Immunopharmacology,* **2**:201-219.

Weiss, M. E., Nyhan, D., Zhikang, P., Harrow, J. C., Lowenstein, E., Hirshman, C., and Adkinson, N. F., Jr. (1989). Association of protamine IgE and IgG antibodies with life-threatening reactions to intravenous protamine. *N. Engl. J. Med.,* **320**:886-892.

Wheeldon, E. B., and Hansen-Flaschen, J. H. (1986). Intravascular macrophages in the sheep lung. *J. Leukocyte Biol.,* **40**:657-661.

Winkler, G. C., and Cheville, N. F. (1985). Monocytic origin and postnatal mitosis of intravascular macrophages in the porcine lung. *J. Leukocyte Biol.,* **38**:471-480.

Wonders, T., Huttemeier, P., Berry, D., Schuette, A., Kong, D., Watkins, W. D., and Zapol, W. M. (1983). Complement depletion prevents pulmonary hypertension and leukopenia in sheep extracorporeal membrane oxygenation. *Trans. Am. Soc. Artif. Intern. Organs,* **29**:210-213.

Zapol, W. M., and Snider, M. T. (1977). Pulmonary hypertension in severe acute respiratory failure. *N. Engl. J. Med.,* **296**:476-480.

22

Lung Transplantation

LARRY R. KAISER and JOEL D. COOPER

Washington University School of Medicine
St. Louis, Missouri

I. Introduction

Developments in pulmonary transplantation continue to command the most attention within the specialty of thoracic surgery despite significant advances in other areas. Essentially all of the current activity in pulmonary transplantation has occurred within the past 6 years, though we are currently riding the crest of a wave of exciting and important developments rapidly pushing our knowledge forward, with changes taking place almost on a weekly basis. Initially, however, the pace of activity in this area moved somewhat more slowly. Having performed the first successful single lung transplant in 1983, it was not until 1 year later that the Toronto Lung Transplant Group carried out a second transplant. To this group goes the credit for establishing lung transplantation as a viable therapeutic alternative.

The development of lung transplantation is as a superb example of problem-solving or goal-oriented research, a type of investigation for which surgeons are particularly well suited (Cooper, 1989). It requires observation of a clinical problem, formulation of appropriate questions to attempt to answer in the laboratory, the development of a model with which to answer these questions, and finally, application of the new knowledge to the clinical situation. Cooper and colleagues recognized that poor bronchial anastomotic healing caused, or at least contributed significantly to, the death of most patients undergoing lung transplantation and set out to solve the problem in an animal model. Through a series of elegant experiments they learned that steroids greatly inhibited bronchial wound healing, cyclosporin did not, and a pedicled omental flap wrapped around the bronchial anastomosis restored blood supply (Lima et al., 1981; Goldberg et al., 1983; Dubois et al., 1984; Morgan et al., 1982). Using this knowledge, they performed a series of lung transplantations in dogs and demonstrated excellent bronchial healing. After perfecting the technique in the autopsy room, they decided to embark on a cautious clinical program. Their success, of course, is by now well known. Since this pioneering work, numerous other centers around the world have begun lung transplant programs. Compared to transplantation of other organs, lung transplantation remains in its infancy though its development is proceeding rapidly.

II. History of Lung Transplantation

Despite the fact that the Western world remained unaware of his work, Demikhov, a Russian physiologist, successfully performed homografts on individual canine pulmonary lobes as early as 1947 (Demikhov, 1962). Bellinazzo and Pulin performed autografts and allografts of canine pulmonary lobes in 1950 (Staudacher et al., 1950). The allografts underwent rejection in 6-8 days while the autografts maintained function for longer periods. Metras first published the technique of canine pulmonary allotransplantation in 1950 and showed remarkable foresight, describing a technique of harvesting and anastomosing the left bronchial artery to provide systemic blood supply to the airway. In addition, he described a left atrial anastomosis rather than separate pulmonary venous anastomoses. Many early investigators documented deterioration of allograft function which caused death in recipient animals at 7 days, an observation attributed to rejection. Hardy's initial attempts at alleviating rejection employed methotrexate and subsequently azathioprine or azathioprine plus hydrocortisone, which resulted in a marked prolongation in graft survival (Hardy et al., 1963a,b).

Having accumulated considerable technical experience in dogs, J. D. Hardy, at the University of Mississippi, was ideally suited to perform the first human lung transplantation in 1963 (Hardy et al., 1963c). His patient, a 58-year-old convict serving a life sentence, had a squamous carcinoma almost completely obstructing the left mainstem bronchus. The patient was not a candidate for pneumonectomy because of underlying emphysema; in addition, he had mild preexisting renal insufficiency and nephrotic syndrome. On June 11, 1963, Hardy performed a left lung transplant, having harvested the donor lung postmortem from a patient who sustained cardiac arrest following a massive mycocardial infarction. The recipient operation presented numerous difficulties beginning with the finding of multiple pulmonary abscesses, secondary to the obstructing carcinoma. Further complicating the effort was the finding of metastatic disease in subaortic lymph nodes. A pulmonary arteriogram on the first postoperative day confirmed perfusion of the transplanted lung, and the patient survived 18 days; death was attributed to renal failure and malnutrition. This effort established the technical feasibility of lung transplantation and demonstrated that a transplanted lung could indeed function in the human. This attempt was soon followed by others (Magovern and Yates, 1964; White et al., 1966). The only recipient during that period to actually leave the hospital was a young man with silicosis who received a lung transplant in an operation performed by Derom (Derom et al., 1971). The patient survived 10 months, spending most of that time in the hospital.

The lack of clinical progress stimulated further laboratory investigation into the technical and physiologic aspects of lung transplantation. Questions concerning pulmonary physiology following lung transplantation, the effects of ischemia, denervation, loss of lymphatics, and loss of bronchial circulation on the transplanted lung needed to be answered. The first successful heart transplantation in 1967 further stimulated general interest in the field of thoracic transplantation (Barnard, 1967). By 1978 another 13 human lung transplant attempts had been reported, and all had been unsuccessful. During this time, however, considerable advancement occurred in the care of patients with acute respiratory failure—specifically, improvements in ventilatory support and hemodynamic monitoring, extracorporeal membrane oxygenator support, and fiberoptic bronchoscopy. Simultaneously significant progress occurred in transplantation of other organs.

An unsuccessful attempt at transplantation at the University of Toronto led to a close review of the experience of others. Of 20 patients surviving more than 7 days following lung transplantation, 16 had major complications related to the bronchial anastomosis (Wildevuur and Benfield, 1970). It was postulated that this failure of bronchial healing was due to either ischemia, rejection, immunosuppressive medication, or a combination of these factors. This led to a major effort to define and obviate the problems of bronchial healing. The ultimate outcome was the elimination of steroids during the early posttransplantation period and the use of an omental pedicle flap to wrap the bronchial anastomosis. The utility of the omentum to revascularize had previously been demonstrated by others (Goldsmith et al.,

1968). In a series of elegant experiments, the capability of the omentum to revascularize a totally ischemic bronchus was demonstrated by the Toronto Group (Morgan et al., 1982). Collateral vessels from the omentum provided blood supply to the bronchus within 4 days. Until these collaterals develop, the donor bronchus is entirely dependent on collaterals from the pulmonary arterial circulation. The omentum also offers a margin of safety to prevent the development of a bronchovascular or bronchopleural fistula in the event that bronchial healing is compromised.

Encouraged by these experimental results, the Toronto Group resumed clinical lung transplantation and focused their efforts on those patients with end-stage pulmonary fibrosis in whom life expectancy was deemed to be only a matter of months. Pulmonary fibrosis seemingly offers an ideal situation for single lung transplantation since the fibrotic lung has decreased compliance and some degree of increased pulmonary vascular resistance. Ventilation and perfusion, therefore, would be expected to go preferentially to the more compliant, transplanted lung which also has a lower pulmonary vascular resistance. On November 7, 1983, a right lung transplant was performed on a 58-year-old man with end-stage pulmonary fibrosis utilizing the omentopexy technique. Prednisone was eliminated from the immunosuppression regimen until 3 weeks following the procedure. Six weeks following transplantation the patient left the hospital and 6 years later remains active, works regularly, and has shown no significant deterioration of lung function.

This initial success with single lung transplantation for pulmonary fibrosis stimulated interest in transplantation for other lung pathology, where single lung transplant would be contraindicated. Despite the success of combined heart-lung transplantation, it became apparent that the majority of patients with end-stage interstitial lung disease had adequate or reversible right heart function. Replacing a recipient's otherwise normal heart not only exposed the recipient to the acute and long-term problems associated with cardiac transplantation, but also prevented use of the donor heart for another recipient. Cadaver dissection confirmed the feasibility of performing en bloc bilateral lung transplantation via a median sternotomy with the use of cardipulmonary bypass. Further experiments in primates confirmed these observations, and subsequently a successful double lung transplant was performed in a 42-year-old woman with end-stage emphysema caused by alpha-1 antitrypsin deficiency. Three years later this recipient also remains in excellent health.

Currently much effort centers around defining the appropriate indication for each type of lung transplantation. Much has been learned in the short time since lung transplantation became a clinical reality and the knowledge continues to expand rapidly.

III. Indications for Lung Transplantation

With few exceptions, the indication for lung transplantation is the presence of irreversible, progressively disabling end-stage pulmonary disease. We have offered transplantation when, in our judgment, life expectancy is limited to 12-18 months. For most lung disease, however, specific clinical factors that allow for survival prediction are lacking and one must make a judgment as to when to intervene.

For purposes of discussing appropriate transplant operations, it is convenient to classify end-stage lung disease according to predominant physiology: restrictive, obstructive, infective, or increased pulmonary vascular resistance. Selection of the appropriate transplant operation depends on underlying individual recipient factors and the pathophysiology of the end-stage disease process. The technical ease of performing a single lung transplant, routinely done without cardiopulmonary bypass, must be weighed against any potential problems caused by retention of the opposite native lung. The double lung operation, as originally described (Patterson et al., 1988b), is much more complicated and we reserved it for those in whom single lung transplant was contraindicated. Currently our "double lung" operation involves bilateral single lung transplants, which has eliminated many of the problems associated with the double lung procedure. Indications for each operation continue to evolve.

A. Restrictive Lung Disease

Until recently, most single lung transplants had been performed for idiopathic pulmonary fibrosis or other restrictive disorders. The diagnosis of pulmonary fibrosis is usually established with a transbronchial lung biopsy or open lung biopsy performed in a patient with a history of progressive respiratory insufficiency, typical chest X-ray findings, and pulmonary function tests which demonstrate a significant reduction of lung volumes with preservation of flows. Diffusing capacity is usually markedly reduced. Idiopathic pulmonary fibrosis is associated with a 40-80% mortality within 5 years of diagnosis (Kern et al., 1988). A profile of the first 11 patients with pulmonary fibrosis whom we transplanted shows a mean vital capacity of 41% predicted, a mean total lung capacity of 45% predicted, and diffusing capacity of 37% predicted (Toronto Lung Transplant Group, 1988). It is particularly difficult in this group of patients to predict length of survival as there is a wide variation in progression of symptoms among patients. This makes it especially difficult to decide when to intervene with transplantation. It is helpful to follow the progress of these patients in a supervised program of pulmonary rehabilitation. A steady reduction in exercise tolerance or an increasing requirement for supplemental oxygen to prevent desaturation is an ominous sign, signifying further reduction in an already limited pulmonary reserve, and is an indication for intervention assuming that the patient is otherwise a transplant candidate.

B. Obstructive Lung Disease

The majority of these patients have emphysema but the occasional chronic bronchitic is seen (Reid, 1988). By conservative estimates there are over 10,000,000 Americans with some form of obstructive lung disease; it is the fifth leading cause of death in the United States (Higgins, 1984). While many of these patients are elderly, especially those whose disease is related to chronic cigarette smoking, a considerable number could potentially benefit from transplantation.

Severe life-threatening emphysema may occur in the fourth and fifth decades of life in individuals with alpha-1 antitrypsin deficiency. There are over 30 different biochemical variants of the alpha-1 protease inhibitor. Emphysematous changes have been associated with the homozygous type Z variant. The prevalence of homozygous type Z is estimated to range from 1 in 1600 to 1 in 5000, but only a minority of these—usually those who are smokers (Hutchison, 1988)—present with end-stage obstructive respiratory disease. Deficiency of alpha-1 protease inhibitors is associated with a lack of protection against neutrophil elastase in the lower respiratory tract (Gadek et al., 1981). Patients with this disorder may be excellent lung transplant candidates because of their relatively young age and lack of other organ system involvement. It is not yet clear what effect the persistence of the alpha-1 antitrypsin-deficient state will have on the transplanted lung and whether recently available replacement therapy will be of value (Wewers et al., 1987).

We have also seen patients who present in the same age range with premature end-stage emphysema of a similar pattern who have normal serum levels of alpha-1 antitrypsin. There are heterozygous phenotypes of alpha-1 protease inhibitor that increase the risk of developing emphysema (Hutchison, 1988), and there may be other, as yet undescribed, proteases that are important in protecting the pulmonary parenchyma from enzymatic destruction. Obstructive disease has been the underlying disorder in the majority of patients who have had double lung transplantation. The first six patients undergoing double lung transplantation for chronic obstructive pulmonary disease (COPD), in our experience, had a mean vital capacity of 47% predicted, a mean FEV-1 of 22% predicted, a mean total lung capacity of 145% predicted, and a mean diffusing capacity of 23% predicted (Cooper et al., 1989a).

As mentioned above, we initially felt that patients with obstructive lung disease were not candidates for a single lung transplant. The prospect of preferential ventilation of the remaining emphysematous, overly compliant lung causing air trapping with resultant compression of the lung graft was felt to be a distinct possibility. As perfusion will preferentially be directed to the transplanted lung, because of its relatively normal pulmonary vascular resistance, a significant ventilation-perfusion imbalance might result. Early investigators reported that single lung transplantation for obstructive lung disease resulted in progressive alteration in the ventilation:perfusion ratio, but the extent to which the V/Q mismatch contributed to the patients' demise remains unclear (Stevens et al., 1970). Wildevuur and Benfield (1970) reported on two patients who developed compression of their transplanted lung by the native emphysematous lung. Veith et al. (1971a) also described two emphysema patients who underwent single lung transplantation, both of whom demonstrated radiographic evidence of a mediastinal shift toward the transplanted side. A summary of this early experience with single lung transplantation for chronic obstructive pulmonary disease is shown in Table 1.

Table 1 Selection Criteria for Lung Transplant Recipients

End-stage lung disease with evidence of progression of disease and life expectancy < 12-18 months	
No other systemic disease	
No significant coronary artery disease	
No evidence of right ventricular (RV) failure (tricuspid regurgitation, ascites, hepatomegaly, poor RV contractility)	
Able to move to transplant center and maintain self plus support person for 3-6 months	
Demonstrated compliance with medical regimens	
No contraindication to immunosuppression	
Psychologically stable; no history of alcohol or drug abuse or psychosis	
Mobility—must be ambulatory with O_2 as required	
Must *not* be on systemic steroids	
Single lung Tx	*Double lung Tx*
Age < 60 years	Age < 50 years
No chronic infectious lung disease (e.g., chronic bronchitis, bronchiectasis, cystic fibrosis)	No prior major thoracic surgery or pleurodesis

All of these transplants were performed in the precyclosporin era, and the contribution of rejection and infection to the poor outcome remains unclear.

Recently we have reassessed the application of single lung transplantation for obstructive lung disease after Mal and co-workers (Mal et al., 1989) in Paris reported several successes in patients with this disorder. Following this lead, we and others have performed single lung transplants in certain patients with emphysema with excellent results. We feel that this approach is justified in selected cases, particularly in those situations where double lung transplantation might be especially risky, such as in the patient over age 50 or in an individual who has previously undergone unilateral thoracotomy or pleurodesis. We do, however, continue to utilize a modified double lung transplant procedure for patients with end-stage emphysema under the age of 50 in the absence of contraindications, until such time as the additional accrual of data indicates which procedure produces the best long-term survival and functional result.

C. Infectious End-Stage Lung Disease

The primary focus of lung transplantation for this group centers around those individuals with cystic fibrosis, a lethal inherited disease with an incidence of 1 in 2000 live births in the United States. More than 98% of patients with cystic fibrosis die from pulmonary-related complications (Scanlin, 1988). In the lung the production of abnormally viscous mucous results in frequent infections beginning at an early age. Despite aggressive attempts at pulmonary toilet, the cumulative effect of these repeated episodes is a progressive bronchiectasis/atelectasis accompanied by destruction of lung tissue and a gradual and irreversible decrease in pulmonary function. Airway destruction exceeds that of parenchyma, so that the pulmonary pathophysiology is largely obstructive in nature.

Patients with cystic fibrosis present particularly challenging problems to the transplant surgeon. In addition to the sequelae of chronic respiratory insufficiency, these individuals often manifest nutritional depletion resulting from exocrine pancreatic dysfunction, as well as from chronic infection. Because of the chronic ongoing pulmonary sepsis and colonization of the airways with antibiotic-resistant, gram-negative organisms, single lung transplantation is felt to be contraindicated. Chronic sinusitis is a constant feature in cystic fibrosis patients and the potential for contamination and infection of the lower respiratory tract after transplantation is ever-present.

Nevertheless the experience of several groups suggests that these problems are not insurmountable. Yacoub and co-workers have performed 22 heart-lung transplants in patients with cystic fibrosis and have achieved a 70% 1-year survival (M. Yacoub, personal communication). The Papworth group has reported six heart-lung transplants for cystic fibrosis with five operative survivors (Scott et al., 1988). Because the heart in most of these patients retains reasonable function, we believe a double lung transplant offers the most rational approach, as it preserves the recipient's own heart and eliminates the acute and chronic problems associated with cardiac transplantation. Furthermore, the donor heart can be used for an appropriate heart transplant candidate. Yacoub and others have favored the so-called "domino procedure" where the cystic fibrotic patient receives a heart-lung transplant and donates his heart to another recipient (Cavarocchi and Badellino, 1989).

D. Pulmonary Hypertension

For patients with pulmonary hypertension and cor pulmonale a combined heart-lung transplant has generally been advocated. However, intervention with an isolated lung transplant even after the development of severe right heart failure, may prove to be a rational approach.

Primary pulmonary hypertension (PPH), a disorder of unknown etiology where the primary defect is increased pulmonary vascular resistance, usually strikes young, otherwise healthy individuals (female to male 1.7:1) (Rich, 1988). The natural history of PPH is quite variable, but the typical mean survival is 2-3 years from the time of diagnosis (Fuster et al., 1984). Occasional patients survive for longer periods, but sudden death is not an infrequent manifestation of this disorder (Ackerman and Edwards, 1987; Suarez et al., 1979). The course of this disease is progressive right heart failure which ultimately results in the patient's demise. The traditional transplant approach for this group of patients has been combined heart-lung transplantation pioneered by the Stanford University Group (Reitz et al., 1982). The major issue in assessing patients with pulmonary hypertension for transplantation is the variability in survival. This was further confirmed by the Stanford Group, who reported on a group of patients with PPH awaiting heart-lung transplantation (Glanville et al., 1987b). In a cohort of 90 patients mean survival from diagnosis was 42.9 months. Fourteen of these underwent heart-lung transplant, a mean of 24 months following diagnosis.

Since this disease is primarily a problem of increased afterload on the right ventricle, the question arises as to the degree of reversibility of the right ventricular dysfunction. Specifically, we have considered the possibility of single lung transplantation for patients with primary pulmonary hypertension based on experimental and clinical evidence that a significant degree of right ventricular failure is reversible (Hsieh et al., submitted; Daily et al., 1987). We feel that single lung transplantation may indeed be the operation of choice for many patients with PPH. Exact parameters of right ventricular function to allow for prediction of reversibility remain to be determined, but our current thinking favors the concept that most of the dysfunction, no matter how severe, reverses once the afterload is reduced by inserting a new lung.

Those patients with secondary pulmonary hypertension resulting from volume overload of the lungs as a result of congenital left-to-right shunts make up a second group who potentially could be considered for lung transplantation. The pulmonary vascular lesions seen in this group are similar to those seen in PPH (Haworth, 1983). Typically these patients are seen late in their course when reversal of flow to right to left through a shunt occurs. As long as right ventricular function is reasonably compensated, it would be feasible, in our opinion, to attempt single lung transplant and repair of the cardiac defect.

In summary, we believe that candidates for lung transplantation should have end-stage disease with significant functional impairment that interferes with activities of daily living. Most of these patients require oxygen 24 hr a day. To further support the need for transplantation there should be documented evidence of disease progression with an anticipated life expectancy of 12-18 months or less without transplant intervention. Potential candidates need to be extremely well motivated to cope with the stresses associated with the pre- and postoperative period, and with the lifelong care they require after transplantation. The complete selection criteria are summarized in Table 1.

IV. Evaluation and Management of Potential Candidates

Records of patients referred for transplantation consideration are reviewed in an initial screening process. Information required for this initial assessment is summarized in Table 2. Once beyond this initial screening, acceptable candidates must come for an inpatient evaluation, the details of which are summarized in Table 3. Right heart function is assessed by right heart catheterization. Serial radionuclide right ventriculograms allow continued assessment of RV ejection fraction in patients selected for transplant. All patients over the age of 40 have left heart catheterization and coronary arteriography.

The 6-min walk test is a useful indicator of functional status and overall performance. Oxygen is administered as required, and oxygen saturation is monitored with a portable pulse oximeter. We measure the total distance traveled and the maximal heart rate achieved while assessing whether oxygen saturation decreases with exercise. The patients are also rated on stair-climbing ability and are asked to score their perceived dyspnea level during this activity.

Systemic steroids must be discontinued prior to consideration for lung transplantation because of the adverse effects of steroids on bronchial healing (Lima et al., 1981). It is often a lengthy and difficult process to wean these patients off steroids, and in some cases withdrawal of steroids may not be possible.

Table 2 Screening Data

Medical
History
Nature and progression of lung disease
Smoking
Prior surgery, especially abdomen, thorax
Health in general
Medications, including steroid history
Exercise tolerance
Physical examination
Laboratory
Arterial blood gases
Complete blood count
Electrolytes—blood urea nitrogen—creatinine—liver function tests
Chest x-ray
Pulmonary function tests
Psychosocial data

Patients who are accepted for transplantation move to the area and enroll in an outpatient pulmonary rehabilitation program. While awaiting transplantation, patients have often doubled their distance on the 6-min walk test. It has been our experience that the conditioning provided by the pulmonary rehabilitation program allows for earlier weaning from the ventilator and facilitates ambulation following transplantation. Every effort is made to transplant only those patients who are well enough to function in an outpatient setting, and we currently do not consider transplantation in patients on mechanical ventilators. Contraindications to lung transplantation also include advanced age, the presence of active systemic disease, renal insufficiency, the presence of significant coronary artery disease, psychologic instability, or perceived inability to comply with the complex postoperative medication regimen.

In the first 11 months of our lung transplant program at Washington University, St. Louis, there were 210 referrals for transplant consideration. A summary of referrals by disease is presented in Table 4. Approximately 10% were accepted for transplantation. The main reasons for refusal are advanced age, steroid dependence, poor cardiac function, or technical considerations.

Table 3 Lung Transplantation In-patient Evaluation

- Pulmonary assessment
  - PFT's
  - V/Q scan
  - CT scan when indicated
- Cardiac assessment
  - MUGA
  - 2-D echo
  - Rt. heart catheterization—if suspect
    - Increase PA pressure
  - Coronary angiography
    - All patients over 40
    - All double lung candidates >30
- Evaluation by social worker
- Consultation with clinical psychologist
  - Psychologic testing
- Assessment by physical therapist
  - Define O_2 requirement at rest and with exercise
  - Define exercise tolerance
    - 6-min walk
    - Treadmill — supervised with O_2 sat.
    - Stair climbing — monitor
- Assessment by pulmonary rehabilitation
  - Effective chest PT
- Assessment by dietitian
  - Ideal body weight
  - Caloric intake

V. The Pulmonary Donor

One of the limiting factors to the widespread application of lung transplantation remains the scarcity of suitable lungs for implantation. It is estimated that organs are retrieved from only 20-30% of potential organ donors because of religious, social, or other reasons (Bart et al., 1981). Probably only 5-10% of available donors have lungs that are currently considered acceptable for transplantation.

Motor vehicle trauma is a common cause of fatal head injury, but blunt chest trauma with resultant pulmonary contusion is a frequent accompani-

Table 4 Summary of Referrals for Lung Transplantation: Distribution of Diagnoses

Diagnosis	Number of referrals
Chronic obstructive lung disease	85
Alpha-1 antitrypsin deficient	24
Cystic fibrosis	29
Bronchiectasis	8
Lymphangioleiomyomatosis	2
Idiopathic pulmonary fibrosis	37
Sarcoidosis	10
Eosinophilic granuloma	2
Other interstitial lung disease	10
Primary pulmonary hypertension	6
Secondary pulmonary hypertension	8

ment. Aspiration is a constant hazard following head injury or any condition affecting the level of consciousness. Potential donors have endotracheal tubes in place and are being supported by mechanical ventilation, a situation often associated with rapid bacterial colonization of the airway which can lead to infection. Following brain death, pulmonary dysfunction (Popp et al., 1982) and pulmonary edema are frequent occurrences, the latter possibly related to the outpouring of catecholamines (Novitzky et al., 1984).

Because of these factors, many potential donor lungs become unsuitable either before or after brain death has been declared. To reduce this loss it is essential that optimum pulmonary care be administered from the time a potential donor is identified. This includes postural drainage, suctioning of the airway, judicious fluid administration, frequent monitoring of chest X-ray and blood gases, sputum smear and culture, and if not contraindicated, 5 cm of positive end-expiratory pressure (PEEP) to replace normal physiologic PEEP which is lost with intubation. All of these "lung protective" measures in no way conflict with the optimal care of the patient who does not become a donor or with the procurement of other organs, should brain death occur.

Our criteria for acceptance of donor lungs are, by design, somewhat rigid (Boychuk and Patterson, 1988) and are summarized in Table 5. When contacted about a potential donor we request information regarding the chest X-ray and evidence of adequate gas exchange, as evaluated by a Pa_{O_2}

Table 5 Lung Donor Criteria

Age < 55 years
Normal chest x-ray
Pa_{O_2} 300 mmHg on F_{IO_2} 1.0, PEEP 5 cm, for 5 min
Bronchoscopically clear with no evidence of purulent secretions or aspiration
No significant chest trauma or pulmonary contusion
No previous thoracic surgery on side of harvest

of ≥300 mmHg on 100% oxygen and 5 cm PEEP. We ask that repeat arterial blood gases be performed every 2 hr. We hesitate to accept lungs when the arterial PO_2 continues to drop over time. Thoracic dimensions that we find useful are depicted in Figure 1 and are taken from a standard chest radiograph.

In general, we attempt to provide a prospective recipient with donor lungs that would be an appropriate size for that individual in the absence of lung disease. For patients with pulmonary fibrosis, a lung larger than the native lung is chosen, since considerable mediastinal shift occurs, the diaphragm lowers, and the thorax expands to accommodate the new, normal lung (Fig. 7). In contrast, patients with COPD have an overexpanded chest cavity that will decrease in size when air trapping is no longer a clinical problem; hence lungs that are smaller, by as much as 5-10 cm in vertical height and 5 cm in horizontal chest diameter, have been utilized (Figs. 8 and 9). If the *predicted* total lung capacity and vital capacity of the donor and recipient are similar, based on height, age, and sex, a satisfactory size match usually results for either single or double lung transplant.

As for other organ transplants, lung transplantation requires ABO compatibility. We currently do not require HLA matching since no evidence exists that the results of such matching significantly influence the long-term outcome, as is apparent for renal transplantation (Sanfillipo et al., 1984).

Our recommendations for management of multiorgan donors are presented in Table 6. Management of the multiorgan donor is a complex problem, and one constantly needs to balance various pharmacologic interventions among the requirements of each donor team. From the standpoint of the lungs, fluid replacement should be kept to a minimum, as the lungs easily become edematous. We advocate the judicious use of vasopressors or low-dose dopamine to maintain blood pressure in the presence of adequate filling pressures. Because pulmonary function in the immediate posttransplant period is precarious, we do not feel that utilization of wet lungs is safe and would

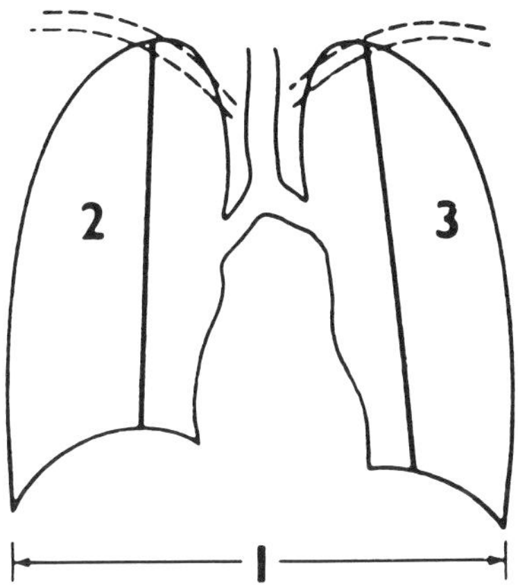

1 HORIZONTAL MEASUREMENT
— Costaphrenic angle to costaphrenic angle

2 RIGHT VERTICAL
— Peak of diaphragm to highest apical point on x-ray

3 LEFT VERTICAL

** Measure in centimeters please

Figure 1 Chest measurements necessary for assessment of a pulmonary donor (Boychuk and Patterson, 1988).

Table 6 Guidelines for Management of Multiple Organ Donors

Maintain mean arterial BP > 70
CVP not to exceed − 10 cm H_2O and/or PCWP not to exceed − 12 mmHg
Vasopressor support is preferable to massive infusion of fluid to maintain blood pressure
Dopamine 2.5-10 μg/kg/min
Phenylephrine, 0.06-0.18 mg/min
Treat diabetes insipidus with vasopressin (5-10 units every 8 hr IV) or DDAVP (0.3 μg/kg IV over 30 min)
Fluid replacement—previous hour's urine output plus 100 ml
Maintain output 1-2 ml/kg/hr
Replace electrolyte losses
Maintain normothermia (35-37 °C)
Pa_{O_2} > 100 on lowest FI_{O_2} possible
Maintain 5 cm PEEP
Strict pulmonary toilet
ABG's every 2 hr
Elevate head of bed if possible

prefer to abandon the proposed transplant if the alveolar-arterial oxygen gradient deteriorates during preparations for retrieval. Diabetes insipidus can be successfully controlled, in most cases, by the administration of vasopressin or DDAVP. Recent reports of improved donor stability utilizing pharmacologic doses of thyroid hormone are intriguing, but to date we have had only limited experience with such therapy (Novitzky et al., 1987).

Once the retrieval team reviews the chest radiograph and finds it acceptable, flexible fiberoptic bronchoscopy is performed. The presence of purulent secretions or evidence of aspiration contraindicates the use of the lungs. Material is obtained for culture and gram stain at the time of this initial bronchoscopy. Results of the gram stain are used as a guide to antibiotic therapy in the recipient. Additional cultures of the donor airway are obtained at the time of implantation. The final assessment of the donor lungs is direct inspection after opening both pleural spaces. The presence of a major pulmonary contusion or significant intrapleural adhesions would preclude lung donation. Only after this inspection does anesthetic induction of the recipient proceed. Though lung procurement in no way precludes other organ harvest, some delays are inevitable in any multiple organ retrieval. Close coordination with the recipient team is mandatory to minimize both the ischemic time of the donor lungs and the anesthetic time of the recipient.

With current preservation techniques we strive to keep total donor ischemic time under 6 hr. This constraint limits flying time between donor and recipient hospitals to 2 hr.

VI. Retrieval of the Donor Lung

We have developed and described a method of lung extraction which allows the heart to be utilized for a separate recipient (Todd et al., 1988). Cardiectomy is completed prior to removal of the lung bloc, which allows the heart retrieval team to leave promptly.

The key features of the donor operation include a precisely placed left atrial incision designed to leave an adequate cuff for both the heart and lung bloc, and appropriate division of the pulmonary artery. To facilitate the left atrial division, the interatrial groove is completely dissected in the full, beating heart (Fig. 10). This increases the margin between the right pulmonary veins and the atrial septum and facilitates the left atrial incision. The left atrial division is begun at the midpoint between the left pulmonary veins and the coronary sinus with the heart retracted up and out of the pericardium and with the apex directed toward the right shoulder (Fig. 11). The orifices of the pulmonary veins can then be visualized from the inside, and care is taken to preserve a cuff of left atrium on the heart side as well as the lung side.

Recognizing that the pulmonary artery proceeds in a posterolateral direction to the left allows for accurate placement of a transverse incision. The site of division is approximately halfway between the pulmonary valve and bifurcation of the pulmonary artery. The initial incision is made in the anterior wall, after which the pulmonary valve and bifurcation may be visualized and used to guide the remainder of the incision. The left atrial cuff and pulmonary artery stump that remain following transplant cardiectomy are shown in Figure 2.

We flush the lungs via the pulmonary artery with cold electrolyte solution to produce rapid cooling and cytoprotection. The site of cannula placement in the pulmonary artery coincides with the site of the subsequent division of the artery. The perfusate runs in under low pressure with the bag elevated no more than 30 cm above the level of the patient. Prior to flushing with electrolyte solution, PGE-1 (500 μg) is given, over 60 sec, by injection into the pulmonary artery. During the flush, the tip of the left atrial appendage is excised to allow for venting of the left heart, while the right heart is vented via the cut in the inferior vena cava. We clamp the inferior vena cava above the diaphragm. During instillation of the pulmonary artery flush, both pleural spaces are flooded with cold Eurocollins solution. To allow more uniform distribution of the perfusate, the lungs are ventilated during the pulmonary artery flush.

The trachea is dissected and divided as far above to the carina as possible. Division of the innominate artery and vein facilitates this dissection. We divide the trachea between staple lines to prevent flooding when the lungs are immersed for transport back to the recipient center. No attempt is made to dissect around the carina or at the level of either main bronchus. Both lungs are removed as a bloc which contains a left atrial cuff and the pulmonary artery bifurcation. The specimen is immersed in cold Eurocollins solution and packed for transport. Taken in this fashion the bloc may then be prepared for two separate single lung transplants or kep intact for a double lung transplantation. Currently, we use both lungs either for simultaneous single lung transplants in two recipients or for bilateral single lung transplants in one recipient. If we do not use both lungs, we attempt to place one of the lungs with another transplant center. Therefore, our donor retrieval operation does not vary and we routinely take both lungs as a single bloc to try to achieve maximal utilization of all donor organs.

The technique described adds very little time to the extraction process, and most of the dissection is accomplished after removal of the heart so that cardiac extraction is not delayed. The actual retrieval of the lung bloc, once

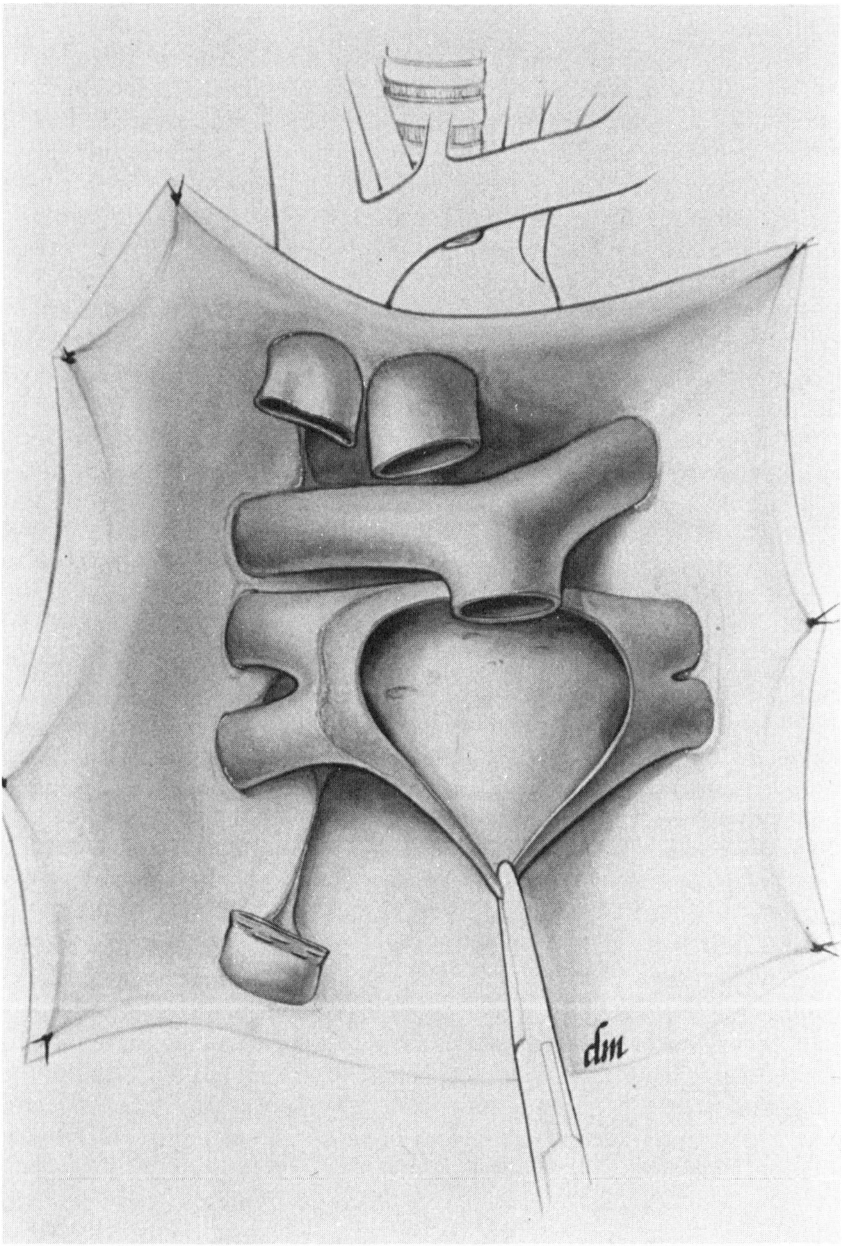

Figure 2 Lung bloc following cardiectomy, showing left atrial cuff and divided pulmonary artery.

the heart is removed, takes an additional 15 min and is done while the liver and kidney teams continue working.

VII. Lung Preservation

Since the maximal safe cold ischemic time for lung was not known, initial lung transplants were carried out with the donor and the recipient in adjacent operating rooms in minimize the ischemic period. This requirement greatly limited access to donor organs and significantly complicated the logistics of the procedure. From animal experiments, it was apparent that cold ischemia, using simple immersion of the lung, was well tolerated for periods of 4-6 hr. Subsequent clinical application of this technique proved satisfactory, and the ability to retrieve donor lungs from distant centers greatly improved donor availability.

The ability to safely preserve lungs for periods longer than 6 hr would have a significant impact on lung transplantation. Numerous experimental studies of lung preservation have been conducted, though with conflicting results (Haverich et al., 1985; Toledo-Pereyra et al., 1977). Efforts have focused on whether the lung should be inflated and with what gas mixture, the optimum preservation temperature, organ perfusion vs. flushing of the pulmonary circulation, and the constituents of the flush solution. Methods used to determine the quality of lung preservation include lung weight, measurement of lung water, histology, radiographic appearance, biochemical and metabolic changes, pulmonary vascular resistance, and, most commonly, assessment of gas exchange and overall survival following transplantation.

Despite the development of various animal models, no standard method of assessing lung preservation currently exists, a situation that contributes greatly to the inconclusive or conflicting nature of may previous reports. Nonetheless, occasional graft survival with reasonable function occurs in animals after 24 hr of preservation, demonstrating the potential ability to prolong ischemic time (Rabinovitch et al., 1983; Hoyer et al., 1980; Pinsker et al, 1979; Toledo-Pereyra and Condie, 1978). Of particular interest are recent reports by Fujimura and co-workers (1987) of successful 48-hr preservation in a dog model using a flush solution of extracellular electrolyte composition containing a high concentration of phosphate buffer.

In an animal model, it is difficult to assess function of a single transplanted lung since a normal contralateral lung remains. However, exclusion of the contralateral lung diverts all of the cardiac output through the transplanted lung, placing an abnormal burden on both this lung and the right ventricle. Furthermore, contralateral pneumonectomy or pulmonary artery ligation carries a high mortality in dogs, unrelated to adequacy of preservation of the transplanted lung. Assessment of lung function following replacement of both lungs is ideal, but requires primates for survival experiments since other species cannot maintain adequate ventilation after bilateral pulmonary denervation.

To address this problem we developed a canine model that allows for in vivo, interval assessment of the function of a single transplanted lung (Jones et al., 1988). We position an inflatable pulmonary artery cuff around the right pulmonary artery at the time of left single lung transplant. The inflatable cuff attaches to a subcutaneously placed reservoir, allowing for easy cuff inflation and temporary occlusion of the opposite pulmonary artery so that assessment of gas exchange and pulmonary artery pressure may be made with the normal, contralateral lung excluded. We have documented acceptable gas exchange immediately following and at 3 days posttransplant in dogs after 12 hr of donor lung ischemia following preservation by flushing with a solution similar to that proposed by Fujimura (Keshavjee et al., 1989).

The importance of inflation or ventilation of ischemic lungs remains unclear. Several authors claim that ischemia is better tolerated at normothermia if the lung is ventilated or inflated (Veith et al., 1971b; Stevens et al., 1973). At cold temperatures, ventilation with 100% oxygen may be detrimental (Veith, 1974), but recent experience with a rabbit lung model in our laboratory suggests that inflation with 100% oxygen may be superior to inflation with room air. Furthermore, storage of the lung in hyperbaric oxygen has also been reported as beneficial for preservation (Garzon et al., 1968; Karlson et al., 1970).

It is known that kidneys flushed with hypertonic solutions of intracellular electrolyte composition may be stored for 48 hr (Collins et al., 1969; Sacks et al., 1973). This knowledge prompted the use of similar solutions with a high potassium content for pulmonary flushing experiments. Adequate long-term lung function has been sporadically achieved after ischemic periods up to 24 hr with use of this type of solution (Pinsker et al., 1981). Similar success occurred in a canine allotransplant model using Sacks solution (Crane et al., 1975; Veith et al., 1976). Primates undergoing heart-lung transplantation following pulmonary flushing with Eurocollins solution and cold ischemia for 5-6 hr also demonstrated adequate pulmonary function (Reichart et al., 1987; Starkey et al., 1986).

Several centers report safe preservation of human lungs for periods up to 4 hr utilizing a cold electrolyte flush solution preceded by injection of prostacycline or prostaglandin E1 into the pulmonary artery. The latter substances are pulmonary vasodilators and probably improve the uniformity and efficiency of distribution of the cold electrolyte flush solution (Wallwork et al., 1987). PGE-1 may also decrease pulmonary vascular permeability (Fantone et al., 1980).

Either flushing donor lungs with Eurocollins solution or core cooling with an extracorporeal circuit without flushing provides acceptable gas exchange following heart-lung transplantation in dogs (Wahlers et al., 1986). However, of the two methods, core cooling results in lower pulmonary vascular resistance immediately posttransplant. Core cooling is a reasonable method of preservation for calf lungs for up to 4 hr of ischemia prior to transplantation (Kontos et al., 1987) and has been used widely in England by Yacoub and co-workers (1989) for clinical heart-lung transplantation.

Autoperfusion of the heart-lung bloc is an alternate method of heart-lung preservation (Ladowski et al., 1985). Early animal experiments with this method were encouraging and pulmonary function following calf heart-lung transplantation compared favorably to pulmonary function following hypothermic flushing with Collins solution in the same model (Adachi et al., 1987). Clinically, however, this method is inconsistent and complicated, and therefore, it is no longer utilized.

It is currently believed that lung injury in donor organs results not only from the ischemic insult, but also from injury occurring at the time of reperfusion of blood through the preserved organ. Several experimental models of acute lung injury implicate oxygen-free radicals in the genesis of reperfusion injury (Parks et al., 1983; McCord, 1985). A variety of mediators, including prostaglandin metabolites, pay a role in the vascular and bronchial smooth muscle response to injury in the lung (Demling, 1982). It is likely that some of these mediators are also important in the lung's response to ischemia. Ischemia-reperfusion injury in other organs is associated with lethal calcium influx, and thus calcium channel blockers, such as Verapamil, may offer some protection against warm ischemia in canine lungs (Hachida and Morton, 1988). Enhanced tolerance to ischemia also results from infusion of prostacycline analog (PGI 2) in a model of in situ canine lung ischemia and autotransplantation (Yamashita et al., submitted). Prostacycline infusion improved pulmonary function in acute heart-lung transplants in dogs (Jurman et al., 1987). Ischemic injury in isolated, perfused canine lobes is reduced after pretreatment with superoxide dismutase (SOD) (Koyama et al., 1987) or SOD and catalase given upon restoration of blood flow (Paull et al., 1989a). SOD has been shown to enhance preservation in an acute model of canine heart-lung transplantation (Bando et al., 1989). Similarly, the free radical scavenger glutathione added to Eurocollins flush solution reduced the increase in lung water that usually accompanies canine pulmonary autotransplantation (Bryan et al., 1989), and dimethylthiourea has been shown to have a beneficial effect as well (Paull et al., 1989b).

Despite satisfactory results with the dog transplant model, such a model is expensive, time consuming, and less than ideal as a screening method for testing the many factors relating to lung preservation. We have developed an isolated, perfused rabbit lung model to rapidly screen preservation techniques, such as storage temperature and perfusate composition (Wang et al., 1989). With this model we demonstrated that lung preservation at 10°C is significantly better than preservation at 4°C. Others note that this storage temperature may be optimum for cardiac preservation as well (Keon et al., 1988). Using a model of isolated perfused rabbit lungs, Breda and coworkers (1985) demonstrated that lung function was improved if preserved lungs were reperfused with leukocyte-depleted blood or if the perfusate contained methoprednisolone (Hall et al., 1988).

Most experimental studies in lung preservation to date have been largely empiric, looking at the effect of various preservation techniques on subsequent lung function. These are summarized in Table 7. Further progress requires a more detailed understanding of events at the cellular level during ischemia and reperfusion so that a rational approach to reduce or eliminate

Table 7 Methods of Lung Preservation

Hypothermic immersion
With atelectasis
With inflation
With ventilation
With hyperbaric oxygen
Normothermic perfusion
Autoperfused heart-lung preparation
Hypothermic perfusion
Core cooling, with or without perfusion
Flushing
ECF solutions
Lpd
Fujimura
Ringer's, saline
Plasma, blood
Rheomacrodex
ICF solutions
Collins
Sacks
Pharmacologic additives
Prostaglandins—PGI-2
Calcium channel blockers
Free radical scavengers
SOD, catalase, glutathione, DMSO

these changes may evolve. Satisfactory preservation techniques must protect not only cell structure and metabolism, but also functional integrity of the lung as a whole, so as to maintain normal gas exchange. In addition, methods that allow for prolongation of ischemic time must also preserve the viability and microcirculation of the airway to prevent the subsequent development of airway healing complications. Given the current ability to safely preserve livers and kidneys for 24 hr or more, it seems likely that lung preservation for periods up to 12 hr will become a reality in the near future.

VIII. Technique of Lung Transplantation

A. Unilateral Lung Transplant Operation

Our technique of lung transplantation approximates that initially reported by Metras in France in 1950 and subsequently by Hardin and Kittle (1954) in the United States, with the addition of bronchial omentopexy as previously noted. We applied these techniques initially in the animal laboratory and in multiple cadaver procedures before implementing our clinical program. We have previously published our techniques (Cooper et al., 1987; Patterson et al., 1988b) but minor revisions are constantly occurring. Transplants have been performed on either side with equal success. We provide here a brief review of the technical features. The choice of which side to transplant depends on several factors: (1) prior major thoracotomy—transplant nonoperated side; (2) significant disproportion of ventilation and perfusion to one side—transplant the worse side; (3) donor factors—transplant the best donor lung, if there is concern as to radiologic or bronchoscopic findings of one of the lungs.

Anesthetic Technique

Our anesthetic management for single lung transplant recipients has recently been outlined (DeMajo, 1990). Preoperatively, a pulmonary artery catheter is positioned on the side opposite that to be transplanted. Additional monitoring includes pulse oximetry, arterial pressure, and continuous end-tidal CO_2. An extracorporeal bypass circuit incorporating a membrane oxygenator is primed and available in the room on a standby basis, should partial bypass prove necessary while the patient is being supported by only one lung. For most transplants this has not been required. Patients undergoing left lung transplant have a bronchus blocking balloon positioned, with bronchoscopic guidance, in the left mainstem bronchus. For patients undergoing right lung transplant, we insert a left endobronchial tube and confirm the placement with a pediatric flexible bronchoscope.

The patient is placed in the lateral decubitus position and the chest, abdomen, and ipsilateral groin area are prepared and draped. Previously we began the procedure by performing the omental mobilization with the patient in the supine position, followed by abdominal closure and repositioning the patient. We now prefer the lateral decubitus position for the entire procedure.

Surgical Technique

Through an upper midline abdominal incision we mobilize the gastrocolic omentum off the transverse colon. The apex of the omentum is placed in the retrosternal region for subsequent positioning into the pleural space. The thoracotomy is performed and the main pulmonary artery is isolated and temporarily clamped. If the trial clamping of the pulmonary artery causes a significant rise in pulmonary artery pressure, infusion of a pulmonary vasodilator such as nitroprusside or PGE-1 is used in an attempt to reduce the pulmonary vascular resistance and right heart strain. If this is not well tolerated, the femoral vessels are prepared for subsequent partial venoarterial bypass during replacement of the lung. If the trial clamping of the pulmonary artery is well tolerated, the clamp is removed and the remaining hilar structures exposed. The pulmonary artery clamp is then replaced and the pulmonary artery is divided just distal to the first branch. The artery is trimmed back at the time of pulmonary artery anastomosis. The pulmonary veins are divided between ligatures outside the pericardium (Fig. 3). The bronchus is divided just proximal to the upper lobe takeoff. The inflated bronchus blocking balloon maintains a sealed airway. Alternatively, the bronchus can be divided just distal to a staple line with subsequent resection of the staple line and inflation of the balloon at the time of the bronchial anastomosis (Fig. 4).

After the lung has been removed, the pericardium is opened around the pulmonary veins and a left atrial clamp placed as centrally as possible without impinging on the contralateral pulmonary veins. The previously placed ligatures are removed from the stumps of the two pulmonary veins and a suitable left atrial cuff is prepared, by incising between the two venous orifices.

Preparation of the donor lung commences prior to implantation, with division of the bronchus two rings above the upper lobe takeoff and division of the pulmonary artery at its origin from the common pulmonary artery. A cuff of left atrium remains around the pulmonary veins from the time the donor heart was extracted prior to lung extraction. The lung, wrapped in cold, moist laparotomy sponges, is placed posteriorly in the chest. The posterior wall of the atrial anastomosis is performed first, with subsequent completion of the anterior wall. The donor and recipient arteries are trimmed to

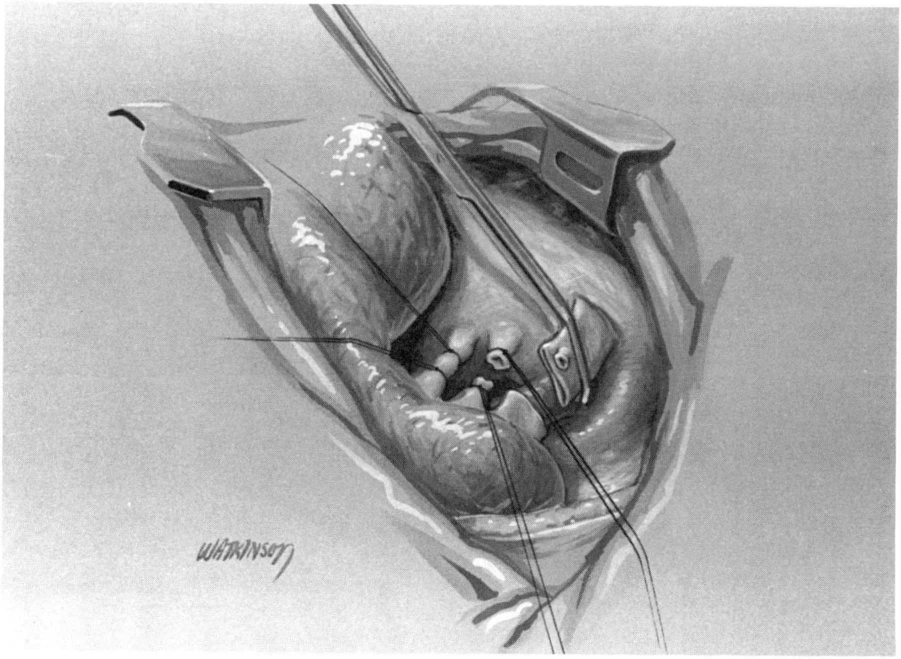

Figure 3 The left pulmonary artery is divided distal to its first branch and the left pulmonary veins are taken extrapericardially for the recipient pneumonectomy.

suitable lengths and an end-to-end anastomosis is performed with running monofilament suture. Upon completion, the pulmonary artery anastomosis is left untied, temporarily. The bronchial anastomosis is performed with interrupted absorbable sutures. The left atrial clamp is then gradually removed and the pulmonary artery anastomosis is observed for back-bleeding, which usually occurs after 3-4 min. Gentle inflation of the lung may assist this process. When back-bleeding occurs, or after several minutes if no back-bleeding results, the pulmonary artery clamp is gradually removed as the pulmonary artery suture is tied. The bronchial suture line is tested for air leaks and the omentum is withdrawn from its position in the anterior mediastinum, brought inferior and posterior to the hilum of the lung, and completely wrapped around the bronchus (Fig. 5).

B. Double Lung Transplant Operation

The double lung procedure, as first described, was done via median sternotomy, and required total cardiopulmonary bypass with a period of aortic

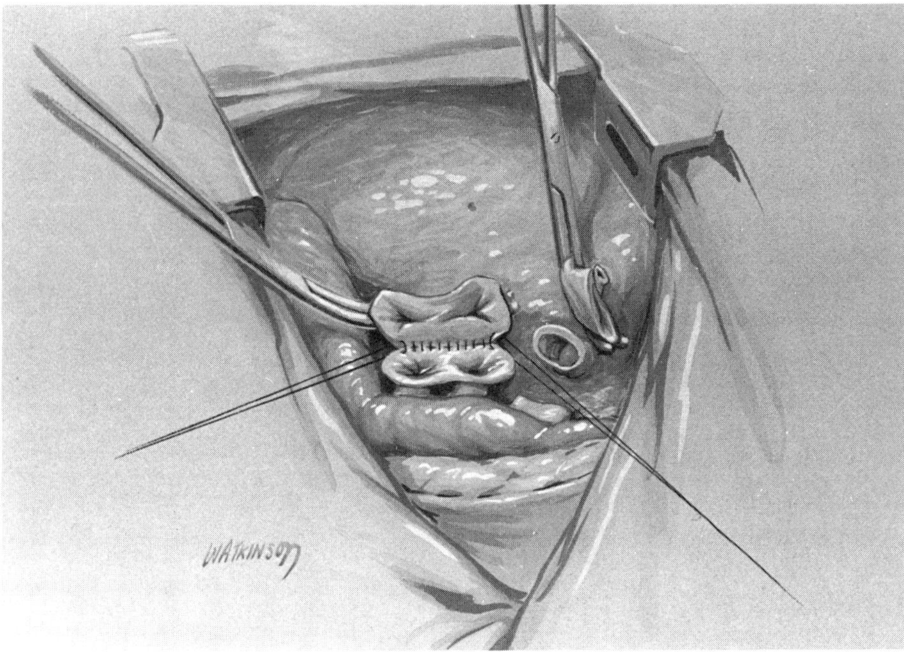

Figure 4 After the donor lung is oriented in the left chest, the left atrial anastomosis is performed with running prolene suture. The bronchus is occluded with a bronchus-blocking balloon in its lumen.

cross clamping and myocardial protection (Patterson et al., 1988b). The double lung bloc was positioned behind the heart, and left atrial, pulmonary artery, and tracheal anastomoses completed. Initial results with this technique were encouraging (Patterson et al., 1988a), but almost 50% of patients experienced problems with airway healing, some fatal (Patterson et al., 1990). Also, because of the lung cardiopulmonary bypass time and significant cross-clamp time, we noted problems with cardiac function, either intraoperative or in the immediate postoperative period. Because of our dissatisfaction with aspects of this operation, but our belief in double lung replacement for certain recipients, we sought to develop an alternative operation.

There is evidence, in dogs, that the pulmonary circulation contributes to the blood supply of the main bronchi, but the contribution to the distal trachea is considerably less (Barman et al., 1988; Michelassi et al., 1987). This may partially explain the observed higher incidence of airway complications following the double lung operation.

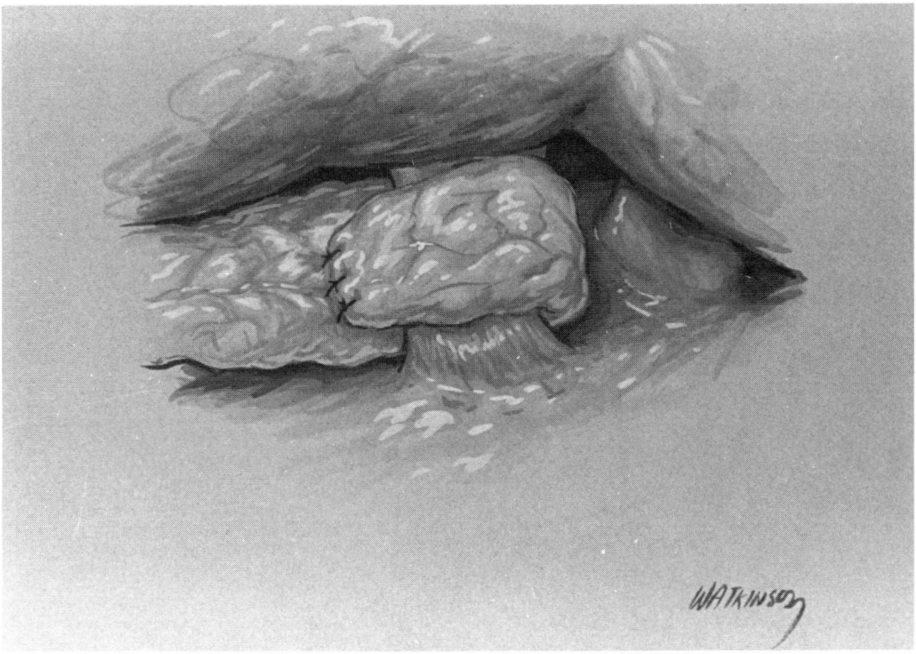

Figure 5 Following completion of the bronchial anastomosis, the omentum is completely wrapped around the bronchus and secured loosely.

Initially a modification of the technique utilizing double bronchial anastomoses, in lieu of a tracheal anastomosis, was tried and proved quite satisfactory. Noiclerc, in Marseilles, recently reported on a series of patients utilizing this technique with excellent results (Noiclerc et al., in press). This procedure still required total cardiopulmonary bypass and was done via median sternotomy. For patients with obliterated pleural spaces, the dissection to remove the lungs, especially posteriorly, is particularly difficult via median sternotomy. Large areas must be dissected without benefit of direct visualization. This usually leads to significant bleeding following heparinization for cardiopulmonary bypass.

Once performing double bronchial anastomoses, we reasoned that bilateral, single lung transplants might be a reasonable alternative. After several cadaver dissections, we realized that bilateral, fifth-interspace, anterolateral thoracotomy with transverse division of the sternum provides maximal exposure, greatly facilitating dissection in a fixed pleural space.

The patient is placed in the supine position and the omentum is mobilized after an upper abdominal midline incision is made. Following the simultaneous

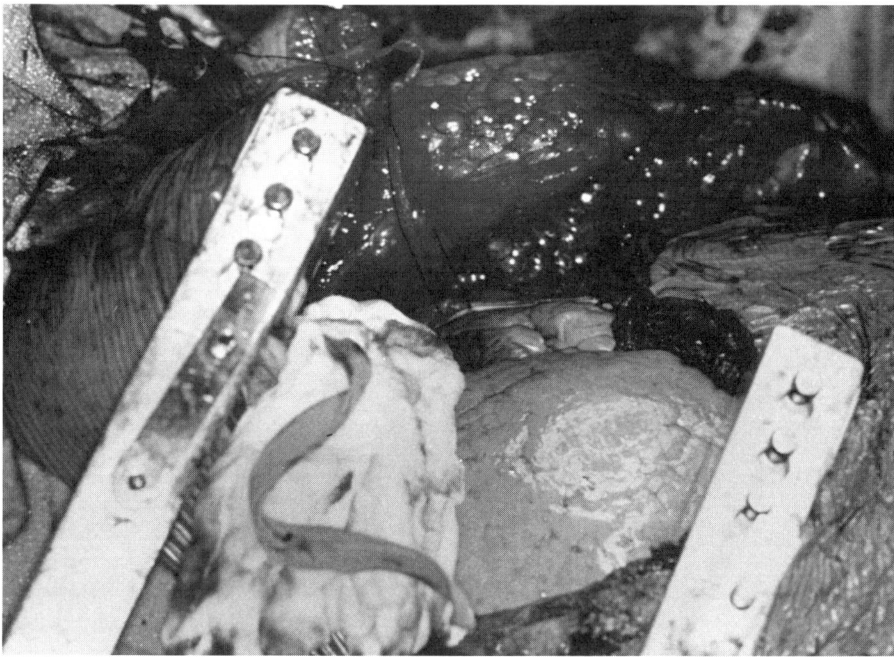

Figure 6 Operative photograph showing the newly implanted right lung with the native left lung still in place. Note the exposure provided by the bilateral thoracotomies with transverse division of the sternum.

performance of the bilateral thoracotomies and mobilization of hilar structures, the right lung is removed. The new right lung is implanted by first completing the bronchial anastomosis following by the atrial and pulmonary artery anastomoses (Fig. 6). Partial cardiopulmonary bypass is then instituted, after cannulation of the ascending aorta and right atrium. We employ "low dose" heparin (initial 1.5-2.0 mg/kg) and maintain the activated clotting time between 250 and 400 sec, based on our experience with long-term extracorporeal membrane oxygenation (Egan et al., 1988) and recent animal data (Cardosa et al., in press). The left lung is then removed and the new one implanted in the same fashion as described for the right lung. Cardiopulmonary bypass is then discontinued, having been required usually for about 1 hr. An omental pedicle is used to wrap each bronchial anastomosis.

IX. Postoperative Course Following Lung Transplantation

The first hours following surgery may be marked by a high arterial-alveolar (Aa) gradient. We reviewed the early Aa gradient as a function of donor

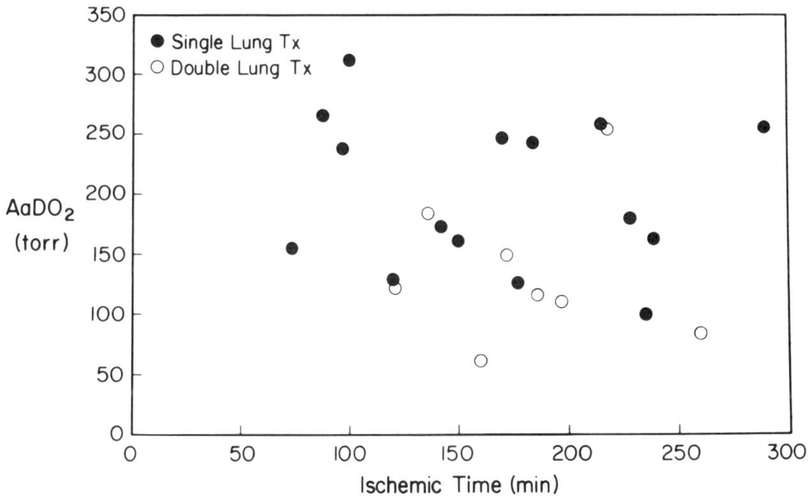

Figure 7 Scattergram of postoperative Aa gradient vs. ischemic time for 23 lung transplants. Using simple atelectasis and cold immersion as a method of preservation, there was no apparent relationship between ischemic time and early lung function as assessed by Aa gradient.

ischemic time following transplantation and found no relationship between Aa gradient and duration of donor lung ischemia. The results are shown graphically in Figure 7. The transplanted lung is susceptible to fluid overload, perhaps because of the total disruption of pulmonary lymphatics combined with the increase in extravascular lung water that accompanies reimplantation (Cowan et al., 1976). We employ low-dose pressor support rather than volume infusion, once adequate filling pressures have been established. Transcutaneous oximetry, arterial pressure, and pulmonary artery pressures are continuously monitored. Cardiac output and mixed venous saturation are measured at appropriate intervals.

Intraoperative and postoperative hemorrhage has been a problem in some double lung transplant recipients, especially those with inflammatory disease such as cystic fibrosis or bronchiectasis. We suspect that prolonged postoperative hemorrhage and hypotension may be significant contributing factors to subsequent fatal ischemic airway problems.

Patients are weaned from ventilatory support as early as possible. We feel that this is facilitated by the preoperative rehabilitation program. Clearly, the longer intubation is required, the higher the likelihood of developing pneumonia. This is of particular concern in patients with infective end-stage lung disease whose upper and lower airways are colonized at the time of transplantation.

We monitor the airway with frequent bronchoscopies, usually performing the initial one on the first postoperative day. It is important to assess the airway anastomosis and to obtain appropriate cultures if indicated. We utilize bronchial washings, bronchoalveolar lavage (BAL), and protected brush specimens with quantitative culture techniques (Chastre et al., 1988; Kahn and Jones, 1987; Thorpe et al., 1987). Bronchoscopy is performed prior to extubation and again at 2-3 weeks to assess airway healing prior to adding maintenance prednisone to the immunosuppressive regimen. As with other surgical procedures on the airway, ischemic injury may not be apparent until the third postoperative week.

We have noticed that many patients have a prolonged ileus following lung transplantation, out of proportion to what might be anticipated following omental mobilization. Whatever the cause, the end result is that the gut is often not useful as a route of alimentation in these patients, and gastric distention necessitates nasogastric tube suction for a prolonged period postoperatively. This prolonged ileus frequently mandates the use of postoperative intravenous total parenteral nutrition. Patients walk as early as possible, using supplemental oxygen as necessary and monitoring transcutaneous oxygen saturation. Vigorous chest physiotherapy is essential for optimal mobilization of secretions.

Our immunosuppression protocol consists, at the outset, of cyclosporin (4 mg/hr) and azathioprine (2 mg/kg/day), given intravenously. We start the intravenous cyclosporin at the conclusion of the transplant operation. Therapy is monitored by whole blood radioimmunoassay utilizing a monoclonal antibody technique. We attempt to achieve a whole blood level in the range of 300-400 ng/ml during intravenous therapy. When the gastrointestinal tract appears to be functioning, oral cyclosporin is administered and adjusted to provide trough levels in this range. We previously avoided routine daily use of steroids for the first 3 weeks because of the deleterious effect on bronchial wound healing, but now start them 1 week after operation.

Suspected rejection episodes are treated with bolus doses of steroids, although the diagnosis of rejection is difficult. Early acute rejection has been an almost constant feature of isolated lung transplantation, with two or three rejection episodes usually occurring within the first month. These episodes are well managed with pulsed steroid therapy. Clinical signs include a temperature elevation which may be as slight as 0.5 °C, a deterioration in gas exchange as seen by a decrease in Po_2, or a decrease in exercise tolerance. Radiographically the appearance of a fluffy hilar infiltrate is quite suggestive of a rejection episode especially if it occurs during days 4-6. However, we recognize that these same changes may be seen with infection, and as previously noted, bronchoscopy is helpful to rule out infection. We consider radiographic changes to be late signs of rejection, and thus we maintain a low threshold for giving an initial bolus of steroid (500 mg methylprednisolone sodium succinate). The diagnosis of rejection is frequently confirmed by virtue of the response to a bolus dose of steroids. Significant resolution of the infiltrate is usually seen within 12 hr of the first dose of steroid. If there has been a clear-cut clinical or radiologic response to the initial steroid bolus, it is followed by two subsequent doses of steroids on the succeeding 2 days (250-500 mg of methylprednisolone sodium succinate).

In single lung recipients, rejection is usually accompanied by a reduction in perfusion to the transplanted lung documented on quantitative radionuclide scan to determine the percent of total blood flow to each lung. Despite the sensitivity of this technique, is not necessarily specific. This redistribution of perfusion is promptly reversed with a pulse dose of steroids. With few exceptions, a rejection episode occurs during the first 4-6 days following transplant. This corresponds to classical first-set rejection and is the same time frame in which rejection develops in untreated laboratory animals after a lung allograft (Veith et al., 1972; Kondo et al., 1974). A second rejection episode is also a frequent occurrence between 2 and 3 weeks postoperatively.

Because of the frequency of rejection episodes despite "triple therapy," we explored the use of the murine monoclonal antibody OKT-3 for initial prophylaxis, an agent for which there is favorable experience in cardiac transplant patients (Bristow et al., 1987; Sweeney et al., 1987). We found, however, that there was a significant price to pay. There was no decrease in number or severity of rejection episodes, and all four patients treated with OKT-3 developed significant cytomegalovirus (CMV) infections. Episodes of rejection after the first month following successful transplantation are unusual. However, two of our recipients have died with a picture of chronic rejection.

Experience with airway complications following lung transplantation has been recently reviewed (Schafers et al., in press; Patterson et al., 1990). Of 17 single lung transplants, airway necrosis caused one death. This was the only patient transplanted while still on steroids. Two patients required insertion of silastic stents for anastomotic stenoses, a technique previously described (Cooper et al., 1989b) (Fig. 8). One of these patients subsequently died from chronic rejection while the other remains alive and well nearly 5 years following the transplant. Of 16 double lung recipients in our experience, there have been three perioperative deaths, leaving 13 patients at risk for airway complications. Of these, three patients died from complications directly related to airway necrosis or dehiscence, and two additional patients have had placement of silastic airway stents (Fig. 9).

Infectious complications following lung transplantation have also recently been reviewed (H. Vellend, personal communication). In the first 30

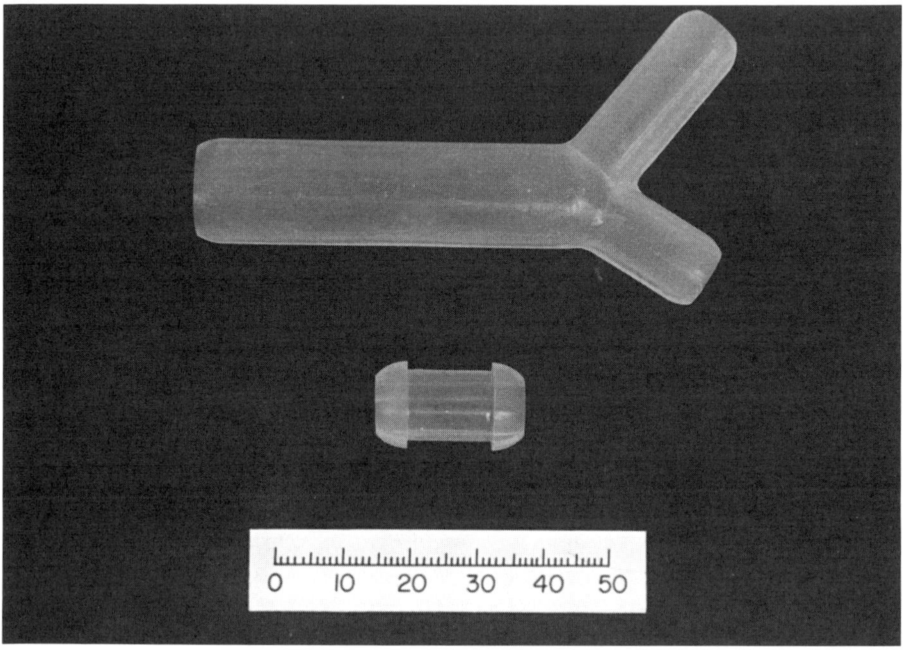

Figure 8 Intraluminal airway stents fashioned from silastic; they can be inserted endoscopically.

single or double lung transplants performed by the Toronto Lung Transplant Group, 32 infections occurred in 19 patients, most within 6 months of transplantation. Twenty of thirty-two infections involved the chest. Seven patients who were seronegative for CMV received seropositive lungs. Two of these patients seroconverted but had no evidence of clinical infection. The only patient who developed fatal CMV pneumonia was seropositive and received a seronegative graft. We routinely employ pneumocystic prophylaxis with Septra in all our patients as well as herpes prophylaxis with acylovir.

X. Clinical Results of Lung Transplantation

A report detailing results in our first 11 single lung transplant recipients has been published (Toronto Lung Transplant Group, 1988). The experience of the senior author (JDC) includes 28 single lung transplants performed since 1983 with an absolute survival rate of 70% and the longest survivor at 6.0 years. We have performed nine single lung transplants for emphysema with

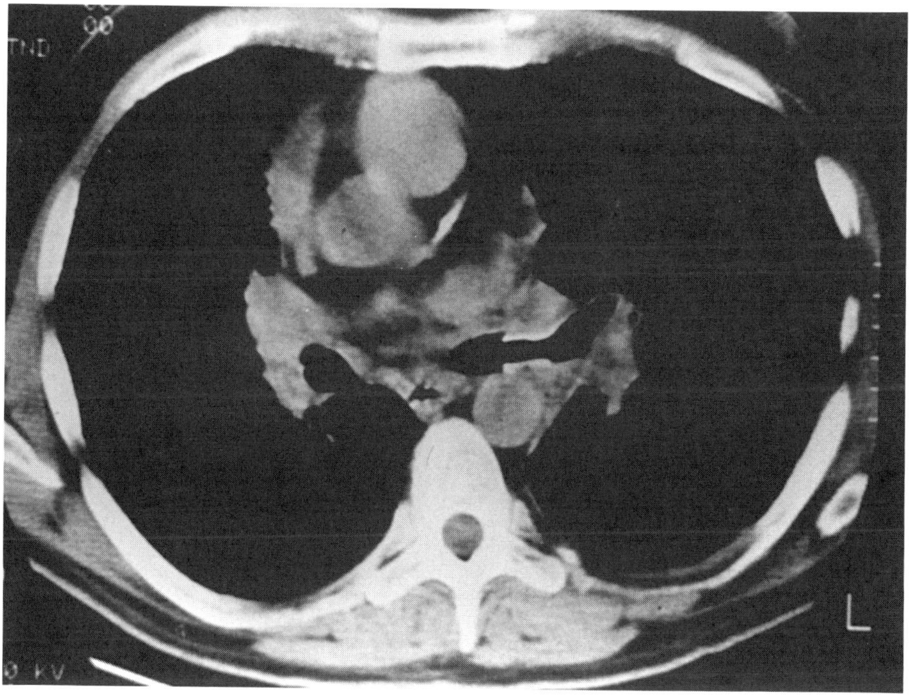

Figure 9 Computed-tomography scan showing a silastic stent in the left mainstem bronchus of a double lung transplant recipient. (From Cooper et al., 1989b.)

no mortality and without significant problems resulting from air trapping or mediastinal shift. These patients all are off oxygen and are able to live a relatively normal existence. As expected, almost all have an element of ventilation-perfusion mismatch, as the native emphysematous lung continues to receive a significant portion of the ventilation. The transplanted lungs receive a mean of 48% of the ventilation and 69% of the perfusion. Long-term functional assessment remains to be determined. Initial exercise testing shows a decrease in V_D/V_T, indicative of a shift in ventilation toward the transplanted lung.

We have recently performed our first single lung transplant for primary pulmonary hypertension. Pulmonary pressure immediately decreased and right ventricular ejection fraction improved significantly, as assessed by a right ventricular ejection fraction catheter.

We recently established a Registry of Lung Transplantation, and as of October 1989 we have reports of 144 single lung transplants performed worldwide since 1983 with 97 (67%) of all recipients currently alive and well.

Our initial experience with double lung transplantation has also been reported (Cooper et al., 1989a). The senior author's (JDC) personal experience involves 14 recipients with nine (65%) long-term survivors, including four patients alive at 2 years or greater and one cystic fibrosis patient at 14 months following transplantation. Fatal airway complications occurred in three patients and an additional three patients developed late airway stenosis requiring dilatation and/or silastic stent insertion. Data from the Lung Transplant Registry show 73 double lung transplants, with 40 (55%) surviving. As mentioned above, our double lung operation has been modified significantly. We have now performed bilateral single lung transplants in two patients with excellent results. One patient, with cystic fibrosis, was discharged from the hospital by the middle of the third postoperative week. We are excited about the prospects for this operation and it currently is our procedure of choice for patients requiring double lung replacement.

Following successful single lung transplantation there is a progressive increase in blood flow to the transplanted lung as documented by serial perfusion lung scans (Grossman et al., 1990). In our experience the mean perfusion to the transplanted lung is 66% at 1 week, 72% at 3 weeks, with subsequent gradual increase (Toronto Lung Transplant Group, 1988). In some cases where there is increased pulmonary vascular resistance in the native lung, perfusion to the transplanted lung has been in excess of 80% in the first 24 hr.

Improvements in ventilation and lung function for single and double lung recipients are shown in Figures 10 and 11. The improvement in measured volumes is accompanied by a marked increase in exercise capacity in these patients (Figs. 12 and 13) (Grossman et al., 1990). Improvement in lung function and exercise capacity has been sustained in all of our isolated lung transplant patients with the exception of the two who developed chronic rejection. We currently are treating one double lung recipient, 14 months following transplant, for obliterative bronchiolitis.

To date no patient has demonstrated reinnervation of a transplanted lung, as determined by the absence of cough upon stimulation of the transplanted airway at the time of bronchoscopy. There is evidence that autonomic reinnervation may occur in dogs following pulmonary reimplantation (Lall et al., 1973; Edmunds et al., 1971). Higenbotham (1989) showed that in humans the pattern of breathing following heart lung transplantation is normal during rest and exercise despite pulmonary denervation. Carbon dioxide response curves and sleep studies have been done in patients following single lung, double lung, and combined heart-lung transplantation and have been found to be normal.

We have demonstrated airway hyperreactivity in patients undergoing single lung and combined heart lung transplantation suggesting that denervation

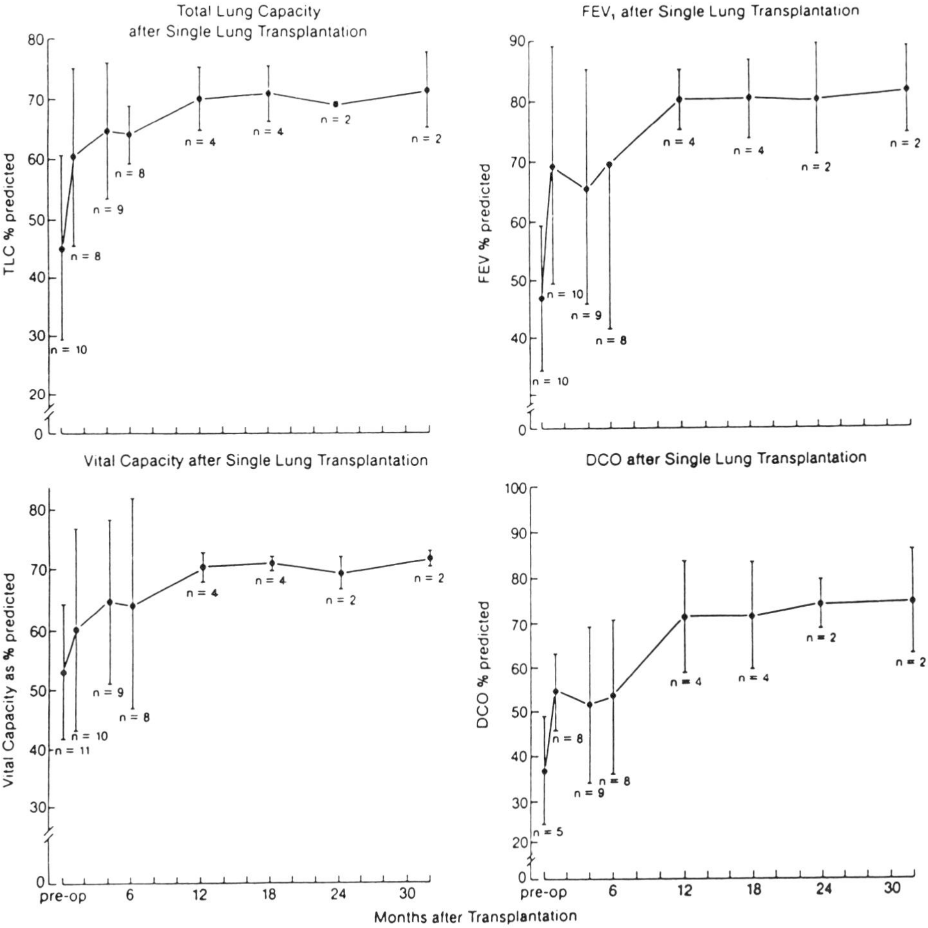

Figure 10 Improvements in total lung capacity (upper left), FEV_1 (upper right), vital capacity (lower left), and diffusing capacity for carbon monoxide (lower right) following single lung transplantation. (From Grossman et al., 1990.)

may play a role in airway hyperresponsiveness in humans (Maurer et al., 1987). Increased airway hyperreactivity in the denervated lung has also been reported by others following combined heart lung transplant (Glanville et al., 1987a).

We measured mucociliary clearance and ciliary beat frequency in five patients, 6-12 months following single lung transplantation for pulmonary fibrosis (Dolovich et al., 1987). Mucociliary clearance was measured over

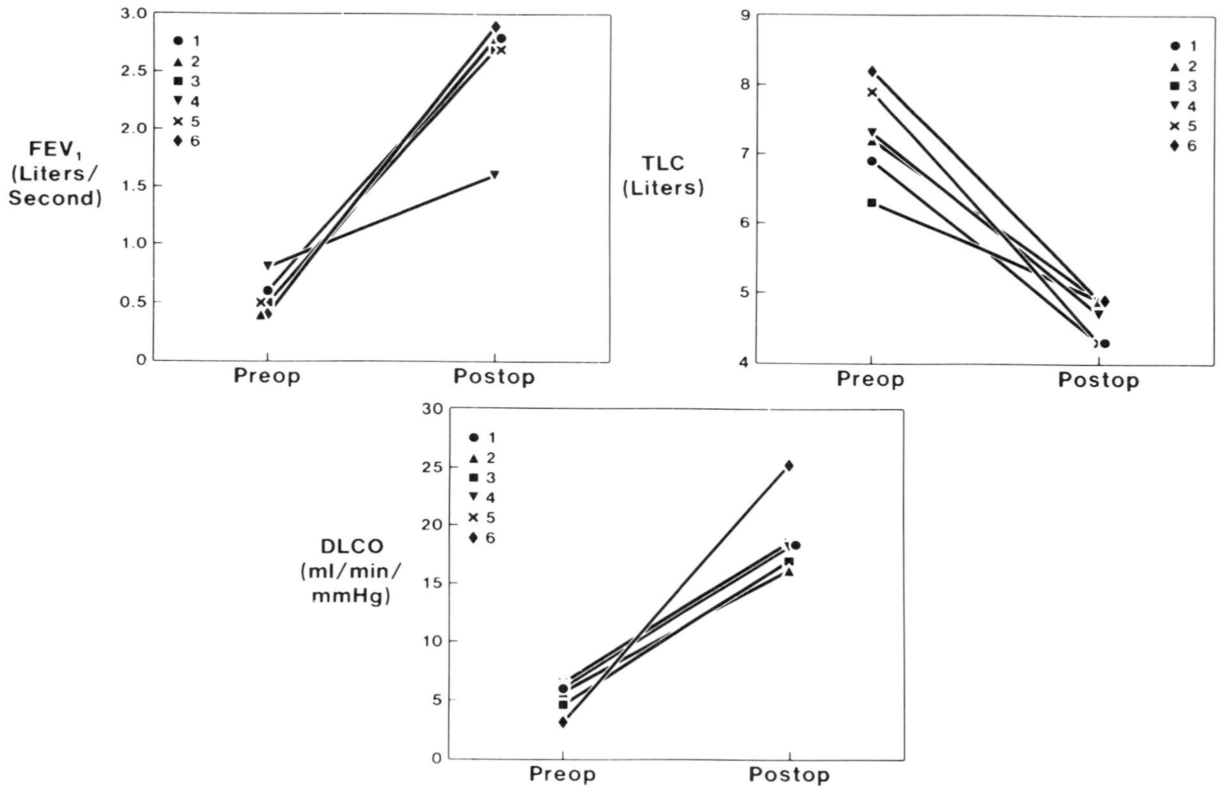

Figure 11 Improvement in FEV$_1$ (upper left), total lung capacity (upper right), and diffusing capacity for carbon monoxide (lower middle) following double lung transplantation in the first six double lung recipients performed by the Toronto Lung Transplant Group.

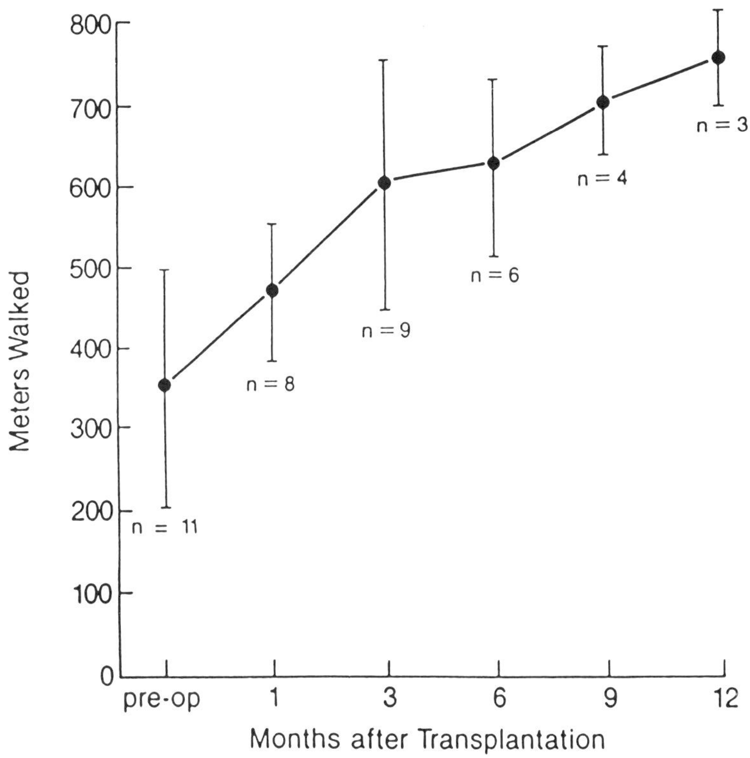

Figure 12 Improvement in exercise performance as assessed by meters walked in 6 min following single lung transplantation. (From Grossman et al., 1990.)

6 hr by monitoring the disappearance of an inhaled 99m Tc-sulfur colloid aerosol. The clearance rate of the aerosol from the transplanted lung was less than 50% of that in the opposite, native lung. Bronchial biopsies were taken from both native and transplanted lungs to measure ciliary beat frequency using phase contrast light microscopy. In all specimens ciliary activity appeared normal. We concluded that the abnormality in mucociliary clearance was unrelated to ciliary beat frequency but might reflect a quantitative or qualitative defect in mucous or periciliary fluid composition following transplantation. Edmunds also demonstrated impaired mucociliary clearance using tantalum bronchography in a canine lung transplant model (Edmunds et al., 1969).

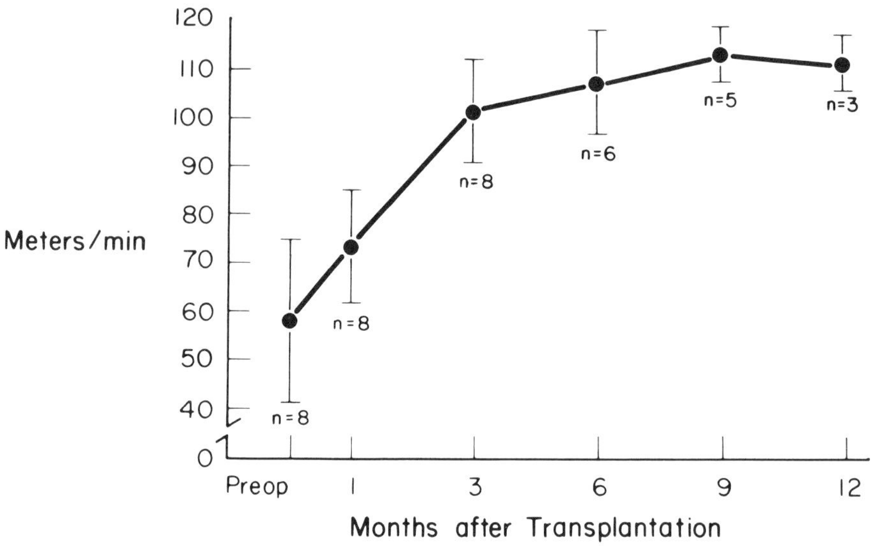

Figure 13 Improved performance in 6-min walk following double lung transplantation. (From Frost et al., 1988.)

We did not anticipate that the double lung transplant procedure would affect cardiac innervation but recent studies show a variable degree of denervation following this procedure (Schafers et al., 1988). Evaluation of maximal heart rate after carotid sinus massage, Valsalva maneuver, intravenous atropine, and during the first 3 min of rest following a standardized exercise test was performed in four double lung recipients and revealed a normal response in two patients. However the other two patients had minimal response indicating at least some degree of cardiac denervation.

To date recurrence of the original lung disease for which patients received a single lung, double lung, or heart-lung transplant has not been observed. This includes patients transplanted for idiopathic pulmonary fibrosis, cystic fibrosis, and primary pulmonary hypertension.

XI. Summary and Conclusions

The supply of donor organs remains extremely limited, and improved methods to maintain the lungs of potential donors to allow for transplantation must be developed. Currently the upper limit of donor lung ischemia even with our "best" preservation techniques is approximately 4-6 hr. Improved methods for preservation will increase the supply of suitable lungs and considerably simplify the logistics of transplantation, just as has occurred with liver transplantation. In the meantime we continue to strive to utilize donor organs in the most efficient manner. On two occasions, within the past 3 months, we have performed two simultaneous single lung operations and are prepared either to do this as a routine or to offer a lung not used by us to another center.

Sufficient progress has been achieved to date to warrant continued application of lung transplantation for end-stage pulmonary disease. With increasing experience, one can anticipate refinement of techniques, and broader application of these procedures. Single lung transplantation, initially restricted to patients with end-stage pulmonary fibrosis, has now been successfully applied to patients with emphysema, pulmonary hypertension, and other conditions.

Though currently transplantation can offer real benefit only to a limited number of individuals, it can create hope for many others. An additional benefit may prove to be the interest and attention that transplantation focuses on patients with end-stage lung disease and on the pathophysiology of chronic respiratory failure. Knowledge gained may ultimately result in the prevention of many of the disorders for which lung transplantation currently offers the only hope.

References

Ackerman, D. M., and Edwards, W. D. (1987). Sudden death as the initial manifestation of primary pulmonary hypertension. *Am. J. Med. Pathol.,* **8**:97-102.

Adachi, H., Fraser, C. D., Kontos, G. J., Borkon, A. M., Hutchins, G. M., Galloway, E., Braun, J., Reitz, B. A., and Baumgartner, W. A. (1987). Autoperfused working heart-lung preparation versus hypothermic cardiopulmonary preservation for transplantation. *J. Heart Transplant.,* **6**:253-260.

Bando, K., Tago, M., Teraoka, H., Seno, S., Senoo, Y., and Teramoto, S. (1989). Extended cardiopulmonary preservation for heart-lung transplantation: A comparative study of superoxide dismutase. *J. Heart Transplant.,* **8**:59-66.

Barman, S. A., Ardell, J. L., Parker, J. C., Perry, M. L., and Taylor, A. E. (1988). Pulmonary and systemic blood flow contributions to upper airways in canine lung. *Am. J. Physiol.* (*Heart Circ. Physiol.,* **24**) **255**: H1130-H1135.

Barnard, C. N. (1967). A human cardiac transplant. *S. Afr. Med. J.,* **41**: 1271-1274.

Bart, K. J., Macon, E. J., Humphries, A. L., Baldwin, R. J., Fitch, T., Pope, R. S., Rich, M. J., Langford, D., Teutsch, S. M., and Blount, J. H. (1981). Increasing the supply of cadaveric kidneys for transplantation. *Transplantation,* **31**:383-387.

Boychuk, J. E., and Patterson, G. A. (1988). Assessing heart and lung donors. *Diagnosis,* **5**:165-173.

Breda, M. A., Hall, T. S., Stuart, R. S., Baumgartner, W. A., Borkon, A. M., Brawn, J. D., Hutchins, J. M., and Reitz, B. A. (1985). Twenty-four hour lung preservation by hypothermia and leukocyte depletion. *Heart Transplant.,* **4**:325-329.

Bristow, M. R., Gilbert, E. M., Renlund, D. G., DeWitt, C. W., Burton, N. A., and O'Connell, J. B. (1987). Use of OKT3 monoclonal antibody in heart transplantation: Review of the initial experience. *J. Heart Transplant.,* **7**:1-11.

Bryan, C. L., Cohen, D. J., Dew, A., Lawrence, R. A., and Jenkinson, S. G. (1989). Glutathione decreases the pulmonary reimplantation response in canine lung autotransplants (abstract). *Am. Rev. Respir. Dis.,* **139**:A45.

Cardosa, P. F. G., Yamazaki, F., Keshavjee, S., Schaffers, H. F., Hsieh, C. M., Wang, L. S., Glynn, M. F. X., Patterson, G. A., and Cooper, J. D. (in press). Re-evaluation of heparin requirements for safe cardiopulmonary bypass. *J. Thorac. Cardiovasc. Surg.*

Cavarocchi, N. C., and Badellino, M. (1989). Heart/heart-lung transplantation. The domino procedure. *Ann. Thorac. Surg.,* **48**:130-133.

Chastre, J., Fagon, J. Y., Soler, P., Bornet, M., Domart, Y., Trouillet, J. L., Gibert, C., and Hance, A. J. (1988). Diagnosis of nosocomial bacterial pneumonia in intubated patients undergoing ventilation: comparison of the usefulness of bronchoalveolar lavage and the protected specimen brush. *Am. J. Med.,* **85**:499-506.

Collins, G. M., Bravo-Shugarman, M., and Terasaki, P. I. (1969). Kidney preservation for transportation: initial perfusion and 30 hours ice storage. *Lancet* **2**:1219-1222.

Cooper, J. D. (1989). Lung transplantation. *Ann. Thorac. Surg.,* **47**:28-44.

Cooper, J. D., Pearson, F. G., Patterson, G. A., Todd, T. R. J., Ginsberg, R. J., Goldberg, M., and DeMajo, W. A. P. (1987). Technique of successful lung transplantation in humans. *J. Thorac. Cardiovasc. Surg.,* **93**:173-181.

Cooper, J. D., Patterson, G. A., Grossman, R., Maurer, J., and the Toronto Lung Transplant Group (1989a). Double-lung transplant for advanced chronic obstructive lung disease. *Am. Rev. Respir. Dis.,* **139**:303-307.

Cooper, J. D., Pearson, F. G., Patterson, G. A., Todd, T. R. J., Ginsberg, R. J., Goldberg, M., and Waters, P. (1989b). Use of silicone stents in the management of airway problems. *Ann. Thorac. Surg.,* **47**:371-378.

Cowan, G. S., Staub, N. C., and Edmunds, L. H. (1976). Changes in the fluid compartments and dry weights of reimplanted dog lungs. *J. Appl. Physiol.,* **40**:962-970.

Crane, R., Torres, M., Hagstrom, J. W. C., Koerner, S. K., and Veith, F. J. (1975). Twenty-four hour preservation and transplantation of the lung without functional impairment. *Surg. Forum,* **26**:111-113.

Daily, P. O., Dembitsky, W. P., Peterson, K. L., and Moser, K. M. (1987). Modifications of techniques and early results of pulmonary thromboendarterectomy for chronic pulmonary embolism. *J. Thorac. Cardiovasc. Surg.,* **93**:221-233.

DeMajo, W. A. P. (1990). Anaesthetic technique for single lung transplantation. In *The Transplantation and Replacement of Thoracic Organs.* Edited by D. K. C. Cooper and D. Novitzky. Lancaster, UK, Kluwer Academic Publishers.

Demikhov, V. P. (1962). *Experimental Transplantation of Vital Organs.* New York, Consultants Bureau Enterprises.

Demling, R. H. (1982). Role of prostaglandins in acute pulmonary microvascular injury. *Ann. NY Acad. Sci.,* **384**:517-534.

Derom, F., Barbier, F., Ringoir, S., Versieck, J., Rolly, G., Berzsenyi, G., Vermiere, P., and Vrints, L. (1971). Ten month survival after lung homotransplantation in man. *J. Thorac. Cardiovasc. Surg.,* **61**:835-846.

Dolovich, M., Rossman, C., Chambers, C., Grossman, R. F., Newhouse, M., Toronto Lung Transplant Group, and Maurer, J. (1987). Muco-ciliary function in patients following single lung or lung/heart transplantation (abstract). *Am. Rev. Respir. Dis.,* **135**:A363.

Dubois, P., Choiniere, L., and Cooper, J. D. (1984). Bronchial omentopexy in canine lung allotransplantation. *Ann. Thorac. Surg.,* **38**:211-214.

Edmunds, L. H., Stallone, R. J., Graf, P. D., Sagel, S. S., and Greenspan, R. H. (1969). Mucus transport in transplanted lungs of dogs. *Surgery,* **66**:15-22.

Edmunds, L. H., Graf, P. D., and Nadel, J. A. (1971). Reinnervation of the reimplanted canine lung. *J. Appl. Physiol.,* **31**:722-727.

Egan, T. M., Duffin, J., Glynn, M. F. X., Todd, T. R. J., DeMajo, W., Murphy, E., Fox, L., and Cooper, J. D. (1988). Ten-year experience with extracorporeal membrane oxygenation for severe respiratory failure. *Chest,* **94**:681-693.

Fantone, J. C., Kunkel, S. I., Ward, P. A., and Zurier, R. B. (1980). Suppression by prostaglandin E_1 of vascular permeability induced by vasoactive inflammatory mediators. *J. Immunol.,* **125**:2591-2596.

Frost, A., Dear, C. L., Grossman, R. F., Cooper, J. D., Maurer, R., and Toronto Lung Transplant Group (1988). Exercise tolerance in patients undergoing double lung transplant for end stage pulmonary disease (abstract). *Am. Rev. Respir. Dis.,* **137**:336.

Fujimura, S., Handa, M., Kondo, T., Ichinose, T., Shiraishi, Y., and Nakada, T. (1987). Successful 48-hour simple hypothermic preservation of canine lung transplants. *Transplant. Proc.,* **19**:1334-1336.

Fuster, V., Steele, P. M., Edwards, W. D., Gersh, B. J., McGoon, M. D., and Frye, R. L. (1984). Primary pulmonary hypertension: natural history and the importance of thrombosis. *Circulation,* **70**:580-585.

Gadek, J. E., Fells, G. A., Zimmerman, R. L., Rennard, S. I., and Crystal, R. G. (1981). Antielastases of the human alveolar structures: Implications for the protease-antiprotease theory of emphysema. *J. Clin. Invest.,* **68**:889-898.

Garzon, A. A., Cheng, C., Pangan, J., and Karlson, K. E. (1968). Hypothermic hyperbaric lung preservation for twenty-four hours with replantation. *J. Thorac. Cardiovasc. Surg.,* **55**:546-554.

Glanville, A. R., Burke, C. M., Theodore, J., Baldwin, J. C., Harvey, J., Vankessel, A., and Robin, E. D. (1987a). Bronchial hyper-responsiveness after human cardiopulmonary transplantation. *Clin. Sci.,* **73**:299-303.

Glanville, A. R., Burke, C. M., Theodore, J., and Robin, E. D. (1987b). Primary pulmonary hypertension: Length of survival in patients referred for heart lung transplantation. *Chest,* **91**:675-681.

Goldberg, M., Lima, O., Morgan, E., Ayabe, H. A., Luk, S., Ferdman, A., Peters, W. J., and Cooper, J. D. (1983). A comparison between cyclosporin A and methylprenisolone plus azathioprine on bronchial healing following canine lung autotransplantation. *J. Thorac. Cardiovasc. Surg.,* **85**:821-826.

Goldsmith, J. S., Kiely, A. A., and Randal, H. T. (1968). Protection of intrathoracic esophageal anastomoses by omentum. *Surgery,* **63**:464-466.

Grossman, R. F., Frost, A., Zamel, N., Patterson, G. A., Cooper, J. D., Dear, C. L., Maurer, J. R., and Toronto Lung Transplant Group (1990). Results of single-lung transplantation for bilateral pulmonary fibrosis. *N. Engl. J. Med.,* **322**:727-732.

Hachida, M., and Morton, D. L. (1988). The protection of ischemic lung with verapamil and hydralazine. *J. Thorac. Cardiovasc. Surg.,* **95**:178-183.

Hall, T. S., Borkon, A. M., Gurtner, G. C., Brawn, J., Hutchins, G. M., Reitz, B. A., and Baumgartner, W. A. (1988). Improved static lung preservation with corticosteroids and hypothermia. *J. Heart Transplant.,* **7**:348-352.

Hardin, C. A., and Kittle, C. F. (1954). Experiences with transplantation of the lung. *Science,* **119**:97-98.

Hardy, J. D., Eraslan, S., and Dalton, M. L. (1963a). Autotransplantation and homotransplantation of the lung: further studies. *J. Thorac. Cardiovasc. Surg.,* **46**:606-615.

Hardy, J. D., Eraslan, S., Dalton, M. L., Alican, F., and Turner, M. D. (1963b). Re-implantation and homotransplantation of the lung. *Ann. Surg.,* **157**:707.

Hardy, J. D., Webb, W. R., Dalton, M. L., and Walker, G. R. (1963c). Lung homotransplantation in man. *JAMA,* **186**:1065-1074.

Haverich, A., Scott, W. C., and Jamieson, S. W. (1985). Twenty years of lung preservation—A review. *Heart Transplant.,* **4**:234-240.

Haworth, S. G. (1983). Primary pulmonary hypertension. *Br. Heart J.,* **49**: 517-521.

Higenbottam, T. (1989). Physiology of the transplanted lung and the results. In *Heart and Heart-Lung Transplantation.* Edited by J. Wallwork. Philadelphia, W.B. Saunders, pp. 533-544.

Higgins, M. (1984). Epidemiology of COPD: State of the art. *Chest,* **85** (suppl.):3S-8S.

Hoyer, J., Garbe, L., Delpierre, S., Prieur, A., Macquart-Moulin, G., and Noiclerc, M. (1980). Functional evaluation of the transplanted lung after long-term preservation. *Respiration,* **39**:323-332.

Hsieh, C. M., Mishkel, G., Rakowski, H., Dunn, S., Gresser, C., Butany, J., Jones, M. T., Schafers, H. J., Wang, L. S., Yoshikawa, K., Weisel, R. D., Patterson, G. A., and Cooper, J. D. (submitted). Production and reversibility of right ventricular hypertrophy and right ventricular failure in dogs.

Hutchison, D. C. S. (1988). Natural history of alpha-1-protease inhibitor deficiency. *Am. J. Med.,* **84** (suppl. 6A):3-12.

Jones, M. T., Hsieh, C., Yoshikawa, K., Patterson, G. A., and Cooper, J. D. (1988). A new model for assessment of lung preservation. *J. Thoracic. Cardiovasc. Surg.,* **96**:608-614.

Jurman, M. J., Dammenhayn, L., Schafers, H. J., Wahlers, T., Fieguth, H. G., and Haverich, A. (1987). Prostacyclin as an additive to single crystalloid flush: Improved pulmonary preservation in heart-lung transplantation. *Transplant. Proc.,* **19**:4103-4104.

Kahn, F. W., and Jones, J. M. (1987). Diagnosing bacterial respiratory infection by bronchoalveolar lavage. *J. Infect. Dis.,* **155**:862-869.

Karlson, K. E., Garzon, A. A., Goldstein, S., Motlagh, F., and Torres, R. (1970). Functional evaluation of immediately replanted and 24 hour preserved and replanted lungs after longer than one year. *Bull. Soc. Int. Chirurg.,* **3**:175-181.

Keon, W. J., Hendry, P. J., Taichman, G. C., and Mainwood, G. W. (1988). Cardiac transplantation: The ideal myocardial temperature for graft transport. *Ann. Thorac. Surg.,* **46**:337-341.

Kern, J. A., and Fishman, A. P. (1988). End stage fibrotic lung disease: treatment and prognosis. In *Pulmonary Diseases and Disorders.* Edited by A. P. Fishman. New York, McGraw-Hill, pp. 2237-2250.

Keshavjee, S. H., Yamazaki, F., Cardoso, P. F., McRitchie, D. I., Patterson, G. A., and Cooper, J. D. (1989). A method for safe 12 hour pulmonary preservation. *J. Thorac. Cardiovasc. Surg.,* **98**:529-534.

Kondo, Y., Cockrell, J. V., Kuwahara, O., and Hardy, J. D. (1974). Histopathology of one-stage bilateral lung allografts. *Ann. Surg.,* **180**: 753-759.

Kontos, G., Adachi, H., Borkon, A. M., Cameron, D. E., Baumgartner, W. A., Hall, T. S., Hutchins, G., Brawn, J., and Reitz, B. A. (1987). Successful four-hour heart-lung preservation with core cooling on cardiopulmonary bypass: a simplified model that assesses preservation. *J. Heart Transplant.,* **6**:106-111.

Koyama, I., Toung, T. J. K., Rogers, M. C., Gurtner, G. H., and Traystman, R. J. (1987). O2 radicals mediate reperfusion lung injury in ischemic O2 ventilated canine pulmonary lobe. *J. Appl. Physiol.,* **63**:111-115.

Ladowski, J. S., Kapelanski, D. P., Teodori, M. F., Stevenson, W. C., Hardesty, R. L., and Griffith, B. P. (1985). Use of autoperfusion for distant procurement of heart-lung allografts. *Heart Transplant.,* **4**:330-333.

Lall, A., Graf, P. D., Nadel, J. A., and Edmunds, L. H. (1973). Adrenergic reinnervation of the reimplanted dog lung. *J. Appl. Physiol.,* **35**:439-442.

Lima, O., Cooper, J. D., Peters, W. J., Ayabe, H., Townsend, E., Luk, S. C., and Goldberg, M. (1981). Effects of methylprednisolone and azathioprine on bronchial healing following lung transplantation. *J. Thorac. Cardiovasc. Surg.,* **82**:211-215.

Magovern, G. J., and Yates, A. J. (1964). Human homotransplantation of left lung: Report of a case. *Ann. NY Acad. Sci.,* **120**:710-728.

Mal, H., Andreassin, B., Pamela, F., Duchatelle, J. P., Rondeau, E., Dubois, F., Baldeyrou, P., Kitzis, M., Sleiman, C., and Pariente, R. (1989). Unilateral lung transplantation in end-stage pulmonary emphysema. *Am. Rev. Respir. Dis.,* **140**:797-802.

Maurer, J. R., McClean, P. A., Zamel, N., and Cooper, J. D. (1987). Airway hyperreactivity in patients undergoing single lung and lung/heart transplantation (abstract). *Am. Rev. Respir. Dis.,* **135**:A475.

McCord, J. M. (1985). Oxygen-derived free radicals in postischemic tissue injury. *N. Engl. J. Med.,* **312**:159-163.

Metras, H. (1950). Note preliminaire sur la greffe totale du poumon chez le chien. *C. R. Acad. Sci. (Paris)*, **231**:1176-1178.

Michelassi, F., Schuette, A., Landa, L., Zapol, W. M., and Grillo, H. C. (1987). Pulmonary and systemic contribution to canine tracheobronchial blood flow. *Ital. J. Surg. Sci.,* **17**:105-112.

Morgan, E., Lima, O., Goldberg, M., Ferdman, A., Luk, S. K., and Cooper, J. D. (1982). Successful revascularization of totally ischemic bronchial autografts with omental pedicle flaps in dogs. *J. Thorac. Cardiovasc. Surg.,* **84**:204-210.

Noiclerc, M., Metras, D., Vaillant, A., Cambouilives, J., Couvely, J. P., Pannetier, A., Garby, O., Chazalette, J. P., Goudard, A., and Carcassone, M. (in press). Technique chiururgicale de la transplantation bipulmonaire. *J. Lyon Chirurg.*

Novitzky, D., Wicomb, W. N., Cooper, D. K. C., Rose, A. G., Fraser, R. C., and Barnard, C. N. (1984). Electrocardiographic, hemodynamic, and endocrine changes occurring during experimental brain death in the chacma baboon. *J. Heart Transplant.,* **4**:63-69.

Novitzky, D., Cooper, D. K. C., and Reichart, B. (1987). Hemodynamic and metabolic responses to hormonal therapy in brain-dead potential organ donors. *Transplantation,* **43**:852-854.

Parks, D. A., Bulkley, G. B., and Granger, D. N. (1983). Role of oxygen free radicals in shock, ischemia, and organ preservation. *Surgery,* **94**: 428-432.

Patterson, G. A., Cooper, J. D., Dark, J. H., Jones, M. T., and Toronto Lung Transplant Group (1988a). Experimental and clinical double lung transplantation. *J. Thorac. Cardiovasc. Surg.,* **95**:70-74.

Patterson, G. A., Cooper, J. D., Goldman, B., Weisel, R. D., Pearson, F. G., Waters, O. F., Todd, T. R., Scully, H., Goldberg, M., and Ginsberg, R. J. (1988b). Technique of successful clinical double-lung transplantation. *Ann. Thorac. Surg.,* **4**:626-633.

Patterson, G. A., Todd, T. R., Cooper, J. D., Pearson, F. G., Winton, T. L., Maurer, J., and Toronto Lung Transplant Group (1990). Airway complications following double lung transplantation. *J. Thorac. Cardiovasc. Surg.,* **99**:14-20.

Paull, D. E., Keagy, B., Kron, E. J., and Wilcox, B. R. (1989a). Reperfusion injury in the lung preserved for 24 hours. *Ann. Thorac. Surg.,* **47**:187-192.

Paull, D. E., Keagy, B., Kron, E. J., and Wilcox, B. R. (1989b). Improved lung preservation using a dimethylthiourea flush. *J. Surg. Res.,* **46**: 333-338.

Pinsker, K. L., Montefusco, C., Yipintsoi, T., Kamholz, S. L., Norin, A., and Veith, F. J. (1979). Total in vivo functional adequacy of canine lung autografts after 24-hour preservation. *Transplant. Proc.,* **11**:599-602.

Pinsker, K. L., Kamholz, S. L., Montefusco, C., and Veith, F. J. (1981). Long-term functional adequacy of canine lung autografts after 24-hour preservation. *Transplant. Proc.,* **13**:715-717.

Popp, A. J., Shah, D. M., Berman, R. A., Paloski, W. H., Newell, J. C., Cooper, J. A., Rahm, R. L., Gottlieb, M. E., Bourke, R. S., and Malik, A. B. (1982). Delayed pulmonary dysfunction in head-injured patients. *J. Neurosurg.,* **57**:784-790.

Rabinovitch, J., Kirpikov, S., and Morosova, M. (1983). Conservation pulmonaire pendant 24 heures avec autogreffe retardee. *Ann. Chir.: Chir. Thorac. Cardiovasc.,* **37**:572-576.

Reichart, B. A., Novitsky, D., Cooper, D. K. C., Cunningham, M. S., and Rose, A. G. (1987). Successful orthotopic heart-lung transplantation in the baboon after five hours of cold ischemia with cardioplegia and Collins' solution. *J. Heart Transplant.,* **6**:15-22.

Reid, L. M. (1988). Chronic obstructive pulmonary diseases. In *Pulmonary Diseases and Disorders.* Edited by A. P. Fishman. New York, McGraw-Hill, pp. 1247-1272.

Reitz, B. A., Wallwork, J. L., Hunt, S. A., Pennock, J. L., Billingham, M. E., Oyer, P. E., Stinson, E. B., and Shumway, N. E. (1982). Heart-lung transplantation: Successful therapy for patients with pulmonary vascular disease. *N. Engl. J. Med.,* **306**:557-564.

Rich, S. (1988). Primary pulmonary hypertension. *Prog. Cardiovasc. Dis.,* **31**:205-238.

Sacks, S. A., Petrisch, P. H., and Kaufman, J. J. (1973). Canine kidney preservation using a new perfusate. *Lancet,* **1**:1024-1028.

Sanfillipo, F., Vaughan, W. K., Spees, E. K., Light, J. A., and LeFor, W. M. (1984). Benefits of HLA-A and HLA-B matching on graft and patient outcome after cadaveric-donor renal transplantation. *N. Engl. J. Med.,* **311**:358-364.

Scanlin, T. F. (1988). Cystic fibrosis. In *Pulmonary Diseases and Disorders.* Edited by A. P. Fishman. New York, McGraw-Hill, pp. 1273-1294.

Schafers, J. H., Frost, A. E., Waxman, M. B., Maurer, J. R., Grossman, R. F., Patterson, G. A., and Toronto Lung Transplant Group (1988). Cardiac innervation following double lung transplantation (abstract). *Am. Rev. Respir. Dis.,* **137**:245.

Schafers, H. J., Todd, T. R., Ginsberg, R. J., Goldberg, M. J., Patterson, G. A., Pearson, F. G., and Cooper, J. D. (in press). Bronchial complications following single lung transplantation. *J. Thorac. Cardiovasc. Surg.*

Scott, J., Higenbottam, T., Hutter, J., Hodson, M., Stewart, S., Penketh, A., and Wallwork, J. (1988). Heart-lung transplantation for cystic fibrosis. *Lancet,* **2**:192-194.

Starkey, T. D., Sakakibara, N., Hagberg, R. C., Tazelaar, H. D., Baldwin, J. C., and Jamieson, S. W. (1986). Successful six-hour cardiopulmonary preservation with simple hyperthermic crystalloid flush. *J. Heart Transplant.,* **5**:291-297.

Staudacher, V., Bellinazzo, P., and Pulin, A. (1950). Primi rilievi su tentativi di reimpianti autoplstici e di trapianti omoplastici di lobi polmonari. *Chirurgia* (*Milan*), **5**:223-227.

Stevens, G. H., Sanchez, M. M., and Chappell, G. L. (1973). Enhancement of lung preservation by prevention of lung collapse. *J. Surg. Res.,* **14**: 400-405.

Stevens, P. M., Johnson, P. C., Bell, R. L., Beall, A. C., and Jenkins, D. E. (1970). Regional ventilation and perfusion after lung transplantation in patients with emphysema. *N. Engl. J. Med.,* **282**:245-249.

Suarez, L. D., Seindaro, E. E., Llera, J. J., and Perosio, A. M. (1979). Long term follow up and primary pulmonary hypertension. *Br. Heart J.,* **41**: 702-708.

Sweeney, M. S., Sinnott, J. T., Cullison, J. P., and Weinstein, S. S. (1987). The use of OKT3 for stubbord heart allograft rejection: An advance in clinical immunotherapy? *J. Heart Transplant.,* **6**:324-328.

Thorpe, J. E., Baughman, R. P., Frame, P. T., Wesseler, T. A., and Staneck, J. L. (1987). Bronchoalveolar lavage for diagnosing acute bacterial pneumonia. *J. Infect. Dis.,* **155**:855-861.

Todd, T. R., Goldberg, M., Koshal, A., Menkis, A., Boychuk, J., Patterson, G. A., and Cooper, J. D. (1988). Separate extraction of cardiac and pulmonary grafts from a single organ donor. *Ann. Thorac. Surg.,* **46**:356-359.

Toledo-Pereyra, L. H., Hau, T., Simmons, R. L., and Najarian, J. S. (1977). Lung preservation techniques. *Ann. Thorac. Surg.,* **23**:487-494.

Toledo-Pereyra, L. H., and Condie, R. M. (1978). Lung transplantation. Hypothermic storage for 24 hours in a colloid hypoosmolar solution. *J. Thorac. Cardiovasc. Surg.,* **76**:846-852.

Toronto Lung Transplant Group (1988). Experience with single lung transplantation for pulmonary fibrosis. *JAMA,* **259**:2258-2262.

Veith, F. J. (1974). Preservation of the lung. *Transplant. Proc.,* **6**:323-328.

Veith, F. J., Koerner, S. K., Siegleman, S. S., Torres, M., Bardfield, P. A., Attai, L. A., Boley, S. J., Takaro, T., and Griedman, M. L. (1971a). Single lung transplantation in experimental and human emphysema. *Ann. Surg.,* **178**:463-476.

Veith, F. J., Sinha, S. B. P., Graves, J. S., Boley, S. J., and Dougherty, J. C. (1971b). Ischemic tolerance of the lung—The effect of ventilation and inflation. *J. Thorac. Cardiovasc. Surg.,* **61**:804-810.

Veith, F. J., Sinha, S. B. P., Blumcke, S., Dougherty, J. C., Becker, N. H., Siegleman, S. S., and Hagstrom, J. W. C. (1972). Nature and evolution of lung allograft rejection with and without immunosuppression. *J. Thorac. Cardiovasc. Surg.,* **63**:509-520.

Veith, F. J., Crane, R., Torres, M., Colon, I., Hagstrom, J. W. C., Pinsker, K., and Koerner, S. K. (1976). Effective preservation and transportation of lung transplants. *J. Thorac. Cardiovasc. Surg.,* **72**:97-105.

Wahlers, T., Haverick, A., Fieguth, H. G., Schafers, H. J., Takayama, T., and Borst, H. G. (1986). Flush perfusion using Euro-Collins solution vs cooling by means of extracorporeal circulation in heart-lung preservation. *J. Heart Transplant.,* **5**:89-98.

Wallwork, J., Jones, K., Cavarocchi, N., Hakim, M., and Higenbottam, T. (1987). Distant procurement of organs for clinical heart-lung transplantation using a single flush technique. *Transplantation,* **44**:654-658.

Wang, L. S., Yoshikawa, K., Miyoshi, S., Nakamoto, K., Hsieh, C. M., Yamazaki, F., Cardoso, P. F. G., Schafers, H. J., Brito, J., Keshavjee, S. H., Patterson, G. A., and Cooper, J. D. (1989). The effect of ischemic time and temperature on lung preservation using a simple exvivo rabbit model for functional assessment. *J. Thorac. Cardiovasc. Surg.,* **98**:333-342.

Wewers, M. D., Casolaro, M. A., Sellers, S. E., Swayze, S. C., McPhaul, K. M., Wittes, J. T., and Crystal, R. G. (1987). Replacement therapy for alpha-1 antitrypsin deficiency associated with emphysema. *N. Engl. J. Med.,* **316**:1055-1062.

White, J. J., Tanser, P. H., Anthonisen, N. R., Wynands, J. E., Pare, J. A. P., Becklake, M. R., Munro, D. D., and MacLean, L. D. (1966). Human lung homotransplantation. *Can. Med. Assoc. J.,* **94**:1199-1209.

Wildevuur, C. R., and Benfield, J. R. (1970). A review of 23 human lung transplantations by 20 surgeons. *Ann. Thorac. Surg.,* **9**:489-515.

Yacoub, M. H., Khaghani, A., Banner, N., Tajkarimi, S., and Fitzgerald, M. (1989). Distant organ procurement for heart and lung transplantation. *Transplant. Proc.,* **21**:2548-2550.

Yamashita, C., Oobo, H., Tsuji, F., Satoshi, T., Nakamura, K., Itoo, H., and Ejiri, K. (submitted). Lung transplantation: Effects of PGI2 analogue on reimplantation response.

AUTHOR INDEX

Italic numbers give the page on which the complete reference is listed.

Aaron, D., 452, 453, 454, 470, *483*
Aasen, A. O., 329, *330, 348*
Abendschein, D. R., 266, 267, 268, 269, *276*
Abernethy, K., 403, *406*
Abrams, L. M., 452, 453, 454, 470, *483*
Abrams, M. E., 385, *395*
Abrans, W., 386, *391*
Abrarus, W., 328, *333*
Abrouk, F., 150, *156*, 255, 257, 270, 271, 272, *278, 282*
Abston, S., 326, *334*
Adam, A., 307, 316, 323, 324, 326, *336, 342*
Adam, Y. G., 55, *60*
Adams, D. F., 425, 426, *430*
Adams, D. O., 314, 323, 324, 326, *330*
Adams, H. R., 263, *279*
Adachi, H., 511, *534*
Adkinson, N. F., Jr., 452, 481, *490*
Afshari, M., 258, *277*
Agostoni, A., 446, *448*
Agostoni, E., 170, *194*
Agusti-Vidal, A., 31, 33, *36, 55, 63*
Ahluwalia, B., 215, *220*
Aiegler, E. J., 401, *405*
Aiken, B. M., 312, *333*
Ailion, D. C., 417, 418, 419, 420, 421, 422, 423, 427, *428, 429, 430, 431*
Akerback, D., 142, *158*
Akesbi, A., 81, *87*
Akhtari, M., 422, 423, 427, *430*
Akins, C. W., 453, 472, 473, *486*
Albert, J. D., 86, *89*, 263, 264, *282*
Albert, R. K., 155, *156*, 434, *446, 447*
Albertine, K. H., 461, *482, 487*
Alberts, W. M., 53, *59*
Alderman, E. L., 269, 272, *275*

Alexander, R. S., 71, *74*
Ali, J., 446, *447*
Ali, M., 464, *486*
Alican, F., 492, *533*
Allan, R. M., 216, 217, *221*
Allen, P. S., 425, *429, 431*
Allison, R. C., 353, 358, 361, 362, 364, *365, 366*
Al-Mondhiry, H., 456, *482*
Alomram, A., 326, *330, 335, 339*
Alperovitch, A., 52, *61*
Altman, L. C., 311, *330*
Altose, M. D., 164, *194*
Amamou, M., 144, *159*
Amin, D., 71, *75*
Amundsen, E., 329, *348*
Andersen, J. M., 397, *408*
Andersen, R. W., 28, *34*
Anderson, B. D., 326, *339*
Anderson, D. J., 306, 315, *332*
Anderson, D. L., 3, 4, *19*
Anderson, P. S., 320, *341*
Anderson, R. R., 2, *18*, 306, *330*
Anderson, R. W., 226, *250*, 266, *281*
Andrada, L., 122, *136*
Andreassin, B., *534*
Andrews, C. P., 40, 42, 55, *59*, 81, *87*, 377, *378*
Andrivet, P., 255, *282*
Annat, G., 69, *73*, 188, *198*
Ansfield, M. J., 385, *391*
Ansquer, J. C., 144, 149, *159*
Anthonisen, N. R., 493, *538*
Antic, R., 115, *134*
Appel, P., 6, *21*
Appert, H., 320, *347*
Arakawa, K., 453, *485*
Archer, G. T., 314, *330*
Arens, J. F., 155, *158*
Arentzen, C. E., 226, *250*, 266, *281*
Argersinger, R. E., 424, 425, 426, *429*
Armanganidis, A., 155, *156, 276*
Arnold, K. F., 401, *406*
Arora, N. S., 178, *197*
Artigas, A., 45, 47, 48, 49, 50, 52, 53, 55, 56, *59, 60, 62*
Ashbaugh, D. G., 2, *18*, 23, 24, *33 35*, 37, 39, 54, *59*, 80, *87*, 139, 143, *156, 160,* 199, *219,* 286, *302, 304,* 305, *330, 346,* 367, *379,* 381, *391*
Astrand, P., 66, 71, *73*
Atlan, G., 144, 146, 147, 149, 154, *159*
Atlas, S. A., 309, *348*
Attai, L. A., 497, *537*
Aubier, M., 163, *194, 198*
Audran, R., *348*
Austen, K. F., 324, *337, 347*
Austen, W. G., 452, 453, 454, 456, 457, *485*
Auyama, T., 465, *482*
Avalli, L., 144, 146, 146, 150, 154, *157,* 423, *430*
Avery, D. M., 452, *489*
Avery, M. E., 145, *160*, 433, *449*
Avioli, L. V., 265, *276*
Ayabe, H., 429, 500, *532, 534*
Axler, O., 255, *282*
Ayars, G. H., 311, *330*

Bacalzo, L. V., 70, *75*
Bacharach, S. L., 263, *279*
Bache, R. J., 260, *276*
Bachmann, M., 50, 51, *62*, 316, *343*
Bachofen, H., 55, *59*, 147, 153, *156*, 445, *448*
Bachofen, M., 2, *19*, 55, *59*, 441, *447*
Back, U., 404, *406*
Badke, F. R., 226, *250*
Baehrendtz, S., 155, *156*
Baer, R. W., 261, *275*
Baggiolini, M., 311, *335, 344*
Baglioni, S., 150, 152, *157, 158, 211, 213, 214, 215, 220*
Bagniewski, A., 368, *380*
Bailey, G. L., 316, *349*
Baird, J. M., 65, *74*
Baird, M., 80, *88*, 305, *336*, 368, *378*
Baker, S. P., 313, *331*
Balder, A. E., 326, *339*
Baldeyrou, P., *534*
Baldwin, J. C., 510, 525, *532, 537*

Baldwin, S. R., *391*
Balk, R. A., 312, *352*
Ballantyne, H. K., 263, *279*
Balldin, G., 320, *345*
Banda, M. J., 314, 325, *338, 351*
Banerjee, C. M., 145, *160*
Banner, M. J., 188, 189, *194*
Banner, N., 511, *538*
Barabe, J., 309, *346*
Barash, P., 258, *277*
Barash, P. G., 266, 267, *274, 281*
Bardfield, P. A., 497, *537*
Baretta, G., 309, *332*
Barie, P. S., 320, *349*
Barlai-Kovach, M., 256, 260, 268, *277*
Barnard, C. N., 503, 506, *535*
Barnes, R. W., 452, 453, 454, 455, 457, *484*
Barr, H. A., 434, *449*
Barr, P. J., 324, *347*
Barrett, A. J., 306, 325, 326, 328, *331, 347*
Barry, B. E., *429*, 453, 461, *489*
Bar-Shavit, Z., 314, 325, *351*
Bartelt, D. C., 325, *346*
Bartlett, R. A., 109, 112, 115, *136*
Bartlett, R. G., Jr., 165, *194*
Bartlett, R. H., 253, *274*, 368, 370, 376, 377, *378, 380*
Basarab, R. M., 456, *482*
Base, W., 427, *430*
Basilico, E., 154, *157*
Baskin, T. L., 54, *62*
Bass, J. A., 82, *89*
Basset, G., 437, 438, 439, 441, 443, 444, 445, 446, *447, 449*
Bassi, F., 150, *157*
Batcher, S., 385, 388, *394*
Bates, D. V., 146, *159*
Bates, J. H. T., 116, 118, *133, 134*
Baugh, R., 311, 323, 324, *350*
Baughman, R. P., 520, *537*
Baumann, W., 305, *331*
Baumgartner, J.-D., 264, 274, *401*, 402, *405, 406*
Baumgartner, W., 234, 237, 238, *250*
Baumgartner, W. A., 511, *532, 534*
Bave, A. E., 70, *74*
Baydur, A., 120, 121, *134*, 171, *194*
Bazin, M., 50, *61*
Beall, A. C., 497, *537*
Beaton, M. K., 226, *250*
Bechard, D. E., 30, *34*
Becker, J., 147, 148, *159*
Becker, N. H., 521, *538*
Becker, V., 316, *331*
Becklake, M. R., 493, *538*
Beel, R. J., 328, *335*
Befus, D., 426, *432*
Begin, P., 105, 114, 118, *136,* 142, *160*
Begley, C. J., 288, 289, 290, 293, 294, 295, 296, *302, 304*
Behrakis, P. K., 120, 121, *134*,, 171, *194*
Bell, D. R., 71, *74*
Bell, R. C., 24, 25, 26, 31, 32, *33, 36*, 40, 42, 44, 48, 55, *59*, 65, *73*, 77, 78, 79, 81, *87*, 93, *103*, 263, *274*, 305, *331*, 368, 376, 377, *378*
Bell, R. L., 497, *537*
Bellemare, F., 178, *194*
Bellinazzo, P., 492, *537*
Bellman, S. M., 18, *19*
Bellows, C. F., 462, *489*
Bemis, C., 258, *277*
Benavente, A., 324, *334*
Bender, B. S., 83, 85, *87*
Bendixen, H. H., 144, *156*
Benfield, J. R., 493, 497, *538*
Benhamou, D., 122, *134*
Benito, S., 142, 145, 147, 148, 154, *156, 159*
Ben Lakhal, S., 150, *156*
Bennett, E. J ., 368, *379*
Benson, B. J., 383, 385, *391*
Benson, K., 305, *337*
Benson, K. N., 31, *34*, 45, 48, *60*, 65, *74*, 80, *88*, 305, *336*, 368, *378*
Benson, K. T., 453, *485*
Berberick, S., 84, *88*

Berg, R., 84, *88*
Berg, R. A., 321, *342*
Bergel, D. H., 239, *250*
Berger, H. J., 71, *73*
Berger, H. W., 55, *61*
Berggren, P., 387, *391*
Bergman, N. A., 120, 127, *134*, 173, *194*
Beri, J. E., *343*
Berman, D. S., 258, *278*
Berman, R. A., 503, *536*
Bernard, G. R., 24, 32, *33*, 186, *198*, 286, 288, 296, 297, 298, 299, *302*, 427, *429*, 468, *482*
Bernard, H., 85, *89*
Bernardi, L., 248, *250*
Bernasconi, M., 105, 106, 110, 114, 118, 119, *134*
Berninger, R. W., 315, *344*
Bernito, S., 193, *194*
Berry, D., 385, 388, *391*, 459, 464, 467, *490*
Berry, L. C., 286, *302*
Bertram, T. A., 461, 462, *482, 483, 484*
Bertrand, O., 188, *198*
Besbes, M., 255, *282*
Best, N., 461, 464, *483*
Beutler, B., 86, *87, 89,* 263, 264, *274, 282*
Bhat, R., 387, *394*
Bhattacharya, J., 217, *219*
Bianco, J. A., 272, *281*
Bierman, M., 452, 457, *484*
Bieth, J. G., 312, 313, 323, 325, 326, *331, 332, 345*
Bigelow, D. B., 2, *18*, 23, *33*, 37, 39, 54, *59*, 139, *156*, 199, *219*, 286, *302*, 305, *330*, 381, *391*
Bigelow, D. D., 80, *87*
Bigland-Ritchie, B., 167, *194*
Bihardi, B., 71, *73*
Bihari, D., 263, *274*
Billingham, M. E., 529, *536*
Binion, J. T., 265, *275*
Bion, J. F., 102, *103*
Biondi, J. W., 266, 267, *274, 281*
Bismuth, H., 101, *104*
Bitran, D. D., 464, *486*
Bitterman, P. B., 425, *429*
Bizzari, D. V., 66, 67, *75*
Black, L. F., 179, *194*
Blackburn, C. W., 427, *430*
Blackstone, E. H., 307, *333*, 377, *379*
Blackstone, E. W., 464, *486*
Blair, I., 288, *302*
Blaisdell, F. W., 31, *34*, 367, *378*
Blake, L. H., 446, *447*
Blanc, P. L., 149, *158*
Blanch, L., 193, *194*
Blank, N. E., 202, *220*
Blatter, D. D., 417, 418, 420, 421, 427, *428, 429, 431*
Bleifeld, W. H., 258, *279*
Blinc, R., 425, *430*
Blomqvist, G., 270, *275*
Bloom, B., 387, *393*
Blumcke, S., 521, *538*
Blumenstock, F. A., 85, *89*, 320, *349*
Bode, J., 115, *134*
Bodson, L., 226, 306, 307, 316, 323, 324, *335, 336, 341, 342*
Bogard, W. C., 403, *408*
Bogard, W. C., Jr., 403, *406*
Boggis, C., 259, *282*
Bog-Hansen, T. C., 404, *406*
Bohnsack, J. F., 83, 85, *87*
Boisante, L., 226, *250*, 256, 260, 266, 267, 270, *277*
Boisvert, D. P. J., 425, *429*
Bolcerzak, S. P., 288, *304*
Bolds, J. M., 288, *303*
Boley, S. J., 497, 510, *537*
Bombeck, C. T., 368, *379*
Bombino, M., 144, 145, 146, 150, 152, *157, 158,* 211, 213, 214, 215, *220*, 423, *430*
Bond, J. S., 307, 311, 321, *331*
Bone, R. C., 32, *33*, 144, *156*, 307, 309, 311, 321, *331*
Border, D., 315, *332*
Border, J. R., 315, *332*
Bore, C. F., 424, 425, *432*
Borg, T., 17, *19*, 306, *332*

Borgström, A., 320, *345*, 452, 453, 458, 463, 467, *486*

Borkon, A. M., 234, 237, 238, *250*, 511, *532, 534*

Borman, K. R., 300, 307, *304, 350*

Borovetz, H. S., 2, *20*

Borst, H. G., 511, *538*

Boswell, D. R., 323, *333*

Bottomley, P. A., 424, 425, 426, *429*

Bouchama, A., 81, *87*

Bouffard, J. A., 452, 453, 454, 456, 460, *489*

Bouma, B. N., 309, *332*

Bourdarias, J. P., 226, *250*, 256, 260, 266, 267, 270, *277*

Bourke, R. S., 503, *536*

Bouwman, D. L., 316, *350*

Bove, A. A., 239, *249*, 261, *275*

Bowen, J., 311, 323, 324, *350*

Bowers, R. E., 288, 300, *302*, 306, *332*

Bowman, C. M., 286, *304*

Boxer, L. A., *391*

Boychuk, J., 506, *537*

Boyco, W. J., 17, *21*, 306, *349*

Boylen, C. T., 305, *331*

Bradenberg, C. E., 28, *34*

Bradley, R., 296, 297, 298, 299, *302*

Brady, T. J., 413, *432*

Brain, J. D., 306, *332*, 453, 461, 462, *489, 490*

Brainwald, E., 177, *197*

Brasch, R. C., 424, 427, *431, 432*

Bratton, D. L., 312, 314, *338*

Braude, A. I., 264, *283*, 400, 401, 402, 403, *406, 407, 409, 410*

Braum, M., 316, *341*

Braun, M., 306, 307, 316, *335*

Braun, N. M. T., 178, 183, *194, 197*

Braunwald, E., 265, *275*

Braverman, B., 140, *156*

Brawn, J., 511, *532, 534*

Bredengerg, C. E., 384, 388, *394*, 434, *447*

Brendel, W., 452, 453, 454, 455, 457, 458, 463, 464, *483, 485*

Brennan, S. O., 323, *333*

Brenner, M., 263, *282*

Brent, B. N., 71, 73

Bretz, U., 311, *335, 344*

Brigham, K. L., 37, *62*, 286, 288, 289, 290, 291, 292, 293, 294, 295, 296, 297, 298, 299, 300, 302, 303, 304, 305, 306, *338*, 427, *429*, 446, *447*, 464, 468, 471, 472, *482, 483, 487*

Brimioulle, S., *282*

Brinker, J. A., *249*

Brinker, P. A., 370, 377, *378*

Brito, J., 511, *538*

Brochard, L., 189, *194*

Brodrick, J. N., 326, *342*

Brody, A. R., 461, *482, 483*

Brody, A. W., 120, 124, *134*

Bromberg, P. A., 125, *136*

Bromberger-Barnea, B., 239, 248, *250*, 254, 268, *280, 281, 283*

Brower, R. G., 248, *249*

Brown, E., 16, *19*

Brown, M. A., 326, 328, *331*

Brown, R., 226, *250*, 268, 272, *281*

Brubach, H. F., 165, *194*

Bruce, E. W., 167, 171, *196*

Bruch, M., 325, *332*

Bruins, S. C., 400, 401, *407*

Brun, P., 81, *87*

Brun-Buisson, C., 53, *61*, 144, 147, 148, 149, 150, *156, 159*, 255, 257, *282*

Brunet, F., 155, *156*, 256, 258, 266, 270, *276*

Bryan, A. C., 446, *448*

Bshouty, Z., 446, *447*

Buchser, E., 55, 57, *59*

Buckberg, G. D., 316, *349*

Buckingham, P. D., 217, *220*

Buda, A. J., 226, *249*, 269, 272, *275*

Budinger, T. F., 413, *429*

Bueschine, W. J., 461, *484*

Buford, T. H., 23, *34*

Bulkley, G. B., 511, *535*

Bundsen, P., 323, *347*

Bunn, J., 193, *195*

Buonanno, F. S., 413, *432*

Burbank, B., 23, *34*
Burch, C., 263, 264, *279*
Burchard, K. W., 306, *348*
Burger, E. J., 145, *156*
Burgess, B. F., Jr., 124, *134*
Burke, R. A., 84, *88*
Burke, R. A., 84, *88*
Burns, S. R., 69, *74*
Burrowes, C. E., 324, *333*
Busuito, M. J., 316, *350*
Butany, J., *533*
Butler, J., *20*, 45, 48, *62*, 254, 258, 267, 268, *275, 278, 279, 282,* 434, *446, 447, 448*
Butler, P. E., 307, 311, 321, *331*

Cain, S. M., 66, 67, 71, *73*
Calaf, N., 142, *159*
Calandra, T., 402, *406*
Calandrino, F. S., 306, 315, *332*
Caldini, P., 268, *281*
Calindrino, F. S., Jr., 3, 4, *19*
Callahan, L., 403, *407*
Calore, J., 323, *352*
Calore, J. D., 323, *333*
Calvano, S., 263, 264, *282*
Calverley, P. M. A., 105, 114, 118, 123, 124, 129, *135, 136,* 142, *160*
Calvin, J. E., 261, 266, 268, *275*
Cambouilives, J., 517, *535*
Cameron, D. E., 511, *534*
Cameron, J. L., 82, *87*
Campbell, E. J., 312, 314, 325, 326, *332, 348, 351*
Campbell, E. J. M., 183, *195*
Campisi, D. J., 70, *75*
Campos, R. A., 93, *104*
Cane, R. D., 139, *160*
Canet, J., 126, *136*
Canizaro, P. C., 255, *278*
Cantin, A. M., 323, *339*
Capper, M. W., 177, 189, *195*
Capps, J. S., 170, *196*
Carcassone, M., 517, *535*
Cardoso, P. F., 510, 511, *534, 538*
Carey, L. S., 424, 426, *432*
Carli, F., 123, 124, 129, *135*
Carlon, G. C., 155, *159*
Carlson, C. J., 266, 267, 268, 269, *276*
Caroll, G. C., 140, *156*
Carp, H., 311, 323, *332, 340*
Carrell, R., 324, *332*
Carrell, R. N., *337*
Carrell, R. W., 323, *333*
Carrico, C. J., 3, 4, 6, 7, 8, *20*, 24, 25, 26, 28, 30, 31, 32, 33, *35*, 38, 40, 42, 44, 45, 47, 48, 51, *62*, 77, 78, *88, 89*, 253, 255, 263,, *278, 279,* 305, 316, *343, 345,* 368, 370, 376, *379*
Carrico, C. T., 101, *104*
Carrico, L. J., 297, *304*
Carrico, S. C., 65, *75*
Carroll, F. E., 424, 425, 426, 427, *429, 431*
Carson, J., 139, *156*
Carson, S. D., 266, 268, *276*
Carvalho, A. A., 306, 309, *333*
Carvalho, A. C. A., 18, *19*, 306, 310, *347*, 452, 454, 457, 458, 460, 463, *487*
Case, T. A., 417, 418, 419, 420, 421, 422, 423, 427, *428, 429, 430*
Casolari, M. A., 324, 329, *351*, 496, *538*
Cassidy, S. S., 265, 268, 270, *275*
Cassiman, J. J., 328, *350*
Castella, J., 50, *59*
Casthely, P. A., 452, 453, 454, 470, *483*
Castorena, G., 264, *279*
Castro, M. E., 425, *429*
Catanazaro, A., 385, 388, *394*
Caubergh, M., 126, *135*
Caughey, G., 386, *394*
Cavarocchi, N. C., 464, *483*, 510, *538*
Celli, B. R., 84, *88*
Cengiz, M., 55, 57, *60*
Cenotti, L., 270, 271, 272, *278*
Centor, R. M., 30, *34*

Cerami, A., 86, *87, 89,* 263, 264, *282*
Cerami, A. C., 264, 265, *274, 282*
Cerra, F. B., 305, *333*
Cerretelli, P., 68, *75*
Chadwick, L. E., 139, *160*
Chan, J. Y. C., 324, *333*
Chan, M. K. W., 86, *87*, 263, *279*
Chance, B., 69, *73*
Chandler, A., 384, *391*
Chang, H. K., 114, *134*
Chang, S.-W., 452, 453, 457, *483*
Chapman, H. A., 314, 325, *333*
Chappel, G. L., 510, *537*
Chastre, J., 31, *34*, 81, *87*
Chaudry, I. H., 70, *74*
Chazalette, J. P., 517, *535*
Chedid, L. A., 404, *410*
Chedid, L. C., 399, *409*
Chelucci, G. L., 155, *156*
Chen, V., 444, *448*
Cheng, C., 258, *280*, 510, *532*
Chenoweth, D. E., 307, *333, 350*, 377, *379,* 454, 455, 456, 457, 458, 459, 463, 464, 465, 467, 468, 475, *483, 486, 487*
Cherniack, R. M., 165, *195*
Cheung, A. K., 464, *483*
Cheung, H., 256, 260, *281*
Cheville, N. F., 461, *490*
Chiles, C., 202, *220*
Chiolero, R., 55, 57, *59*, 264, *274*, 401, *405*
Chmielewski, R., 80, *89*
Cho, K., 314, *349*
Christer, P., 328, *333*
Christman, J., 306, *347*
Christner, P., 386, *391*
Christou, N. V., 81, *88*
Chung, H., 211, *221*
Cimason, G., 314, *340*
Civetta, J. M., 140, 141, *157, 158, 160,* 255, *276*
Clark, A., 323, *352*
Clark, B. J., 69, *73*
Clark, E. J., 325, *338*
Clark, J. M., 312, *333*
Clark, R. A., 323, *333*
Clarkson, S., 461, *488*
Clasen, C., 329, *333*
Claus, D. R., 464, *483*
Claypool, W. D., 384, *391*
Clement, J., 146, *157*
Clements, J. A., 122, *134*, 145, *156*, 383, 384, 389, *392, 395,* 434, *449*
Clemmer, T. P., 32, 33, *34*
Cluff, L. E., 399, *406*
Clyman, R. I., 389, *392*
Coalson, J. J., 24, 26, *33, 35,* 42, 44, 48, *59*, 65, *73*, 77, 78, 79, 80, 81, 82, 86, *87, 88,* 93, *103,* 263, *274*, 305, *331*, 368, 376, 377, *378*
Cochrane, C. G., 309, 311, 323, 324, 328, *333, 334, 341, 352,* 383, 384, 386, 388, 389, *392, 393, 394, 395*
Cockrell, J. V., 521, *534*
Coffano, B., 206, *220*
Coffey, J. W., 211, *221*
Coggeshall, J. W., 193, *195*
Cohen, A. B., 323, *334, 347,* 386, *393*
Cohen, A. T., 367, *379*
Colditz, I. G., 263, *279*
Coleridge, H. M., 270, *275*
Coleridge, J. C. G., 270, *275*
Collee, G. C., 364, *365*
Colley, C. M., 315, 323, *334, 336*
Collier, C., 154, *160*
Collins, J. A., 28, *34*, 367, *378*
Collins, J. C., 427, *429*
Colman, R. W., 309, 323, 324, *334, 335, 337, 347*
Colocousis, J., 255, *278*
Colon, I., 510, *538*
Compean, R., 226, 239, *251*, 268, *282*
Comroe, J. H., Jr., 120, *134*
Condie, R. M., *537*
Conklin, J. J., 263, *279*
Connolly, N. L., 314, *348*
Constantian, M. B., 326, 329, *334*

Conzen, P. F., 452, 453, 454, 455, 457, 458, 463, 464, *483, 485*
Cook, C. D., 147, *156*
Cook, J. A., 306, *346*
Cook, R., 314, *349*
Cooper, D. K. C., 503, 506, 510, *535, 536*
Cooper, J. A., 437, *447*, 503, *536*
Cooper, J. D., 464, *486*, 492, 494, 495, 500, 506, 510, 511, 513, 516, 521, 524, 528, 532, 533, *534, 535, 536, 537, 538*
Cooper, S. W., 307, *337*
Cooperland, S. R., 326, *334*
Cope, D. K., 353, 361, 362, 364, *365*
Corbeil, L. B., 402, *407*
Cott, G. R., 383, *393*
Cotta, L. A., 306, 307, *348*
Cottrell, T. S., 440, 441, *447*
Cournand, A., 265, *275*
Courtney, M., 323, 324, *334, 339*, 383, 389, *394*
Couvely, J. P., 517, *535*
Cox, S. C., 305, *334*
Craddock, P. R., 286, *303*, 306, 307, *338*
Craig, J. M., 147, *156*
Crandall, E. D., 437, *448*
Crane, R., 510, *538*
Crapo, J. D., *429*, 462, 469, *484, 485*
Crapo, R. D., 55, *60*
Craven, D. E., 84, *88*, 400, 401, *407*
Craven, K. D., 254, *275*
Crawford, M. H., 470, *486*
Crocker, S. H., 461, *484*
Crockford, G., 403, *408*
Crooks, L., 413, 424, *430*
Crosher, G. A., 427, *431*
Crottogini, A., 261, *280*
Crutchley, D. J., 315, *334*
Crystal, R., 323, *339*
Crystal, R. G., 312, 324, 329, *337, 334, 351*, 425, *429*, 438, 439, *449*, 496, *538*
Cullison, J. P., 521, *537*
Cuddy, T. E., 66, 71, *73*
Culver, B. H., 170, 174, 188, 193, *196, 197*, 254, 267, 268, *275, 278*
Cunningham, D. D., 325, *341*
Cunningham, D. G., 211, *221*, 256, 260, *281*
Cunningham, L. W., 328, *334*
Cunningham, M. S., 510, *536*
Cunnington, P. G., 400, *407*
Cunnion, R. E., 264, *276*
Curd, J. G., 464, *486*
Curien, N., 256, 260, 266, 267, 270, *277*
Curreri, P. W., 310, *342, 343*
Curstedt, T., 387, 390, *391, 394*
Cury, J. D., 314, *348*
Cutillo, A., 425, *430*
Cutillo, A. G., 416, 417, 418, 419, 420, 421, 422, 423, 427, *428, 429, 430, 431*
Cutz, E., 446, *448*
Cybulsky, M. I., 86, *87*, 263, *279*
Cymerman, A., 66, *75*
Czer, L. S. C., 6, *21*

Dagoett, W. M., 453, 472, 473, *486*
Dall'Ava-Santucci, J., 155, *156*
Dalton, M. L., 492, *533*
Da Luz, P. L., 25, 31, *34*
Damas, F., 316, *335*
Damas, P., 306, 316, 323, 324, 326, *335, 341, 342*
D'Ambra, M., 453, 472, 473, *486*
Damia, G., 446, *448*
Dammenhayn, L., 511, *533*
Damske, B. A., 263, *279*
Danek, S. J., 66, 69, *74*, 140, *157*
Dang, A. Q., 252, 254, 259, 463, 467, 470, *484*
Dangott, L. J., 328, *334*
Daniels, J. C., 326, *334*
Danilowicz, R., 461, *482*
Dannmiller, F. J., 140, *158*
Dantzker, D. R., 66, 67, 69, *74*, 140, *157*
Dargent, F., 50, 51, *62*, 316, *343*

Dark, J. H., *535*
Dart, C. H., 316, *345*
Daszkiewsicz, O. K., 425, *430*
Dauber, J. H., 306, *347*
Dauge, M., 81, *87*
Daughters, G. T., II., 269, 272, *275*
David, J. K., 215, *220*
Davie, E. W., 309, *334*
Davies, P., 259, *282*
Davis, B., 306, *350*
Davis, C. E., 400, 401, *406, 410*
Davis, J. W., 226, *250*, 266, *281*
Davis, W. B., 2, *19*, 306, *339*
Dawson, C. A., 356, *365*
Dawson, H., 316, *340*
De Agostini, A., 324, *335*
Deanfiled, J., 216, 217, *221*
de Anta, M. T. J., 31, 33, *36*
Dear, C. L., 525, *532*
Dearing, R., 311, *340*
Debanne, M. T., 328, *335*
De Bos, M., 402, *406*
Deby, C., 306, 316, *335, 341*
Deby-Dupont, G., 306, 316, 319, 323, 324, 326, *335, 336, 341, 342*
de Camp, M. M., 462, *490*
De Camp, M. M., Jr., 461, 462, *489*
De Campo, T., 255, *276*
Decker, S. A., 461, *482*
de Deckker, F. A., 404, *410*
Degges, R. D., 452, 454, 459, 463, 467, *470*
De Gournay, J. M., *276*
Degryse, E., 383, 389, *394*
Dehring, D. J., 462, *484*
Deitch, E. A., 84, *88*, 315, *335*
De Jongh-Leuvenink, J., 402, *406*
de la Bellacasa, J. P., 31, 33, *36*
De Latoree, F. J., 48, *59, 60*
Delavault, E., 126, *134*
Del Guercio, L. R., 263, *281*
Dellinger, E. P., 94, 100, 101, *103*
De Los Santos, R., 33, *35*
Delpierre, S., 509, *533*
DeMars, D., 321, *341*
Demedts, M., 146, *157*
Demers, R. R., 186, *195*
Desfond, P., 50, *61*
Desrochers, P. E., 323, *335*
Devall, L. J., *391*
Devaux, J. Y., 256, 258, 266, 270, *276*
Dewald, B., 311, *335*
Dewater, R., 325, *335*
Dhainaut, J. F., 155, *156*
Diamond, J. M., 316, *335*
Dietschy, J. M., 399, 400, 402, *408*
Dijkman, J. H., 325, *335*
De Lisio, R., 29, *36*
Dimcheff, D. G., 54, *63*
Dinarello, C. A., 263, *279*, 404, *408*
Dine, N. L., 54, *60*
Di Prampero, P. E., 68, *75*
Dobb, G. J., 142, 157
Dobbs, L., 383, 389, *395*
Dobbs, L. G., 383, *392, 393*
Doherty, K., 234, 237, 238, *250*
Dollery, C. T., 255, *283*
Dolovich, J., 328, *335*
Dolovich, M. B., 145, *160*
Domart, Y., 33, *34*
Domingue, G. J., 402, *408*
Don, H. F., 142, 157
Donnelly, P. K., 326, *330, 335*
Dorinsky, P. M., 71, *75*, 139, *157*, 265, *276*, 306, *350*
Dorph, S., 261, *280*
Dosman, J., 115, *134*
Dougherty, J. C., 510, 521, *537, 538*
Douglas, H., 264, 283, 400, 401, 402, 403, *406, 407, 409, 410*
Douglas, M. E., 54, *60*
Downey, J., 360, 361, *365*
Downs, J. B., 54, *60*, 140, *158*
Doyle, T., 311, *330*
Draper, E. A., 31, *35*, 92, 93, 94, 95, 101, *103, 104*
Drazen, J. M., 114, *135*
Dreyfuss, D., 437, 438, 441, 443, 444, 445, 446, *447*
Driedger, A. A., 2, *18, 21,* 256, 260, 266, *275, 281,* 306, *330, 346*

Driks, M. R., 84, *88*
Drinker, P. A., 368, *380*
Drugge, U., 452, 453, 454, *488*
Druml, W., 427, *430*
Dubois, A. B., 122, 124, *134, 135*
Dubois, F., 525, *534*
Dubourg, O., 256, *277*
Du Buy, J. B., 400, 403, *406*
Duchateau, J., 14, 15, 16, *19,* 306, 307, 316, 326, *335, 336, 341*
Duchatelle, J. P., *534*
Duke, J. T., 452, 470, *484*
Duke, S., 288, *303*
Duke, S. S., 288, *303*
Dumond, M. E., 361, 362, *365*
du Moulin, G. C., 83, *88*
Duncan, C. A., 305, *334*
Dunn, D. L., 403, *406*
Dunn, J. T., 309, *341*
Dunn, S., *533*
Durand, D. J., 389, *392*
Durney, C. H., 417, 418, 419, 421, 422, 423, 427, *429, 430, 431*
Durst, A. L., 316, *345*
Duswald, K. H., 314, 326, *336, 340*
Dutton, R. E., 254, *278, 280*

Eaton, R. J., 265, *276*
Eberle, D. J., 65, *74*, 80, *88*, 305, *336*, 368, *378*
Eckert, C., 254, *278*
Eckstein, E., 80, *89*
Eddeland, A., 325, *336*
Eddy, D. O., 461, *484*
Edlin, S. A., 102, *103*
Edmunds, L. H., 368, *380*, 524, *534*
Effros, R. M., 211, *219*, 306, *336*
Egan, E. A., 384, *393*, 435, 436, 445, *447*
Egbert, L. D., 144, *156*
Ehrenfreund, C., 403, *407*
Ehrlich, Y. D., 321, *341*
Eiseman, B., 80, *89*
Eisenstein, R., 464, 467, *488*
Ejiri, K., *538*
Elam, J. O., 122, *134*

El-Etr-A.A., 269, 270, 272, *279*
El Hag, A., 323, *333*
Eling, T. E., 461, *482, 483*
Eliott, E. A., 114, *135*
Eliraz, A., 44, 48, *60*, 80, *88*
Elliott, C. G., 55, 57, *60*
Ellner, J. J., 80, *89*
Ellsworth, M. L., 71, *74*
Engler, R., 325, *345*
Englert, M., 54, *63*
English, D., 291, 292, 293, 294, *304*
English, D. K., 291, *303*
English, M., 254, *278*
Enhorning, G., 384, 387, 389, *392*
Enzan, K., 461, *488*
Eraslan, S., 492, *533*
Erdmann, J., 215, *220*
Erdös, E. G., 470, *488, 489*
Ertel, N., 464, 467, *488*
Esbenshade, A. M., 288, *303*
Eschenbacher, W. L., 270, *275*, 306, *343*
Esmon, C. T., 315, *336*
Esnard, F., 325, *345*
Estopa, R., 48, 55, *59, 60, 63*
Evans, B. H., 367, *378*

Fadali, M. A., 452, 470, *484*
Fagon, J.-Y., 33, *34*
Fahey, T. J., III., 86, *89*, 263, 264, *282*
Fairley, H. B., 141, 142, 148, 154, *158, 161*, 253, *274*, 368, 370, 376, *378*
Fairman, R. P., 452, 457, *484*
Faling, L. J., 31, 33, *34*
Falke, K. J., 139, 143, 154, *157, 159,* 211, *219*
Fallat, R. J., 48, 54, *60, 61,* 305, *336,* 368, *380*
Fantone, C., 311, *336*
Fantone, J., 286, *303*
Farber, H. W., 84, *88*
Farcot, J. C., 226, *250*, 256, 260, 266, 267, 270, *277*
Faridy, E. E., 145, *157,* 433, 434, *447*

Farre, R., 126, *136*
Faymonville, M. E., 306, 307, 316, 319, 323, 324, 326, *335, 336, 341, 342*
Fazio, F., 216, 217, *221*
Fearon, D. T., 324, *336*
Feeley, T. W., 202, *220*, 427, *431*
Fehr, J., 452, 458, 459, 464, *484*
Fein, A., 2, *19*, 26, *34*, 306, 328, *333, 336,* 386, *391*
Fein, A. M., 44, 48, *60*, 80, *88*, 328, *342*
Feinstein, G., 314, *336*
Fells, G. A., 312, 323, *337, 339*
Fenn, W. O., 139, *157, 160*
Ferdman, A., 492, 494, *532, 535*
Fernandez, H. N., 459, *484*
Fernandez, R., 193, *194*
Ferrari, B. T., 316, *349*
Ferris, B. G., 153, *157*
Fessler, H. E., 248, *249*
Feuth, H., 325, *339*
Fewell, J. E., 266, 267, 268, 269, *276*, 452, 453, 454, 455, 457, *484*
Fick, R. B., 314, *344*
Fiedel, B. A., 464, *484, 488*
Fieguth, H. G., 511, *533, 538*
Fields, A., 68, *74*
Fierer, J., 264, *283*, 401, *410*
Fiers, W., 265, *278*
Filiatrault, S., 118, *134*
Finegold, D. S., 80, *89*
Fink, M. P., 263, *279*
Finkelstein, J. N., 385, 388, *393*
Fiorica, N. O., 437, *447*
Fiser, W. P., 452, 453, 454, 455, 457, *484*
Fisher, A. B., 384, *391*
Fisher, B. J., 30, *34*
Fisher, C. J., 32, *33*
Fisher, M. M., 464, *483*
Fishman, A. P., 261, *283*, 440, 441, *447*, 495, *534*
Fittschen, C., 312, 314, *338*
Fitzgerald, M., 511, *538*
Fitzgibbon, C., 452, 454, 455, 456, 457, 458, 459, 460, 463, 465, *486, 487*
Fitzpatrick, F. A., 470, *486*
Fleck, A., 315, *336*
Flesk, A., 323, *334*
Fletcher, J. R., 265, *281*
Fleury, B., 181, 184, 190, 191, *195*
Flick, M. R., 2, 4, *20*, 38, *51*, 286, 303, 306, 316, *336, 344,* 370, *379*, 459, 460, *484, 487*
Flynn, J. T., 459, 464, 467, *485, 487, 489*
Foda, H. D., 471, 472, *488*
Fong, Y., 263, 264, 265, *282*
Fontcuberta, J., 50, *59, 60*
Forkert, P. G., 446, *448*
Forrest, J. B., 433, *448*
Forrester, J. S., 258, *278*
Forse, R. A., 31, *35*, 79, *88*
Foscue, H. A., *429*
Foster, M. A., 427, *431*
Foster, M. E., 452, 454, 459, 463, 467, 470, *484*
Foster, T. H., 424, 425, 426, *429*
Fowler, A. A., 3, 7, 8, *19*, 24, 26, 28, 30, 31, 32, *34, 35,* 40, 44, 45, 48, *60*, 65, *74*, 80, *88*, 263, *277*, 305, 336, 337, 340, 368, *378*
Fowler, S. R., 83, *89*
Fox, D. K., 453, *485*
Fox, U., 446, *448*
Fraki, J. I., 314, *349*
Frame, P. T., 520, *537*
Franchimont, P., 316, 323, 324, 326, *335, 341, 342*
Francica, P., 462, *484*
Francis, D. M., 326, *330, 335*
Francis, P. B., 309, *331*
Frank, L., 425, *430*
Frank, M. M., 83, 85, *87*
Frank, N. R., 147, *156*
Franken, C., 325, *335*
Franks, J. J., 310, *338*
Fransen, J., 325, *335*
Franzblau, C., 323, *333, 352*

Fraser, R. C., 503, 506, *535*
Fraser, R. G., 146, *159*
Frazer, D. G., 145, *157*
Fredberg, J. J., 125, *134*
Frederick, T. M., 263, *279*
Freedman, H. H., 403, *406*
Freeman, B. A., 469, *485*
Freeman, G. L., 452, *489*
Fridhandler, L., *343*
Fridy, W. W., Jr., 146, *158*
Friedman, A. S., 265, *280*
Fritsch, A., 326, *351*
Fritts, L. L., 314, *344*
Fritz, H., 314, 326, 329, 331, 336, 337, 340
Froese, A. B., 446, *448*
Froment, M., 69, *73*
Frost, A., 524, *532, 536*
Fry, D. E., 31, *34*, 78, 84, *88*
Fujikawa, K., 309, *334*
Fujita, M., 465, *482*
Fujiwara, T., 389, *392*
Fukuzaki, M., 425, *432*
Fulkerson, W. J., 291, 292, 293, 294, 303, 304
Fullerton, G. D., 413, *430*
Fullton, J. M., 126, *134*
Fulton, R. L., 31, *34*, 78, *88*, 367, *379*
Fumagalli, R., 150, 152, *157, 158,* 206, 211, 213, 214, 215, *220,* 444, *448*
Fung, W. P., 325, *337*
Fyman, P. N., 452, 453, 454, 470, *483*

Gaar, K. A., 354, 360, *365*
Gabel, J. C., 155, *158*
Gadek, J. E., 2, *19*, 71, *75*, 306, 312, *337, 339, 350, 351*
Gadian, D. G., 68, *74*
Gagnon, J., 308, *340*
Gallagher, T. J., 140, *157*
Gallimore, M., 306, *350*
Gammon, M. T., 403, *407*
Ganesan, K., 422, 423, 427, *430*
Gann, D. S., 306, *348*
Garbe, L., 509, *533*
Garbisa, S., 315, *341*
Garby, O., 517, *535*
Garcia, J., 316, *340*
Gardiner, M., 265, *281*
Garrison, R. N., 84, *88*
Garvin, G. M., 84, *88*
Garzon, A. A., 510, *532, 533*
Gateau, O., 148, *161*
Gattinoni, L., 144, 145, 146, 150, 152, 154, *157, 158,* 202, 204, 206, 208, 211, 212, 213, 214, 215, 218, *219, 220,* 377, *379,* 423, *430,* 446, *448*
Gauthier, F., 325, *345*
Gavazzeni, V., 206, *220*
Gavrilovic, J., 325, *338*
Gawryl, M. S., 306, 307, 309, *342*
Gee, I. B., 314, *344*
Gee, M. H., 459, 464, 467, *485, 487, 489*
Geffin, B., 2, *20*, 139, 143, 154, *157, 159,* 211, *219*
Gehr, P., 445, *448*
Genell, S., 320, *345*
Geokas, H. C., 326, *342*
Geokas, M. C., 326, *347*
George, R. B., 55, *61*
Georges, R., 126, *134*
Gerard, M., 144, *161*
Gerdin, B., 306, *332*
Geroulanos, S., 264, *274,* 401, *406*
Gewurz, H., 464, 467, *483, 484, 488*
Ghebrehiwet, B., 309, 337, *341*
Gibney, R. T. N., 188, *195*
Giclas, P. C., 310, *338*
Gielas, P. C., 309, *352*
Gigli, I., 316, *337*
Gigliotti, F., 403, *406*
Gil, J., 425, *430,* 445, *448*
Gilbert, C., 33, *34*, 81, *87*
Giles, P. J., 311, 323, 324, *350*
Gillan, J. E., 446, *448*
Gilluly, J. J., 260, *276*
Gimbrere, J. S. F., 306, *337*
Gimson, A., 70, *73*, 263, *274*

Ginsberg, R. J., 495, 513, 516, 521, 528, *535, 536*
Giotto, G., 270, 271, 272, *278*
Gitlin, J. D., 387, *392*
Giuntini, C., 202, *220*, 417, *431*
Gjerde, G. E., 188, *195*
Glaister, D. H., 146, 154, *158*
Glantz, S. A., 261, *275*
Glanville, A. R., 499, 525, *532*
Glaser, B., 315, *341*
Glass, D. D., 155, *158*
Glatzl, A., 386, *394*
Glauser, F. L., 54, *60*, 452, 457, *484*
Glauser, M. P., 264, *274*, 283, 401, 402, *405, 406, 410*
Glazier, J. B., 239, *250*, 266, *276*
Gluck, L., 385, *392*
Gmaz-NiKulin, E., 316, *337, 338*
Göber, I., 316, *337*
Goerge, P. M., *337*
Goetz, A. E., 452, 453, 454, 455, 457, 458, 463, 464, *483, 485*
Goetzl, E. J., 306, *343*
Gold, F. L., 260, *276*
Goldbach, P., 70, *75*
Goldberg, A. L., 265, *278*
Goldberg, H. S., 265, *276*
Goldberg, M., 492, 494, 495, 500, 506, 513, 516, *532, 534, 535, 537*
Goldberg, M. J., 521, 528, *536*
Goldberg, N. B., 144, 153, 160
Goldberg, S., 328, *333*, 386, *391*
Goldberg, S. K., 44, 48, *60*, 80, *88*
Golde, D. W., 306, *339*
Goldfarb,, R. D., 71, *74*
Goldin, M., 140, *156*
Goldman, B., 495, 513, 516, *535*
Goldman, B. S., 452, 453, 454, 456, 457, *485*
Goldman, M., 126, *135*
Goldman, M. R., 413, *432*
Goldsmith, J. S., 493, *532*
Goldstein, I. M., 306, 307, 309, 337, 339, 346, 351, 459, 460, 461, *484, 485, 487, 488*
Goldstein, S., 510, *533*
Gomez, P., 33, *35,* 81, 82, *88*
Gonzalez, R., 383, *392*
Good, J. J., 65, *74*
Good, J. T., 3, 7, 8, *19*, 40, 44, *60*, 80, *88*, 305, *336*, 368, *378*
Goode, A. W., 323, *334*
Gooding, C. A., 427, *431*
Goodman, K., 452, 453, 454, 470, *483*
Goodman, M., 56, *63*
Goodman, P. C., 255, *278*
Goralnick, B. S., 399, *407*
Gordon, R., 314, 326, *351*
Gordon, S., 314, *350, 351*
Goree, A., 385, *393*
Goris, J. A., 314, *344*
Goris, R. J. A., 306, *337*
Gote, T., 426, *432*
Goto, H., 453, *485*
Gottfried, S. B., 105, 106, 110, 114, 118, 123, 124, 126, 128, 129, 130, *134, 135, 136,* 142, *160,* 173, 174, 185, 186, *195, 197*
Gottlieb, M. E., 503, *536*
Goudard, A., 517, *535*
Gourin, A., 452, 453, 454, *485*
Goutier, R., 306, *335*
Grace, W. J., 28, *35*
Graes, B. M., 66, *75*
Graf, P. D., 524, *534*
Graham, R. C., 80, *89*
Graham, W., 125, *135*
Grammatica, L., 320, *341*
Granelli-Peperno, A., 314, *337*
Granger, D. N., 511, *535*
Grassino, A., 105, 114, 118, 126, 128, 129, 130, *136,* 142, *160,* 167, 178, 183, *194, 195*
Graves, J. S., 510, *537*
Green, L. H., 268, *281*
Green, M. V., 263, *279*
Green, N. M., 68, *74*
Green, R., 259, *282*
Greene, E. M., 452, 454, 455, 456, 457, 458, 459, 460, 463, 465, *486, 487*
Greene, L., 325, *346*

Greenfield, J. C., 241, *251*
Greenspan, M., 263, *281*
Greineder, J. K., 452, 453, 454, *485*
Greisman, S. E., 399, 400, 403, *406, 407*
Gresser, C., *533*
Griedman, M. L., 497, *537*
Griffen, G. L., 321, *348*
Griffin, J. H., 309, 323, *332, 333*
Griffith, B. P., 2, *20*, 511, *534*
Grillo, H. C., 516, *535*
Grimby, G., 125, *135*, 193, *195*
Grissman, J. D., 29, *36*
Groenveld, A. B. J., 71, *74*
Gross, D., 167, *195*
Gross, J. L., 315, *337*
Gross, M. D., 452, 453, 454, 456, 460, *489*
Grossman, G., 16, *21*, 387, *391*
Grossman, J. E., 83, *88*
Grossman, R. F., 26, *34*, 306, *336*, 524, *532, 536*
Grover, F. I., 452, *489*
Grubb, A., *331*
Grudzinskas, J. G., 464, *483*
Grum, C. M., *391*
Guenther, S. M., 164, *198*
Gueret, P., 226, *250*, 256, *277*
Guerin, C., 149, *158*
Guerrero, A., 306, *350*
Guiguet, M., 33, *34*
Gumnay, R. S., 306, *352*
Gurtner, G. C., 511, *532, 534*
Guthaner, D. F., 202, *220*
Gutierrez, G., 67, 69, 70, *74, 75*
Gutmann, R., 452, 453, 454, 455, 458, 463, 464, *483*
Guyton, A. C., 260, *276*, 354, 360, 363, 364, *365*, 384, *392*
Guz, A., 226, *250*
Gyzander, E., 323, *347*

Haas, M., 14, 15, 16, *19*, 306, 307, 316, *335*
Habazettl, H., 452, 453, 454, 455, 458, 463, 464, *483*
Habel, F. H., 324, *333*
Hachida, M., 511, *532*
Haddon, W., 313, *331*
Hagberg, R. C., 510, *537*
Hagstrom, J. W. C., 510, 521, *538*
Haida, M., 425, *432*
Hakim, M., 510, *538*
Hakim, T. S., 356, *365*
Hakki, A.-H., 258, *277*
Hales, C. A., 215, *220*
Hall, C. L., 399, 400, 402, *408*
Hall, P. K., 323, *347*
Hall, T. S., 511, *532, 534*
Haller, J., 427, *430*
Hallewell, R. A., 324, *347*
Hallgren, R., 17, *19*, 306, *332*
Hallman, M., 2, *19*, 382, 383, 384, 385, 386, 387, 388, 389, *392, 393, 394*
Halperin, B. D., 202, *220*
Halperin, M. L., 68, *74*
Halushka, P. V., 306, *346*
Halvey, A., 55, *60*
Hamilton, P. P., 446, *448*
Hamilton, R. L., 383, *395*
Hamilton, T. A., 314, 323, 324, 326, *330*
Hamlin, R. L., 125, *136*
Hamman, R. F., 3, 7, 8, *19*, 24, 26, 28, 30, 31, 32, *34*, 40, 44, 45, 48, *60*, 65, *74*, 80, *88*, 305, *336, 337*, 368, *378*
Hammer, C., 16, *19*
Hammerschmidt, D. A., 306, 307, *338*
Hammerschmidt, D. E., 14, *19*, 29, *36*, 286, *303*
Hammerschmidt, D. H., 307, *340*
Hammon, J. W., Jr., 226, *250*, 266, *281*
Hanahan, D. J., 470, *486*
Hance, A. J., 33, *34*, 425, *429*
Hancock, R. E. W., 403, *408*
Handler, J. B., 265, *280*
Hanley, J. A., 102, *103*

Hanning, C. D., 56, *60*
Hanover, J. A., 328, *338*
Hansen-Flaschen, J. H., 461, *490*
Hantler, C. B., 452, 453, 454, 456, 457, 458, 459, 460, 467, *489*
Hardesty, R. L., 2, *20*, 511, *534*
Hardin, C. A., 513, *533*
Hardy, J. D., 492, 521, *533, 534*
Harel, S., 311, *340*
Harf, A., 122, *134*, 144, 145, 146, 147, 148, 149, 154, *156, 158, 159,* 193, *196*
Hariri, R. J., 86, *89*
Harken, A. M., 70, *74*
Harlan, J. M., 14, 16, *20*
Harlan, W. R., Jr., 145, *160*
Harpel, P. C., 326, *338*
Harrell, J. H., 2, *19*, 385, *392*
Harris, G. D., 25, 26, 31, 32, *36*
Harris, T., 296, 297, 298, 299, *302*
Harris, T. M., 139, *156*
Harris, T. R., 427, *429*
Harrison, R. A., 139, *160*
Harrow, J. C., 452, 481, *490*
Harry, R. R., 116, *136*, 147, *160*
Hart, A. K. E., 434, *447*
Harvey, J., 525, *532*
Haslett, C., 306, *352*
Hassett, J., 315, *332*
Hasty, D. L., 312, *342*
Hasty, K. A., 312, *338*
Hatterslea, P. G., 453, *485*
Hau, T., 509, *537*
Hauley, M. E., 312, *352*
Haupt, H. M., 29, *34*
Haverich, A., 509, 511, *533, 538*
Havill, A. M., 464, 467, *487*
Havill, J. H., 101, *104*
Hawgood, S., 383, 386, 389, *391, 392, 394, 395*
Haworth, S. G., 500, *533*
Hayes, C. E., 425, *430*
Hayes, D. A., 126, *134*
Hayes, E., 403, *407*
Haynes, J., 306, *332*
Haynes, J. B., 266, 268, *276*, 310, *338*
Heath, T., 461, *487*
Hechtman, H. B., 267, 268, *278*, 306, *338*, 464, *486*
Hedenstierna, G., 155, *156*
Hedley-Whyte, J., 83, *88*, 144, *156*
Heflin, A. C., 286, *303*, 306, *338*
Hegewald, G., 316, *338*
Heideman, M., 323, *347*
Heimbach, D., 255, *278*
Heisterkamp, C. A., 28, *34*
Hendee, W. R., 412, 413, *430, 432*
Henderson, J. A. M., 145, *160*
Henderson, L. W., 464, *483*
Hendry, P. J., 512, *534*
Hennel, J. W., 425, *430*
Henning, R. J., 266, 268, *277*
Henson, J. E., 306, 312, 314, *338, 352,* 452, 453, 457, *483*
Henson, P. M., 16, *20*, 309, 311, 312, 314, *338, 352,* 459, 470, *484, 485, 490*
Heran, C. L., 452, 463, 464, *488*
Herbert, J. M., 403, *409*
Hernandez, L. A., 435, 445, *448*
Herron, G. S., 325, *338*
Herzyk, D. J., 312, *351*
Hesse, B., 329, *339*
Hesse, D. G., 263, 264, 265, *282*
Hesterberg, T., 387, *393*
Heyman, A., 398, *407*
Heymann, M. A., 389, *392*
Hibbs, M., 314, *339*
Hibbs, M. S., 312, 314, *338, 339*
Hida, W., 146, *158*
Higenbottam, T., 499, 510, 524, *533, 536, 538*
Higgins, C. B., 424, 426, 427, *431, 432*
Higgins, M., 496, *533*
Higgins, S., 296, 297, 298, 299, *302*
Higgs, B. D., 105, 114, 118, 120, 121, 123, 124, 126, 128, 129, 130, *134, 135, 136,* 142, *160,* 186, *195*
Higuchi, J. H., 81, 82, *88*
Hildebrandt, J., 115, *135*, 147, 153, *156, 158,* 434, *446*

Hilgard, P., 452, 454, 456, 459, 467, *486*
Hill, D. E., 452, 453, 454, 455, 457, *484*
Hill, J. D., 38, 39, *63*, 368, 370, 377, *378, 380*
Hill, R. D., 264, *279*, 364, *365*
Hill, R. N., 370, 377, *378*
Hines, R. L., 266, *274*
Hinshaw, D. B., 386, *395*
Hirsh, J. G., 314, *330*
Hirsh, R., 253, *274*, 368, 370, 376, *378*
Hirshman, C., 452, 481, *490*
Hitashi, K., 453, *485*
Hobbhahn, J., 452, 453, 454, 455, 457, 458, 463, 464, *483, 485*
Hochachka, P. W., 68, *74*
Hochgesand, K., 325, *339*
Hochstrasser, K., 325, *339*
Hocking, W. G., 306, *339*
Hodges, M., 140, *158*
Hodson, M., 499, *536*
Hoeffel, J. M., 459, 460, *484, 487*
Hoffat, J. D., 2, *21*
Hoffman, J. I. E., 260, *282*
Hogg, J. C., 145, *159*, 306, *349*
Hoidal, J. R., 314, *339*
Holcomb, K., 387, *393*
Holcroft, J. W., 263, *277*
Holland, L., 268, *281*
Holle, R. H. O., 165, *196*
Holliday, R. L., 2, *18, 21,* 306, *330*
Holloway, H., 360, 361, *365*
Holm, B. A., 385, 388, *392, 393*
Holter, J. F., 2, *19*, 306, *339, 350*
Holtman, D., 78, *89*
Holtman-Reus, D., 6, 7, 8, *20*, 305, *345*, 368, 370, 376, *379*
Holtzman, H., 44, 48, *60*, 80, *88*
Holzapfel, L., 149, *158*
Holzman, H., 328, *342*
Homburger, H. A., 464, *483*
Hong, S. R., 459, *490*
Horie, T., 115, *135*
Horn, J. K., 307, *339*, *346,* 460, *484*
Horn, R., 81, *88*
Horovitz, J. H., 255, *278*
Horrow, J. C., 452, 453, *485*
Horton, E. H., 316, *339*
Hosea, S., 16, *19*
Hougland, M. W., 315, *348*
Houston, C. S., 66, *75*
Hovi, T., 326, *339*
Howard, J. M., 320, *347*
Howell, J. B. L., 434, *448*
Howland, W. S., 155, *159*
Hoyer, J., 509, *533*
Hsiao, H. S., 116, *136*, 147, *160*
Hsieh, C., 510, 511, *533, 538*
Hubbard, R. C., 323, *339*
Hubbard, W. J., 326, *339*
Huber, D. J., 425, 426, *430*
Huber, G. L., 385, *393*
Hudson-Civetta, J., 141, *160*
Hudson, L., 16, *21*
Hudson, L. D., 3, 4, 7, 8, 10, 13, 14, *19, 20,* 24, 25, 26, 28, 30, 31, 32, 33, *35*, 38, 53, 55, *60, 61, 62,* 65, *75*, 77, 78, *88, 89*, 101, *104*, 253, 263, 266, *279, 280,* 297, *304*, 305, 306, 307, *338, 345,* 368, 370, 376, *379*
Hufnagel, H. V., 70, *74*
Hughes, J. M. B., 145, *158*, 217, *220,* 266, *276,* 437, *449*
Hugli, T. E., 307, *333*, 459, *483, 484*
Hunt, S. A., 529, 536
Hunter, I. W., 118, *134*
Hurford, W. E., 256, 259, 260, 268, 273, *277*
Hurley, J. V., 440, 441, *448*
Hurst, J. M., 306, 307, *348*
Huseby, J., 258, *282*
Hussain, S. N. A., 263, *277*
Hussein, A., 286, *302*
Hutchins, G. M., 29, *34*, 511, *532, 534*
Hutchison, A. A., 288, *302*
Hutchison, D. C. S., 496, *533*
Huttemeier, P. C., 39, 42, *62*, 305, *346*, 367, *379*, 459, 464, 467, *490*

Hutter, J., 499, *536*
Huyghebaert, M.-F., 256, 258, 266, 270, *276*
Hwang, K. K., 368, *379*
Hyatt, R. E., 170, 179, *194*
Hyde, R. W., 54, *61*, 437, *447*
Hyers, T., 305, *337*
Hyers, T. M., 30, *34, 35,* 45, 48, *60*, 65, *74*, 80, *88*, 263, 266, 268, *276, 277,* 305, 310, *336, 338, 340,* 368, *378*
Hyslop, P. A., 386, *395*

Ibanez, J., 218, *220*
Ikegami, M., 381, 387, 388, 389, *391, 393*
Ilebekk, A., 266, *282*
Iliff, L. D., 434, *448*
Ingbar, D. H., 53, *61*
Ingels, N. B., 269, 272, *275*
Ingels, N. B., Jr., 226, *249*
Ingram, J., 401, *410*
Ingram, R. H., Jr., 146, *158*, 185, *198*, 268, *281*
Innes, J. A., 226, *250*
Ino, Y., 465, *482*
Inoue, H., 146, *158*
Interiano, B., 54, *61*
Inthorne, D., 326, *340*
Iotti, G., *276*
Isemura, S., *331*
Isenberg, M. D., 141, 142, 148, 154, *161*
Ishikawa, J., 314, *340*
Iskandrian, A., 258, *277*
Itoo, H., *538*
Ivankovich, A. D., 140, *156*
Iwanaga, S., 325, *344*

Jackman, H., 470, *488, 489*
Jackson, A. C., 122, *135*
Jackson, J., 403, *407*
Jacob, H. S., 29, *36*, 306, 307, *338, 340*
Jacobs, E. R., 312, *352*
Jacobs, H. K., 140, *161*
Jacobs, M. R., 80, *89*
Jacquemin, D., 307, 316, 326, *336*
Jacques, L. B., 452, *485*
Jaffe, E., 315, *343*
Jaffe, E. A., 312, 315, *337, 340*
Jallat, S., 323, 324, *334, 339*
James, A. E., Jr., 413, 424, *431*
James, H. L., 323, *347*
James, P. M., 28, *34*
Jamieson, S. W., 509, 510, *537*
Janicki, J. S., 261, *283*
Jann, B., 401, *407*
Jann, K., 401, *407*
Janney, C. D., 144, *158*
Janoff, A., 311, 314, 323, 326, *332, 336, 340, 351*
Jardin, F., 50, *61*, 226, *250*, 256, 260, 266, 267, 270, *277*
Jarvenpaa, A. L., 387, *392*
Jarvinen, M., *331*
Jasper, A. C., 71, *75*
Jastrzebski, J., 452, 454, 456, 459, 467, *486*
Javaheri, S., 215, *220*
Jayamanne, D. S., 55, *61*
Jeffrey, J. A., 389, *395*
Jenkins, D. E., 497, *537*
Jenkins, P. A., 389, *395*
Jenkinson, S. G., 55, *61*
Jenson, P. M., 306, *352*
Jeppsson, J. O., 323, *333*
Jesmok, G., 288, *303*
Jewell, M., 403, *407*
Jobe, A., 381, 388, *391, 393*
Jobsis, F. F., 66, *74*
Jochum, M., 314, 326, 329, *333, 336, 340, 352*
Johanson, G., 42, *59*
Johanson, W. G., 305, *331,* 368, 376, 377, *378*
Johanson, W. G., Jr., 24, 25, 26, 31, 32, 33, 35, 36, 42, 44, 48, *59,* 65, 73, 77, 78, *79*, 80, 81, 82, 83, *87, 88, 89,* 93, *103,* 263, *274,* 377, *378*

Johns, M., 400, 401, 402, *407*
Johnson, D., 311, 321, 323, 324, *345, 349, 350*
Johnson, D. A., 314, 315, *348, 349*
Johnson, D. M. A., 308, 323, *340*
Johnson, F. N., 144, 153, *160*
Johnson, J. E., 288, *303*
Johnson, J. H., 326, *342*
Johnson, K. J., 16, *21*, 311, *349, 350*, 399, *407*
Johnson, P., 67, *74*
Johnson, P. C., 497, *537*
Johnson, R. L., Jr., 268, 270, *275*
Johnson, R. P., 122, *134*
Johnson, S. A., 417, 418, 421, 427, *430, 431*
Johnson, W. C., 316, *340*
Johnston, A. R., 399, *409*
Johnston, C. A., 399, *407*
Johnston, R. B., 306, *340*, 459, *490*
Johnston, R. B., Jr., 311, *338*
Johnston, W. E., 453, 472, 473, *486*
Joison, J., 452, 453, 454, 456, 457, *485*
Joka, T., 31, *35*, 306, 315, *341*
Jolles, H., 288, *303*
Jones, C. E., 367, *379*
Jones, H. A., 217, *220*
Jones, J. G., 26, *34*, 306, *336*
Jones, J. M., 520, *533*
Jones, K., 510, *538*
Jones, M. S., 316, *340*
Jones, M. T., 510, *533, 535*
Jones, P. A., 314, *351*
Jones, R. T., 316, *340, 341*
Jones, S. R., 265, *281*
Jones, T., 217, *220*
Jonson, B., 142, *158*
Jonsson, S., 385, *393*
Jordening, H., 261, *280*
Joris, M., 444, *448*
Judson, J. A., 101, *104*
Jung, R. C., 305, *331*
Junod, A., 316, *343*
Junot, A. F., 50, 51, *62*
Jurman, M. J., 511, *533*
Kacmarek, R. M., 187, *195*
Kagan, H. M., 312, *333*
Kahn, F. W., 520, *533*
Kahn, R. J., *282*
Kalebic, T., 315, *341*
Kaltreider, H. B., 385, *391*
Kamani, G., 312, 314, *338*
Kamholz, S. L., 509, 510, *535, 536*
Kampanani, W., 387, *394*
Kandel, M. J., 326, *331*
Kane, S. P., 311, 314, *341*
Kaneko, K., 145, *160*
Kang, A. H., 312, 314, 315, 325, *338, 339, 342, 343, 346*
Kang, A. M., 314, *339*
Kania, S., 400, 402, *408, 409*
Kant, J., 69, *73*
Kapelanski, D. P., 511, *534*
Kaplan, A. P., 309, 324, *337, 341, 348*
Kaplan, H. S., 403, *409*
Kaplan, K. B., 459, *485*
Kaplan, R. L., 48, *61*, 368, *379*
Karam, M., 226, *250*
Kariman, K., 69, *74*, 296, 297, 298, 299, *302*, 427, *429*
Karlik, S. J., 426, *432*
Karlson, K. E., 510, *532, 533*
Katz, J. A., 152, 153, 154, *158*, 188, *195*
Kaufman, J. J., 510, *536*
Kaufman, L., 413, 424, *430*
Kay, H. R., 258, 266, *274, 277*
Kazemi, H., 215, *220*
Keagy, B., 511, *535*
Keinecke, H.-O., 31, *35*, 306, 315, *341*
Kelly, W. J., 385, *393*
Kendall, T., 16, *21*
Keogh, B. A., 425, *429*
Keon, W. J., 512, *534*
Kern, J. A., 495, *534*
Keshavjee, S. H., 510, 511, *534, 538*
Kesiel, W., 309, *334*
Kester, A. D. M., 71, *74*
Ketai, L. H., *391*

Ketchem, P. A., 400, *409*
Kettelhut, I. C., 265, *278*
Khaghani, A., 511, *538*
Kiely, A. A., 493, *532*
Kierulf, P., 329, *330*
Kigashiyama, S., 325, *345*
Kiil, F., 266, *282*
Kilgarriff, C., 403, *406*
Kilgore, W. T., 116, *136*, 147, *160*
Kim, K. J., 437, *448*
Kimball, W. R., 173, *195,* 268, *278*
Kimbel, P., 328, *342*
Kimura, T., 321, *342*
Kindahl, H., 459, *485*
Kindred, M. K., 226, 239, 243, *250, 251,* 268, *282*
King, C. H., 80, *89*
King, G. A., 294, 295, 296, *304*
King, L. S., 288, *303*
King, R. G., 383, *393*
Kirby, R. R., 140, *157, 158*
Kirk, W., 434, *446, 447*
Kirkland, T. N., 400, 402, *406, 407*
Kirklin, J. K., 377, *379*, 464, *486*
Kirklin, J. W., 307, *333*, 377, *379,* 464, *486*
Kirpikov, S., 509, *536*
Kistler, J. P., 413, *432*
Kitain, E. M., 453, 464, 465, 475, *487*
Kittle, C. F., 513, *533*
Kitzis, M., *534*
Klain, M., 248, *250*
Klauber, M. R., 264, *274*, 401, *405*
Klausner, J. M., 464, *486*
Klebanoff, S. J., 311, 323, *341*
Klein, E. F., 140, *158*
Klein, J. J., 54, *61*
Kleinberger, G., 427, *430*
Klose, R., 149, *159*
Knapp, M., 462, *484*
Knauer, D. J., 325, *341*
Knaus, W. A., 31, *35*, 92, 93, *94*, 95, 101, 102, *103, 104*
Knights, C. V., 404, *409*
Knudson, R. J., 126, *135*
Kobayashi, T., 291, 292, 293, 294, *304*
Kobzik, L., 464, *486*
Kochi, T., 130, *135*
Koeniger, E., 48, *61*
Koerner, S. K., 71, *75*, 497, 510, *537, 538*
Kohl, F. V., 2, *21*
Kolobow, T., 444, 446, *448*
Komatsu, T., 66, 67, *75*
Kondo, Y., 521, *534*
Kong, D., 459, 464, 467, *490*
Konno, M., *276*
Kontos, G., 511, *534*
Koo, P. H., 326, *341*
Kornecki, E., 321, *341*
Korthuis, R. J., 356, *366*
Koshal, A., 506, *537*
Koshiyama, Y., 465, *482*
Koss, M., 305, *331*
Kotb, K., 368, *379*
Koyama, I., 511, *534*
Kozin, F., 309, 324, *341*
Kraemer, R. W., 188, *195*
Kramps, J. A., 325, *335*
Kreil, E., 452, 454, 455, 456, 457, 458, 459, 460, 463, 468, *486, 487*
Kreisberg, J. I., *341*
Kreit, J. W., 177, *189*
Kremers, W., 468, *488*
Kreuzfelder, E., 31, *35*, 306, 315, *341*
Krog, H. H., 404, *406*
Kron, E. J., 511, *535*
Kronberg, G. M., 255, *278*
Kubal, K., 66, 67, *75*
Kubo, K., 288, *303*
Kumar, A., 139, *159*, 211, *219*
Kumar, H., 139, 143, 154, *157*
Kumar, V., 66, 67, *75*
Kunches, L. M., 84, *88*
Kundel, H. L., 424, *432*
Kung, G. Y., 102, *104*
Kung, P. C., 403, *406*
Kunkel, J. L., 311, *336*

Kunkel, R., 16, *21*, 311, *349*
Kunze, H., 329, *339*
Kuo, G. C., 265, *282*
Kurachi, K., 309, 325, *334, 345*
Kushihashi, T., 453, *485*
Kuwahara, O., 521, *534*
Kveder, M., 425, *430*
Kvetan, V., 155, *159*
Kvietys, P. R., 425, *432*
Kwaan, H. C., 320, *341*
Kwang, M. S., 384, *393*
Kyei Aboagye, K., 433, *449*

Labrousse, J., 148, *161*, 254, *278*
La Buglio, A. F., 288, *304*
Lachmann, B., 387, *391, 394*
Ladowski, J. S., 511, *534*
La Duca, J., 315, *332*
La Force, F. M., 385, *393*
Laggner, A., 427, *430*
Lahajnar, G., 425, *430*
Lakner, K., 202, *221*
Lakshminarayan, S., 53, 54, *61*, 180, *197*, 434, *446, 447*
Lallemand, D. P., 427, *431*
Lamb, V., 170, 171, 172, 175, 176, 179, 180, 181, 182, *196, 198*
Lampert, M. B., 323, *349*
Lams, P. M., 288, *303*
Lamy, M., 48, *61*, 306, 307, 316, 319, 323, 324, 326, *335, 336, 341, 342*
Landa, L., 264, *279*, 516, *535*
Landser, F. J., 126, *127*
Landy, M., 399, *407*
Lane, S., 173, *198*
Langenstein, H., 141, *161*
Langer, M., 204, 206, *220,* 446, *448*
Langlois, P. F., 306, 307, 309, *342*
Lankisch, P. G., 329, *339*
Lanore, J. J., *276*
Lappas, D. G., 453, 472, 473, *486*
Laragh, J. H., 309, *348*
Largman, C., 326, *342*
Larrick, J. W., 403, *408*
Larson, D. L., 326, *334*
Laskin, D. L., 321, *342*
Lassen, N. A., 71, *74*
Lasson, A., 320, 321, *342*
Latty, A., 215, *220*
Laurell, C. B., 323, *333*
Lauterbur, P. C., 424, *431*
Lavelle, R. F., Jr., 54, *63*
Lavere, M. B., 139, 143, 154, *157*, 211, *219*, 254, 261, 265, 268, *278, 280*
Lawrence, D., 92, *103*, 325, *344*
Lawrence, E. C., 385, *393*
Laws, A. K., 139, 140, *159*
Lazar, N. M., 437, *448*
Lecart, M. P., 306, *335*
Lecocq, J. P., 324, *334*
Lecossier, D., 438, 439, *449*
Ledbetter, M., 452, 470, *484*
Lederman, M., 80, *89*
Ledingham, E., 56, *60*
Ledingham, I., Mc A., 56, *60*, 102, *103*
Lee, A. T., 265, *282*
Lee, C. T., 328, *342*
Lee, D., 311, *340*
Leech, A. R., 66, 68, *75*
Leechawengwong, M., 55, *61*
Lefcoe, M., 2, *18*, 306, *330*
LeFor, W. M., 504, *536*
Le Gall, J. R., 52, 53, *61,* 93, 101, *103*
Leight, J. S., 69, *73*
Leith, D. E., 139, 143, 154, *157,* 173, *195,* 211, *219,* 268, *278*
Lejeune, P., *282*
Lemaire, F., 144, 145, 146, 147, 148, 149, 150, 154, *156, 158, 159,* 189, 193, *194, 196,* 255, 257, 270, 271, 272, *278, 282*
Lennox, P. M., 142, *160*
Lennox, S., 105, 114, 118, *136*
Lenox, R. H., 321, *341*
Lentnek, A. L., 286, *303*
Lenz, K., 427, *430*
Leslie, C. C., 383, *393*
Leuenberger, C., 316, 326, *344*

Leuenberger, P., 55, 57, *59*
Levine, B. E., 2, *18*, 23, *33*, 37, 39, 54, *59*, 80, *87*, 305, *330*
Levine, O. R., 440, 441, *447*
Lew, w. Y. W., 464, *483*
Le Winter, M., 464, *483*
Lewis, D. H., 124, *134*
Lewis, F., 427, *431*
Lewis, G. P., 294, *303*
Lewis, R. A., *347*
Lichtenstein, L. M., 315, *344*
Lieberman, P., 55, *63*
Liebman, P. R., 267, 268, *278*
Liebow, C., 316, *342*
Lien, D. C., 311, *352*
Light, J. A., 504, *536*
Light, R. W., 54, *62*
Lijnen, H. R., 324, *335*
Lillo, R. S., 70, *74*
Lim, L., 140, *161*
Lima, O., 492, 494, 500, *532, 534, 535*
Lindauer, J. M., 255, *278*
Lindblad, B., 452, 453, 454, 456, 457, 458, 459, 460, 463, 467, *486, 489*
Lindsey, A. W., 260, *276*, 363, 364, *365*
Line, B. R., 437, *447*
Linehan, J. H., 356, *365*
Linhardt, G., 316, *340*
Linhardt, G. E., *341*
Liotta, L. A., 315, *341*
Lipavsky, A., 437, *448*
Lippman-Hand, A., 102, *103*
Lippmann, M., 44, 48, *60*, 80, *88*, 328, *333, 342,* 386, *391*
Lipton, J. M., 400, 402, *408*
Lisbon, A., 83, *88*
Lischer, P., 141, *161*
Lissac, J., 148, *161*, 254, *278*
Little, W. C., 452, *489*
Lixfield, W., 268, *281*
Llamas, R., 54, *61*
Llera, J. J., 499, *537*
Lloyd, J. E., 427, *429*
Lockhard, A., 155, *156*
Logas, W. G., 140, *156*
Logon, W. B., 313, *331*
Loirat, P., 52, 53, *61*
Longoni, F., 446, *448*
Loring, S. H., 114, *135*, 167, 171, *196*
Lorino, A. M., 122, *134*
Lorino, H., 122, *134*, 144, *158*
Losi, P., 315, *332*
Loskutoff, D. J., 325, *344*
Lowenstein, E., 2, *20*, 254, 256, 260, 264, 265, 268, 273, *277, 279, 280,* 452, 453, 454, 457, 458, 459, *460,* 463, 465, 467, 468, 472, 473, 481, *486, 490*
Lowery, B. D., 461, *484*
Lowry, S. F., 86, *89*, 263, 264, 265, *282*
Loyd, J. E., 37, *62*, 288, 291, *302, 303*
Lozman, J., 254, *278*
Lubas, B., 425, *430*
Luce, J. E., 296, 297, 298, 299, *302*
Luce, J. M., 2, 4, *20*, 24, 32, *33, 35,* 38, 51, *62*, 254, 255, 265, *278,* 316, *344*, 367, 370, *378, 379,* 437, *448*
Lucht, J. E., 288, *302*
Lucht, W. D., 468, *482*
Luck, J. C., 270, *275*
Luethy, R., 264, *274*, 401, *405*
Luk, S., 492, 494, 500, *532, 534, 535*
Lunt, J. A., 425, *429*
Luterman, A., 255, *278*, 310, *342*
Lynch, J. M., 470, *485*
Lynch, J. P., 66, 69, *74*, 140, *157*
Lynch, K., 256, 268, 273, *277,* 452, 454, 457, 458, 460, 463, *487*
Lynch, K. E., 364, *365*

Macartney, H. W., 325, *342*
Mac Beth, M. C., 383, *393*
Mac Gregor, D., 268, *281*
Mac Gregor, R. R., 286, *303*
Machado, M., 316, *345*

Machiedo, G. W., 315, *342*
Machin, S. J., 306, *350*
Mac Intyre, N., 189, *196*
Mackie, I., 306, *350*
Macklem, P. T., 115, 125, *134, 135,* 145, 146, *156, 159,* 178, 183, *195, 197*
MacLean, L. D., 493, *538*
MacLennan, F. M., 427, *431*
Macquart-Moulin, G., 509, *533*
Macquin-Mavier, I., 270, 271, 272, *278*
Mac Vittie, T. J., 263, *279*
Maddahi, J., 258, *278*
Magovern, G. J., 493, *534*
Mahler, D. A., 71, *73*
Mahutte, C. K., 165, *197*
Maier, G., 226, *250*, 266, *281*
Maillot, J. P., 147, 148, *159*
Mainardi, C. L., 312, 314, *338, 339, 342, 343*
Mainwood, G. W., 512, *534*
Mal, H., *534*
Malconian, M. K., 66, *75*
Malik, A. B., 306, *349*, 437, *447* 503, *536*
Malmsten, C. L., 459, *485*
Maloney, J. E., 239, *250*, 266, *276*
Man, D., 320, *343*
Mancebo, J., 45, 47, 48, 49, 50, 52, *59, 62,* 142, 154, *159*
Mancini, M. C., 2, *20*
Mankikian, B., 145, 147, 148, 154, *156, 159*
Mannick, A., 326, *334*
Mannick, J. A., 326, 329, *334*
Manning, M., 84, *88*
Manny, J., 267, 268, *278*
Manogue, K. R., 263, 264, 265, *282*
Mansfield, P., 413, 424, 425, *431*
Mantey-Stiers, F., 84, *89*
Manwaring, D., 310, *342, 343*
Manyak, C. L., 403, *407*
Marcelis, J. H., 402, *406*
Marco, D., 254, *278*
Marcolin, R., 150, 152, *157, 158,* 204, 206, 211, 213, 214, 215, *220*
Margairez, A., 50, *61*, 256, 260, 266, 267, 270, *277*
Marglin, S. I., *20*, 45, 48, *62*, 446, *448*
Margulis, A. R., 413, 424, *429, 430*
Marini, J. J., 170, 171, 172, 173, 174, 175, 176, 177, 178, 184, 185, 186, 188, 191, 192, 193, *195, 196, 197, 198,* 254, 255, 267, 268, *275, 278, 279, 280*
Marino, J., 80, *89*
Maris, J., 69, *73*
Marks, J. D., 24, 32, *35*, 437, *448*
Marks, M. I., 402, *407*
Marshall, B., 424, *432*
Marshall, J. C., 81, *88*
Marshall, R., 115, 122, 131, *135,* 144, *159*
Martin, G. R., *350*
Martin, M., 154, *159*
Martin, P., 404, *409*
Martin, P. G., 438, 439, *449*
Martin, R., 115, *134*
Martin, V., 326, *349*
Mascheroni, D., 150, 154, *157*, 202, 204, 206, 211, 212, 213, 214, 215, *219, 220,* 377, *379,* 444, *448*
Maseri, A., 216, 217, *221*
Mason, G. R., 306, *336*
Mason, J. W., 324, *337*
Mason, R. J., 2, *19*, 383, *393*
Massa, G., 206, *220*
Massabie, P., 254, *278*
Massi, G., 321, *344*
Matalon, S., 388, *393*
Matamis, D., 144, 149, 154, *159,* 193, *196*
Matheson, N. R., 323, *343*
Mathey, D. G., 258, *279*
Mathison, J. C., 399, 405, *407, 409*
Mathru, M., 269, 270, 272, *279*
Mathur-De Vre, R., 424, 426, *431*
Matsuoka, D. T., 258, *278*
Matthay, M. A., 2, 4, 14, 15, 16, 18, *19, 20, 21,* 38, 51, 53, *61, 62,* 71, *73,* 306, 307, 316, *343, 344, 351,* 370, *379*

Matthay, R. A., 266, 267, *274, 281,* 314, *344*
Matthews, K. P., 470, *486*
Matuschak, G. M., 248, *250,* 316, *343*
Maunder, R., 16, *21*
Maunder, R. J., 3, 10, 13, 14, 16, *19, 20,* 45, 48, *62*, 202, *220,* 446, *448*
Maurer, J. R., 516, 525, *532, 535, 536*
Maxwell, D. L., 437, *449*
Mc Adam, K. P. W. J., 405, *409*
Mc Cabe, S., 102, *103*
Mc Cabe, W. R., 84, *88*, 400, 401, 402, *407*
Mc Carthy, J., 446, *449*
Mc Cord, J. M., 315, *343, 347*
Mc Culloch, P. R., 446, *448*
Mc Cutchan, A., 264, *283*
Mc Cutchan, J. A., 264, *274*, 401, *405, 410*
McDonald, J. K., 306, 325, *331*
Mc Donald, J. W. D., 464, 470, *486 488*
Mc Guire, W. W., 309, 323, *334, 352,* 386, *393*
Mc Hale, P. A., 226, 241, *250, 251,* 266, *281*
Mc Hugh, J. W., *20*, 45, 48, 62, 202, *220*, 446, *448*
Mc Illroy, M. B., 109, 112, 115, 120, *135, 136*
Mc Intosh, J. D., 102, *104*
Mc Intyre, R. W., 139, 140, *159*
Mc Keen, C. R., 288, 300, *302*
Mc Kerrow, C. B., 109, 112, 115, *136*
Mc Lean, A. P., 31, *35*, 79, *88*
Mc Lean, R. F., 102, *104*
Mc Manus, L. M., 470, *486*
Mc Namara, M. T., 424, 427, *432*
McPhaul, K. M., 496, *538*
Mc Rae, B. J., 314, *349*
Mc Ritchie, D. I., 510, *534*
Mead, J., 109, 112, 115, 122, 125, 126, 131, *134, 135, 136,* 147, 153, 154, *156, 160,* 193, *195*
Meakins, J. L., 31, *35*, 79, 81, *88*, 94, 100, 101, *103*
Mecham, R. P., 321, *348*
Medegard, A., 323, *347*
Mela, L., 70, *75*
Mengeot, P. M., 123, 124, 129, *135*
Menkis, A., 506, *537*
Menon, R. S., 425, *431*
Menzoian, J. O., 326, 329, 334
Mergenhagen, S. E., *350*
Mergner, W., 316, *340*
Merrill, W. W., 314, *344*
Merritt, T. A., 382, 383, 384, 386, 387, 388, 389, 390, *392, 393, 394*
Merryweather, J., 86, *89*
Metras, D., 517, *535*
Metz, C. A., 24, 32, *35*
Meyrick, B., 2, *20*, 286, 288, 289, 290, 291, 292, 293, 294, *302, 303, 304,* 464, 471, 472, *483, 487*
Micheels, J., 307, 316, 326, *336*
Michelassi, F., 264, *279*, 516, *535*
Michels, A., 126, *135*
Mielke, C. H., Jr., 305, *336*
Mihm, F. G., 202, *220*, 427, *431*
Miles, L. A., 309, *332*
Milhorn, H. T., Jr., 122, *135*
Milic-Emili, J., 105, 106, 110, 114, 116, 118, 119, 120, 121, 123, 124, 129, 130, *133, 134, 135, 136, 137,* 142, 145, 154, *158, 160,* 167, 172, 184, *195, 196*
Millan, J. L., 325, *344*
Miller, E., 29, *36*
Miller, L. D., 70, *75*
Miller, R. G., 368, *380*
Milligan, S. A., 459, 461, *487, 488*
Mills, B., 315, *332*
Milne, B., 452, 453, 454, 455, 457, *488*
Milne, E. N. C., 202, *220*, 417, *431*
Milsark, I. W., 86, *89*, 264, *274*
Miner, K. M., 403, *407*
Miniati, M., 202, *220*, 417, *431*
Minta, J. O., 320, *343*

Mintun, M. A., 3, 4, *19*, 306, 315, *332*
Mishkel, G., *533*
Mitchell, J. H., 265, *275*
Mitchell, M. D., 461, *487*
Mitchell, R. A., 6, 11, *21*, 368, *380*
Mitzner, W., 211, *220*
Miyamoto, K., 461, *487*
Miyoshi, S., 511, *538*
Mizer, L. A., 71, *75*
Modell, J. H., 140, *158*
Modig, J., 306, *332*
Moffatt, D. F., 384, *392*
Mogensen, T., 261, *280*
Mohammed, J. R., 306, *350*
Mohsenifar, Z., 70, 71, *75*
Molho, M., 55, *63*
Molina, R. M., 461, 462, *489, 490*
Monsallier, J. F., 155, *156*, 256, 258, 266, 270, *276*
Montalescot, G., 452, 454, 455, 456, 457, 458, 459, 460, 463, 465, *486, 487*
Montefusco, C., 509, 510, *535, 536*
Montgomery, A. B., 24, 25, 26, 31, 32, 33, *35*, 65, *75*, 77, 78, *88*, 101, *104*, 165, *196*, 305, 316, *343*
Montgomery, A. S., 253, 263, *279*
Montgomery, B., 40, 42, 44, 45, 47, 48, 51, *62*
Montz, R., 258, *279*
Moon, R. G., 69, *75*
Moore, C., 403, *409*
Moore, E. E., 16, *20*
Moore, E. H., 424, 425, 426, 427, *431*
Moore, G. W., 29, *34*
Moreau, S. C., 403, *407*
Morel, D., 50, 51, *62*
Morel, D. R., 316, *343*, 452, 453, 454, 457, 458, 459, 463, 464, 465, 467, 468, 475, *487*
Moreno, L. F., 72, *75*
Moretti, M. P., 444, *448*
Morgan, A. P., 316, *349*
Morgan, C. J., 413, *430*
Morgan, E., 464, *486*, 492, 494, *532, 535*
Morgan, K. A., 398, *408*
Morgan, W. K. C., 426, *432*
Morgan, W. L., Jr., 265, *275*
Morii, M., 324, *350*
Morin, F. C., III., 387, 389, *395*
Morosova, M., 509, *536*
Morris, A. H., 55, 57, *60*, 253, *274*, 368, 370, 376, *378*, 417, 418, 419, 420, 421, 422, 423, 425, 427, *428, 429, 430, 431*
Morris, H. G., 461, 467, *489*
Morris, P. G., 413, 424, 425, *431*
Morrissey, R., *343*
Morse, P. A., 437, *447*
Mortillaro, N., 358, *365*
Mortola, J. P., 114, *134*
Morton, D. L., 511, *532*
Moscattelli, D., 315, *337, 343*
Moser, K. M., 53, *59*, 385, *392*
Mosesson, N. W., 326, *338*
Mosher, D. F., 326, 328, *339, 343*
Moss, J., 453, 464, 465, 475, *487*
Motin, J., 69, *73*
Motlagh, F., 510, *533*
Motley, H. L., 265, *275*
Mott, P. D., 403, *410*
Movat, H. Z., 86, *87*, 263, *279*, 320, 324, *333, 343*
Moxham, J., 165, 167, 178, *197*
Moyer, E. D., 326, *346*
Muehlen, E., 264, *274*, 401, *405*
Mueller-Esterl, W., 325, 329, *333, 344*
Mulholland, J. H., 403, *410*
Mullan, N. A., 400, *407*
Muller, B. R., 323, *334*
Muller-Eberhard, H. J., 307, *344*
Muller, N., 424, 425, 426, 427, *431*
Mullins, C. B., III., 83, *89*
Mundth, E. D., 258, *277*
Munford, R. S., 399, 400, 402, *408*
Munn, E. A., 326, *331*
Munro, D. D., 493, *538*
Munster, A. M., 85, *89*

Murata, G. H., 265, *280*
Murciano, C., 181, 184, 190, 191, *195*
Murphy, G., 311, 325, *344*
Murphy, K., 226, *250*
Murray, J. F., 2, 4, 18, *20, 21,* 24, 26, 32, *34, 35,* 38, 51, *62,* 266, 267, 268, 269, *276,* 306, 307, 316, *336, 344, 351,* 370, *379,* 437, *448*
Murthy, S. K., 316, *339*
Musher, D. M., 385, *393*
Musiani, P., 321, *344*
Mutharia, L. M., 403, *408*
Myer, M. A., 323, *334*
Myers, M. A., 315, *336*
Myers, M. L., 2, *21*
Myers, T. M., 31, *34*
Myerson, D. A., 54, *60*
Myerson, P. J., 54, *60*
Mygind, T., 261, *280*
Myhrman, R., 464, *484, 488*

Nadel, J. A., 120, *135*, 524, *534*
Naftel, D. C., 464, *486*
Nagel, E. L., 266, *281*
Naimark, A., 255, *283*
Najarian, J. S., 509, *537*
Najarian, R. C., 324, *347*
Nakahara, K., 217, *219*
Nakamoto, K., 511, *538*
Nakamura, K., *538*
Nakaninski, S., 325, *344*
Nakanishi, I., 325, 328, *345*
Nakhosteen, J., 306, 315, *341*
Namikawa, C., 325, *345*
Narayana, P., 69, *74*
Nasbeth, D. C., 316, *340*
Nastri, G., 150, *157*
Natanson, C., 71, *75*, 263, 264, *276, 279*
Natarjan, J. K., 226, *250*
Naulart, Ll., 55, *63*
Nauta, J. J. P., 71, *74*
Navajas, D., 126, *136*
Navarro, L., 305, *331*
Neagley, S. R., 165, *196*
Nellenbogen, J., 383, 389, *392*
Nelles, M. J., 403, *408*
Nelson, D. H., 286, *303*
Nelson, L. D., 141, *160*
Nelson, R. D., 306, 307, *348*
Nelson, R. M., 435, 436, *447*
Net, A., 154, *159*
Neuhof, H., 385, *395*
Neurath, H., 307, *344*
Nevalainen, T. J., 320, *344*
Newball, H. H., 315, *344*
Newell, J. C., 72, *75*, 503, *536*
Newham, D., 167, *197*
Newhouse, J. H., 413, *432*
Newman, J. H., 37, *62*, 193, 195, 288, 291, 292, 293, 294, *302, 303, 304,* 367, *379*
Newsholme, E. A., 66, 68, *75*
Newsome, P. M., 400, *407*
Ngeow, Y. K., 211, *220*
Nicholas, T. E., 434, *449*
Nicholson, R. L., 424, *432*
Nicod, L., 316, 326, *344*
Nicolas, F., 53, *61*
Niedemeyer, M. E., 288, *302,* 468, *482*
Niederman, M., 2, *19*
Niederman, M. S., 314, *344*
Nielsen, S. L., 71, *74*
Nieman, G. F., 384, 388, *394*, 434, *447*
Nienaber, C. A., 258, *279*
Niewoehner, D. E., 154, *160*
Nikulin, A., 316, *337, 338*
Nimberg, R. B., 326, 329, *334*
Nims, R. G., 120, *134*
Nioka, S., 69, *73*
Nisell, O. I., 120, *134*
Niswander, C. A., 403, *408*
Nixon, J. V., 270, *275*
Noel, F. X., 306, 307, *335*
Noiclerc, M., 509, 517, *533, 535*
Nolop, K. B., 437, *449*
Nolop, K. E., 427, *429*
Norcross, J. F., 300, *304,* 307, *350*

Nordström, L., 142, *158*
Norin, A., 509, *535*
Norman, J. R., 122, *135*
Norris, S. E., 452, *489*
Norton, J. F., 226, *251*
Norwood, S., 315, *334*
Notter, R. H., 381, 384, 385, 387, 388, 389, 390, *392, 393, 394, 395*
Novick, R. J., 452, 453, 454, 455, 456, 457, *489*
Novitsky, T. J., 399, 400, 404, *408, 409*
Novitzky, D., 503, 506, 510, *535, 536*
Nozaki, M., 387, *393*
Nunn, J. F., 367, *379*
Nuytinck, J. K. S., 306, 314, *337, 344*
Ny, T., 325, *344*
Nyhan, D., 452, 481, *490*

Oates, J., 288, *302*
Obenant, R. N., 461, *484*
Oberdoerster, G., 437, *447*
Obertacke, U., 306, 315, *341*
Obladen, M., 387, *394*
O'Brien, T. X., 402, *406*
O'Cain, C. F., 146, *158*
O'Connor, N., 253, *274*, 368, 370, 376, *378*
Oda, M., 465, *482*
Oden, M., 323, *347*
O'Donnell, K. M., 438, 439, *449*
O'Flaherty, J. T., 470, *487*
Ogawa, M., 325, *344*
Ogletree, M. L., 288, 289, 290, 291, 293, 294, 295, 296, *302, 303, 304,* 452, 463, 464, 468, *482, 488*
Ogushi, F., 323, *339*
O'Hara, P. J., 316, *350*
Ohkubo, I., 325, *345*
Ohlsson, K., 320, 321, 325, 326, 336, 342, 345, 349
Ohlsson, K. K., 311, 314, *345*
Ohning, B., 389, 390, *394*
Ohta, Y., 425, *432*
Okada, Y., 325, 328, *345*
Okubo, S., 118, 130, *134, 135*
Older, T., 254, *278*
Olsen, C. O., 226, *250*, 266, *281*
Olsen, G. N., 54, *60*
Olsson, I., 314, *345*
Olsson, I., 311, 314, *345*
Olsson, P., 452, 453, 454, 457, 458, 460, *488*
Olsson, S. G., 142, *158*
Olver, R. E., 435, 436, *447*
Onayemi, A., 446, *448*
O'Neill, B., 313, *331*
O'Neill, W. W., 368, *379*
Ong, R., 307, *339, 346*
Oobo, H., *538*
Oppenheimer, L., 266, 268, 270, *280*
Op'Tholt, T., 155, *161*
O'Quin, R., 174, 193, *197*, 254, 255, *279*
O'Reilly, R. A., 452, *487*
O'Rourke, R. A., 470, *486*
Orszulak, T. A., 464, *483*
Ortiz, X., 312, *352*
Osbakken, M., 452, 470, *484*
Osborn, M. J., 399, *407*
Osmand, A. P., 464, *483*
Ossanna, P. J., 323, *349*
Osswald, P. M., 149, *159*
Otani, A., 459, *484*
Otis, A. B., 109, 112, 115, 122, *136*, 139, *160*, 165, 171, 172, *197*
Overby, L. H., 461, *482*
Overland, E., 26, *34*, 306, *336*
Owen, M. C., 323, *333*
Owens, D. H., 116, *136*, 147, *160*
Owens, L. J., 354, 360, *365*
Oyarzun, M. J., 434, *449*
Oyer, P. E., 529, *536*
Oza, N. B., 309, *348*
Ozanne, G. M., 152, 153, 154, *158*
Ozeki, M., 465, *482*
Ozier, Y., 50, *61*

Paar, D., 306, 315, *341*
Pacht, E. R., 2, *19*, 306, *339*
Pacifico, A. D., 377, *379*
Padrines, M., 313, 323, *345*
Pagano, M., 325, *345*
Paglioni, S., 208, 218, *220*
Paliotta, J., 114, *136*
Palm, T., 71, *74*
Palmer, G. H., 400, *407*
Palmier, B., 149, *158*
Paloski, W. H., 503, *536*
Pamela, F., *534*
Panebianco, A. C., 316, *345*
Pangan, J., 510, *532*
Pannell, R., 321, *345*
Pannetier, A., 517, *535*
Papacostas, C. A., 452, 470, *484*
Parad, R. B., 387, *392*
Pare, J. A. P., 493, *538*
Pariente, R., 525, *534*
Parker, J. C., 356, 358, 364, *365, 366,* 425, *432,* 434, 435, 444, 445, *448, 449*
Parker, J. L., 263, *279*
Parker, M. M., 71, *75*, 263, 264, *276, 279, 282*
Parker, R. E., 424, 425, 426, *431*
Parks, D. A., 511, *535*
Parmentier, J. L., 353, 361, 364, *365*
Parrillo, J. E., 263, 264, *276, 279, 282*
Parsons, P. E., 16, *20*
Partain, C. L., 413, 424, *431*
Paskanik, A. M., 434, *447*
Pastan, I., 328, *338*
Paterson, D. G., 83, *88*
Patiota, J., 186, *195*
Patten, M. T., 267, 268, *278*
Patterson, G. A., 495, 506, 510, 511, 513, 516, 521, 524, 528, *532, 533, 534, 535, 536, 537, 538*
Paul, G. W., 2, *20*, 145, *160*, 385, *394*
Paull, D. E., 511, *535*
Pavek, K., 464, *487*
Pearlstein, L., 31, *34*, 78, *88*
Pearson, D., 2, *21*
Pearson, F. G., 495, 513, 516, 528, 528, *535, 536*
Pearson, M. G., 426, *432*
Peevy, K., 435, 445, *448*
Peirce, E. C., 368, *380*
Pejaudier, L., 326, *349*
Pelizzola, A., 446, *448*
Pelot, D., *343*
Pendergrass, R. E., 316, *340*
Penketh, A., 499, *536*
Penn, I., 316, *345*
Pennock, J. L., 529, *536*
Pepe, P. E., 6, 7, 8, *20*, 24, 26, 28, 30, 32, 35, 38, 40, 44, 48, *62*, 78, *89*, 173, 185, *197*, 268, *280*, 297, *304*, 305, *345*, 368, 370, 376, *379*
Peppin, G. J., 312, *346, 351*
Percival, C., 69, *73*
Perel, A., 306, *336*
Perez, H. D., 307, *339, 346*
Perez, W., 164, *198*
Perkins, G., 426, *432*
Perkowski, S. Z., 464, 467, *485, 487*
Permutt, S., 145, *157*, 211, *220*, 226, 248, *249, 250, 251,* 254, 268, 272, *280, 281, 283,* 433, 434, *447, 448, 449*
Perret, C., 316, 326, *344*
Perrin, F., 149, *158*
Perry, M., 360, 361, *365*
Perry, M. A., 425, *432*
Peru, A., 286, *303*
Pesenti, A., 144, 145, 146, 150, 152, 154, *157, 158,* 208, 211, 213, 214, 215, 218, *220,* 377, *379,* 423, *430,* 446, *448*
Peslin, R., 122, *136*
Peter, K., 452, 453, 454, 455, 457, 458, 463, 464, *483, 485*
Peters, J., 223, 225, 243, *250*
Peters, R., 254, *283*
Peters, R. M., 171, 181, *197*
Peters, T. J., 311, 314, *341*
Peters, W. J., 492, 500, *532, 534*
Peterson, N., 126, *135*
Petkau, A. J., 264, *279*

Petras, K., 464, *483*
Petrisch, P. H., 510, *536*
Petry, N. A., 452, 453, 454, 456, 460, *489*
Petty, T. L., 2, 4, *18, 20,* 23, 24, *33, 35,* 37, 39, 48, 54, *59, 61,* 65, *74,* 80, *87, 88,* 139, 143, 145, *156, 160,* 180, *197,* 99, *219,* 286, *302, 304,* 305, 310, *330, 336, 338, 346,* 367, 368, *278, 379,* 381, 385, *391, 394*
Pfeifer, L. M., 424, 425, 426, *429*
Piantelli, M., 321, *344*
Pick, R. A., 265, *280*
Pierce, A. K., 80, 82, *88*, 268, *275,* 309, *331*
Pierce, W. S., 456, *482*
Pierre, J., 33, *34*, 81, *87*
Pifarre, R., 269, 270, 272, *279*
Piiper, J., 68, *75*
Pimmel, R. L., 125, 126, *134, 136*
Pincemail, J., 306, 316, *335, 341*
Pinckard, R. N., 470, *486*
Pinkston, P., 438, 439, *449*
Pinsker, K. L., 509, 510, *535, 536, 538*
Pinsky, M. R., 226, 248, *249, 250,* 269, 270, 272, *275, 280*
Piper, P. J., 294, *303*, 464, *487*
Pison, U., 386, *394*
Pistolesi, M., 202, *220*, 417, *431*
Pitt, B., 256, *280*
Pitts, L., 26, *34*, 306, *336*
Pixley, R. A., 324, *335*
Pizzo, S. V., 324, *346*
Plamena, P., 316, *337*
Ploysongsang, Y., 29, *36*, 105, 106, 110, 114, *134*
Pluskwa, F., 189, *194*
Pluth, J. R., 464, *483*
Podgorski, G. T., 424, 425, 426, *431*
Pohil, R. J., 69, 70, *74*
Pohl, D., 25, 26, 31, 32, *36*
Pohost, G. M., 265, *278*, 413, *432*
Polk, H. C., Jr., 84, *88*
Pollack, M., 403, *408*
Pollard, D. S., 153, *157*
Pomerleau, C. M., 177, 189, *195*
Pontoppidan, H., 2, *20*, 39, 42, *62*, 139, 143, 154, *157*, 188, *195*, 211, *219*, 253, 254, 265, 268, *274, 280*, 305, *346*, 367, 368, 370, 376, *378, 379*
Popp, A. J., 503, *536*
Porter, R. R., 307, 324, *346*
Possmayer, F., 387, 389, 390, *392, 395*
Postlethwaite, A. E., 314, 315, 325, *346*
Potkin, R. T., 6, 7, 8, *20*, 24, 26, 28, 30, 32, *35*, 40, 44, 48, *62*, 78, *89*, 266, *280*, 305, *345*, 368, 370, 376, *379*
Poulis, D., 307, *339*
Powanda, M. L., 326, *346*
Powe, J. E., 306, *346*
Powers, J. C., 314, *349*
Powers, S. R., 71, *74*
Powers, S. R., Jr., 85, *89*, 254, *278, 280*
Pratap, K. S., 155, *161*
Prato, F. S., 424, *432*
Prato, P., 444, *448*
Pratt, C. W., 324, *346*
Pratt, P. C., 56, *62*, 368, *380*
Prewitt, R. M., 266, 268, 270, *280,* 446, *449*
Price, R. R., 413, 424, *431*
Priest, G. R., 53, *59*
Prieur, A., 509, *533*
Prihoda, T. J., 40, 55, *59*
Primiano, F. P., 154, *160*
Prockop, D. J., 425, *432*
Proctor, D. F., 122, *136*, 145, *159*, 434, *448*
Proctor, H. J., 368, *380*
Prommas, D. C., 266, *281*
Prost, J. F., 50, *61*, 226, *250*
Proud, G., 326, *330, 335*
Proud, G. M., 326, *339*
Pubols, J. E., 325, *346*
Puette, D., 328, *334*
Pulin, A., 492, *537*
Pykett, I. L., 413, *432*

Quan, S. F., 255, *278*
Quentin, M., 326, *349*
Quinn, D., 258, *280*
Quinn, D. A., 39, 42, *62*, 305, *346*, 367, *379*
Quinn, T. C., 83, 85, *87*
Qvist, J., 254, 261, 265, 268, *280*

Rabinovitch, J., 509, *536*
Rabson, J., 265, 268, *276, 281*
Radegran, K., 452, 453, 454, 457, 458, 460, *488*
Radford, E. P., Jr., 109, 112, 115, 131, *135, 136,* 147, 153, *160*
Radoux, L., 306, 307, *335*
Ragsdale, C., 312, *351*
Rahm, R. L., 503, *536*
Rahn, H., 139, *160*
Rajagopalan, B., 258, *280*
Raju, T. K., 387, *394*
Rakowski, H., *533*
Raleigh, J. A., 468, *488*
Ramachandran, P. R., 139, 140, *159*
Rambo, W., 306, *346*
Ramsay, G., 102, *103*
Randal, H. T., 493, *532*
Rankin, J. S., 226, *250*, 266, *281*
Ranson, J. H. C., 307, *339*
Rao, T. L. K., 269, 270, 272, *279*
Rapaport, E., 266, 267, 268, 269, *276*
Rapin, M., 146, 147, 154, *159*
Rasmussen, B., 55, *60*
Rattenborg, C., 116, *136*
Raubitschek, A. A., 403, *408*
Rauric, J. M., 218, *220*
Rauss, A., 255, 257, *282*
Rauvala, H., 385, *394*
Read, R. C., 452, 453, 454, 455, 457, 459, 463, 467, 470, *484*
Redl, H. R., 314, *344*
Rees, A. J., 306, *352*
Reese, L., 424, *432*
Reeves, J. T., 66, *75*
Reeves, T. G., 464, *486*
Regoli, D., 309, *346*
Reich, E., 314, *337, 350*
Reichart, B., 510, *535, 536*
Reid, B., 2, 18, *306, 330*
Reid, B. A., 2, *21*
Reid, K. B. M., 307, 308, 324, *340, 346*
Reid, L., 259, *282*
Reid, L. M., 496, *536*
Reilly, C. F., 311, 323, 324, *350*
Reines, H. D., 306, *346*
Reitz, B. A., 511, 529, *532, 534, 536*
Rekik, N., 255, *282*
Rennard, S., 16, *21*, 425, *429*
Rennard, S. I., 438, 439, *449*
Rent, R., 464, 467, *484, 488*
Repine, J. E., 286, *304*, 311, *349*, 461, 467, *489*
Reus, D. H., 24, 26, 28, 30, 32, *35*, 40, 44, 48, *62*
Revak, S., 383, 384, 386, 387, 388, 389, *392, 393, 394*
Revak, S. D., *334*
Rey, F., 316, 326, *344*
Reynaert, M., *335*
Reynolds, H. Y., 314, *344*
Reynolds, J., 82, *87*
Reynolds, J. J., 311, 325, *344*
Revak, S. D., 309, 311, 323, 328, *333, 334*
Rhodes, C. G., 216, 217, *220, 221*
Ribaudo, C. A., 28, *35*
Rich, S., 499, *536*
Richards, D. W., Jr., 265, *275*
Richards, J. H., 69, *75*
Richardson, J. V., 54, *62*
Riches, D. W. H., 312, 314, *338*
Richman, P., 385, 388, *394*
Richman, P. S., 390, *394*
Rickway, D. A., 356, *365*
Rieuf, P., 154, *159*
Rifkin, D. B., 315, *337, 343*
Righetti, A., 266, 270, *282*
Riley, D. J., 321, *342*
Riley, R. L., 433, 434, *447, 448*
Rinaldo, J., 296, 297, 298, 299, *302*

Rinaldo, J. E., 2, 13, *20*, 24, *35*, 40, 41, 42, *62*, 305, 306, 316, *343, 346*
Rinderknecht, H., 326, *347*
Rinehart, J. J., 288, *304*
Rippe, B., 356, 358, *365, 366,* 434, 435, 444, *449*
Risberg, B. O., 323, *347*
Ritzman, S. E., 326, *334*
Rivara, D., 144, 146, 147, 154, *159*
Riveau, G. R., 404, *408, 410*
Rivolta, M., 152, *158*, 208, 211, 213, 214, 215, 218, *220*
Robbins, R., 16, *21*
Robert, D., 144, 149, *158, 161*
Roberts, R. C., 323, *347*
Robertson, B., 387, 390, *391, 394*
Robertson, C. H., 268, *275*
Robertson, C. H., Jr., 270, *275*
Robertson, O. H., 82, *89*
Robin, E. D., 66, *75*, 499, 525, *532*
Robins, A. G., 173, *195*, 268, *278*
Robinson, D., 452, 454, 455, 456, 457, 458, 459, 463, 465, *486*
Robinson, D. R., 452, 453, 454, 457, 458, 460, 463,464, 475, *487*
Robinson, P. C., 383, *393*
Robotham, J. L., 223, 225, 226, 234, 237, 238, 239, 243, 248, *250, 251,* 254, 265, 268, 269, 272, *281, 282, 283*
Robson, J. G., 146, *157*
Rochester, D. F., 178, *197*
Rock, P. B., 66, *75*
Rocker, D. M., 2, *21*
Rodmark, O., 459, *485*
Rodriguez-Roisin, R., 31, 33, *36*, 55, *63*
Rodriguez, R. M., 170, 171, 175, 176, *196*
Rodvien, R., 305, *336*
Rogers, K., 452, 453, 454, 455, 457, *488*
Rogers, M. C., 511, *534*
Rohr, H., 452, 458, 459, 464, *484*
Rogers, R. M., 13, *20*, 42, *62*, 305, 306, *346, 347*
Rohrer, F., 114, 116, *136,* 187, *197*
Rollo, F. D., 413, 424, *431*
Rommelsheim, K., 202, *221*
Rondeau, E., *534*
Roos, A., 266, *281*
Rose, A. G., 503, 506, 510, *535, 536*
Rosen, F. S., 399, *407*
Rosen, H., 311, *330*
Rosenberg, R. D., 324, *348*
Rosenberg, S., 324, *347*
Rosenthal, M. H., 427, *431*
Rosenzweig, D. Y., 145, *158*
Roskos, K. V., 306, 307, *351*
Roslansky, P. F., 399, 400, 404, *408, 409*
Ross, W. R. D., 167, 173, 174, 185, *195, 197*
Rossi, A., 105, 114, 116, 118, 119, 123, 124, 126, 128, 129, 130, *133, 134, 135, 136, 137, 142, 160*, 186, *195*
Rossi, F., 144, 145, 146, 150, 152, *157, 158,* 211, 213, 214, 215, *220,* 423, *430*
Rossi, G. P., 150, *157*, 206, 211, 213, 214, 215, *220*, 446, *448*
Rotget, M., 126, *136*
Rothma, S. S., 316, *342*
Rotman, H. H., 54, *63*
Roussos, C., 163, 165, 167, 178, *194, 197,* 263, *277*
Roussos, C. H., 178, *197*
Roy, R. J., 254, *278*
Roy, R. S., 315, *347*
Royston, D., 437, *449*
Rozkovec, A., 216, 217, *221*
Rozmanith, J. S., 320, *347*
Rubenstein, M., 403, *410*
Rubin, D. B., 18, *21*
Ruhmann-Wennhold, A., 286, *303*
Russell, J. A., 17, *21*, 306, *349*
Rutllant, M., 50, *59*
Ruud, T. E., 329, *330*
Ryan, J. W., 309, *348*
Ryan, U. S., 315, *347*

Saba, T. M., 85, *89*
Sabiston, D. C., Jr., 226, *250*, 266, *281*
Sacks, S. A., 510, *536*
Sadoff, J. C., 264, *283*, 401, *410*
Sagawa, K., 182, *197*, 226, *251*
Sagone, A. L., 288, *304*
Sahn, S. A., 48, *61*, 180, *197*, 368, *379*
Said, S. I., 145, *160*, 471, 472, *488*
Saidel, G. M., 154, *160*
Sakakibara, N., 510, *537*
Sakakibara, S., 321, *342*
Saklad, M., 114, *136*
Sakulramrung, R., 402, *408*
Sala, N., 50, *60*
Salata, R., 80, *89*
Saldeen, T., 309, 310, *347*
Salerno, T. A., 452, 453, 454, 455, 456, 457, *488, 489*
Salmon, R. B., 154, *160*
Saltin, B., 66, 71, *73*
Saltzman, H. A., 423, *432*
Salvador, R. A., 211, *221*
Salvesen, G. S., 326, *347*
Samuelsson, B., 459, *485*
Samuelson, P. N., 464, *486*
Sanchalla, V., 66, 67, *75*
Sanchez, M. M., 510, *537*
Sanfillipo, F., 504, *536*
Sanford, J. P., 80, 82, *88*
Santamore, W. P., 239, *249*, 261, *275*
Sarnoff, S. J., 177, *197*, 265, *275*
Sasaki, M., 325, *345*
Sasaki, T., 146, *158*
Saskela, O., 326, *343*
Sassoon, C. S. H., 165, *197*
Satake, K., 320, *347*
Sato, T., 465, *482*
Satoh, P. S., 306, 307, *348*
Satoshi, T., *538*
Saullo, V. J., 18, *19*
Saumon, G., 126, *134*, 437, 438, 441, 443, 444, 445, 446, *447*
Saunders, N., 226, *250*, 268, *281*
Sawdey, M., 325, *344*
Sayers, C. A., 326, 328, *331*
Scanlin, T. F., 498, *536*
Schaer, G. L., 264, *276*
Schafers, H. J., 511, 521, 528, *533, 536, 538*
Schaff, H. V., 464, *483*
Schapira, M., 323, 324, *335, 347*
Scharf, S. M., 185, *198*, 226, *250*, 265, 268, 269, 272, *281*
Schaufstatter, I. U., 386, *395*
Scheiermann, N., 306, 315, *341*
Schellekens, J., 402, *406*
Schenep, J. L., 398, *408*
Scherzinger, A. L., 412, 413, *432*
Schever, R., *352*
Schlagg, G., 314, *344*, 386, *394*
Schlesinger, T., 263, *282*
Schlobohm, R. M., 255, *278*, 367, *378*
Schmid, K., 326, 329, *334*
Schmidt, G. B., 368, *379*
Schmidt, H. C., 424, 426, 427, *432*
Schmidt-Neuerberg, K. P., 306, 315, *341*
Schneider-Pozzer, M., 313, 323, *345*
Schneider, R. C., 306, 310, *347*, 413, 453, 472, *486*
Schnell, W. A., Jr., 464, *483*
Schnells, G., 386, *394*
Schnieder, H., 382, 388, *392*
Schoene, R. B., 4, *21*
Schonfeld, S. A., 29, *36*, 55, *63*
Schramm, W., 314, *336*
Schraufstatter, I. U., 386, *395*
Schreiber, G., 325, *337*
Schreiner, G. L., 147, *156*
Schreyen, H., 14, 15, 16, *19*, 306, 307, *335*
Schroeder, W. R., 461, 467, *489*
Schroter, R. C., 154, *158*
Schuette, A., 459, 464, 467, *490*, 516, *535*
Schuette, W., 263, 264, *279*
Schulman, D. S., 266, 267, *274, 281*
Schultz, E., 461, *487, 488*
Schultz, E. L., 461, *482*
Schulz, F., 326, *351*
Schumacher, W. A., 452, 463, 464, *488*

Schuster, D. P., 3, 4, *19*, 306, 315, *332*
Schuyler, M., 323, *343*
Schwaber, J. R., 126, *135*
Schwartz, G. G., 241, *251*
Schwartz, L. B., *347*
Schwendener, R., 141, *161*
Scott, C. F., 323, 324, *347*
Scott, J., 499, *536*
Scott, S. M., 316, *345*
Scott, W. C., 509, *533*
Scovill, W. A., 85, *89*
Scully, H., 495, 513, 516, *535*
Seal, R. M. E., 316, *339*
Sealy, J., 309, *348*
Seeger, W. G., 385, *395*
Segovia, L., 54, *60*
Seibel, R., 315, *332*
Seidenfeld, J. J., 25, 26, 31, 32, 33, *35, 36,* 83, *89*
Seindaro, E. E., 499, *537*
Sellers, S. E. 496, *538*
Selverstone, N. J., 109, 112, 115, *136*
Senior, R. M., 314, 321, 325, *348, 351, 440, 441, 447*
Senor, R. M., 312, 314, *332*
Serafin, W., 288, *302*
Sergysels, R., 54, *63*
Sessler, C. N., 452, 457, *484*
Seydoux, C., 316, 326, *344*
Seyer, J. M., 312, 314, *342, 343*
Shabetai, R., 226, *251*
Shah, D. M., 503, *536*
Shah, P. K., 71, *75*
Shale, D. J., 2, *21*
Shapiro, B. A., 139, *160*
Shapiro, D. L., 387, 389, 390, *394, 395*
Sharma, O. M., 305, *331*
Sharp, J. T., 122, *134*, 144, 153, *160*
Shaw, R. A., 55, *63*
Shear, M. J., 399, *407*
Shelburne, J., *429*
Shelhamer, J. H., 71, *75*, 263, 264, *279*
Shellburne, J. D., 56, *62*
Sheller, J. R., 288, *302*
Shenep, J. L., 403, *406*
Shennan, A., 387, 389, *392*
Shenton, B. K., 326, *330, 335, 339*
Shepard, R. J., 124, *136*
Shepro, D., 306, *338*, 464, *486*
Sherer, S. D., 306, *332*
Sherman, J. E., 401, *410*
Shibutani, K., 66, 67, *75*
Shiokawa, H., 325, *345*
Shioya, S., 425, *432*
Shires, G. T., 86, *89*, 263, 264, *282*
Shlaes, D., 80, *89*
Shoemaker, W. C., 6, *21*, 140, *161*
Short, A., 306, *346*
Short, A. K., 211, *221*
Short, B. L., 265, *281*
Shroff, S., 261, *283*
Shubin, H., 25, 31, *34*
Shuman, W. P., *20*, 45, 48, *62*, 202, *220*, 446, *448*
Shumway, N. E., 529, *536*
Shurter, H. J., 54, *61*
Sibbald, W. J., 2, *18, 21*, 211, *221,* 256, 260, 266, 268, *275, 281,* 296, 297, 298, 299, *302,* 306, 330, 346
Siber, G. R., 399, 400, 402, 404, *408, 409*
Siegel, J., 464, *483*
Siegel, J. H., 263, *281*
Siegleman, S. S., 497, 521, 537, 538
Sigal, N. H., 403, *407*
Silberberg, M., 309, *341*
Sillye, G., 163, *198*
Silverberg, M., 309, *337*
Silvers, G. W., 2, *20*, 145, *160*, 385, *394*
Simmons, D. L., 28, *34*
Simmons, R. L., 509, *537*
Simon, R. H., 18, *21*, 306, *348, 391*
Simoneau, G., 144, 146, 147, 154, *159*
Simonneay, G., 254, *278*
Simpson, D. L., 56, *63*
Sinha, S. B. P., 510, 521, *537, 538*
Sinnott, J. T., 521, *537*
Sinosich, M. J., 464, *483*

Siraganian, R. P., 314, 315, *348*
Sirik, Z., 55, *60*
Skalina, S., 424, *432*
Skarnes, R. C., 399, 403, *407, 408*
Skehill, A., 401, 402, *407*
Skidgel, R. A., 470, *488, 489*
Skillman, J. J., 80, *89*
Sklar, L. A., 386, *395*
Skor, D., 464, *483*
Sleiman, C., *534*
Slotman, G. J., 306, *348*
Sludson, L. D., 305, 316, *343*
Sly, P. D., 118, *134*
Smadja, C., 101, *104*
Smallbone, B. W., 470, *488*
Smedegard, G., 464, *487*
Smith, D., 69, *73*, 254, *283*
Smith, F. W., 427, *431*
Smith, J. D., 42, 44, 48, *59*, 65, *73*, 77, 78, 79, 81, *87*, 93, *103*, 263, *274*, 305, *331*, 368, 376, 377, *378*
Smith, J. J., 315, *348*
Smith, J. P., 24, 26, *33*
Smith-Erichsen, N., 329, *348*
Smith, P. K., 226, *250*, 266, *281*
Smith, T. C., 172, 176, 179, 180, 181, 182, 191, 192, *196, 198*
Smith, W. R., 54, *60*
Smithies, M., 70, *73*, 263, *274*
Smyth, J. A., 446, *448*
Snapper, J. R., 286, 288, 289, *302, 304,* 427, *429,* 468, *482*
Snider, G. L., 323, *352*
Snider, M. T., 38, 39, *63*, 259, *283*, 368, *380*, 451, *490*
Snyder, W. H., 368, *380*
Snyder, W. H., III, 6, 11, *21*, 300, *304*
Soldau, K., 405, *409*
Soler, P., 437, 438, *447*
Solitto, R., 424, 425, 426, 427, *431*
Soll, R. F., 387, *392*
Solomkin, J. S., 306, 307, *348*
Sommer, G., 427, *430*
Soufer, R., 266, 267, *274, 281*
Sourlis, S. H., 83, 85, *87*
Spagnaolo, P. J., 286, *303*
Spaulding, S., 452, 453, 454, 456, 460, *489*
Specht, H., 165, *194*
Spees, E. K., 504, *536*
Spector, S. L., 56, *63*
Spielmann, R. P., 258, *279*
Spiro, D., 440, 441, *447*
Spitznagel, J. K., 311, 314, *345*
Spragg, R., 2, *19*
Spragg, R. G., 311, 323, 328, *334,* 385, 386, 390, *392, 393, 394, 395*
Sprangers, L., 306, 307, *335*
Sprung, C. L., 24, 32, *33*, 296, 297, 298, 299, *302*
Stager, M. A., 25, 26, 31, 32, 33, *35*, 40, 42, 44, 45, 47, 48, 51, *62*, 65, *75*, 77, 78, *88*, 101, *104*, 253, 263, *279*, 305, 316, *343*
Stahl, W. M., 323, *348*
Staneck, J. L., 520, *537*
Stanescu, D. C., 146, *157*
Stanfor, R. E., 54, *61*
Stanford, R. E., 145, *160*, 385, *394*
Stankus, K. E., 258, *278*
Stanley, J. C., 452, 453, 454, 456, 457, 458, 459, 460, 463, 467, *486, 489*
Starkey, P., 326, *331*
Starkey, T. D., 510, *537*
Staub, N. C., 26, *34, 36*, 216, 217, *219, 221,* 286, *303*, 306, *336,* 426, *432,* 446, *447,* 461, *482, 487, 488*
Staudacher, V., 492, *537*
Stead, N., 324, *348*
Steele, P., 266, 268, *276*
Stefani, L., 383, 389, *394*
Stefaniszyn, H. J., 452, 453, 454, 455, 456, 457, *489*
Steg, G., 270, 271, 272, *278*
Steinberg, S., 315, *332*
Steinbuch, M., 324, 326, *348, 349*
Stenberg, J., 66, 71, *73*
Stengel, P. W., 145, *157*
Stevens, G. H., 510, *537*

Stevens, P., 401, *410*
Stevens, P. M., 497, *537*
Stevens, R. M., 80, *89*
Stevenson, W. C., 511, *534*
Stewart, R. W., 307, *333*
Stewart, S., 499, *536*
Stiff, E. J., 125, *136*
Stinnett, H. O., 270, *281*
Stinson, E. B., 269, 272, *275*, 529, *536*
Stohr, G., 385, *395*
Stollhoff, K., 316, *331*
Stone, O. L., 314, 325, *333*
Stone, P. J., 323, *333*
Stone, P. S., 323, *352*
Straton, H. H., 72, *75*
Stratton, C.J., 383, *395*
Strauss, D. C., 82, *89*
Strauss, H. W., 256, 258, 260, 265, 268, 273, *277, 278, 280*
Strayer, D., 387, *393*
Streisand, R. L., 452, 453, 454, *485*
Stricklin, G. P., 325, *349*
Stuard, I. D., 54, *61*
Stuart, R. S., 234, 237, 238, *250*
Stuckey, J. H., 452, 453, 454, *485*
Suarez, L. D., 499, *537*
Sudlow, M. F., 154, *158*
Suffredini, A. F., 263, *282*
Sugahara, K., 383, *393*
Sullivan, M., 114, *136*
Sullivan, M. J., 186, *195*
Summer, W. R., 226, *251*, 270, *280*
Suratt, P. M., 116, *136*, 147, *160*
Suter, P. M., 50, 51, *62*, 141, 142, 148, *161*, 266, 268, 270, *282*, 316, *343*
Sutherland, J. B., 266, 268, *280*
Sutton, J. R., 66, *75*
Suzuki, S., 465, *482*
Suzuki, Y., 387, *395*
Swan, H. J. C., 258, *278*
Swayze, S. C., 496, *538*
Sweeney, M. S., 521, *537*
Sykes, M. K., 452, 454, 456, 459, 467, *486*
Szczepkowski, T. W., 425, *430*
Taeusch, H. W., Jr., 433, *449*
Tahamont, M. V., 306, 320, *349*, 459, 464, *485, 489*
Taichman, G. C., 512, *534*
Tajkarimi, S., 511, *538*
Takaro, T., 497, *537*
Takasowa, T., 325, *345*
Takayama, T., 511, *538*
Takishima, T., 125, *135*, 146, *158*
Talamo, C., 181, 184, 190, 191, *195*
Talamo, R. C., 315, *344*
Talucci, R. C., 14, 16, *20*
Tan, F., 470, *488, 489*
Tan, L., 386, *394*
Tanaka, T., 314, *349*
Tanser, P. H., 493, *538*
Tashkin, D. P., 70, *75*
Tate, R. M., 16, *20*, 286, 296, 297, 298, 299, *302, 304,* 311, *349*, 461, 467, *489*
Tate, W. J., 400, *409*
Taxman, R. M., 265, *276*
Taylor, A. E., 353, 354, 356, 358, 360, 361, 362, 364, *365, 366,* 425, *432*, 434, 435, 444, *449*
Taylor, D. G., 424, 425, *432*
Taylor, F. B., 385, *395*
Taylor, G. A., 452, 453, 454, 457, 458, 460, *488*
Taylor, M. R., 326, *330*
Taylor, N. E., 470, *488*
Taylor, R. F., 176, *198*
Taylor, R. L., 452, *489*
Taylor, R. M., 326, *335*
Tazelaar, H. D., 510, *537*
Te, T. T., 165, *197*
Teboul, J.-L., 255, 257, 270, 271, 272, *278, 282*
Teger-Nilsson, A. C., 323, *347*
Teisner, B., 464, *483*
Teitelbaum, S. L., 314, 325, *351*
Tenaillon, A., 148, *161*, 254, *278*
ten Boekhorst, T. P. A., 306, *337*
ten Cate, J. W., 84, *89*
Teng, N. N. H., 403, *409*
Tenney, S. M., 71, *75*
Teodori, M. F., 511, *534*

Teplitz, C., 211, *221*, 440, 441, *449*
Teres, D., 86, *89*
Tesseire, B., 146, 147, 154, *159*
Tessier, L. H., 324, *334*
Test, S. T., 31;2, 323, *349, 351*
Theodore, J., 499, 525, *532*
Thigpen, J., 434, 435, 444, *449*, 461, *483*
Thijs, L. G., 71, *74*
Thirion, M., *282*
Thomas, A. N., 368, *380*
Thomas, G. D., 80, 82, *88*
Thomas, L., 144, *161*
Thomas, L. J., 266, *281*
Thomas, S. J., 453, 464, 465, 475, *487*
Thommasen, H. V., 17, *21*, 306, *349*
Thompson, R. C., 325, *349*
Thonar, E. J., 312, *352*
Thorpe, J. E., 520, *537*
Thorvaldson, J., 266, *282*
Thupari, J. N., 85, *89*
Tierney, D. F., 120, *135*, 384, *392*, 437, 442, 446, *449*
Till, G. O., 16, *21*, 311, *349*
Tilney, N. L., 316, *349*
Tinker, J., 263, *274*
Tobias, P. S., 404, 405, *409*
Tobin, M. J., 146, *161*, 164, *198*
Todd, T. R., 495, 506, 513, 516, 521, 528, *535, 536, 537*
Toledo-Pereyra, L. H., 509, *537*
Tomashefski, J. F., Jr., 259, *282*
Tompkins, R. K., 316, *349*
Tonnensen, A. S., 155, *158*
Tonnesen, M. G., 311, *352*
Tooker, J., 258, *282*
Toossi, Z., 80, *89*
Toresin, A., 152, *158*
Torres, A., 31, 33, *36*, 306, *350*, 452, 454, 457, 458, 460, 463, *487*, 497, 510, *537, 538*
Torres, R., 510, *533*
Torresin, A., 150, *157*, 202, 204, 206, 211, 212, 213, 214, 215, *219, 220*
Toung, T. J. K., 511, *534*
Tow, D. E., 272, *281*
Townsend, E., 492, 500, *534*
Townsend, E. R., 464, *486*
Townsley, M. I., 356, 358, *365, 366*, 434, 435, 444, *449*
Tracey, K. J., 86, *89*, 263, 264, 265, *282*
Trai, I., 211, *221*
Trapani, R.-J., 399, *407*
Traverso, L. W., 316, *349*
Travis, D., 323, *340*
Travis, J., 311, 321, 323, 324, 325, 328, *332, 337, 343, 345, 349, 350*
Traystman, R. J., 511, *534*
Treiber, E. O., 425, *429*
Trelstad, R. L., 211, *221*
Treves, S., 258, *280*
Trinkle, J. K., 452, *489*
Trippenbach, T., 163, *194*
Trobaugh, G., 266, *280*
Trop, D., 145, *160*
Trouillet, J.-L., 33, *34*
Trubovich, R. V., 101, *104*
Trump, B. F., 316, *340, 341*
Trunet, P., 53, *61*
Truwit, J. D., 172, 176, 177, 184, *198*
Tryba, M., 84, *89*
Tsai, M. J., 125, *136*
Tsay, D.-G., 424, 426, 427, *432*
Tschesche, H., 325, *342*
Tsuji, C., 425, *432*
Tsuji, F., *538*
Tucker, H. J., 54, *60*
Tuman, K. J., 140, *156*
Tumen, J., 286, *302*
Turino, G. M., 425, *432*
Turley, K., 260, *282*
Turner, J., 24, 32, *35*
Turner, M. D., 492, *533*
Tuxen, D. V., 173, *198*
Tweardy, D., 80, *89*
Tyson, G. S., 226, *250*, 266, *281*
Tytgat, G. N. J., 84, *89*

Ulevitch, R. J., 399, 402, 404, 405, *407, 409*
Unkeless, J. C., 314, *350*
Utell, M. J., 437, *447*
Uziel, L., 446, *448*

Vadas, P., 17, *21*
Vaheri, A., 326, 328, *339, 343*
Vaillant, A., 517, *535*
Valeri, C. R., 306, *338*, 464, *486*
Valigorsky, J., 316, *340*
Van Den Berghe, 328, *350*
Van Der Zee, H., 437, *447*
van Deventer, S. J. H., 84, *89*
Van Erck, J., 316, *341*
Van Haeringen, J. R., 54, *61*
Vankessel, A., 525, *532*
Van Leuven, F., 328, *350*
Van Lith, P., 144, 153, *160*
vanMelle, G., 264, *274*, 316, 326, *344*, 401, *405*
Van Muijen, G. N., 325, *335*
Van Munster, P. J., 314, *344*
van de Woestijne, K. P., 126, *135*, 146, *157*
Vassalli, J. D., 314, *337*
Vassary, M. J., 263, *277*
Vaugham, L., 323, *333*
Vaughan, D. W., 312, *333*
Vaughan, W. K., 504, *536*
Vavrin, Z., 314, *333*
Veith, F. J., 497, 509, 510, 521, 535, *536, 537, 538*
Velsaco, F., 306, *350*
Venge, P., 17, *19*, 314, *345*
Venstrom, K., 383, 389, *392*
Venus, B., 140, 155, *161*
Verhoef, J., 402, *406*
Vesconi, S., 150, *157*, 446, *448*
Viale, J. P., 69, *73*, 188, *198*
Viau, F., 81, *87*
Vidyasagar, D., 387, *394*
Viires, N., 163, *198*
Villemant, D., 256, 258, 266, 270, *276*
Vincent, J.-L., *282*
Vinitski, S., 424, 426, *432*
Viquerat, C. E., 266, 270, *282*
Virgilio, R., 254, *283*
Visser, M. C. M., *337*
Vitale, G., 208, 218, *220*
Vlahakes, G. J., 260, *282*
Voelkel, N. F., 452, 453, 457, *483*
Vogt, M., 264, *274*, 401, *405*
Voigt, W. H., 386, *394*
Volmer, R. T., 56, *62*
von Neergaard, K., 115, 122, *136*
von Wichert, P., 2, *21*
Vreede, R. W., 402, *406*
Vuilleumier, P., 122, *137*

Wachter, E., 325, *339*
Wachter, R. M., 367, *378*
Wager, R. E., 383, 389, *395*
Wagner, D. P., 92, 93, 94, 95, 101, *103, 104*
Wagner, H. W., 226, *250*
Wagner, P. D., 31, *35*, 66, *75*, 92, *103*, 423, *432*
Wahl, L. M., *350*
Wahl, S. M., *350*
Wahlers, T., 511, *533, 538*
Wakefield, T. W., 452, 453, 454, 456, 457, 458, 459, 460, 463, 467, *486, 489*
Walker, G. R., 492, *533*
Walker, L., 80, *89*
Walker, R. I., 265, *281*
Walkinshaw, M., 140, *161*
Wallis, T., 226, 239, *251*
Wallis, T. W., 268, *282*
Wallwork, J. L., 499, 510, 529, *536, 538*
Walsh, K. A., 307, *344, 350*
Walshe, K., 306, *350*
Waltemath, C. L., 120, 127, *134*
Walter, S. D., 66, *75*
Wang, D. L., 384, *391*
Wang, L. S., 511, *533, 538*
Wang, T., 461, *488*
Ward, P., 286, *303*
Ward, P. A., 306, 311, *348, 349*, 399, *407*

Ward, S. B., 403, *410*
Warley, A. R., 67, *74, 75*
Warner, A. E., 453, 461, 462, *489, 490*
Warp, P., 311, *336*
Warp, P. A., 311, *350*
Warren, H. S., 399, 400, 402, 404, *408, 409, 410*
Warren, J. S., 311, *350*
Warshaw, A. L., 316, *350*
Warshawski, F. J., 211, *221*
Wasmus, G., 258, *279*
Wasserman, M. A., 464, *485*
Watanabe, F., 422, 423, 427, *430*
Watanabe, S., 325, 328, *345*
Waters, O. F., 495, 513, 516, *535*
Watkins, W. D., 264, *279*, 459, 464, 467, *490*
Waxman, A. D., 258, *278*
Waxman, M. B., *536*
Wead, W. B., 226, *251*
Weaver, D. W., 316, *350*
Weaver, L. J., 14, *19*, 266, *280*, 306, 307, *338*
Webb, H. H., 437, 442, 446, *449*
Webb, W. R., 424, 425, 426, 427, *431*, 492, *533*
Weber, C. J., 263, *277*
Weber, K. C., 145, *157*
Weber, K. T., 261, *283*
Webler, W., 258, *277*
Webster, N. R., 367, *379*
Webster, R. O., 14, 15, 16, *21*, 30, *34*, 306, 307, *351*, 459, *490*
Wedel, S. A., 84, *88*
Weg, J. G., 66, 69, *74*, 140, *157*
Wei, H., 263, 264, *282*
Weibel, E. R., 2, *19*, 441, 445, *447, 448*
Weigelt, J. A., 6, 11, *21*, 307, *350*, 368, *380*
Weigfelt, J. A., 300, *304*
Weil, M. H., 25, 31, *34*
Weiland, J. E., 2, *19*, 306, *339, 350*
Weinbaum, G., 328, *333, 342*, 386, *391*
Weinberg, P. F., 14, 15, 16, 18, *21*, 306, 307, *351*
Weiner, J., 440, 441, *447*
Weiner-Kronish, J. P., 2, *19*
Weinstein, D. B., 399, *409*
Weinstein, S. S., 521, *537*
Weisel, R. D., 495, 513, 516, *533, 535*
Weiss, J., *249*
Weiss, M. E., 452, 481, *490*
Weiss, S. J., 311, 312, 314, 323, 325, 327, 328, *335, 346, 351*
Weissman, G., 459, *485*
Welch, G. H., 177, *197*
Welgus, H. G., 312, 314, 325, *332, 348, 349, 351*
Welther, H., 326, *340*
Wendt, P., 326, *351*
Werb, Z., 314, 325, *338, 344, 351*
Werko, L., 265, *275*
Wertz, M. J., 94, 100, 101, *103*
Wesbey, G. E., 427, *431*
Wesseler, T. A., 520, *537*
West, J. B., 255, 266, *276, 283*, 423, *432*
Wetaby, S., 377, *379*
Westcott, J. Y., 452, 453, 457, *483*
Westhofen, P., 202, *221*
Wetmore, V., 370, 377, *378*
Wewers, M. D., 312, 324, 329, *351*, 496, *538*
Wexler, H. R., 424, *432*
Wheeldon, E. B., 461, *490*
Whitcomb, M. E., 55, *63*, 265, *276*
White, J. G., 286, *303*
White, J. J., 493, *538*
White, R., 311, 314, 326, *340, 351*
Whitehouse, W. M., Jr., 452, 453, 454, 456, 458, 459, 460, 463, 467, *486, 489*
Whitelaw, W. A., 167, *195*
Whitney, W. P., 266, 268, *276*
Whittenberger, J. L., 115, 122, 131, *135*, 147, 153, *160*
Wichterman, K. A., 70, *74*
Wickersham, N., 288, *303*
Wicklund, B., 31, *35*, 79, *88*

Wicomb, W. N., 503, 506, *535*
Widdicombe, J. G., 144, *159*
Wiener-Kronish, J. P., 367, *378*
Wiggins, R. C., 309, *352*
Wilcox, B. R., 511, *535*
Wilcox, P. E., 307, *350*
Wildevuur, C. R., 493, 497, *538*
Wiles, C. M., 167, *197*
Wilkinson, A., 389, *395*
Willems, L. N., 325, *335*
Williams, E., 403, *407*
Williams, M. C., 383, *391*
Willingham, M. C., 328, *338*
Wilson, M. E., 400, *407*
Wilson, R. F., 316, *350*
Wilson, R. S., 188, *195*, 254, 265, 268, *280*
Winchurch, R. A., 85, *89*
Winkler, G. C., 461, *490*
Winterbourne, C. C., *337*
Winterton, J., 84, *88*
Winton, T. L., 516, *535*
Wirz, K., 115, 122, *136*
Wise, R. A., 226, 239, 248, *249, 250*, 254, 268, *280, 283*
Wise, W. C., 306, *346*
Wiseman, M. S., 2, *21*
Wismar, B. L., 461, 462, *484*
Withcomb, M. E., 139, *157*
Witte, J., 326, *340, 352*
Wittes, J. T., 496, *538*
Wohl, M. E., 126, *135*
Wolf, G., 424, *432*
Wolf, H. R. D., 385, *395*
Wolff, G., 141, *161*
Wolff, S. M., 403, *410*
Wolke, S., 86, *89*
Wollmer, P., 216, 217, *221*
Wonders, T., 459, 464, 467, *490*
Wong, P. D., 323, *343*
Wong, P. S., 323, *343*
Wood, L. D. H., 254, 266, 268, 270, *275, 280*, 446, *449*
Woods, D. E., 81, 82, *88, 89*
Wool, N., 140, *156*
Woolverton, W. C., 446, *447*
Worthen, G. S., 16, *20*, 306, 311, *352*
Wright, D. G., 312, *337*
Wright, J. R., 383, 389, *392, 395*
Wright, P., 186, *198*
Wu, J. N., 437, *448*
Wuepper, K. D., 309, *333*
Wunderer, G., 329, *337*
Wunderlich, A., 403, *409*
Wykle, R. L., 470, *487*
Wynands, J. E., 493, *538*
Wyszogrodski, I., 433, *449*

Xaubet, A., 55, *63*

Yacoub, M. H., 511, *538*
Yahav, J., 55, *63*
Yamabayaski, H., 425, *432*
Yamashita, C., *538*
Yamazaki, F., 510, 511, *534, 538*
Yates, A. J., 493, *534*
Yernault, J. C., 54, *63*
Yipintsoi, T., 509, *535*
Yoshikawa, K., 510, 511, *533, 538*
Younes, M., 446, *447*
Young, E. J., 400, 403, *406*
Young, L. S., 401, *410*
Young, P. M., 66, *75*
Young, S. L., 427, *429*
Young, S. W., 413, 424, *432*
Yu, S. H., 389, 390, *395*

Zadoff, A., 288, *302*
Zamel, N., 524, *532*
Zapol, W. M., 18, *19*, 38, 39, *63*, 211, *221*, 256, 258, 259, 260, 264, 268, 270, 271, 272, 273, *277, 278, 279, 280, 282, 283*, 306, 310, *347*, 368, *380*, 451, 452, 453, 454, 455, 456, 457, 458, 459, 460, 463, 464, 465, 467, 468, 475, *486, 487, 490*, 516, *535*
Zaret, B. L., 71, *73*, 267, *281*

Zarins, C., 254, *283*
Zaslow, M. C., 323, *352*
Zenker, B., 452, 453, 454, 457, 463, *485*
Zentella, A., 86, *89*
Zerah, F., 122, *134*
Zerbe, G. O., 31, *34*, 45, 48, *60*, 266, 268, *276*, 305, *337*
Zheutlin, L. M., 312, *352*
Zhikang, P., 452, 481, *490*
Ziccardi, R. J., 307, 324, *352*
Ziegler, E. J., 264, *274*, *283*, 400, 401, 402, *406, 407, 410*
Zimmerman, I., 387, *394*
Zimmerman, J. E., 31, *35*, 92, 93, 95, 101, *103, 104*
Zin, W. A., 116, 120, 121, 130, *134, 135, 137, 171, 194*
Zinn, S. E., 152, 153, 154, *158*
Zocchi, L., 105, 114, 118, 123, 124, 126, 128, 129, 130, *135, 136,* 142, *160,* 173, 174, 185, *197*
Zreika, M., 326, *331*
Zsigmond, E. K., 470, *488, 489*
Zuidema, G. D., 82, *87*
Zupancic, I., 425, *430*
Zweerink, H., 403, *407*

SUBJECT INDEX

Acetylglyceryl ether phosphorylcholine (*see* Platelet activating factor)
Acute lung injury
 circulating mediators or markers for, 14
 lung surfactant functions in, 381-395
  abnormalities of lung surfactant in ARDS, 385
  animal models for evaluation of surfactant therapy, 387-388
  function, 383-385
  possible causes of surfactant abnormalities in ARDS patients, 385-386
  surfactant replacement in ARDS patients, 386-387
  surfactant system of the healthy lung, 382-383
[Acute lung injury]
  surfactants available for therapeutic administration, 388-390
  use of exogenous surfactants in ARDS therapy, 390
Acute pulmonary artery hypertension, effect on cardiovascular function of, 259-262
Adult respiratory distress syndrome (ARDS) lung, model of (derived from CT scanning), 217
Adverse heparin-protamine interactions and the lung, 451-490
 animal models of heparin-protamine-associated pulmonary vasoconstriction, 452-471
  biochemical mediators, 463-467
  cellular elements, 458-463
  other mediators, 470-471

[Adverse heparin-protamine interactions and the lung]
pulmonary vascular physiology, 454-458
reactive oxygen species, 467-469
clinical syndrome of heparin-protamine-associated acute pulmonary vasoconstriction in humans, 472-482
mediators, 474-481
true allergic reactions to protamine, 481-482
heparin-protamine, lipopolysaccharide, and lung injury in sheep, 471-472
Aspiration of gastric contents as major cause of ARDS, 28
Auto-PEEP (intrinsic PEEP), 173-174, 176
dynamic hyperinflation and, 191-193
reduction of, 185

Bacterial infection, 77-89
gastrointestinal tract as source of sepsis in ARDS, 83-86
mechanisms of MOF related to sepsis, 86
overview, 77-80
pneumonia as source of sepsis in ARDS, 80-83
Barotrauma, 433
Blood cell proteases, 310-321
Body positioning
altered, CT changes with, 204-206
prone, changes in lung anatomy and function due to, 215-217
Breathing effort during mechanical ventilation, minimizing, 163-198
quantifying breathing efforts, 164-194
direct measures, 165-180
indirect measures, 164-165
[Breathing effort during mechanical ventilation, minimizing]
minimizing work of breathing during mechanical ventilation, 183-194
work performance of patient, 180-183

Capillary pressure measurement in human lungs, 353-366
capillary pressure and its relation to transcapillary fluid exchange, 354-356
measurement of Ppc using only arterial occlusion, 360-365
measurement of pulmonary capillary pressure in isolated lungs, 356-360
Carboxypeptidase N (CPN), 470
Cardiac cycle in cardiorespiratory interactions, 228
Cardiorespiratory interactions, 223-251
cardiac cycle, 228
circulatory system, 224-225
lung volume and intrathoracic pressure, 224
positive pressure ventilation and cardiopulmonary resuscitation, 246-249
spontaneous ventilation
left ventricle and, 225-227
mitral and aortic flows, 228-238
transient analysis of a negative ITP, 238
transient analysis techniques, 238-246
Cardiovascular function, 253-283
assessing cardiac function during ARDS, 254-259
transmural pressure, 254-255
ventricular pressure, 255-259
during weaning from mechanical ventilation, 270-273
effect of acute pulmonary artery hypertension, 259-262

[Cardiovascular function]
effect of sepsis, 262-265
positive-pressure ventilation and PEEP, 265-270
Circulatory system in cardiorespiratory interactions, 224-225
Clinical predispositions to ARDS, 26, 27-28
Clinical risks, 1-21
criteria for the diagnosis of ARDS, 3
definition of ARDS, 2-4
prediction of ARDS
in cellular and biochemical markers, 13-18
by clinical predispositions, 7-13
by physiologic measurements, 6-7
rationale for identifying patients at risk, 4-5
(*See also* Risk groups)
Clinical studies of ARDS, new directions in, 32-33
Computed tomography (CT) scanning, 199-221
alterations in lung anatomy and function with changing conditions, 214-217
effects of PEEP, 214-215
effects of prone body positioning, 215-217
calculations for estimating pulmonary weight, 218-219
comparing physiological measurements with CT scan anatomy, 211-213
lung morphology, 200-208
comparing CT scans with X-rays, 200-202
CT changes with altered body positioning, 204-206
CT changes in PEEP, 203-204
CT patterns in ARDS, 202-203
model of the ARDS lung derived from CT scans of the lung, 217
quantitative analysis of CT scan images, 208-210
Constant inspiratory flow method for measuring respiratory mechanics, 116, 118-120
Corticosteroids, 285-304
actions of corticosteroids that may be beneficial in ARDS, 286-288
evidence of efficacy of corticosteroids in animal and organ models, 288-293
in vitro versus in vivo effects of, 293-300
Cysteine proteases, inhibitors of, 325

Definitions of ARDS, 2-4, 24-26
Detection of ARDS (*see* Prediction of ARDS)
Diagnosis of ARDS
criteria for, 3
European collaborative study and, 38-42
Double lung transplant operation, 515-518
Dynamic hyperinflation, auto-PEEP and, 185, 191-193

Eicosanoids, 463-464
effects on the lungs of, 287
Endotoxin neutralization, humoral aspects of, 397-410
neutralization of endotoxin by immunoglobulin, 400-403
neutralization of endotoxin by normal serum, 399-400
neutralization of LPs by inflammatory factors in serum, 403-405
European collaborative study (1985-1987), 37-63
diagnosis of ARDS, 38-42
etiology, 42-43
long-term recovery, 53-57
mortality and prognostic factors, 44-50
severity scoring index, 50-53
Extracellular proteases, 307-310

Free-induction decay (FID) in inflated lung, 417-421
Forced oscillation technique for measuring respiratory mechanics, 124-126

Gastric contents, aspiration of, as major cause of ARDS, 28
Gastrointestinal tract as source of sepsis in ARDS, 83-86

Heparin-protamine-associated pulmonary vasoconstriction
  animals models of, 452-471
  in humans, clinical syndrome of, 472-482
High-risk groups, 29-30
Histamine, 470
Humoral aspects of endotoxin neutralization, 397-410
  neutralization of endotoxin by immunoglobulin, 400-403
  neutalization of endotoxin by normal serum, 399-400
  neutralization of LPs by inflammatory factors in serum, 403-405

Identifying patients at risk for ARDS, 4-5
  application to clinical trials, 5
  assuring appropriate diagnosis, 4
  triage and clinical management, 5
  understanding the epidemiology and pathogenesis, 5
Incidence of ARDS, 24
Infectious end-stage lung disease, lung transplant and, 498-499
Inflated lung, unique NMR behavior of, 417-421
Intermittent positive pressure ventilation (IPPV), 225
Interrupter technique for measuring respiratory mechanics, 122-124
Intracellular proteases, 310-321
Intrathoracic pressure (ITP)
  changes in lung volume and, 224
  fall in, 239-246
  negative, transient analysis of, 238
  positive pressure transients in, 246-249
Isovolume method for measuring respiratory mechanics, 115

Leukocytes, 458-460
  proteases of, 311-314
Lipopolysaccharides (LPs), 397-399
  neutralization by inflammatory factors in serum, 403-405
Lung distention, pulmonary edema due to, 433-437, 444-446
Lung mechanics, 139-161
  measurement of the total thoraco-pulmonary compliance, 142-147
    constant flow, 147
    dynamic compliance, 143-144
    effective or quasi-static compliance, 143
    occlusion methods, 142
    static pressure-volume loops, 144-147
  methodologic limitations, 154-155
  recent concepts of the P-V loops, 147-154
    alveolar recruitment versus cardiac output decrease, 150
    correlations between lung mechanics and morphology, 150-152
    early and late ARDS, 147-150
    respiratory system versus lung compliance, 153-154
    time dependence, 152-153
  titration of PEEP, 140-142
Lung morphology, 200-208
  comparing CT scans with X-rays, 200-202
  CT changes in altered body positioning, 204-206

[Lung morphology]
CT changes in PEEP, 203-204
CT patterns in ARDS, 202-203
Lung overinflation, 433-449
pathways for pulmonary edema due to lung distention, 433-437
pulmonary edema due to mechanical ventilation, 437-446
microvascular permeability and cellular alterations during HIPPV edema, 437-441
possible explanations for lung distention edema, 444-446
pulmonary edema after intermittent positive-pressure ventilation, 437
separating the effects of high airway pressures from those of high lung volumes, 441-444
Lung surfactant function in acute lung injury, 381-395
abnormalities of lung surfactant in ARDS, 385
animal models for evaluation of surfactant therapy of acute adult lung injury, 387-388
function, 383-385
possible causes of surfactant abnormalities in ARDS patients, 385-386
surfactant replacement in ARDS patients, 386-387
surfactant system of the healthy lung, 382-383
surfactants available for therapeutic administration, 388-390
use of exogenous surfactants in ARDS therapy, 390
Lung transplantation, 491-538
clinical results of, 522-528
evaluation and management of potential candidates, 500-501
history of, 492-494
indications for, 495-500
[Lung transplantation]
infectious end-stage lung disease, 498-499
obstructive lung disease, 496-498
pulmonary hypertension, 499-500
restrictive lung disease, 495-496
in-patient evaluation, 502
lung preservation, 509-513
postoperative course following, 518-522
pulmonary donor, 502-506
retrieval of the donor lung, 506-509
techniques of, 513-518
double lung transplant operation, 515-518
unilateral lung transplant operation, 513-515
Lung water
NMR of, 416-417
nonspatial distributions of, 422-423

α_2-Macroglobulin, 326-327
Massachusetts General Hospital, ARDS at, 367-380
discussion, 376-378
etiologies of ARF, 370-371
ICU mortality of ARF classified at time of ICU admission, 371-372
mortality rates of highest severity of ARF, 372-374
patients at high risk to develop ARF, 374-376
Measuring respiratory mechanics, 113-126
comparison of the methods, 126-130
constant inspiratory flow and occlusion methods, 116-120
forced oscillation technique, 124-126
interrupter technique, 122-124
single-breath method, 120-121
zero flow and isovolume methods, 115

Mechanical ventilation
cardiovascular function during weaning from, 270-273
minimizing breathing efforts during, 163-198
pulmonary edema due to, 437-446
(*See also* Respiratory elastance and resistance in mechanically ventilated patients)
Metalloprotease inhibitors, 328
Multiple organ failure (MOF), 77-80
mechanisms related to sepsis, 86

National Heart, Lung and Blood Institute, current definition of ARDS used by, 25, 26
Negative ITP, transient analysis of, 238
Nonblood cell proteases, 315
Noncardiac causes of pulmonary edema, 30
Nuclear magnetic resonance (NMR), 411-432
basic NMR phenomena, 413-415
geometric information about lung structure without requiring optical resolution, 423-424
imaging frequency encoding of position, 415-416
nonspatial distribution of lung water, 422-423
of lung water, 416-417
potential applications in ARDS, 426-428
relaxation of times T_1 and T_2, 424-426
unique NMR behavior of inflated lung, 417-421

Obstructive lung disease, lung transplant and, 496-498
Occlusion method for measuring respiratory mechanics, 116-120
Outcome of ARDS, 30-32
Oxygen utilization or consumption (VO_2), 66
(*See also* Tissue oxygen delivery in ARDS patients)

Platelet activating factor (PAF), 470-471
Platelets, 460-461
Pneumonia as source of sepsis in ARDS, 80-83
Positive end-expiratory pressure (PEEP), 139
alterations in lung anatomy and function with changing conditions, 214-215
auto-PEEP, 173-174, 176
dynamic hyperinflation and, 191-193
reducing dynamic hyperinflation, 185
CT changes in, 203-204
positive-pressure ventilation and, 265-270
heart rate, 270
left ventricular afterload, 269-270
left ventricular preload, 267-268
myocardial contractility, 268-269
right ventricular afterload, 266-267
right ventricular preload, 265-266
titration of, 140-142
Postoperative course following lung transplantation, 518-522
Prediction of ARDS
in cellular and biochemical markers, 13-18
by clinical predispositions, 7-13
by physiologic measurements, 6-7
Prognostic factors in the ICU, 91-104
discussion, 100-102
source of patient information, 82-100
data collection, 94-95

[Prognostic factors in the ICU]
patients selected for this study, 95-97
results, 97-100
Prone body positioning, alterations in lung anatomy and function due to, 215-217
Proteases and antiproteases, 305-352
protease-antiprotease imbalance during ARDS, 327-330
proteases involved in ARDS, 306-321
extracellular proteases, 307-310
intracellular proteases, 310-321
regulation of protease activity, role of antiproteases in, 321-327
inhibitors of cysteine proteases, 325
inhibitors of serine proteases, 321-325
α_2-macroglobulin, 326-327
metalloprotease inhibitors, 325
Pulmonary edema
due to lung distention, 433-437
alveolar-capillary barrier alterations, 434-437
increased filtration of fluid, 433-434
due to mechanical ventilation, 437-446
microvascular permeability and cellular alterations during HIPPV edema, 437-441
possible explanations for lung distention edema, 444-446
pulmonary edema after intermittent positive-pressure ventilation, 437
separating the effects of high airway pressures from those of high lung volumes, 441-444
noncardiac causes of, 30
Pulmonary hypertension, lung transplant and, 499-500
Pulmonary intravascular macrophages, 461-463
Respiratory elastance and resistance in mechanically ventilated patients, 105-137
limits of models and methods, 130-133
methods, 133
respiratory models, 130-133
methods for measuring respiratory mechanics, 113-126
comparison of methods, 126-130
constant inspiratory flow and occlusion methods, 116-120
forced oscillation technique, 124-126
interrupter technique, 122-124
single-breath method, 120-121
zero flow and isovolume methods, 115
respiratory models, 107-113
homogeneous respiratory model, 107-109
homogeneous thoracopulmonary model, 109
inhomogeneous respiratory model, 109-113
inhomogeneous thoracopulmonary model, 113
Restrictive lung disease, lung transplant and, 495-496
Risk groups, 26-30
aspiration of gastric contents, 28
high risk groups, 29-30
other sources, 29
sepsis and, 26-28
trauma and, 28-29
(*See also* Identifying patients at risk for ARDS)

Sepsis, 26-28
effect on cardiovascular function of, 262-265
gastrointestinal tract as source of, 83-86
pneumonia as source of, 80-83

Serine proteases, inhibitors of, 321-325
Single-breath method for measuring respiratory mechanics, 120-121
Spontaneous ventilation
left ventricular and, 225-227
mitral and aortic flows, 228-238

Tissue oxygen delivery in ARDS patients, 65-75
normal response to reduced total oxygen delivery (TO_2), 66-69
TO_2-VO_2 relationships in ARDS, 69-72
Total oxygen delivery (TO_2), 66
reduced, normal response to, 66-69
-VO_2 relationships in ARDS, 69-72
Transcapillary fluid exchange, capillary pressure relation to, 354-356
Trauma as major cause of ARDS, 28-29
Tumor necrosis factor (TNF), 86

Unilateral lung disease, 155
Unilateral lung transplant operation, 513-515

X-rays of lung morphology, comparison of CT scans with, 200-202

Zero flow method for measuring respiratory mechanics, 115